Essential

Obstetrics

Textbook for Undergraduates

Essential Obstetrics

Textbook for Undergraduates

Edited by

Asha Oumachigui
Former Director-Professor and Head
Department of Obstetrics and Gynecology
Jawaharlal Institute of Postgraduate Medical Education and Research
Puducherry, India

S Soundara Raghavan
Professor
Department of Obstetrics and Gynecology
Jawaharlal Institute of Postgraduate Medical Education and Research
Puducherry, India

S Habeebullah
Professor and Head
Department of Obstetrics and Gynecology
Jawaharlal Institute of Postgraduate Medical Education and Research
Puducherry, India

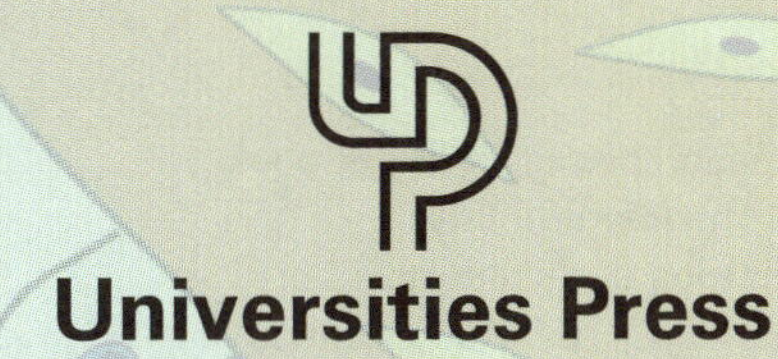

UNIVERSITIES PRESS (INDIA) PRIVATE LIMITED

Registered Office
3-6-747/1/A & 3-6-754/1, Himayatnagar
Hyderabad 500 029 (A.P.), India
info@universitiespress.com; www.universitiespress.com

Distributed by
Orient Blackswan Private Limited

Registered Office
3-6-752, Himayatnagar
Hyderabad 500 029 (A.P.) India

Other Offices
Bangalore / Bhopal / Bhubaneshwar / Chandigarh / Chennai
Ernakulam / Guwahati / Hyderabad / Jaipur / Kolkata
Lucknow / Mumbai / New Delhi / Noida / Patna

ISBN 978 81 7371 735 2

Illustrations by
RK Majumdar

Typeset in Adobe Garamond Pro BT 12/14.4 by
OSDATA, Hyderabad 500 029

Printed in India by
Orion Printers Pvt. Ltd.
Hyderabad 500 004

Published by
Universities Press (India) Private Limited
3-6-747/1/A & 3-6-754/1, Himayatnagar
Hyderabad 500 029 (A.P.), India.

Foreword

Essential Obstetrics: Textbook For Undergraduates has been edited by three very experienced professors from the Jawaharlal Institute of Medical Education and Research, Puducherry: Prof. Asha Oumachigui, Prof. S Soundara Raghavan and Prof. S Habeebullah. They have kept in mind the needs of undergraduate students to help them understand the principles of diagnosis and management of obstetric problems and the necessary details of investigations and methodology of procedures. The complications and solutions to various obstetric problems have been discussed with a practical approach. The basis of physiology and anatomy has been included in each subject. Antenatal care, labour and puerperium are discussed along with useful diagrams.

The first chapter—An Overview gives the standard definitions and national indicators for India. An impressive aspect is the importance given to ethical issues, gender sensitisation as well as communication and counselling. The book covers important subjects such as National Rural Health Mission and its goals and strategies. Each chapter begins with Learning objectives in order to make learning better focused, Key points are summarised clearly at the end, and this is followed by multiple choice questions by answering which the students will benefit.

The medical and surgical complications have included endocrinology, STDs and even psychiatric problems. The editors have covered demography, population control and contraception, subjects of great present day importance. Although the book is for undergraduates, postgraduates will also find it useful.

I wish this book can reach and benefit all the undergraduate medical students. I congratulate the editors and contributors and wish them every success.

Usha R Krishna
Past President— FOGSI
Former Professor KEM Hospital and G S Medical College
Chairperson ICMR— Reproductive Health and Nutrition

Preface

We have always felt that undergraduate students need a textbook that helps them understand the subject in a holistic manner, at the same time keeping the presentation lucid. This book is the result of our conviction, a lot of deliberation, planning and contribution from excellent and committed teachers from different parts of India.

It is important that students learn obstetrics with reference to the national programmes and guidelines. We are of the opinion that students must be aware of the nature of obstetrical problems in India and how socio-cultural factors influence obstetric care. They must also be familiar with the magnitude of maternal and perinatal mortality and morbidity in the country.

Four other issues which have not received the attention they deserve in the undergraduate textbooks are communication, nutrition, gender issues and ethics. A review of the MBBS curriculum shows that maternal nutrition has not been given enough importance. A recent review of some textbooks of obstetrics and gynecology revealed that these books were not 'gender-sensitive', given the current social scenario. It is now clearly established that 'gender bias' influences health care of women significantly. Domestic violence, for example, has an adverse influence on the health of the mother and her unborn child. Medical practitioners of the future need a frame of reference to tackle the 'ethical dilemmas'. As this needs to be dealt with formally at the training level itself, we decided to make a small beginning.

Our aim was to present the subject by integrating basic sciences like anatomy and physiology with situations in obstetrics. We have emphasised what is important for the student to learn. Each chapter starts with Learning Objectives to indicate what the reader could expect to know after reading the chapter. There are Key Points for summary and multiple choice questions at the end of each chapter. This, we hope, would help in consolidation of learning and self-assessment.

We hope that this book will be a valuable resource to the undergraduate students. We thank Padmaja Anant and Ramaa Kishore of Universities Press for their efforts in bringing out this book.

Asha Oumachigui
S Soundara Raghavan
S Habeebullah

Acknowledgement

Ultrasonography has revolutionised the practice of obstetrics. No textbook in the subject can be written without good ultrasound pictures. Dr. S. Suresh, Director, Medscan and Fetal Care and Research Foundation, Chennai, was always willing to help and has provided us with some ultrsonographic pictures from his archives/library. We place on record our heartfelt gratitude to him.

Mr. Pandithurai from the HRRC (ICMR), Department of Obstetrics and Gynecology helped us with his computer skills. We thank him whole-heartedly for his assistance at various stages of writing this book.

Contributors

C Ambuja
Professor and Head, Department of Obstetrics and Gynecology
Osmania Medical College, Hyderabad

N Ananthakrishnan
Professor, Department of Surgery
Mahatma Gandhi Medical College and Research Institute
Puducherry and Former Director-Professor and Head, Department of Surgery
JIPMER, Puducherry

Asha Oumachigui
Former Director-Professor and Head, Department of Obstetrics and Gynecology
JIPMER, Puducherry

Asmita Rathore
Professor, Department of Obstetrics and Gynecology
Maulana Azad Medical College, New Delhi

S Habeebullah
Professor and Head, Department of Obstetrics and Gynecology
JIPMER, Puducherry

Kamala Ganesh
Former Director-Professor,
Department of Obstetrics and Gynecology
Maulana Azad Medical College, New Delhi

Kapila E Bharucha
Former Professor-Head, Department of Obstetrics and Gynecology
BJ Medical College, Pune

Lakshmi Seshadri
Professor, Department of Obstetrics and Gynecology
Christian Medical College and Hospital, Vellore

Lavanya Rai
Professor and Head, Department of Obstetrics and Gynecology
Kasturba Medical College, Manipal

S Mahadevan
Professor, Department of Pediatrics
JIPMER, Puducherry

Manorama Purwar
Professor and Head, Department of Obstetrics and Gynecology
Government Medical College, Nagpur

V Mathini
Former Director, Institute of Obstetrics and Gynecology, Chennai

Prema Ramachandran
Director, Nutrition Foundation of India, New Delhi
Formerly Advisor, Reproductive Health and Nutrition Planning Commission
New Delhi

R Raguram
Professor and Head, Department of Psychiatry
Kempegowda Institute of Medical Sciences, Bengaluru
Former Professor, NIMHANS, Bengaluru

Raj Narayan
Assistant Professor and Associate Residency Program Director
Medical College of Wisconsin, Milwaukee, Wisconsin

Raksha Arora
Professor, Department of Obstetrics and Gynecology
Maulana Azad Medical College, New Delhi

M Ravishankar
Professor and Head, Department of Anesthesiology
Mahatma Gandhi Medical College and Research Institute
Puducherry and Former Professor and Head, Department of Anesthesiology
JIPMER, Puducherry

CH Shashindran
Dean, Indira Gandhi Medical College and Research Institute, Puducherry and
Former Director-Professor and Head, Department of Pharmacology
JIPMER, Puducherry

Shyama Kanungo
Professor, Department of Obstetrics and Gynecology
SCB Medical College, Cuttack

Sindhu Nandini Tripathy
Former Professor, Department of Obstetrics and Gynecology
SCB Medical College, Cuttack

S Soundara Raghavan
Professor, Department of Obstetrics and Gynecology
JIPMER, Puducherry

Sudha Rao
Professor and Head, Department of Anatomy
Mahatma Gandhi Medical College and Research Institute
Puducherry and Former Director-Professor and Head, Department of Anatomy
JIPMER, Puducherry

Sundari Ravindran
Professor, Achutha Menon Centre for Health Science Studies, Thiruvananthapuram

N Sundari
Professor, Department of Obstetrics and Gynecology
MS Ramaiah Medical College, Bengaluru

Sunesh Kumar
Professor, Department of Obstetrics and Gynecology
AIIMS, New Delhi

Vinita Salvi
Professor and Head, Department of Obstetrics and Gynecology
Seth GS Medical College, Mumbai

VP Paily
Former Professor, Department of Obstetrics and Gynecology
Thrissur Medical College, Thrissur

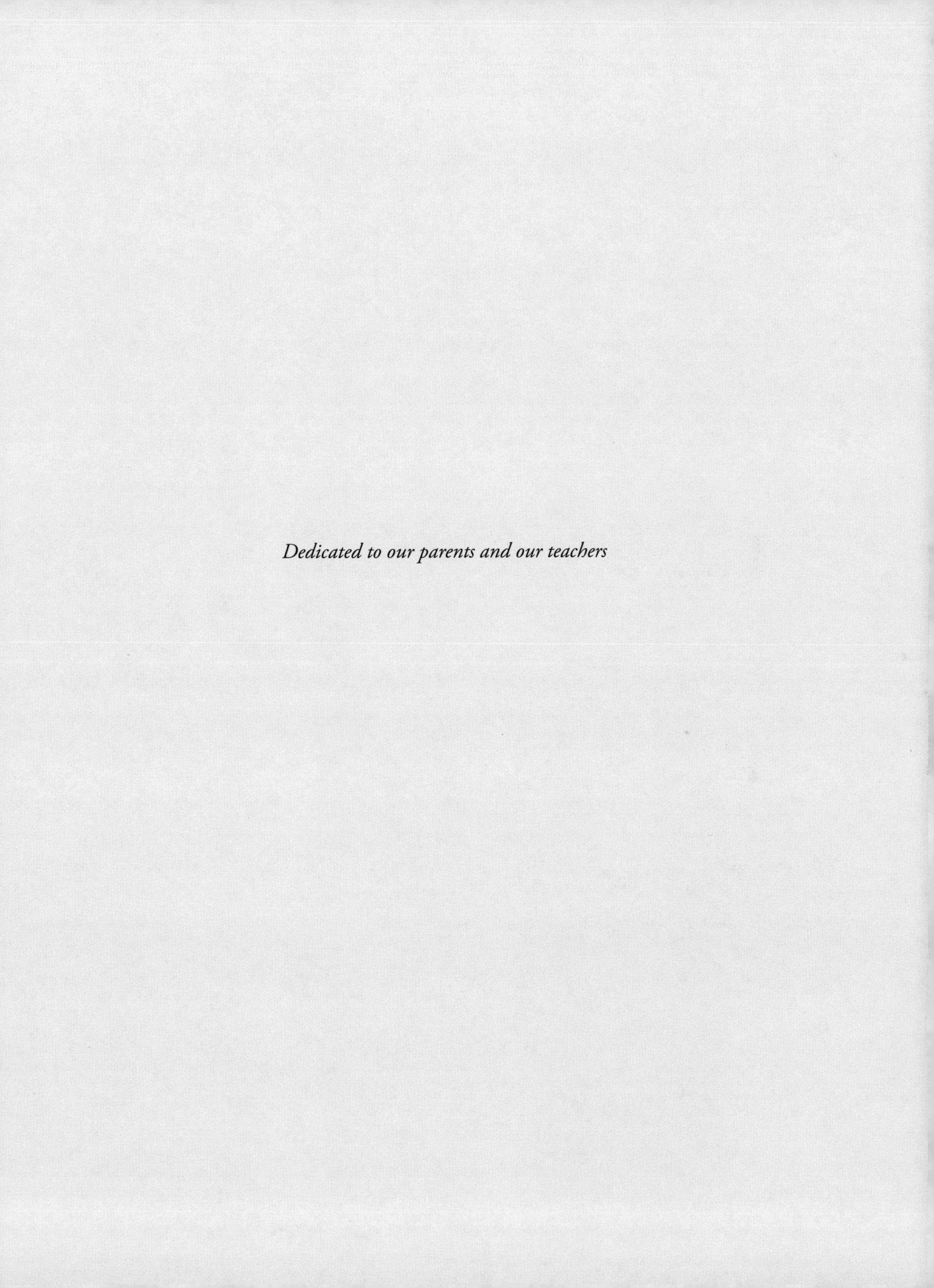

Dedicated to our parents and our teachers

Contents

Part I Perspectives in Obstetrics

Part II Pregnancy

Continued...

Part III Labour

Part IV Puerperium

Part V Complications of Pregnancy

Continued...

Part VII Contraception

Abbreviations

AC	Abdominal circumference
ACE	Angiotensin converting enzyme
ACOG	American College of Obstetricians and Gynecologists
ACTH	Adrenocorticotrophin hormone
ADH	Antidiuretic hormone
AED	Anti-epileptic drugs
AFI	Amniotic fluid index
AFLP	Acute fatty liver of pregnancy
AFP	Alpha feto-protein
AIDS	Acquired immunodeficiency syndrome
AMH	Anti-mullerian hormone
ANM	Auxillary nurse midwife
APH	Antepartum hemorrhage
aPTT	Accelerated partial thromboplastin time
ARDS	Adult respiratory distress syndrome
ARM	Artificial rupture of membranes
ASB	Asymptomatic bacteriuria
ASCUS	Atypical squamous cells of unknown significance
ASD	Atrial septal defect
ASHA	Accredited social health activist
ATT	Antitubercular treatment
AYUSH	Ayurvedic, yoga, unani, siddha, homeopathy (systems of health)
BMI	Body mass index
BPD	Biparietal diameter
BPP	Biophysical profile
BPPS	Biophysical profile scoring
cAMP	Cyclic adenosine monophosphate
CAP	Contraction-associated protein
CC	Conventional contraceptives
cGMP	Cyclic guanine monophosphate
CNA	Community needs assessment
COC	Combined oral contraceptive
CPD	Cephalopelvic disproportion
CRH	Corticotrophin releasing hormone
CRL	Crown–rump length
CS	Cesarean section
CSE	Combined spinal epidural
CSF	Cerebrospinal fluid
CSSM	Child survival and safe motherhood
CST	Contraction stress test
CT	Computerised axial tomography
CTG	Cardiotocography
CVS	Chorionic villus sampling
DFMC	Daily fetal movement count
DHT	Dihydrotestosterone
DIC	Disseminated intravascular coagulation
DIH	Drug-induced hepatitis
DMPA	Depot medroxy progesterone acetate
DVT	Deep vein thrombosis
EC	Emergency contraception
ECG	Electrocardiograph
EDC	Estimated date of confinement
EDD	Expected date of delivery
EE	Ethinyl estradiol
ELISA	Enzyme-linked immunosorbent assay
EP	Ectopic pregnancy
ESR	Erythrocyte sedimentation rate
FDA	Food and drug administration
FDP	Fibrin degradation product
FFP	Fresh frozen plasma
FHF	Fulminant hepatic failure
FIGO	Federation Internationale de Gynecolgie et Obstetrique
FISH	Fluorescent in situ hybridisation
FL	Femur length
FRU	First referral unit
FSH	Follicle stimulating hormone
G6PD	Glucose-6-phosphate dehydrogenase
GA	General anesthesia
GCT	Glucose challenge test
GDM	Gestational diabetes mellitus
GFR	Glomerular filtration rate
GnRH	Gonadotrophin releasing hormone
GS	Gestational sac
GTD	Gestational trophoblastic disease
GTT	Glucose tolerance test
HAART	Highly active antiretroviral therapy
HBV	Hepatitis B virus
HC	Head circumference
hCG	Human chorionic gonadotrophin
HELLP	Hemolysis elevated liver enzymes, low platelets
HFWTC	Health and family welfare training centre
HGSIL	High grade squamous intraepithelial lesions
HIV	Human immunodeficiency virus
HM	Hydatidiform mole
hPL	Human placental lactogen
HPT	Home pregnancy test
HPV	Human papilloma virus
HWY	Hundred woman years
ICDS	Integrated child development services
ICMR	Indian Council of Medical Research

IDD	Iodine deficiency disorders
IDDM	Insulin-dependent diabetes mellitus
IDM	Infants of diabetic mothers
IFMA	Immunofluorometric assay
IHCP	Intrahepatic cholestasis of pregnancy
IM	Intramuscular
IMR	Infant mortality rate
IRMA	Immunoradiometric assay
IUCD	Intrauterine contraceptive device
IUD	Intrauterine death
IUGR	Intrauterine growth restriction
IV	Intravenous
IVF	In vitro fertilisation
IVH	Intraventricular hemorrhage
JSRY	Janani suraksha yojana
LAM	Lactational amenorrhea method
LBW	Low birth weight
LDH	Lactic dehydrogenase
LFT	Liver function tests
LGSIL	Low grade squamous intraepithelial lesions
LH	Luteinising hormone
LHRH	Luteinising hormone releasing hormone
LLMP	Last to last menstrual period
LMA	Left mentoanterior
LMP	Last menstrual period
LNG	Levonorgestrel
LNG-IUCD	Levonorgestrel intrauterine contraceptive device
LOP	Left occipitoposterior
LSA	Left sacroanterior
LSCS	Lower segment cesarean section
LSP	Left sacroposterior
MA	Left mentoanterior
MAP	Mean arterial pressure
MBPP	Modified biophysical profile
MCH	Maternal and child health
MCHC	Mean corpuscular hemoglobin concentration
MCV	Mean corpuscular volume
MIS	Management information systems
MLCK	Myosin light-chain kinase
MMR	Maternal mortality rate
MOHFW	Ministry of Health and Family Welfare
MRI	Magnetic resonance imaging
MSAFP	Maternal serum alpha protein
MT	Mentotransverse
MTP	Medical termination of pregnancy
MVA	Manual vacuum aspiration
MVP	Maximum vertical pocket
NACO	National AIDS Control Organization
NBS	New Ballard score
NEC	Necrotising enterocolitis
NFHS	National Family Health Survey
NFP	Natural family planning
NICU	Neonatal intensive care unit
NIDDM	Non–insulin-dependent diabetes mellitus
NMCP	National Malaria Control Programme
NNF	National Neonatology Forum
NRHM	National Rural Health Mission
NSAID	Non-steroidal anti-inflammatory drugs
NST	Non-stress test
NSV	Non-scalpel vasectomy
NT	Nuchal translucency
NTD	Neural tube defects
NYHA	New York heart association
OA	Occipitoanterior
OCP	Oral contraceptive pills
ODD	Optical density deviate
OP	Occipitoposterior
ORS	Oral rehydration solution
PCEA	Patient-controlled epidural analgesia
PCOS	Polycystic ovarian syndrome
PCR	Polymerase chain reaction
PCV	Packed cell volume
PDA	Patent ductus arteriosus
PFT	Pulmonary function tests
PG	Prostaglandin
PHC	Primary health centre
PID	Pelvic inflammatory disease
PIH	Pregnancy-induced hypertension
PNDT	Prenatal diagnostic technique
POG	Period of gestation
POP	Progestogen-only pill
PPD	Purified protein derivative
PPH	Postpartum hemorrhage
PPROM	Preterm premature rupture of membranes
PROM	Premature rupture of membranes
PSTT	Placental site trophoblastic tumour
PT	Prothrombin time
PTCT	Parent-to-child transmission
PTT	Partial thromboplastin time
PUBS	Percutaneous umbilical blood sampling
RCH	Reproductive and child health
RDA	Recommended dietary allowance
RDS	Respiratory distress syndrome
RIA	Radioimmunoassay
ROA	Right occipitoantterior
ROP	Right occipitoposterior
RTI	Reproductive tract infection
S/D	Systolic-diastolic ratio
SE	Suction evacuation
SFD	Small for date
SLE	Systemic lupus erythematosus
SP	Sacral promontory
SRY	Sex determining region

STD	Sexually transmitted diseases
STI	Sexually transmitted infections
TENS	Transcutaneous electrical nerve stimulation
TORCH	Toxoplasma rubella cytomegalovirus herpes
TPN	Total parenteral nutrition
TRH	Thyrotropin releasing hormone
TSB	Total serum bilirubin
TTTS	Twin-to-twin transfusion syndrome
TVS	Transvaginal sonography
US	Ultrasound
USG	Ultrasonography
UTI	Urinary tract infection
VAST	Vibroacoustic stimulation test
VBAC	Vaginal birth after cesarean section
VSD	Ventricular septal defect
WHO	World Health Organization

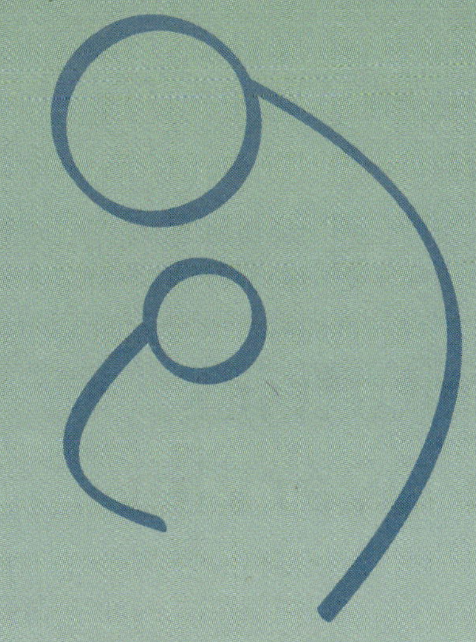

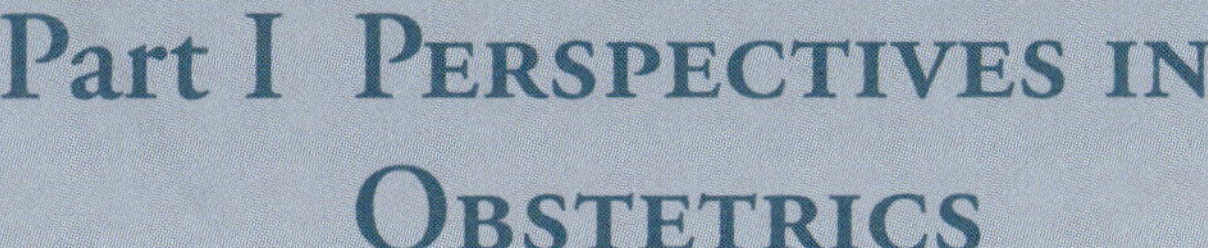

Part I Perspectives in Obstetrics

1

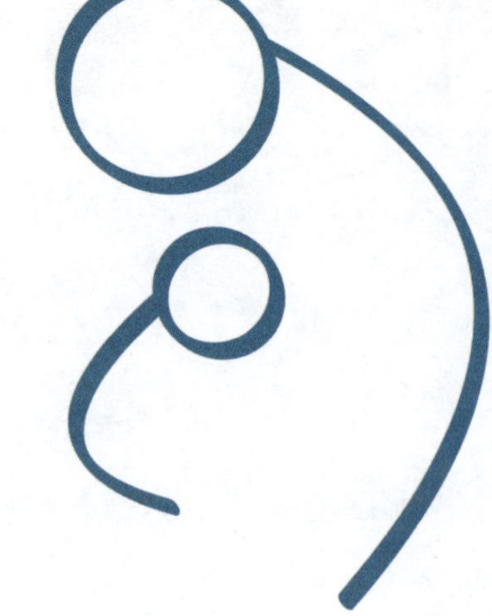

Obstetrics: An Overview

Asha Oumachigui

If you don't ask, you don't know, and if you don't know, you can't act.

N Krieger*

LEARNING OBJECTIVES

At the end of this chapter, the reader should be able to:

- define obstetrics
- define the scope of obstetrics
- appreciate the contribution of good obstetric practice to the health of women and children
- recall the definition of some important terms used in obstetrics
- enumerate and define the indicators that reflect maternal and child health
- enumerate the causes of maternal and perinatal mortality and morbidity
- list some important indicators of maternal and child health in India
- define evidence-based medicine and its role in obstetric practice
- appreciate the rational use of technology in the practice of obstetrics

Introduction

Obstetrics is the branch of medicine concerned with the care of women during pregnancy, childbirth and for a period of six weeks after childbirth. This specialty contributes to the wellbeing of mothers and their infants in a society and is, to a great extent, preventive medicine. The adage 'Good obstetric practice is preventive gynecology' is true even today, as a number of women may see a health care provider only during childbirth and, less frequently, during pregnancy.

The indicators of maternal and child health reflect the quality of obstetric practice. A few decades ago, obstetrics was considered more of an art and less of a science compared to other branches of medicine. But advances in medical science, particularly basic sciences, and technology like ultrasound, electronic fetal monitoring, fetoscopy, prenatal diagnostic and

*from Kreiger N. *Theories of social epidemiology in eco-social perspective.* ije.oxford journals.org/egi/reprint/30/4/668 fetal therapy and genetics have revolutionised the practice of obstetrics. However, with the Consumer Protection Act (CPA) now including medical services, technology is being misused and overused, which is a disadvantage for patients.

Incorporation of **evidence-based medicine** (EBM) has contributed to making obstetrics more scientific. This has immensely helped women and their children in developed countries. In developing countries, however, these benefits have not reached a large part of the population. Therefore, there is wide disparity in maternal and perinatal morbidity and mortality. Moreover, a significant percentage of women in the less developed countries are malnourished or suffer from diseases that were contracted or which existed prior to the pregnancy, with the result that mothers and infants continue to suffer ill health or succumb to it. Family planning also comes within the purview of obstetrics and adopting a right approach will benefit not only women and their families, but also the society and the country.

SCOPE OF OBSTETRICS

The word *obstetrics* is derived from the Latin *obstare,* which means 'to stand by'. It is a surgical specialty that includes the care of the woman during pregnancy, childbirth and the recuperative period of six weeks (**puerperium**). The overarching aim of obstetrics is to ensure that every pregnancy culminates in the delivery of a healthy baby without impairing the health of the mother.

Childbirth is essentially a physiological phenomenon, but complications can arise and an obstetrician needs to foresee and prevent them, or at least control their severity. Therefore, management of pregnancy and labour requires a constant vigil to detect any deviation from the normal. It also involves instituting appropriate measures or deciding on a referral. Besides the management of normal pregnancy and labour, obstetric care includes postpartum evaluation and management of the mother and the newborn.

Care of the woman before conception, or **pre-conception care,** is concerned with the identification of factors that may adversely influence the perinatal outcome. A thorough evaluation of the woman is performed in order to detect incompatible medical, reproductive, genetic and social factors and she is counselled accordingly.

In the last few decades, the availability of ultrasonography and other equipment, improved safety of anesthesia, blood transfusion, aseptic and antiseptic techniques has made pregnancy safer. The use of prenatal diagnosis and therapy has contributed to better neonatal outcome. The use of simple tools like gravidogram and partogram can also contribute to improved outcome for the mother and her child.

STANDARD DEFINITIONS

The use of standard definitions is recommended to remove ambiguity. It enables the smooth collection of obstetrics-related data and comparison between national and international values.

Birth: It refers to the complete expulsion or extraction of a fetus from the mother, irrespective of whether the placenta is attached or the umbilical cord has been cut. In India, fetuses weighing less than 1,000 g are considered as abortuses for statistical purposes.

Live birth: Whenever an infant at birth (or sometimes after birth) breathes spontaneously or shows other signs of life, like heart beat or definite voluntary movement of muscles, it is recorded as a live birth.

Birth rate: It means the number of live births per 1,000 estimated mid-year population in a given year.

Birth weight: It refers to the weight of the infant recorded immediately after delivery or as soon as possible.

Perinatal period: This is defined as commencing from 28 weeks of gestation (20 weeks in developed countries) up to seven days after birth.

Fertility rate: It refers to the number of live births per 1,000 women in the age group 15 years to 44 years.

Stillbirth: It refer to an infant weighing 1,000 g or more who shows no signs of life at or after birth.

Neonatal death: Early neonatal death refers to the death of a live-born infant during the first seven days after birth. Late neonatal death refers to death after seven but before 29 days.

Stillbirth rate: This is the number of stillbirths per 1,000 neonates born, including live births and stillbirths.

Neonatal mortality rate: It refers to the number of neonatal deaths per 1,000 live births.

Perinatal mortality rate: It means the number of stillbirths and early neonatal deaths per 1,000 live births.

Infant mortality: It means the death of a live-born infant any time from birth to 12 months of age.

Infant mortality rate (IMR): It indicates the number of infant deaths per 1,000 live births.

Term baby: It is a baby born any time after 37 completed weeks of gestation and up to 42 completed weeks (200–294 days).

Preterm baby: A baby born before 37 completed weeks of gestation is said to be preterm.

Postterm baby: A baby born after 42 completed weeks of gestation, beginning with day 295, is considered to be postterm.

Abortus: It is a fetus expelled or removed from the uterus before the period of viability, which is 28 weeks, corresponding to a fetal weight of less than 1,000 g. With expert neonatal care, the period has been brought down to less than 20 weeks corresponding to a fetal weight of less than 500 g.

Maternal mortality: The WHO definition of maternal death is 'death of a woman while pregnant or within 42 days of termination of pregnancy, irrespective of the duration and site of pregnancy, from any cause related to or aggravated by the pregnancy or its management but not from accidental or incidental causes.' Maternal mortality can be direct or indirect.

Direct maternal mortality: It means the death of the woman resulting from obstetrical complications of pregnancy, labour or puerperium and from interventions, omissions, incorrect treatment or a chain of events resulting from any of these factors, irrespective of the duration and site of pregnancy. An example is maternal death from massive hemorrhage after delivery.

Indirect maternal mortality: It includes maternal death resulting from a preexisting disease or a disease that developed during pregnancy, labour or puerperium, but which was aggravated by maternal physiological changes of pregnancy. An example is maternal death due to complications of cardiac disease.

Nonmaternal mortality: It refers to death resulting from incidental or accidental causes not related to pregnancy, e.g., death due to a road traffic accident.

Maternal mortality ratio (MMR): It means the number of maternal deaths that result from the reproductive process per 100,000 live births.

Maternal morbidity: It means the deterioration in health attributable to pregnancy, labour and puerperium. It is **direct** if a pregnant mother suffers from complications attributable to pregnancy, for example, eclampsia. It is **indirect** in case of an associated disease like anemia. Vesico-vaginal fistulas are an example of **residual** or **chronic** morbidity.

National indicators for India

In order to improve the quality of obstetric care in a community, it is necessary to find out 'how much' needs to be done and 'how good' it should be. The use of indicators serves this purpose and it is essential to have an idea of the average measurements for India, although there can be wide variation between individual states.

Birth rate and fertility rate: The average birth rate for the country is 23. There are 29 births every minute and every year a population of 15 million is added. At 1.2 billion, India's is the second largest population in the world. The fertility rate is currently 2.7 children per woman (NFHS-3).

Maternal mortality ratio (MMR): It declined from 540 (1998–99) to 301 (2006) and is currently 254 (2009). The national average for this ratio is very high compared to developed countries, where it is around 10. *In India, every year approximately 67,000 women die as a result of childbirth; in other words, one mother dies every 4–8 minutes.* At what point of time during pregnancy and childbirth do mothers die? Maternal deaths are clustered around delivery, and most of them occur on the first two days after delivery, but the maximum deaths are on the first day. A very small percentage of mothers die during pregnancy.

The MMR is the most commonly used indicator to monitor the progress towards the goal of satisfactory maternal health. It considers the number of women dying during pregnancy, childbirth and in the postpartum period (42 days). Late maternal death refers to the death of a woman after 42 days up to one year of childbirth. The period has been extended to one year because the availability of sophisticated life support can facilitate the survival beyond 42 days of a woman who has suffered from complications of childbirth.

Distribution of maternal mortality: According to the year-end evaluation of the National Rural Health Mission (Ministry of Health and Family Welfare 2009), the MMR is 254. It has declined from 301 (Sample Registration Survey and Registrar-General of India 2006). However, India being a large country, the MMR varies amongst the different states. It is highest at 539 in Uttar Pradesh and Uttarakhand and below 150 in some states like Kerala and Tamil Nadu. In fact, of all the maternal deaths, 64.8% occured in Uttar Pradesh, Uttarakhand, Bihar, Madhya Pradesh, Orissa and Rajasthan; these states are now known as 'Empowered Action Group' as enhanced efforts are being made to reduce the MMR there. In contrast, only 10.2% occured in the southern states and 21.7% in other states. In India, the 'lifetime risk' of a woman dying as a result of childbirth is 1 in 100, as compared to 1 in 7,300 in developed countries. **Table 1.1** compares the MMR indicators in India with global values for different categories.

Causes of maternal death: The three leading causes of maternal death continue to be hemorrhage, sepsis and hypertensive disorders (preeclampsia and eclampsia). Others include anemia, unsafe abortion and associated medical and other complications. **Table 1.2** shows the percentage attributable to each of these causes in instances of maternal death.

Reasons for high maternal mortality: They are not far to seek. A large proportion of women deliver without the assistance of a skilled birth attendant. According to the National and Family Health Survey (NFHS-3), only 47% of deliveries in India take place in institutions. The rest are carried out at home, often without skilled assistance.

Non-availability of essential obstetric care in some regions contributes to a large number of maternal deaths. Even where available, for socioeconomic reasons, the women are not able to use the facilities. Some women just cannot afford to pay for the transport and 'hidden costs', although obstetric care is provided free of cost under various government programmes. It is a fact that even in states where facilities for antenatal and intranatal care are good, postnatal care is grossly inadequate. On an average, only 33% of women receive postnatal care. Since a majority of deaths take place in the postnatal period, the overall MMR continues to be high.

Poor public health measures and lack of hygiene affect the health of women adversely and more so during pregnancy, and during and after delivery.

A number of nonmedical factors influence maternal health. Early age at marriage, illiteracy or low level of education, economic dependence and last but not

Table 1.1 Comparison of MMR indicators

Region	No. of maternal deaths	MMR	Lifetime risk: 1 in
World	536,000	400	92
Developed countries	960	9	7,300
Developing countries	533,000	450	75
India	67,000	254	100

(*Source:* Sample Registration Survey and Registrar-General of India 2006)

Table 1.2 Causes of maternal mortality

Cause	Occurrence (%)
Hemorrhage	38
Sepsis	11
Hypertensive disorders	5
Anemia	5
Unsafe abortion	8
Others	33

(*Source:* Sample Registration Survey and Registrar-General of India 2006)

the least, gender bias contribute to poor reproductive health, often resulting in death.

Consequences of maternal death: These are far reaching. A high MMR correlates with a high neonatal death rate. The death of 'under fives' also increases. The disease burden in children increases by almost 20%. The repercussions on the society are significant. There is decreased productivity and earning capacity in the family, leading to poverty. The prospects of children leading a productive life are significantly reduced.

Programmes for reducing maternal deaths: In order to improve maternal health and reduce maternal deaths, several programmes have been launched by the national government in collaboration with nongovernmental organisations and international agencies. They are listed below:

- Safe Motherhood
- Maternal and Child Health (MCH)
- Reproductive and Child Health (RCH I and RCH II)
- Janani Suraksha Yojana (JSRY)
- National Rural Health Mission (NRHM)

Maternal morbidity: Maternal morbidity, that is, ill health or disability resulting from pregnancy, childbirth and puerperium is emerging as an indicator of maternal health. It is estimated that in India it varies widely from 16–238 morbidities to one death.

The first four (hemorrhage, infection, hypertensive disorders and unsafe abortion) are direct causes of maternal mortality; of the indirect causes, anemia is responsible for 5% of deaths. Mothers also succumb to other disorders like infective hepatitis and heart disease. It is very important to recognise that maternal deaths due to direct causes are largely preventable, as also anemia, an indirect cause.

Perinatal mortality rate (PNMR): In India, it is high at 42.5 as compared to 10 in the UK and the USA. It indicates that inadequate obstetric care is provided in a community. Moreover, socioeconomic factors and maternal characteristics also influence the rate.

Causes of perinatal mortality: It is important to remember that about two-thirds of all perinatal deaths occur among infants weighing less than 2,500 g at birth. Very often, the causes may operate through pregnancy to the postnatal period, for example, hypertensive disorders and diabetes mellitus. The common causes may be classified as follows:

- **During pregnancy:** Hypertensive disorders, antepartum hemorrhage, associated medical diseases, intrauterine infections, preterm/postterm pregnancy
- **During labour:** Birth asphyxia, birth injuries
- **After delivery:** Prematurity, intrauterine growth restriction, congenital anomalies

Factors influencing PNMR: The most common factors are listed below:

- maternal age less than 18 years and over 35 years
- poor socioeconomic status
- access to and utilisation of obstetric and neonatal care.

The average infant mortality rate (IMR) for India is 57 (NFHS-3). Although the IMR has declined over the last few decades, it is not satisfactory, as neonatal mortality continues to be unacceptably high. Good obstetric care can reduce stillbirths and early neonatal deaths.

Good practices in obstetrics

It is worth noting that good obstetric practice can contribute tremendously towards reduction in maternal and perinatal mortality and morbidity. Health care providers have access to the latest advances in knowledge and technology. For example, genetics, molecular biology, fetal diagnosis and therapy, intensive care units for the mother and her child have revolutionised the practice of obstetrics. Unfortunately, these mainly benefit the women in urban areas. Excessive and indiscriminate use of such tools provides no additional benefit to the mother and her child. An ultrasound examination performed at every visit in a woman whose pregnancy is normal has no value in its management. Similarly, performing a cesarean section without a genuine indication is of no benefit: a steep rise in this operation has not significantly contributed to a decline in the perinatal mortality rate.

In recent years, there has been a review of studies comparing available options for investigations/ treatment in order to find out which one of these would be the best, so that one could choose the 'best option' that has been scientifically proven. In other words, there is a need to practice **evidence-based medicine**.

'EBM is the conscientious, explicit and judicious use of current best evidence in making decisions about the care of individual patients. The practice of EBM means integrating clinical expertise with the best external clinical evidence from systematic research' (Sackett et al 1996).

Therefore, one must institute the 'best option' for providing desirable obstetric care for the benefit of women, their children and, ultimately, the society.

KEY POINTS

- Obstetrics is the branch of medicine concerned with the care of women during pregnancy, childbirth and a period of six weeks after childbirth.
- Several factors like socioeconomic status, literacy and gender affect the wellbeing of mothers.
- Good obstetric care results in the reduction of maternal and perinatal mortality and morbidity.
- Health indices are useful to assess and compare the quality of health care.
- Appropriate use of technology will help in rendering optimum care.
- Evidence-based approach is useful in obstetric practice.

QUESTIONS

Select the single most appropriate answer:

1. Currently, the maternal mortality ratio (MMR) in India is
   a. 150 to 200　c. 350 to 400
   b. 250 to 300　d. 450 to 500
2. Most maternal deaths occur in which period?
   a. early pregnancy　c. labour
   b. late pregnancy　d. after delivery
3. Which one of the following is the most common cause of maternal mortality?
   a. infection　c. abortion
   b. hemorrhage　d. preeclampsia
4. A baby is said to be at term if it is born after how many weeks of gestation?
   a. 34 weeks　c. 36 weeks
   b. 35 weeks　d. 37 weeks
5. Currently, the average birth rate in India is
   a. 21　b. 23　c. 25　d. 27
6. Early neonatal death refers to the death of the newborn within
   a. 7 days　b. 14 days　c. 21 days　d. 28 days
7. Which one of the following is an indirect cause of maternal death?
   a. septic abortion　c. anemia
   b. hemorrhage　d. eclampsia
8. The lifetime risk of a woman dying as a result of childbirth in India is 1 in
   a. 100　b. 300　c. 600　d. 900
9. The current perinatal mortality rate in India is
   a. 22.5　b. 32.5　c. 42.5　d. 52.5
10. Perinatal mortality rate can be brought down significantly with
    a. liberal use of cesarean section
    b. widespread use of ultrasound
    c. good obstetric practice
    d. use of electronic fetal monitoring
11. A consequence of high maternal mortality can be
    a. high rate of infant mortality
    b. increased disease burden in children
    c. decreased productivity
    d. all of the above
12. The decline in maternal deaths in India in recent years may be attributed to
    a. good obstetric care　c. improved literacy of women
    b. increased age of marriage　d. all of the above

2

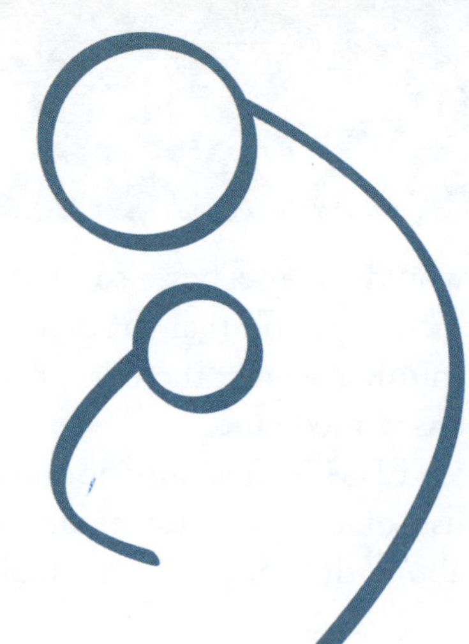

Ethical Issues

S Soundara Raghavan

LEARNING OBJECTIVES

At the end of this chapter, the reader should be able to:

- define medical ethics
- enumerate and define the major principles of ethics
- appreciate the need for following ethical principles
- recognise ethical dilemmas in medical practice
- identify areas with ethical concerns in obstetric practice
- provide suggestions to solve the ethical dilemmas

Introduction

Obstetrics is a specialty dealing with two lives, closely linked, whose interests may not always coincide. Technological advances like assisted reproduction, genetic diagnosis, fetal diagnosis and therapy, endoscopic surgery, interventional radiology and upcoming problems like HIV/AIDS make obstetrics a hotbed of ethical dilemmas. One is expected to learn **medical ethics** from senior practitioners and teachers who are expected to be role models for the students. But, in order to resolve these dilemmas, deliberate effort is required in studying the principles of ethics that govern clinical practice in general and obstetrics in particular.

Rapid advances in technology, changes in economic policies and globalisation have resulted in issues that call for increased attention to ethics in health care. The World Health Organization (WHO) has recommended that ethics should be promoted by formal teaching.

Need for medical ethics: A medical student is expected to gain knowledge, acquire tact, communication and decision-making skills and develop a favourable attitude. Medical ethics is an important pillar of the edifice of medical practice.

Medical ethics can be defined as the study of propriety and moral correctness in health care. While morality in behaviour may be concerned with one's personal convictions and legality the result of what the society considers acceptable, ethicality is often decided by professional consensus. Thus, there is a thin line between what is 'ethical' and what is 'legal'.

It has been rightly said that a doctor who lacks proper 'knowledge' is bound to be a quack. One who has sound knowledge, but lacks 'skills' is dangerous. One with sound knowledge and adequate skills, but found wanting in 'ethics', is deemed a charlatan. Thus, every good doctor should have all the three components, namely, knowledge, attitude and skills.

PRINCIPLES OF ETHICS

Some of the principles that are considered essential for ethical medical practice are given below.

Beneficence: A doctor should always have the best interest of the patient as the supreme consideration.

It requires the doctor to assess objectively and meticulously, all the available diagnostic and therapeutic options and to implement those that protect and promote the interest of the patient by ensuring a balance of good over harm.

Non-maleficence: A doctor must make sure that in the first place, he does no harm.

Autonomy: This principle acknowledges the fact that the patient has a perspective of her interest based on her values and beliefs. One must accept that the patient has the right to choose or refuse treatment.

Justice: Distribution of scarce health resources.

Equality: Social or economic status and religion or race should not be used to discriminate between patients when offering treatment.

Dignity: The patient has the right to dignity.

Honesty: The patient has a right to know the truth about her illness and treatment.

The above principles may not always be in consonance with each other and may sometimes actually contradict each other. Such situations are called **ethical dilemmas**. For example, autonomy and beneficence will clash when a patient refuses a life-saving blood transfusion. Another dilemma is when saving a patient from an attempt to commit suicide.

Ethical dilemmas can be solved by publicly advocating the proposed action. Another suggestion is to formulate a universal prescription in conformance with logic so that the same action can be subscribed to in all circumstances. Sometimes, professional bodies give clear ethical guidelines and good practice statements. A simple method that can often be used is to seek a second or third opinion or better still, where possible, to consult an ethics committee.

For centuries, beneficence was the main guiding principle to decision-making. Too often beneficence-based decisions led to paternalism—the physician overrides the patient's wishes or intentions. The essence of modern medical ethics is a balance between beneficence and autonomy. When there is a conflict, patient autonomy should prevail. If the physician opines that autonomy may harm the patient or such action will offend his professional conscience, he may refuse to carry out the request. Sometimes in issues like medical termination of pregnancy, referring the patient to another physician may assist decision-making.

Ethical Concerns in Obstetric Practice

There are several situations in obstetrics where a doctor is likely to face ethical dilemmas. It would be pragmatic to discuss some of them.

Abortion: Abortion raises a lot of 'heat and dust' during policy discussions. In some countries, elections have been lost on this issue. Hippocrates considered termination of pregnancy as unethical. Times have changed and abortion has been accepted by many societies, the health of the mother being the most important consideration. The autonomy of the woman, the right to decide whether or not to continue the pregnancy is to be respected. In India, abortion was legalised by the Medical Termination of Pregnancy Act in 1972. However, only qualified medical personnel in recognised institutions can terminate a pregnancy under specific circumstances.

Status and rights of the fetus: For a long time, the fetus did not have a legal status or right. These days, the fetus is being conferred individual status and rights. Opponents of abortion often quote the 'right to life' of the fetus. Generally, the woman's right overrides that of her fetus till the period of viability, after which the fetus is bestowed with legal and moral rights in several countries.

In obstetric care, the promotion and protection of the interests of both the pregnant mother and her fetus are foremost. The physician discharges his duties respecting the principles of autonomy and beneficence. The fetus cannot have a perspective on its interest. The pregnant woman may exercise her autonomy, which may not be in the interest of the fetus. For example, administration of insulin to a diabetic mother could prevent fetal macrosomia or sudden intrauterine death, but the mother may refuse to take insulin. In such a case, the physician must bear in mind the need to give more importance to the beneficence-based obligation to the fetus and try to convince the mother.

Assisted reproduction techniques: While moralists question the manipulation of gametes and link sexual intercourse with love, the objections to using the gametes of the partners are generally weak. On the other hand, using donor gametes, surrogate motherhood like lending of uterus, cryopreservation and the use of gametes and embryos often provoke severe criticism. Selective reduction of embryos creates a paradox where embryos are killed to improve the outcome of a treatment of infertility where the primary aim is to achieve pregnancy.

Genetic and prenatal diagnosis: While the objective of the above may appear laudable, conditions like Down syndrome are not incompatible with life and the diagnosis of such conditions leading to termination of the pregnancy is a subject of debate. In such cases, the pregnancy has often been desired and is a deliberately made choice. The question of the severity and treatability of a disability diagnosed antenatally further complicates the matter since the diagnosis may lead to a decision to terminate the pregnancy. When the diagnosis is made after the legally permitted period for the termination of a pregnancy, it becomes an ethical issue.

Use of ultrasound: Ultrasound has become indispensable to obstetric practice. Some of the issues that could pose a dilemma to the obstetrician are the margin of error, who should do the ultrasound, confidentiality of the findings, their disclosure and the use of routine ultrasound for all pregnant women. Misuse of ultrasound and other prenatal diagnostic tests for sex determination has been a bane, and strict laws have been enacted to curb the menace.

Fetal diagnosis and therapy: The expanding possibilities of invasive diagnostic techniques and treating the fetus in utero also raise several ethical concerns. These concerns are who will be the treating physician, detection of the pathological condition and its treatment, and whether to opt for an open or closed method of treatment. One must also consider the risk to the mother versus the benefit to the fetus, logistics of centres, specialists and cost versus benefit and the availability of fetal intensive care units. It is difficult to make decisions in this field, particularly keeping in mind the principles of equality and justice.

Organ donation and transplantation: The obstetrician is involved in this decision because of the possible use of tissues from anencephalic fetuses for the purpose of donation or transplantation. This may extend to fresh stillbirths or very moribund newborns. Currently, several countries including India accept the use of tissues from anencephalic fetuses for therapeutic purposes.

Stem cell research: Stem cells can be obtained from the adult marrow, umbilical cord blood and several tissues. However, those obtained from the inner cell mass of the embryo have totipotent properties, making the embryo an attractive source. Harvesting embryos solely for obtaining stem cells provides grounds for ethical consideration.

Cloning: This means creating an identical copy of the original, and involves somatic cell nuclear transfer. It may be done for '**reproductive**' purposes, but has not found acceptance. On the other hand, cloning of embryos is an attractive alternative to harvesting stem cells for '**therapeutic**' purposes which will obviate the need to destroy embryos resulting from natural conception or assisted reproduction techniques.

HIV/AIDS: The question of routine testing of pregnant mothers in view of the possible benefits of preventing parent-to-child transmission (PTCT) is hotly debated. Though National AIDS Control Organisation has advocated Counselled Voluntary Testing, many institutions resort to routine uninformed testing and referring the HIV-positive mothers to other institutions. HIV-positive mothers are sometimes forced to conceal the information because of social stigma and discrimination, leading to the risk of transmission to the newborn as well as to health care workers and others. Universal precautions, though advised, are often neglected. Informing the status to the spouse/partner and MTP for an HIV-positive mother are areas of concern.

Euthanasia, informed consent and clinical research are areas of enhanced ethical dilemma in obstetric practice as compared to other medical specialties.

A doctor in the practice of obstetrics is likely to face ethical conflicts. Good clinical practice requires the identification of the component of ethical principle in the conflict, and the doctor should work towards making an ethically justifiable decision.

KEY POINTS

- Ethics, with knowledge and skills, forms the foundation of medical practice.
- The basic principles of medical ethics are beneficence, non-maleficence and respect for autonomy.
- Ethical dilemmas should be identified, accepted and decisions should be made based on the principles.
- Obstetric practice is concerned with two lives and therefore lends itself to many ethical considerations and dilemmas.
- Adhering to the basic principles of medical ethics, following good clinical practice guidelines, seeking a second opinion and consultation with ethical committees go a long way in minimising litigations.

QUESTIONS

Select the single most appropriate answer:

1. Ethics are determined by
   a. personal conviction
   b. law of the society
   c. religious leaders
   d. professional bodies' consensus
2. Which of the following domains will ethics be a part of?
   a. scientific knowledge
   b. aptitude for research
   c. attitude
   d. manual skills
3. Which of the following is *not* a basic principle of ethics?
   a. patient autonomy
   b. informed consent
   c. non-maleficence
   d. beneficence
4. Which of the following example is appropriate for overruling patient autonomy?
   a. forcing a patient for tubectomy
   b. refusing termination of pregnancy
   c. refusing to treat because the patient does not agree to the doctor's suggestion
   d. treating a patient who has attempted suicide
5. In case of an ethical conflict, which of the following principles should take precedence over others?
   a. patient autonomy
   b. paternalism
   c. beneficence
   d. justice
6. When facing an ethical dilemma, which of the following is *not* advisable?
   a. taking a second opinion
   b. consulting guidelines from professional body
   c. following one's mind
   d. obtaining peer group advice

3

Gender Sensitisation

Sundari Ravindran

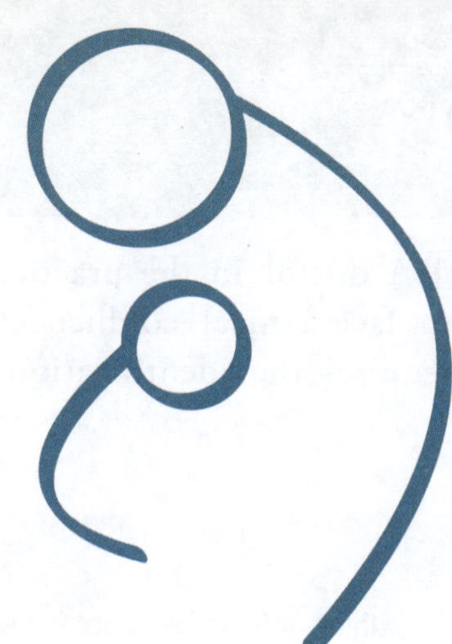

LEARNING OBJECTIVES

At the end of this chapter, the reader should be able to:

- define gender
- list ways in which gender factors influence maternal health in terms of risk and vulnerability to ill health, health-seeking behaviour, utilisation of health services and the ability to successfully access and complete treatment
- list the health consequences of gender-based violence during pregnancy, childbirth and puerperium
- apply the above knowledge to history-taking, clinical examination and diagnosis, treatment and advice given to patients

Introduction

The term **gender** was first used in the 1970s to describe those characteristics of men and women that are socially determined, as against '**sex**', which describes biologically determined characteristics. The lower status of women as compared to men in almost all societies has less to do with the fact that they are biologically different. It has more to do with gender factors such as social and cultural norms about what women and men should and should not do. These, in turn, are derived from the belief that men are inherently superior and that it is the natural order of things that men rather than women be 'in charge' within and outside the home, as heads of families, communities and countries.

Gender factors play a critical role in promoting and protecting, or adversely affecting, women's health. The influence of gender on female health starts even before birth, continues through childhood, well into the reproductive years and into old age. It is important for doctors to understand how gender factors influence a woman's treatment-seeking behaviour and compliance with the medical treatment and advice for her clinical problems. This will help the doctor in making a better diagnosis and providing better care.

Development of gender

Gender refers to those characteristics of women and men which are the result of **socialisation**. In contrast, **sex** refers to characteristics of women and men which are **biologically** determined.

Gender roles are learnt. From very early in life, parents, family members and the community treat boys and girls differently. They are systematically taught to be different from each other, for example, in terms of:

- the way they dress, walk and talk
- the activities and pastimes they are allowed to pursue
- the tasks they perform and the responsibilities they shoulder
- the emotions they should or should not show
- the way they are supposed to behave within the home and in public spaces.

Gender-based discrimination

Although society prescribes specific roles for girls and boys, women and men, it does not treat these different roles and responsibilities as equally valuable. In most societies, girls and women are valued less than boys and men. Studies from many parts of the world show that there is usually lower investment in girls in terms of care given, nutrition and education. Women work longer hours. They are responsible for all domestic work and childcare in addition to income-earning activities. Work that is considered 'women's chore' commands lower wages. Many laws and policies allow women lesser rights.

The **disparity in value** placed on women's roles and responsibilities is the **source of discrimination** of women and accounts for the inferior status given to them in society. Women have **less access to money and other resources**, and also have **less decision-making power** both within the home and outside.

Gender discrimination is perpetuated by a belief system and it is important to remember that **women as well as men play a role in perpetuating it.**

Influence on maternal health

When a woman dies in childbirth, what is noted is the immediate cause of death, which may be eclampsia or hemorrhage. The woman's death is thought to be a misfortune: a chance event that is unavoidable in the process of childbirth. This is a false impression. The outcome of pregnancy, and associated morbidity and mortality, is profoundly influenced by the circumstances of a woman's life. It has been noted that wherever maternal mortality and morbidity rates are high, women's status is low, mainly as a result of gender discrimination. Yet, this connection is rarely perceived and is usually ignored.

Gender-based inequalities and discrimination affect maternal health in many ways. For example, they contribute to enhancing risks and vulnerabilities to maternal health problems and influence health-seeking behaviour, ability to utilise health services or comply with treatment and advice.

Risks and vulnerabilities: The risks and vulnerabilities associated with gender conditioning are grouped as follows:

Nutrition: A large percentage of women are constantly anemic and poorly nourished with or without pregnancy. To some extent, this is a result of poverty and scarcity of nutritious food. However, from infancy and childhood, women receive lesser quantities and less nutritious food. If girls do not have adequate protein, calcium and vitamin D in early childhood, their growth is stunted, subjecting them to a greater risk of contracted pelvis. Gender-based disparity in access to food within households continues into adulthood. More Indian women (41%) than men (34%) suffer from chronic energy deficiency, with a body mass index of 18.5 or less. The deficiency is made worse by pregnancy and breastfeeding.

It is well established that poor nutritional status compromises immunity to infections and healing capacity, making childbirth much more risky in these women than in those who are well-nourished. In India, severe anemia continues to be a major cause of maternal death; it also makes her vulnerable to death from hemorrhage, sepsis, and anesthetic and surgical complications.

Burden of physical labour: Gender-based division of labour is also a major contributor to poor nutrition. In addition to the constant demands of pregnancy, motherhood and childcare, women are almost exclusively responsible for all the domestic work; sometimes they also have to work outside the home.

Gender norms: These refer to values that dictate what is considered 'appropriate' behaviour for girls without prescribing anything similarly for boys. This results in misconceptions, or worse, lack of awareness amongst girls about a range of issues related to their bodies and about reproduction. It leads to many adverse consequences, like vulnerability to sexual abuse, unsafe and/or illegal pregnancy and early childbearing.

Contraception: The woman's unequal position within a marriage is often an important factor that contributes to the non-use of contraception, and to frequent pregnancies, which are either carried to term or end in abortions. Girls often enter into marriage without knowing how to prevent pregnancies. Even the few who do know about contraception may not discuss the issue with their spouses for fear that this would be considered inappropriate. There is also pressure on the newly married woman to bear a child within the first year of marriage, to establish her fertility.

A woman who has recently delivered may not want an immediate pregnancy, but her partner may not be in favour of her using a spacing method of contraception. Very few men use any contraceptive method, and this exposes women to unwanted pregnancy. Women may not be able to enforce periodic abstinence to avoid pregnancy, because men usually enforce sexual rights within the relationship.

Sexual behaviour: Social norms accept men in extramarital or premarital sexual relationships as 'normal' while ostracising the women they partner; women are unable to negotiate safe sex practices, making it difficult to protect themselves from sexually transmitted infections.

Preference for the male child: This gender factor has many negative maternal health consequences. It is very common to see women go through several pregnancies till they give birth to a male child. In recent times, since smaller families are desired, women have been going through sex-selective abortions of the female fetus, till a male child is born. It has been noted that this mindset may also affect mental health in the postpartum period.

Health-seeking behaviour: Gender stereotyping has the following impact on the health-seeking behaviour of women:

- The low educational status of women limits their access to health information. Women have less exposure to the media and fewer opportunities to interact with sources or providers of information. Thus, they are placed at a disadvantage in recognising symptoms of health problems and often postpone seeking appropriate health care.
- Women feel embarrassed to discuss matters related to their reproductive organs even with other women, and more so with their husbands. It is well known that women with white discharge, uterine prolapse and urinary incontinence rarely disclose it to health providers, especially to male doctors, unless the condition becomes unbearable.

Others before self: Since she is brought up to put her-self last, a woman does not perceive that she is entitled to invest in her wellbeing. She feels guilty about taking rest or spending money on herself.

Utilisation of health care services

Women's access to health services is impeded by many factors, most of which are a combination of gender and poverty.

Lack of decision-making power: To begin with, women do not have the power to make decisions about health care, and need the permission of their husbands and other elders in the family. The nature of antenatal and delivery care that women are able to get is thus not within their control. This in turn is influenced by how the woman's health and pregnancy are valued in the family. First pregnancies may be valued more than subsequent ones, and women who have borne many female children may be left to a poorer quality of care. Family members' traditional beliefs and ignorance about danger signs during pregnancy, delivery and postpartum are other formidable barriers.

Restrictions on physical mobility: This is common in many parts of India; thus it may be necessary for women to be accompanied to a health facility by a male or other 'responsible' family members.

Lack of time: Women have very little time to seek health care. A day taken off to go to the health centre or to a referral hospital usually means arranging for someone else to do the household chores; in addition, they may lose the day's income.

Distance: When the health facility is far away and involves considerable travel and time, and when there are long queues at the health facility, patients feel increasingly reluctant to wait and see a doctor.

Case scenario: A third gravida was told to go to the referral hospital by the PHC doctor. Her husband was out of town and she had to wait for him to come back. After he returned, the children were left with relatives, someone was found to take care of the house and a loan was raised. She then went to the referral hospital; 12 days later she delivered a stillborn baby.

Cost of seeking health care: This often discourages many women from going to a doctor or a health facility. Even when there is no formal fee for services, the cost of transport, drugs and supplies and the loss of income can together make health care unaffordable for women.

Domestic violence against women: One tends to think of all pregnancies as happy events and all pregnant women as enjoying the support of their families, especially their husbands. Unfortunately, this is not true for many women who regularly experience violence committed by their husbands or other members of their families.

Types of violence: In many instances, domestic violence is not a chance event but a regular pattern. The violence may be physical or sexual. Less recognised as violence but just as distressing is unpredictable and erratic behaviour on the part of the husband, which causes psychological and emotional distress.

Extent of violence: About 20% of women in the reproductive age group experience physical violence from their husbands. About 22%–28% of pregnant women experience psychological, sexual or physical violence during pregnancy.

Consequences: Women exposed to violence have a higher likelihood of experiencing miscarriages or stillbirths; there is also a significant association between violence during pregnancy and low birth weight babies.

They are also more likely to experience depression during pregnancy and in the postpartum period, injuries, which in the worst case, can result in death.

Case scenario: A 22-year-old primigravida was admitted with antepartum bleeding. She had suffered trauma to the abdomen, which she said was the result of a fall. When taking history it was learnt that she had not had any antenatal care till the third trimester. She had not gained adequate weight, and appeare distressed. On probing, it was learnt that she had been regularly subjected to physical and psychological violence by her husband and in-laws because her family had defaulted on the promised dowry.

Ways to Address Gender Issues in a Pregnant Woman

One may wonder what the physician can do about gender discrimination, which is a larger social problem. It is true that many of the problems cannot be solved by the physician. However, just being aware of the many ways in which gender discrimination affects maternal health can make a significant difference to obstetric practice and health outcome.

Sample questions and guidelines for screening for domestic violence are given in the boxes below. Some principles for addressing gender in obstetric practice include:

- focusing on the woman's life circumstances and the role of gender
- prioritising health education, information and counselling
- respect for the decisions and choices she makes
- upholding the woman's dignity and her safety
- recognising the role and responsibility of husbands/ partners.

How these principles may be put into practice is discussed below.

The first contact

- It must be remembered that the woman may have come to the health facility/provider against great odds. If turned back and asked to come another day, she may never be able to. For example, women seeking abortion services when asked to come later may turn to an unqualified provider, with adverse health consequences. Again, it may be preferable to admit a high-risk patient with 'false' labour pains if her date of delivery is not far away, rather than risk her not returning to the health facility for delivery.
- As far as possible, her health problem must be dealt with in the same visit, and the number of return visits be cut down to the essential minimum.
- The woman should not be blamed for delaying her first visit to the provider or for missing a follow-up visit. She should be treated with understanding and respect.
- If for some reason the service a woman seeks cannot be provided to her, it must be addressed in some other way. For example, a woman seeking sterilisation may be turned down because she could show poor outcome after surgery. But if she is not provided with another method of contraception, she will probably become pregnant again.

- If referring the woman to another facility, it is necessary to ascertain whether the woman will be able to go to the referral facility. If she cannot, other ways of addressing her problem need to be found.

When taking history

- The woman's family circumstances: whether she is part of a joint family, what her workload is, whether she is able to get enough food and so on should be enquired into. These are useful pointers towards her chances of having a healthy pregnancy and delivery.
- Information should be obtained about whether her husband is a migrant worker and is away from home for prolonged periods. This will help assess several risks. Decisions about her health care may be delayed: this is especially crucial when it comes to obstetric emergencies. The woman may also be at risk of STIs and HIV infection.
- If she has had an induced abortion before, find out the circumstances that made her opt for it. This may provide useful insights for contraceptive counselling following the present delivery. It may also indicate whether or not the present pregnancy is a 'wanted' one. Women with unwanted pregnancies tend to neglect their health and not comply with medical advice.
- The sex of her previous children should be noted. A woman with two or more daughters may have had sex-selective induced abortions, which she may not disclose. She may be very stressed about the outcome of the present pregnancy, and may be at risk of prenatal as well as postpartum depression.
- Gently probe for the likelihood of domestic violence. The importance of prenatal screening of women for domestic violence is now widely acknowledged.

When examining the woman

- Explain what is being done and why.
- Many women are especially fearful of vaginal examination, because they have been brought up never to expose themselves. It would help if they are told what to expect and reassured adequately.
- The woman must be treated with dignity. Privacy must be ensured. The woman must not wait with her legs up in the stirrups.
- Unnecessary people should not be around and unwanted conversation should be avoided.
- Her consent should be obtained for students or others to be present during her physical examination.
- If there are any signs of physical injury, these are recorded and the woman is gently questioned to

Introducing screening questions

Asking directly

- Before we discuss contraceptive choices, it might be good to know a little bit more about your relationship with your partner.
- Because violence is common in women's lives, we have begun asking all clients about abuse.
- I don't know if this is a problem for you, but many of the women I see as clients are dealing with tensions at home. Some are too afraid or uncomfortable to bring it up themselves, so I've started asking about it routinely.

Asking indirectly

- Your symptoms may be related to stress. Do you and your partner tend to fight a lot?
- Does your husband have any problems with alcohol, drugs or gambling? How does it affect his behaviour with you and the children?

Source: Heise L, M. Ellsberg and M. Gottemoeller. *Ending violence against women*. Population Reports, Volume XXVI, No. 4, December 1999.

Sample guidelines for screening for domestic violence

1. *Meet the patient alone:* The husband, in-laws, women friends or even staff members from the health facility not trained to maintain confidentiality may not be present.
2. *Ask about violence:* You may ask directly or indirectly, using your judgement to identify women who you consider may be 'at risk'.
3. *If the patient says no, but you suspect violence:* Thank the patient. Tell her that she can get in touch with you any time that she needs to. Give her your contact details.
4. *If the patient says yes:* Tell her it is not her fault. Explain to her that many women experience domestic violence. Make her understand that you take her seriously.
5. *Document in the case sheet:* If you find any symptoms of probable violence, and especially physical injury, document these clearly in the patient's case sheet. This will help in a future visit, to identify whether she has been subjected to violence.
6. *If the patient's health is seriously under threat:* Discuss with the woman ways in which she can be away from the source of violence during pregnancy and delivery.
7. *If needed:* Give the patient information about organisations that offer services for women experiencing violence. Many directories are now available with the Social Welfare Department.

Source: Perinatal domestic violence identification services (PDVIS): A guide to culturally relevant care in health clinics. Washington State Department of Health, April 2004.

determine whether domestic violence could be a cause.

Education and counselling

- At least basic information must be given to the pregnant women on danger signals during pregnancy for which she needs immediate medical attention.
- Relevant health education materials available in the local language may be given to the women.
- Counselling is an important component of health care for women, especially those in very difficult circumstances. Without it, the treatment and advice given may not be adhered to or may be ineffective. For example, many women may not be able to have an institutional delivery. It is then important that they are counselled to find a trained attendant at birth.
- The doctor must speak to the husband and his participation and cooperation must be sought in the care provided to the pregnant woman. It is important that he knows of danger signals during pregnancy, and of preparation for emergency obstetric care and contraception.
- An exception to male involvement is when there is a history of domestic violence. If it is known that the husband is violent, then it is important **not to** disclose to him what his wife may have said in confidence.

Treatment and advice

- Many women find the process of giving birth in a hospital humiliating. This is so because their pain is treated as trivial, the staff members shout at them, and they receive no information on how the labour is progressing and what is being done to them. Women deserve to be treated with honour and dignity throughout the process of labour and delivery. Kind words and reassurance, and keeping them informed of what is happening, will go a long way in making them feel better.
- A woman may not have the resources for expensive or prolonged treatment. Whenever possible, drugs and tests that are less expensive should be used. Interventions should be minimised.
- The potential difficulties in compliance with treatment or advice should be discussed, and alternatives considered.
- When referring a woman for an obstetric emergency, her financial situation must be kept in mind. A referral slip with a summary must be given so that delay in the referral centre is minimised.
- The potential danger of violence to a woman when specific conditions are diagnosed must be remembered. For example, many hospitals

routinely screen antenatal women for HIV status. Disclosure to the husband or family when the woman is confirmed to be HIV-positive may have dire consequences for her.

KEY POINTS

- It is important to address gender issues in obstetric practice.
- Biological risks associated with pregnancy and childbirth interact with gender-based discrimination to affect maternal health.
- Gender factors contribute to increasing health risks, influencing health-seeking behaviour and health outcomes of women during their pregnancy, delivery and postpartum.

QUESTIONS

Select the single most appropriate answer:

1. What is most appropriate about the terms gender and sex?
   a. do not have the same meaning
   b. mean the same
   c. mean the same with differences in some aspects
   d. rarely used interchangeably
2. Gender-based inequalities and discrimination affect maternal health in
   a. the ability to recognise serious problems
   b. utilisation of health services
   c. compliance with treatment and advice
   d. all of the above
3. Gender norms affect boys and girls
   a. equally
   b. unequally, with a greater impact on the wellbeing of girls
   c. all of the above
   d. none of the above
4. Unequal gender power relations within marriage increases the vulnerability of women to all of the following *except*
   a. use of contraception
   b. menstrual disorders
   c. frequent pregnancies
   d. risk of sexually transmitted infections
5. Which of the following factors influences the health-seeking behaviour of women?
   a. socialisation b. cost of seeking health care
   c. both of the above d. None of the above
6. Domestic violence against women can affect
   a. physical health b. mental health
   c. reproductive and sexual health d. all of the above
7. When treating a woman, it is important to know whether the husband is a migrant worker because
   a. Decisions about her health may be delayed.
   b. She may be unable to use effective contraception.
   c. Risk of STI/HIV infection may be elevated.
   d. all of the above
8. Involvement of the husband is *not* advisable during counselling if there is a history of
   a. sexually transmitted infection
   b. poor pregnancy outcome
   c. domestic violence
   d. all of the above
9. Understanding the role of gender factors in women's health is important for
   a. history-taking
   b. treatment
   c. counselling
   d. all of the above
10. Gender-based division of labour contributes to
    a. poor nutrition in women
    b. frequent infections in women
    c. exposure to trauma
    d. none of the above

4

Reproductive and Child Health Programme

Kamala Ganesh

LEARNING OBJECTIVES

At the end of this chapter, the reader should be able to:

- define reproductive health and understand its objectives
- explain why the paradigm shift was introduced in the programme
- enumerate the components of the Reproductive and Child Health (RCH) programme
- describe the package of services offered under each component
- understand the organisational and infrastructure requirements for the implementation of the programme, including special facilities and projects
- appreciate the managerial dimensions of the RCH programme
- enumerate the indicators of quality care
- describe the initiatives for improving the quality of care

Introduction

Poor health status resulting in high mortality and morbidity among women and children has been a major concern in India, even prior to Independence. After 1947, efforts to provide services to this vulnerable section of the population were initiated under the Maternal and Child Health (MCH) services. Major hospitals in urban areas and primary health centres (PHCs) in the rural areas were responsible for rendering these services. Rapid growth in population and its social and economic consequences on the development and quality of life of people resulted in the launch of the National Family Planning Programme. With advances in technology and various other interventions, programmes like immunisation against vaccine-preventable diseases, nutritional interventions like iron and folic acid supplementation and vit A supplementation were initiated.

It was realised that fertility regulation was an extremely important factor in maintaining the health of the mother and child. It was appreciated that couples would accept contraceptive services to prevent pregnancy, only if survival of their existing children was ensured. This realisation of the close relationship between family planning and MCH programmes led to the government's policy decision to integrate family planning with MCH and nutrition services; thus, the Child Survival and Safe Motherhood (CSSM) Programme was launched. These programmes were implemented separately, but concurrently and were significantly beneficial.

At the third International Conference on Population and Development (ICPD) held in

Cairo in 1994, about 180 countries reached a new consensus about how world population issues should be approached. It was agreed that population policies should address social development beyond family planning, especially the advancement of women, and that family planning should be provided in the context of comprehensive reproductive health care. The Cairo Programme of Action (POA) defined the reproductive and child health approach as:

"People have the ability to reproduce and regulate their fertility, women are able to go through pregnancy and childbirth safely, the outcome of pregnancies is successful in terms of maternal and infant survival and wellbeing and couples are to have sexual relations free of fear of pregnancy and contracting diseases." In keeping with the policy of the ICPD, 1994, the RCH programme was launched in India in October 1997.

Objectives of the programme

The objectives of the RCH programme are:

- nationwide improved quality, coverage and effectiveness of RCH services
- improved management performance by:
  a. expanding the existing monitoring system and decentralised participatory planning
  b. institutional strengthening
  c. enhanced programme management capacity
- local capacity enhancement.

Paradigm shift in the programme

The reproductive health approach extends beyond the narrow limits of family planning; it encompasses all aspects of human sexuality and reproductive health needs during various stages of life. A paradigm shift is needed for operationalising the reproductive health programme, a change in focus from the population control approach of reducing numbers to a client-based approach of addressing the reproductive needs of individuals, couples and families, if necessary.

The paradigm shift from the earlier programme is seen in the following aspects:

- target-free approach based on community needs assessment (CNA)
- decentralised participatory planning
- providing integrated RCH package
- state-/district-specific RCH strategy
- emphasis on quality of care
- integrated training at district level
- involvement of the *panchayati raj* system
- increased involvement of non-governmental organisations (NGOs) and corporate sector
- area-specific Information Education and Communication (IEC) campaigns
- incorporating gender concerns
- increased male participation.

Approach based on CNA: Method-specific contraceptive targets and associated incentives were replaced by the achievement of desirable reproductive health indicators. It adopted a CNA based a bottom-up approach, where health personnel assessed the workload and set the goals to be achieved. It was termed target-free approach (TFA) and renamed as the CNA approach in 1997.

Decentralised participatory planning: Planning for the services actually begins at the grassroots level, with health workers carrying out a household survey in the months of January and February each year. Members of the *panchayat* and Mahila Swasthya Sangh (MSS) and other villagers closely interact with the ANM (ancillary nurse-midwife) and male health worker to assess the actual requirement of various family welfare services. This approach improves the sustainability of the programme by generating a sense of involvement and ownership among the community and increases the utilisation of services. It creates a sense of responsibility and accountability among the health workers. The plans prepared for the subcentres are compiled to make the PHC plans, which in turn are aggregated at the district level to prepare the district plan.

State-/District-specific strategy: The main focus of the RCH programme is implementation based on the actual needs of the people. Considering the variation in service requirements among different states and districts in the country, an area-specific approach has been worked out separately for different groups of states and districts.

Emphasis on quality of care: Provision of good quality care is the crux of the RCH programme.

Quality of health is said to be good when the following are incorporated in the delivery of services:

- counselling
- choice of service
- technically competent providers
- maintaining work ethics like confidentiality and privacy
- continued client satisfaction
- increased service utilisation.

Integrated training at district level: A major input in the training of health personnel is the emphasis laid on practical clinical, managerial and communication skills. The training is also imparted to *anganwadi* workers and functionaries from other health-related development sectors. Planning and management of the training programmes are the responsibility of the district health authorities. Central and state governments support the district authorities in training the trainers and in producing training materials.

Involvement of the Panchayati Raj system: The *Panchayati Raj* system is expected to play a significant role in planning, implementing and evaluating RCH services. It is also expected to provide finance and transport for women who have been referred to hospitals for obstetric services.

Involvement of NGOs and the corporate sector: The programme envisages involving NGOs and the corporate sector in the delivery of RCH services as well as in undertaking various types of training activities.

Area-specific IEC campaign: IEC activities play a major role in the RCH programme by demystifying the programme and population issues for the public. The objective is to emphasise the development of local area-specific communication strategies to create more demand for RCH services and to promote informed decision-making on health matters. The use of local traditional media is encouraged so as to increase the acceptance and understanding of the messages; it can thus make an impact and bring about behaviour change.

Gender concerns: All efforts are being made to make the programme as gender-sensitive as possible. Women's groups are involved in its planning and monitoring. In addition, the government has also initiated efforts which trigger changes in societal attitudes towards women.

Increased male participation: There is a need for increased male participation in the RCH programme. It is expected that with specific interventions, men may be ready for responsible parenthood, accept contraception and make an informed decision jointly with female partners regarding reproductive health issues.

Components and Packages of Services

The RCH programme has the following components:

- prevention and management of unwanted pregnancy
- services to promote safe motherhood
- services to promote child survival
- nutritional services for vulnerable groups
- prevention and treatment of reproductive tract infections and sexually transmitted diseases
- prevention and treatment of gynecological problems
- screening and treatment of breast and cervical/uterine cancer
- reproductive health services for adolescents
- health, sexuality and gender information, education and counselling
- establishment of effective referral systems.

Programme Interventions

Following are the interventions to be implemented in all districts:

- safe motherhood interventions
- child survival interventions and facilitation for operationalisation of the CNA approach
- institutional development
- integrated training package
- modified Management Information System (MIS)
- IEC activities and counselling on health, sexuality and gender
- urban and tribal area RCH package

- district subprojects under local capacity enhancement
- opening RTI/STI clinics at district hospitals where not already available
- facility for safe abortions at PHCs by providing equipment and doctors
- enhanced community participation through *panchayats*, women's groups and NGOs
- execution of minor building construction
- provision of laboratory technicians for diagnosis of RTI/STI and for emergency obstetric care, adolescent health and reproductive hygiene.

All the districts in the country have been categorised into A (best performance), B (medium performance) and C (poor performance) on the basis of Crude Birth Rate (CBR) and female literacy rate which reasonably reflect the RCH status in the district. The RCH programme is implemented on a differential approach in order to ensure efficient delivery.

Safe motherhood components: Following are the main components of safe motherhood under the RCH:

- antenatal care
- intranatal care
- emergency obstetric care (EOC)
- postnatal care.

Child survival components: The strategies for improving child survival and development include:

- strengthening essential newborn care
- appropriate management of diarrhea
- appropriate management of acute respiratory infection (ARI)
- sustaining high levels of immunisation coverage
- nutritional intervention like nutrition supplementation, such as vitamin A prophylaxis, supplementary feeding
- improved maternal care
- promotion of birth spacing.

Safe abortion services: Complications of unsafe abortions account for significant maternal mortality and morbidity. Medical termination of pregnancy (MTP) under the MTP Act, 1971, aims to provide safe abortions. The RCH programme places specific emphasis on ensuring women's access to safe abortion services by improving facilities and training people to provide MTP services.

Contraceptive services for eligible couples: Providing contraception services is an important intervention under the RCH programme. Couples are provided assistance in making decisions regarding the right time to have children and are also informed about and ensured access to safe, effective, affordable and acceptable methods of contraception of their choice. There is growing concern among policy makers and planners in India that the overemphasis laid on women as the main target groups, in the past, for accepting contraception services, particularly sterilisation services,is not likely to achieve the desired demographic goal. Hence, more emphasis is now being placed on increasing the choice of available contraceptive methods including reversible ones, for both women and men.

To increase male participation in the acceptance of contraception, facilities for providing non-scalpel vasectomy (NSV) are being expanded. Supportive counselling and follow-up services are also being organised for those willing to adopt contraception.

Prevention and management of RTIs and STIs: Reproductive tract infections (RTIs) and sexually transmitted infections (STIs) form a major group of infections which lead to considerable morbidity among both men and women. These can lead to complications like:

- infertility
- ectopic pregnancy
- irregular menstruation
- cancer of the anus and genitals
- infections in the newborn
- increased risk of vertical transmission of HIV infection.

Screening/Diagnosis of RTIs/STIs is based on identifying groups of easily recognised signs and symptoms (syndromic approach).

Adolescent health services: Adolescents need to be prepared for future parenthood. Since young girls are married very early in many parts of India, adolescent girls are exposed to hazards of pregnancy when they are not emotionally and physically ready for childbearing. It is felt that integrated programmes for family life and reproductive as well as general health, education, employment and other related services need to be provided for this hitherto neglected segment of the population, in order to minimise ill health among adolescent girls and to reduce the risk of low birth weight babies and child mortality.

Cancer and infertility services:

Screening and treatment for cervical cancer and breast cancer: In developing countries, the most common cancers of the reproductive systems are those of the uterine cervix and breast. Screening for these cancers is an important intervention but, at present, the facilities are limited.

Prevention and treatment of infertility: Prevention and proper management of RTI/STI can prevent infertility to a great extent. For further diagnosis and management of infertility, the couple should be referred to institutions where resources are available.

Implementation of the RCH Programme

Implementation of the RCH programme.

Organisational set-up for the delivery of the RCH programme: In the RCH programme, the focus is on active involvement of the community and the local *panchayat* with assistance from the central government through the respective state governments. The emphasis is on improving existing services and making them accessible to the community.

Special facilities and projects under the RCH programme: Special efforts are made to provide the services under the selected components to communities in backward areas.

Twenty-four hour delivery services at PHCs: An important contributor to maternal mortality and morbidity is the lack of trained personnel in rural areas; this is particularly true for deliveries that take place at night. Institutional deliveries are encouraged and attempts are being made to set up 24-hour delivery services in CHCs/PHCs in as many districts as possible.

Referral system and transportation for indigent families through panchayats: In order to ensure timely and appropriate referral services in rural areas, the first referral units (FRUs) have been strengthened and the *panchayat* is expected to provide monetary assistance/transport to economically weak families. The FRUs are being strengthened through the supply of drugs, and equipment and the appointment of contractual staff. Attempts are being made to improve EOC by providing facilities for blood transfusion and having a consultant anesthetist.

Additional programme for urban slums: The following measures are being taken:

- Providing a PHC for each slum with a population of 15,000, with one doctor and 2–3 paramedical workers to provide outdoor services; these would be set up and managed by the concerned urban local body on a project basis.
- For clusters of slums with a smaller population, a mobile clinic is to be sanctioned to provide services in the slum on a fixed day.
- NGOs may be assisted if they set up maternity clinics in or near urban slums.

Special programme for tribal areas: RCH services in tribal areas are being strengthened through the following steps:

- stocking adequate supplies of essential drugs
- providing housing for staff posted at these health centres
- contractual appointment of staff against vacancies by committees at the district level under the chairmanship of the District Magistrate
- district-level committees to assist local NGOs in training and engaging the tribal youth to work within the community for promoting RCH information and to act as a link between the health infrastructure and the community.

RCH camps: These are conducted by a team of specialists and paramedical staff once in two months at specially identified PHCs on pre-fixed dates, with the objective of:

- increasing access to RCH services in remote and underserved areas
- providing good quality RCH services
- increasing the utilisation of underutilised PHCs.

Special programmes for adolescents: Adolescents (10–19 years) constitute a large segment of the population (21.4% of the total estimated population) of India. This programme for adolescents will focus on the reproductive health needs and education of adolescents regarding teenage pregnancy, HIV/AIDS and sex and sexuality.

RCH in the tenth five-year plan

In the tenth five-year plan, there was stress on improving the coverage and quality of services. It was also envisaged to achieve 100% registration of births and deaths to provide a database for decentralised district-based needs assessment, planning, implementation and monitoring of performance. Attempts were made to fill in critical gaps in existing infrastructure (especially CHCs) through reorganisation and restructuring and filling up the vacant posts for health care providers. Special emphasis was on skills upgradation of staff, provision of screening and referral services, essential newborn care and the management of common gynecological problems and infertility at FRUs.

Role of hospitals in the implementation of the RCH programme

Hospitals at various levels are expected to implement the RCH programme. Besides the outpatient and inpatient services, they also provide preventive and curative services and EOC for referred cases. They play an important role in training the health care providers, ensuring registration of births and deaths, rendering health education and managing IEC services. They are involved in conducting research in reproductive health and disease surveillance.

Managerial Dimensions of the RCH Programme

The RCH programme is being implemented all over the country through different institutions and personnel of the health care delivery system at various levels in the hierarchy. Hence, health and hospital personnel need to acquire managerial skills in the following areas:

- participatory, decentralised, CNA-based programme planning
- organising special programmes/schemes/projects under the RCH
- procurement of resources and their efficient management
- ensuring quality of care
- management information system
- monitoring and supervision.

CNA-based decentralised planning: The ANM is provided with a manual that helps her arrive at the appropriate CNA and plan her performance.

Human resource development and capacity-building: The focus is on competency-based training with a view to providing quality services. The following training activities are planned in the RCH programme:

- for functionaries from health and health-related sectors including *panchayat raj* officebearers at the grassroot level on raising awareness in the community
- skill development training courses
- integrated foundation skill-based course for primary health care functionaries at ANM/LHV schools and health and family welfare training centres (HFWTCs)
- specialised skill development courses for procedures like medical termination of pregnancy, laparoscopic and mini-laparoscopic sterilisation, and NSV for doctors, and IUCD insertion for ANM/LHV in selected hospitals
- management training for the state, divisional and district-level programme managers
- training in communication for IEC personnel.

The district shall function as the basic unit and district-based training plans shall be prepared for all types of training activities according to the actual training needs. The district authorities are to be assisted by the collaborating training institutions (CTIs) in this regard. These plans are to be approved by the state RCH Coordination Committee and sent to the national nodal agency, the National Institute for Health and Family Welfare (NIHFW), for release of funds for implementing the training. The district family welfare officer (DFWO), assisted by the district training centres will coordinate with the training institutions to ensure that the health personnel of the district are nominated and relieved for the training regularly. The DFWO will also coordinate with the related departments and the *panchayat raj* system in the district to organise training for functionaries from health-related sectors in generating awareness.

Management of material resources: One of the main responsibilities of health personnel is that of managing different types of material resources, so that effective and efficient services can be provided to the clients. The requirements are estimated for a specified period and are procured on time to ensure their appropriate storage/distribution. Maintenance of proper records and effective monitoring of their use, maintenance of equipment and proper disposal of waste materials are extremely important.

Management information system: The initiation of the CNA approach to the RCH programme involves the collection/generation of data and their use for participatory planning with stakeholders (women and men). The data is used to make reports and for monitoring of the programme. Accordingly, the management information system (MIS) has also been modified and strengthened to provide relevant information on client satisfaction and the impact of the programme on the health status of women and children.

Monitoring of the RCH programme

Monitoring is the process of measuring and observing changes during implementation of the programme; it is also used to assess progress in implementation in relation to the planned schedule. Thus, monitoring will indicate whether:

- the required resources have been provided
- available resources are being optimally utilised
- planned activities are being implemented as scheduled or are in progress
- expected results are being achieved or not
- any unplanned or unforeseen occurrences have taken place.

The measurement of these changes is based on certain predetermined indicators: these could be for inputs (resources), processes (activities), output (performance achievement) or outcomes (effect/ impact). For example:

- health worker-to-population ratio is an input indicator
- frequency of antenatal clinics is a process indicator
- percentage of children receiving measles immunisation is an output indicator
- incidence of neonatal tetanus is an impact indicator.

Service delivery indicators: These reflect the percentage of population that received RCH services like antenatal care, newborn care, contraception and screening for RTI.

Indicators of quality of care reflect the quality of services like:

- percentage of pregnant women who had at least three antenatal checkups
- percentage of laparoscopic sterilisations done adhering to the prescribed protocol
- percentage of ANMs who have undergone skill-based training in IUD insertion
- percentage of men and women with knowledge of the uses and side effects of contraceptive methods
- percentage of users of oral contraceptives receiving follow-up visits from the health worker.

Outcome indicators: These include:

- low birth weight babies per 1,000 live births
- incidence of neonatal tetanus cases
- incidence of anemia in pregnant women.

Monitoring can performed by reviewing the MIS regularly. In addition, direct supervision is carried out by visits to the institutions providing services. Interviews with the community members in the field are an effective means of monitoring the quality of services.

Partnership development, intersectoral cooperation and involvement of NGOs: Under the RCH programme, the Government of India (GOI) has involed the NGOs in both service delivery and in training of health personnel. The NGOs are not only flexible in their procedures, but also enjoy credibility among the public. The GOI encourages NGOs to bring about innovations in the RCH programme and funds such projects.

Improving the quality of services: The RCH programme's main emphasis is on need-based services and ensuring clients' satisfaction. Therefore, measures have been initiated to ensure the quality of services. Standards have been developed for each component of RCH services, training of health personnel is skill-based and proficiency certification of trainees is imperative.

National Rural Health Mission

The National Rural Health Mission (NRHM) was launched in April 2005 by the GOI for a duration of seven years. It seeks to provide effective health care to the rural population throughout the country with special focus on 18 states, which have weak public health indicators and/or weak infrastructure. These states are Arunachal Pradesh, Assam, Bihar, Chhattisgarh, Himachal Pradesh, Jharkhand, Jammu and Kashmir, Manipur, Mizoram, Meghalaya, Madhya Pradesh, Nagaland, Orissa, Rajasthan, Sikkim, Tripura, Uttaranchal and Uttar Pradesh. GOI would provide funding for key components in these 18 high focus states.

The NRHM will cover all the villages in these 18 states through approximately 2.5 lakh village-based Accredited Social Health Activists (ASHA) who would act as a link between the health centres and the villagers. One ASHA will be raised from every village or cluster of villages, across 18 states. The ASHA would be trained to advise village populations about:

- sanitation
- hygiene
- contraception
- immunisation.

The ASHA is to provide primary medical care for diarrhea, minor injuries and fevers. She is to escort patients to medical centres. She would also be expected to deliver direct observed short course therapy for tuberculosis and oral rehydration, to give folic acid tablets and chloroquine to patients and to alert authorities to unusual outbreaks. The ASHA will receive performance-based compensation for promoting universal immunisation, referral and escort services for RCH, construction of household toilets and other health care delivery programmes.

Goals and strategies

The goals of the NRHM include:

- reduction in IMR and MMR
- universal access to integrated comprehensive public health services
- child health, ensure water availability, sanitation and hygiene
- prevention and control of communicable and non-communicable diseases, including locally endemic diseases
- population stabilisation, gender and demographic balance
- revitalise local health traditions and mainstream Ayurvedic, Yoga, Unani, Siddha and Homeopathy (AYUSH) systems of health
- promotion of healthy lifestyles.

The strategies to achieve the goals include:

- train and enhance the capacity of *panchayat raj* institutions (PRIs) to own, control and manage public health services
- health plan for each village through the Village Health Committee of the *panchayat*
- strengthening the subcentre through a joint fund to enable local planning and action (each subcentre will have a fund for local action at ₹ 10,000 per annum). This fund will be deposited in a joint bank account of the ANM and *sarpanch* and operated by the ANM, in consultation with the Village Health Committee and Multipurpose Workers (MPWs)
- provision of 24-hour service in 50% of PHCs by addressing shortage of doctors, especially in high focus states, by mainstreaming AYUSH personnel
- preparation and implementation of an intersectoral District Health Plan prepared by the District Health Mission, including drinking water, sanitation and hygiene and nutrition
- integrating vertical health and Family Welfare programmes at national, state, block and district levels.

By the end of the programme, it is expected that the following will be achieved:

- MMR of 100 per 1,000,000
- infant mortality rate of 30 per 1,000
- TFR of 2.1
- a 50%–100% reduction in mortality caused by kala azar, dengue fever, malaria and Japanese encephalitis
- reduction in the prevalence of tuberculosis, leprosy and filariasis
- the community health centres to be upgraded to Indian public health standards.

KEY POINTS

- Reproductive and Child Health Programme was launched in India in 1997. The programme provides a comprehensive and integrated approach to population issues, including women's development and empowerment.
- A paradigm shift from earlier programmes has been initiated through the CNA approach and decentralisation of functioning with the involvement of stakeholders.
- The services under the comprehensive package aim to ensure the government's commitment to 'Reproductive Health' as defined at the ICPD 1994.
- Efforts have been made to reach the population in rural and tribal areas and urban slums.
- Organisational and infrastructural facilities have been designed to provide EOC and essential newborn care.
- For effective implementation of the RCH programme, a partnership has been developed between GOI and NGOs.
- Special attention has been paid to IEC, MIS and managerial components. Training of all functionaries from health and health-related sectors shall be competency-based.
- In order to improve the quality of the RCH services, gender concern, counselling and follow-up services have been introduced.
- The implementation of NHRM through ASHA is bringing about a rapid improvement in MCH services and health in general.

QUESTIONS

Select the single most appropriate answer:

1. The overall goal of the RCH programme is essentially to
   a. reduce the birth rate
   b. immunise women against tetanus
   c. reduce the incidence of maternal death
   d. adopt a holistic approach to reproductive health
2. The paradigm shift in the RCH programme has been brought about by
   a. adopting community needs assessment
   b. focusing on quality of services
   c. involvement of the *panchayat raj*
   d. all of the above
3. Decentralised participatory planning is done at the level of
   a. primary health centre
   b. subcentre
   c. district hospital
   d. community health centre
4. Provision of quality care services is the crux of the RCH programme. Which of the following best reflects the quality of care?
   a. number of women counselled
   b. competent health care providers
   c. increased utilisation of services
   d. availability of emergency services
5. Which of the following statements is false regarding male participation in reproductive health matters?
   a. men must make a decision with their female partner
   b. men alone must decide about contraception
   c. they should get involved in the health of the female partner
   d. men are responsible for parenthood

6. The recommended package of services under RCH includes
   a. services for unwanted pregnancy
   b. screening for cancer of the cervix and breast
   c. nutritional services for vulnerable groups
   d. all of the above
7. Adolescent health services aim to reduce the hazards of adolescent pregnancy by
   a. imparting family life education
   b. improving general health
   c. promoting health awareness
   d. all of the above
8. In the evaluation of the quality of RCH services, the outcome indicator that is used is
   a. low birth weight babies per 1,000 births
   b. incidence of anemia in pregnant women
   c. number of maternal deaths
   d. incidence of neonatal tetanus
9. The National Rural Health Mission was launched in India in 2005 with the aim of further improving health in rural areas. The main functionary or health care provider in this programme is
   a. auxillary nurse-midwife
   b. accredited social health activist
   c. public health nurse
   d. lady health visitor

5

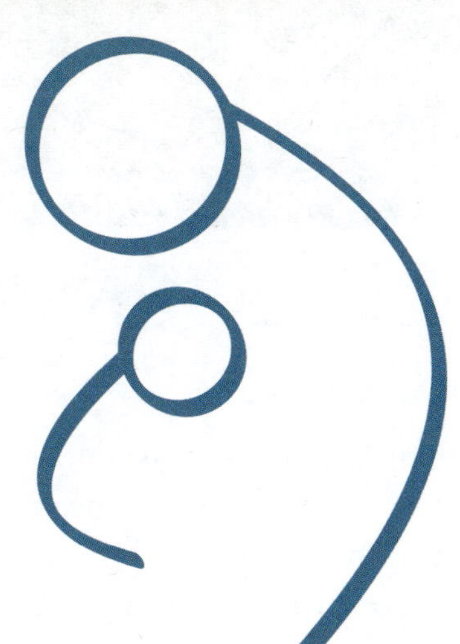

Communication and Counselling

Asha Oumachigui

'Communication is the mother of all existence'

LEARNING OBJECTIVES

At the end of this chapter, the reader should be able to:

- define communication
- enumerate the factors that influence communication
- list the principles of good communication
- appreciate the advantages of good communication
- define the essentials of doctor–patient interaction
- identify the disadvantages of poor communication
- appreciate the need to acquire communication skills for the good practice of obstetrics
- understand the importance of counselling
- state the steps in counselling

Introduction

Communication is an important component of patient care. Both the doctor and the patient need to communicate with each other. The doctor needs to gather information, not only about the patient's medical problems but also about her social background, so that he may arrive at a provisional diagnosis and order appropriate investigations and plan treatment. As Sir William Osler said 'it is more important to know what sort of person has this disease, than what sort of disease this person has'. Currently, across the world, medical practice is becoming 'technology-centred', rather than 'patient-centred', leading to delivery of ineffective health care. It is paradoxical that at a time of global communication, the medical world is faced with a breakdown in communication between patients and doctors, increasing patient dissatisfaction, rising number of complaints and claims for malpractice. The challenges for the new millennium are a greater need for effective communication between the doctor and the patient and an increasing demand from patients for autonomy and participation in medical decision-making. This is all the more true for a specialty like obstetrics where one deals with the pregnant mother and her unborn child.

Communication

Definition

Communication is derived from the Latin word *communis,* which means common. When we communicate, we try to find something common between ourselves and the person(s) with whom we are communicating.

Communication as a process

Communication is a **process.** It is dynamic and changes depending on how the other person responds. It involves the transfer and sharing of meaning.

Components of communication

In order to communicate, one must decide what information or idea is to be shared. This is known as the **message.** Then there is the source of the message: the person who is sending it is known as the **sender.** The person who receives the message is the **receiver.** A **channel** refers to the means by which the message is transmitted to the receiver (**Fig. 5.1**).

Factors influencing communication

It is important to remember that the quality of communication is influenced by factors that affect the four components.

The **sender** and the **receiver** are individuals whose attitude and ability to communicate are influenced by their age, gender, race, nationality, and socioeconomic and educational background. A woman's willingness to communicate depends on the nature of the problem she is suffering from. In many societies, women are expected to be reticent; this reticence is often considered a sign of respect for 'someone superior'. One must be aware that gender influences the doctor–patient interaction to a great extent.

A doctor is educated, but he is not formally trained to communicate with patients in different situations. He often lacks the motivation to communicate with his patients. At times, he believes that it is not possible to communicate with an illiterate patient, particularly if she is from a rural area. The same problem may arise if he is dealing with patients from social strata much higher than his own.

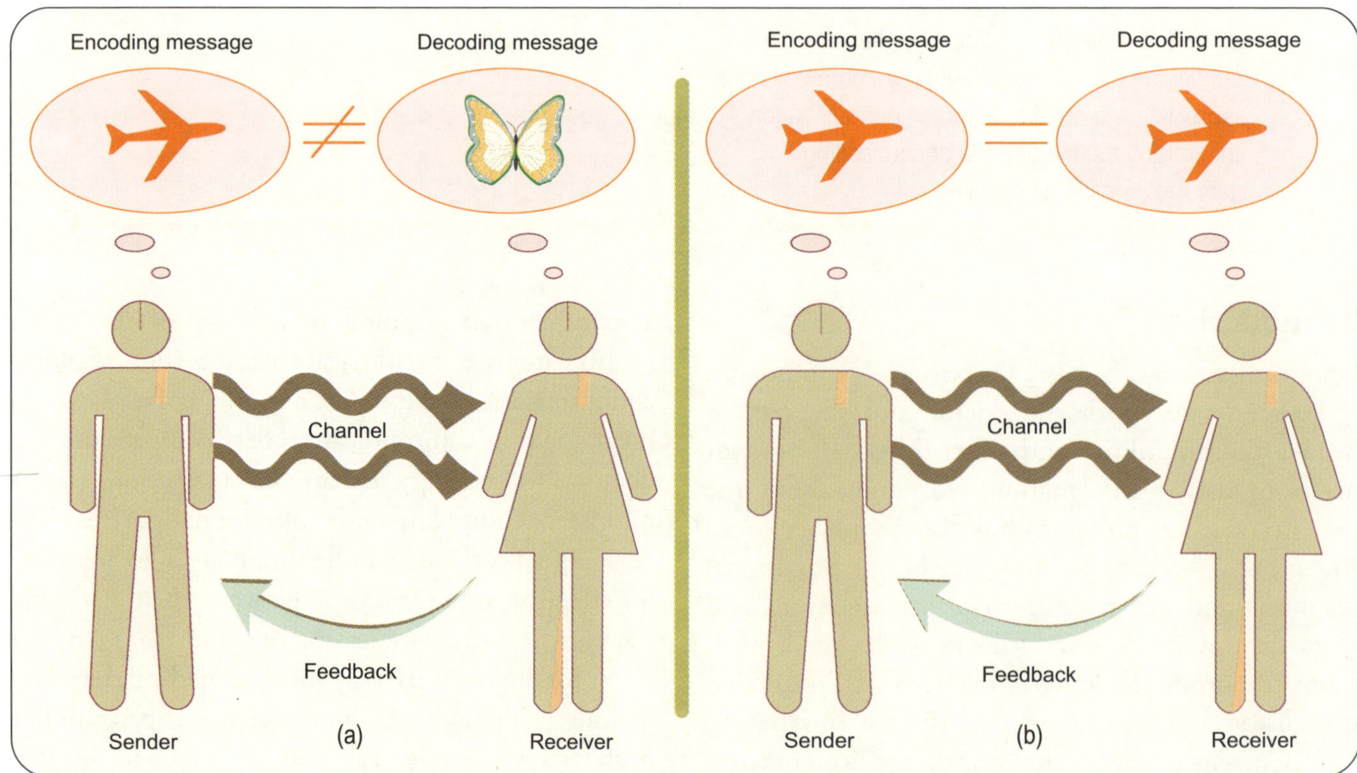

Fig. 5.1 Communication model a: Poor communication b: Good communication.

The message may not be conveyed clearly or accurately. This happens whenever the doctor uses technical words, or speaks a language in which either he or the patient is not proficient, or does not use any illustrations or examples. He may even be reluctant to repeat or clarify the patient's queries.

The most frequently used channel in the doctor–patient interaction is 'a face-to-face exchange'. However, currently some doctors provide pamphlets to educate patients suffering from chronic diseases.

Feedback: It is important to understand that the **response** of the sender or the receiver determines the process of communication. The response, known as **feedback**, helps to improve the interaction between the two individuals. Both positive and negative feedback should be given politely, without hurting the patient. Positive feedback is given to encourage the patient's participation, or to reinforce appropriate actions or ideas. On the other hand, negative feedback helps to clarify doubts regarding the suggested investigations or treatment. It makes the sender aware of how the message is perceived by the receiver. Thus, efforts can be made to change the way the message is given and ensure that both the receiver and the sender are sure of what is being discussed. Thus, feedback helps in the long run to build a good doctor–patient relationship.

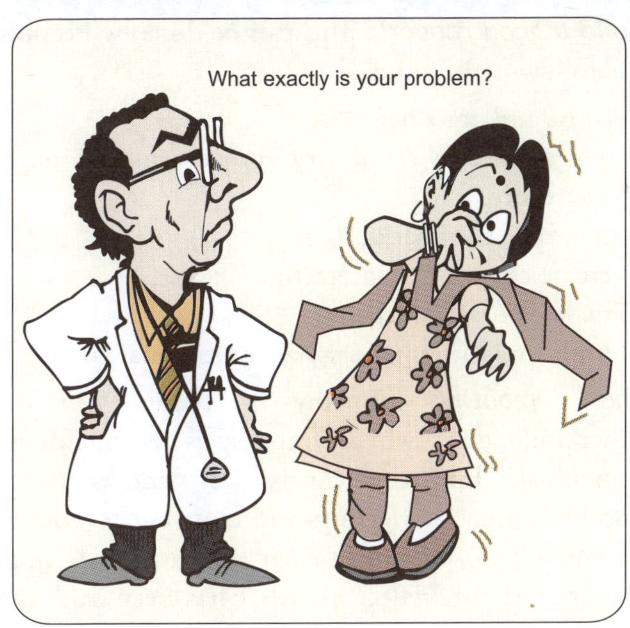

Fig. 5.2 A rude doctor frightens patients away.

In obstetrics and gynecology, the problems are related to the genital tract, sexual function or loss of pregnancy, all of which are not only deeply personal, but are also likely to disturb a woman emotionally. Therefore, it is essential to put the patient at ease, (**Fig. 5.3**) so that she is able to talk explicitly about her problem and participate confidently in its management.

The following elements contribute towards improving communication:

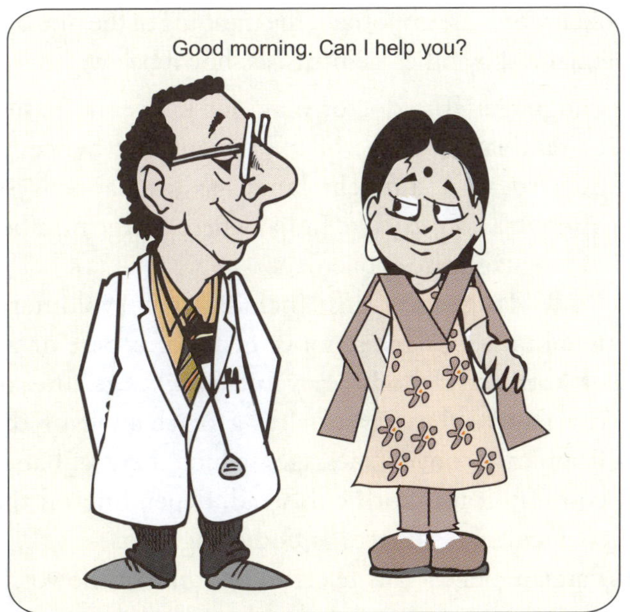

Fig. 5.3 A sympathetic doctor puts the patient at ease.

Principles of good communication

Pregnant mothers often believe that doctors are 'formidable' and in the Indian context 'next to God'. They believe that doctors are extremely knowledgeable, very busy and therefore, one should not talk and waste their time. If the doctor happens to behave rudely they get frightened and are unable to communicate (**Fig. 5.2**). Doctors unfortunately promote this kind of mindset and do not encourage their patients to ask questions and seek clarification. The following example is illustrative:

An educated woman requests delivery by cesarean section as she is afraid of labour pains and the harm of possible instrumental delivery. The doctor gets annoyed at her attitude and shouts 'Why do you make such important medical decisions? Am I the doctor or are you?'

Build a good rapport: This can be done by keeping the following in mind:

- smile and greet her
- address her by name (try and remember/look at the records)
- reinforce the relationship
- create chances for interaction
- make yourself 'attractive'
- find similarities in personal/professional areas.

Show empathy: Empathy is feeling with the other individual, while sympathy is feeling for an individual. Empathy consists of understanding another's situation, feelings and motives. In order to be empathetic, one must elicit the patient's feelings to some extent, reflect on what has been said and encourage the person to speak.

Listen: Listening is by far the most important of all communication skills. Listening differs from hearing in that it is an active mental process. While listening, one first hears, filters what is heard, interprets, evaluates the information gathered and then responds. Then one must probe the hints the patient drops and offer facilitating remarks. Also, the doctor must be responsive, ask open-ended questions, check on accuracy and determine the patient's expectations.

Nonverbal behaviour: In communication, while the spoken words are important, the meaning of the message is enhanced by other elements, as shown below:

- **Language:** The doctor may not know the native or familiar language of the patient and hence he may speak a different language (as happens so often in a country like India, where a large number of languages are spoken).
- **Body language:** This includes any voluntary, involuntary or reflex movements of a part or all of the body. Body movements like gesture of the hands, the way of sitting or shaking of the head can convey messages which may enhance communication or be misread, depending on the sociocultural nuances of body language.
- **Paralanguage:** This refers to the tone of the voice. The words spoken by the doctor may assume a different meaning depending on his tone.
- **Facial expression:** The facial expression may betray the spoken words. A cool and composed personality influences communication positively.
- **Personal appearance:** It refers to the physical features and apperance of the doctor.
- **Dressing and grooming:** Depending on the sociocultural background, patients expect their doctors to be dressed 'appropriately'. This determines initially the respect that the doctor commands from the patient.

Studies support the concept that spoken words convey only a small part of the message, while nonverbal behaviour conveys much more. Fiddling with objects on the table reflects a person's indifference to the patient's narration of her problem.

Role of humour and laughter: Humour and laughter are important components that facilitate communication; they help the patient relax. However, humour should be appropriate in the context of the patient's background. If inappropriate, it is likely to offend patients and their relatives. Laughter is a physiologic response that helps one to feel 'good' and allows one to overcome adverse situations. It is a good mechanism to reduce stress. But one must be careful in some situations and ensure that the patient does not get the impression that the doctor is making fun of her.

This patient-centred approach contributes to better outcome, greater patient satisfaction and development of mutual trust between the doctor and the patient. While the doctor does his best to build a good rapport, he should also ensure he does not get 'over-familiar' with the patient. It is important that no scope is given to misinterpret one's intention to help.

Need for good doctor–patient communication

Communication is an important component of patient care. In the medical world driven by technology and managed care, communication has receded to the background. Doctors seem to be focused on the use of technology to solve the patient's problems; they also strive to see a large number of patients. The end result is indiscriminate use of laboratory investigations and unnecessary medical/surgical interventions. As Sir William Osler said 'Listen to the patient: he is telling you the diagnosis.' Therefore, it is worth listening to the patient so as to find out 'what sort of a person has this disease'.

There are two challenges for the medical profession in the new millennium: a greater need for effective communication and a rapidly rising demand from patients for autonomy and participation in medical decision-making. Patients are more aware of health and disease and would like to be informed about the reason for investigations and the prescribed treatment; many of them seek a second opinion when they are not satisfied with one doctor. It seems reasonable that the doctor make efforts to communicate effectively with the patient in an appropriate manner.

'One of the most vital forces sustaining any successful relationship is the element of trust'. This trust is fundamental to the doctor–patient relationship. It needs to be restored and preserved, regardless of technological and social changes. When doctors communicate properly, they engage patients in their own care, and avoid ordering wasteful tests and treatment. Thus, good doctor–patient communication leads to mutual satisfaction. It is worth mentioning that most medical lawsuits can be avoided if patients are made to participate in medical decision-making.

Attributes of good doctor–patient communication

The main attributes of good communication between a doctor and a patient are listed below:

Invest in the beginning:

- Plan the visit with the patient.
- Create rapport: draw out the patient's concerns.

Elicit the patient's perspectives:

- Ask for the patient's ideas.
- Elicit specific requests.
- Explore the effect on the patient's life.

Demonstrate empathy:

- Be open to the patient's emotions.
- Make at least one empathetic statement.
- Be aware of your own reactions.

Invest in the end:

- Deliver diagnostic information.
- Provide education.
- Involve the patient in decision-making.
- Complete the visit.

Counselling

Patients often seek help from the doctor; it may concern issues like loss of a pregnancy or need for contraception. Counselling is a process, a specialised communication, in which one individual (counsellor) helps another individual to understand and solve a problem. In doing so, the counsellor provides factual information and assists in making a decision about behaviour change. A typical counselling session will involve the following steps (GATHER):

Greet—the client
Ask—about her concerns and expectations
Tell her—facts and options
Help—to clear doubts and make decisions
Explain—the health status and proposed management
Return visits—for reinforcement

The basic principles of good communication should be applied while counselling. In addition, one must stress on the following points:

- principles of counselling
- focusing on the pregnant mother's/patient's needs or concerns
- providing relevant knowledge
- empowering the individual by helping her to decide
- maintaining confidentiality
- obtaining consent if the individual has sought counselling for family planning.

In the present context, with the availability of advanced diagnostic techniques, the pregnant woman must receive a detailed explanation about the need to perform the tests; it will also be necessary to counsel her regarding further management. One must show empathy and take care to counsel her in case of an adverse outcome.

KEY POINTS

- Communication is an important skill required for the practice of medicine in general and obstetrics in particular.
- Good communication helps a doctor to know about the background of the patient/pregnant mother.
- By communicating effectively, a doctor is able to deliver 'patient-centred' care.
- Several factors influence the quality of communication.
- Paying attention to the good principles of communication can help the doctor build a good rapport with the patient.
- Effective communication leads to a relationship of mutual trust; trust is essential to the practice of medicine.
- By acquiring counselling skills, a doctor can help the patient participate in medical decision-making.

QUESTIONS

Select the single most appropriate answer:

1. A doctor can provide effective health care if he
   a. acquires good knowledge c. dresses well
   b. acquires pleasing manners d. communicates well
2. With regard to communication, which of the following statements is false?
   a. reduces malpractice suits
   b. improves patient compliance
   c. helps the patient to relax
   d. is a static process
3. For communication to be clear, the sender must focus on which of the following?
   a. channel c. receiver
   b. message d. all of the above
4. To empathise with a patient means to
   a. feel for the patient c. pity the patient
   b. feel with the patient d. agree with the patient

Select the appropriate answers using the following key:

a. if only responses 1, 2 and 3 are correct
b. if only 1 and 3 are correct
c. if only 2 and 4 are correct
d. if only 4 is correct
e. if all are correct

5. Nonverbal behaviour in communication includes
   1. body movements 3. physical appearance
   2. facial expression 4. tone of the voice
6. If a doctor talks on the phone for a long time while the patient is sitting in front of him, the patient is likely to feel that the doctor
   1. is very popular
   2. will not listen to her
   3. is very competent
   4. has no concern for her

In the following questions, there are two statements. Select the appropriate answers using the following key:

a. if both statements are true and causally related
b. if both statements are true but not causally related
c. if the first statement is true and the second is false
d. if the first statement is false and the second is true
e. if both statements are false.

7. Most women consulting a gynecologist are hesitant to talk to the doctor *because*
   Most women's problems are related to the genital tract.
8. It is not necessary for a doctor to talk to his patients to make a diagnosis *because*
   Advanced technology is available for diagnosis.

Mark true (T) or false (F) against each statement:

9. In order to build a good relationship with the patient, the doctor must
   a. smile c. talk a lot
   b. appear busy d. listen
10. While counselling a patient, the doctor must
    a. greet her
    b. not allow her to speak
    c. keep talking
    d. need not look at her

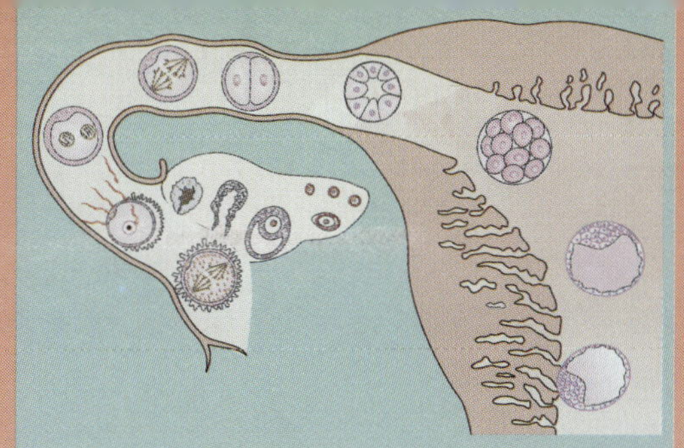

Part II Pregnancy

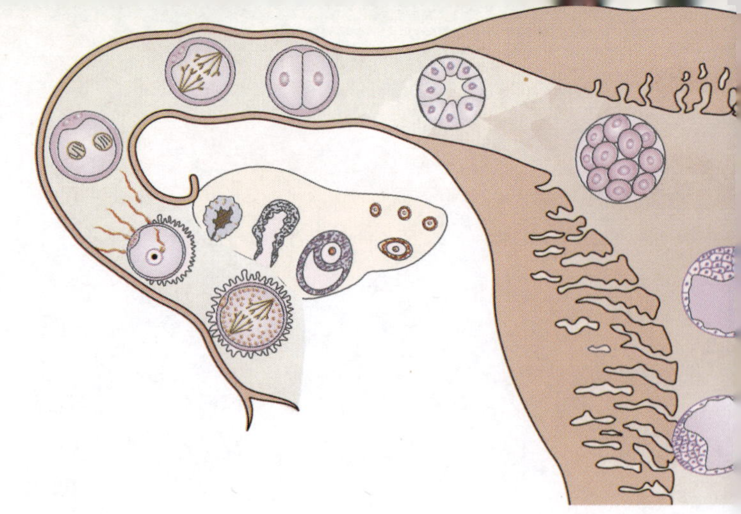

6

Elements of Reproduction and Embryology

Sudha Rao

LEARNING OBJECTIVES

At the end of this chapter, the reader should be able to:

- describe the mechanism of ovulation
- list the important factors that influence sperm transport
- list the steps in the fertilisation of the ovum and its further development
- outline the process of implantation
- list the salient features of the development of the embryo

Introduction

Reproduction is a physiologically well-orchestrated neuroendocrine process, perfectly timed to result in conception and continuation of pregnancy.

A recapitulation of the basics of ovulation, fertilisation and implantation is essential to understand deviations from normal, as seen in infertility, abortion and genetic disorders.

Ovulation

During each menstrual cycle, in the follicular phase, under the influence of the follicle stimulating hormone (FSH) released by the pituitary gland, several graafian follicles develop in the ovary. One (occasionally more) of the predetermined follicles develops to full potential; it is called the **dominant follicle** from which the ovum is released. The stimulated follicles synthesise and secrete 17-β estradiol; its serum concentration rises to peak around midcycle. This leads to a positive feedback to the hypothalamus and pituitary, resulting in a sudden 'surge' in the luteinising hormone (LH). This LH surge further stimulates the growth of the largest and most mature follicle, which by this time has pushed through the ovarian stroma and lies just under the ovarian capsule. **This event occurs 14 days before the next menstrual period.**

In the days immediately preceding ovulation, under the influence of FSH and LH, the dominant follicle grows rapidly to a diameter of about 25 mm. Coincident with the final development of the dominant follicle, there is an abrupt increase in LH that causes the primary oocyte to complete the first meiotic division and the follicle to enter the preovulatory stage. In the meantime, the surface of the ovary begins to bulge, and due to the LH surge and local muscular contraction, the follicle ruptures, and the ovum surrounded by granulosa cells (corona radiata) is released into the peritoneal cavity; this event is known as **ovulation**. The follicle then collapses and its cells, under the influence of LH, are altered and synthesize 17-β estradiol and progesterone; it forms the **corpus luteum**.

The ovum measures about 100 μm in diameter 24–48 hours after ovulation. In the centre is the small nucleus which has reached the metaphase of the second maturation division and is surrounded by a yellowish cytoplasm, the **vitellus**, which contains carbohydrates and amino acids. The ovum has already undergone the first meiotic division, which has reduced its chromosome complement followed by the appearance of the secondary oocyte and the first polar body. **A second meiotic division will occur after the sperm penetrates the egg, with the production of a second polar body.**

The freed ovum is swept by the microfilaments projecting from the cells of the mucosa of the fimbrial end of the fallopian tube. The passage of the oocyte in the fallopian tube is promoted by the ciliary movements and rhythmic muscular contraction of the tube into its lumen. The ovum is now surrounded by the zona pellucida, a homogenous membrane rich in glycoprotein, measuring 5–10 μ in thickness. The ovum at this time is ready for fertilisation; if fertilisation does not occur within 36 hours, it will degenerate. The effective lifespan of the ovum is, therefore, short and fertilisation can only take place within two days of ovulation.

Corpus Luteum

After ovulation, the granulosa cells remaining in the wall of the ruptured follicle together with cells from the theca interna are vascularised by the surrounding vessels. Under the influence of LH, these cells develop a yellowish pigment and change into luteal cells (which form the corpus luteum) and secrete progesterone, which along with estrogen converts the endometrium to the progestational or secretory phase in preparation for implantation of the embryo. If the oocyte is fertilised, the corpus luteum is known as the **corpus luteum of pregnancy** and remains functionally active, producing increasing amounts of progesterone: the woman remains amenorrheic. The corpus luteum supports pregnancy for the first 14–16 weeks. If the ovum is not fertilised, the corpus luteum begins to degenerate from day 22 of the menstrual cycle; the progesterone level drops and menstruation results.

Sperm Transport

Normally, millions of spermatozoa are ejaculated in the semen which bathes the cervix and upper vagina. At the time of ovulation, under the influence of estrogen, the cervical mucus becomes thin, facilitating the passage of spermatozoa through the cervical canal. The sperms move from the cervix to the uterine tube primarily by the flagellation of their tails. In addition to this, uterine aspiratory movements or reverse peristalsis in the smooth muscle of the cervix helps to draw the sperms towards the tubal ostia. At the time of ovulation, the sperms swim up more rapidly under the influence of a chemoattractant produced by the cells surrounding the ovum, and reach the ampulla, where fertilisation takes place. Of the millions of sperms reaching the cervix, only 300–500 reach the site of fertilisation; of these, only a few succeed in penetrating the corona radiata and only one enters the ovum proper, traversing the vitellus and fusing with the female pronucleus.

Fertilisation

Fertilisation is the process by which the pronuclei of the male and female gametes fuse. This fusion occurs in the ampullary part of the fallopian tube. Before the sperm can fertilise the oocyte, it must undergo a structural change known as **capacitation**. This involves an increase in the DNA concentration in the nucleus and increased permeability of the lipoprotein coat of the plasma membrane of the sperm head, allowing the release of hyaluronidase from the acrosomal cap. Only capacitated sperms can pass through the corona radiata (**Figs 6.1a, b**) and undergo an acrosomic reaction, which occurs after sperms bind to the zona pellucida. This ability appears to reside in a protein in the head of the sperm and a glycoprotein on the surface of the zona pellucida. Release of the acrosomal enzyme allows the sperm to penetrate the zona. The permeability of the zona pellucida changes when the head of the sperm comes in contact with the oocyte

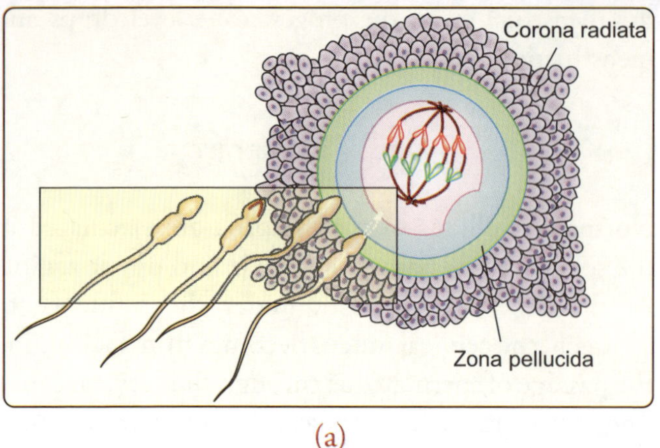

(a)

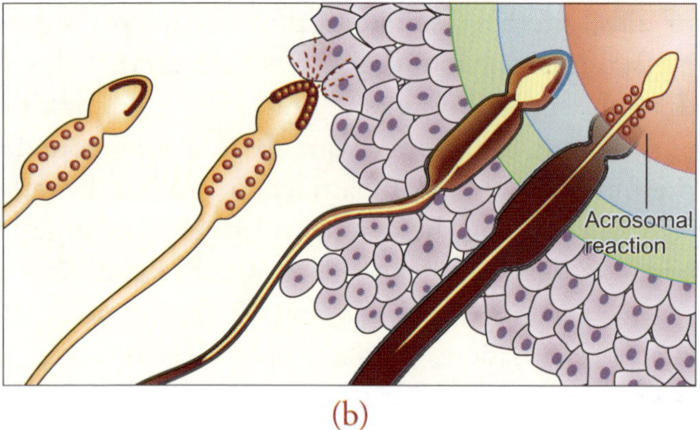

(b)

Fig. 6.1 Fertilisation a: Penetration of the ovum by the sperm b: Sperm capacitation and acrosomal reaction.

surface which releases lysosomal enzymes from the cortical granules lining the plasma membrane of the oocyte. These enzymes alter the property of the zona pellucida which helps to inhibit penetration by other sperms. The following are the results of fertilisation:

- completion of the second meiotic division of the secondary oocyte
- restoration of the normal diploid number of chromosomes (46)
- determination of the sex of the fetus
- initiation of cleavage.

Development of the Embryo

First week

During its passage along the uterine tube, the zygote undergoes **cleavage** (a series of mitotic cell divisions), which results in the formation of smaller cells called **blastomeres.** About three days after fertilisation, a ball of blastomeres, called **morula**, enters the uterus. A cavity soon forms in the morula and partially separates the cells of the morula into an outer cell mass known as **trophoblast** and an inner cell mass known as **embryoblast.**

The trophoblast encloses the embryoblast and blastocystic cavity and later forms extraembryonic structures and the fetal part of the placenta. After fertilisation, the zona pellucida is shed and the trophoblast adjacent to the embryoblast attaches to the endometrial epithelium. The trophoblast adjacent to the embryonic pole differentiates into two layers, an outer syncytiotrophoblast (multinucleated mass without distinct cell boundaries) and an inner cytotrophoblast (multilayer cells). The syncytiotrophoblast invades the endometrial epithelium and, by the end of the first week, the blastocyst is superficially implanted in the endometrium (**Fig. 6.2**).

Second week

Rapid proliferation and differentiation of the trophoblast are important features of the second week. These processes occur as the blastocyst completes its **implantation** in the endometrium. The various endometrial changes resulting from the adaptation of these tissues to implantation are known as the **decidual reaction.** Concurrently, the primary yolk sac forms and an extraembryonic mesoderm arises from the endoderm of the yolk sac. The extraembryonic celom forms spaces that develop in the extraembryonic mesoderm. The extraembryonic celom later becomes the chorionic cavity. The primary yolk sac becomes smaller and gradually forms the secondary or definitive yolk sac (**Fig. 6.3**). The amniotic cavity appears as a space between the trophoblast and the inner cell mass or embryoblast (**Fig. 6.4**). The inner cell mass differentiates into a bilaminar embryonic disc consisting of an epiblast (ectoderm), related to the amniotic cavity, and hypoblast, adjacent to the blastocyst cavity. The prechordal plate develops as a localised thickening of the hypoblast (primary

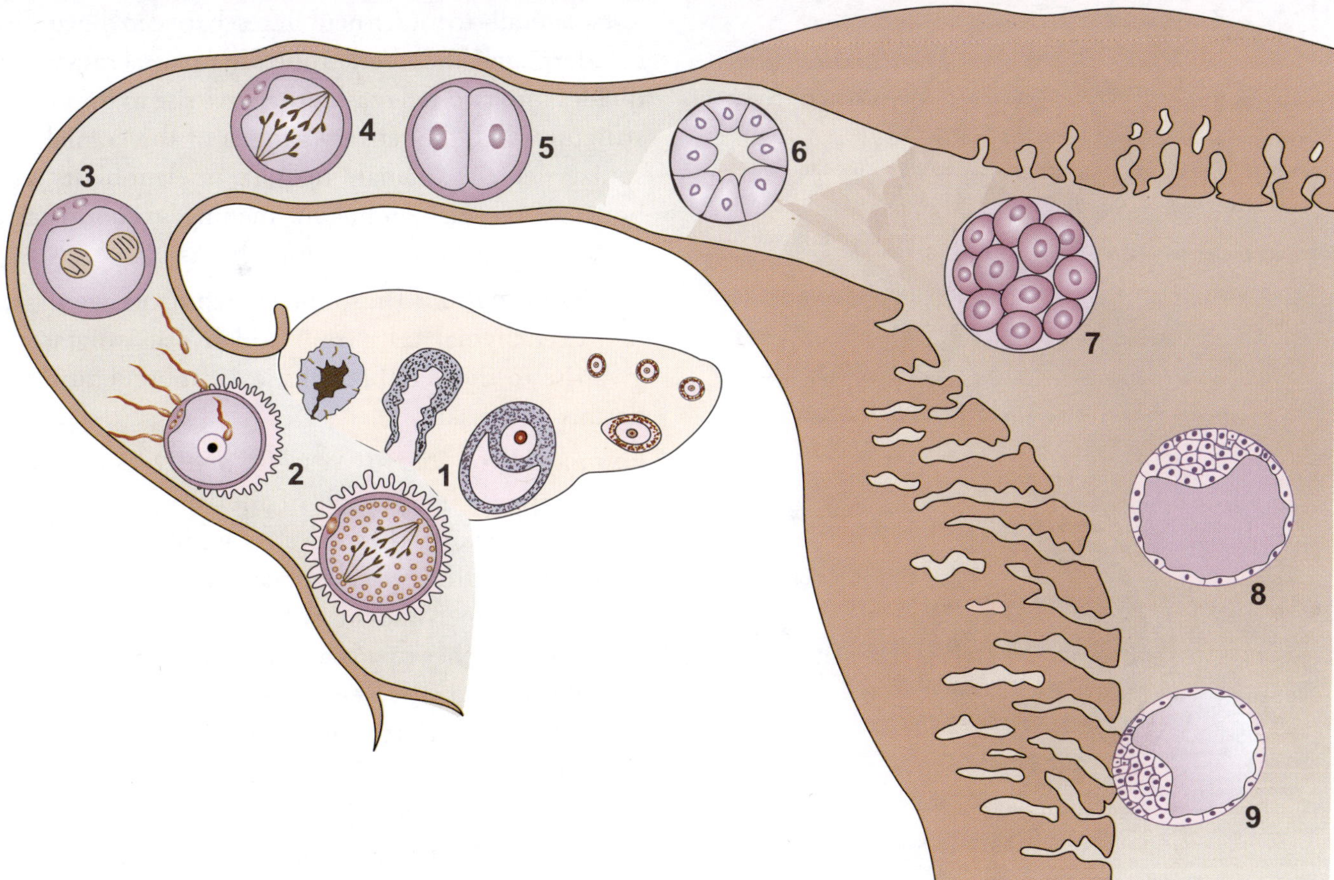

Fig. 6.2 Ovulation to implantation. 1. Release of ovum 2. Fertilisation 3. Pronuclei 4. Cell division 5. Two-cell stage 6. Eight-cell stage 7. Morula 8. Blastocyst 9. Implantation.

endoderm), which indicates the future cranial region of the embryo and the future site of the mouth. The prechordal plate is also an important organiser of the head region.

Fig. 6.3 Early development of the embryo.

Third week

The most characteristic event occurring during the third week of gestation is **gastrulation**, the process that establishes all the three germ layers. Gastrulation begins with the formation of the primitive streak.

Primitive streak: It appears at the beginning of the third week as a localised thickening of the epiblast at the caudal end of the embryonic disc. Invagination of the epiblastic cells from the primitive streak gives rise to mesenchymal cells that migrate cranially, laterally and caudally between the epiblast and hypoblast and give rise to the intraembryonic mesoderm, except in the region of the buccopharyngeal membrane and cloacal membrane.

Notochord formation: Early in the third week, mesenchymal cells arising from the primitive node of

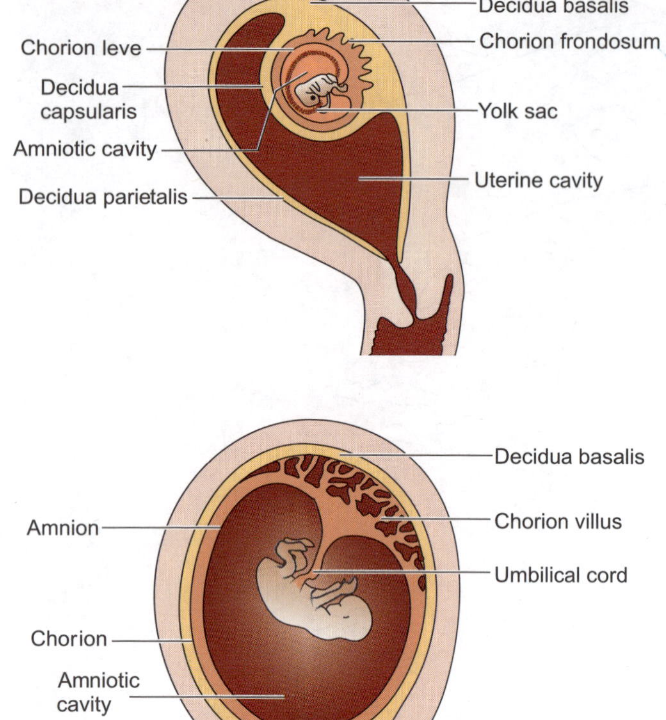

Fig. 6.4 Development of the amnion and chorion.

the primitive streak form the notochord process, which extends cranially from the primitive node as a rod of cells between the embryonic ectoderm and endoderm. A primitive pit extends into the notochordal process and forms a notochordal canal, the floor of which coalesces to form the notochordal plate; it then folds inwards to form the notochord which gives rise to the central axis of the body; in the adult, it persists as the nucleus pulposus of the intervertebral disc.

Neural tube formation: The neural plate appears as a thickening of the embryonic ectoderm, cranial to the primitive node. A longitudinal neural groove develops in the neural plate, which is flanked by the neural folds. Fusion of the folds forms the neural tube: the primordium of the central nervous system.

Neural crest formation: As the neural folds fuse to form the neural tube, neuroectodermal cells migrate dorsolaterally to form a neural crest between the surface ectoderm and the neural tube. The neural crest soon divides into two cell masses that give rise to important structures like the sensory ganglia of the cranial and spinal nerves, adrenal medulla, melanoblasts and bones of the face and skull, meninges, conotruncal septum in the heart and odontoblasts.

Somite formation: The somites are compact aggregates of mesenchymal cells from which cells migrate to give rise to the vertebra, ribs, axial musculature and dermis of the skin.

Formation of blood vessels and blood: Blood vessels appear in the wall of the yolk sac, allantois and the chorion. They develop within the embryo shortly thereafter. Spaces appear within aggregations of mesenchyme, known as blood islands, which in turn fuse together to give rise to blood vessels. By the end of the third week, endothelial heart tubes fuse to form a tubular heart that is joined to vessels in the embryo, yolk sac, chorion and connecting stalk to form a primitive cardiovascular system.

Completion of chorionic villi formation: Trophoblasts differentiate into villi which are finger-like structures. Primary chorionic villi, which are solid, become secondary villi as they acquire mesenchymal cores. When the secondary villi get blood vessels in the mesenchymal core, they are called tertiary villi. The rapid development of chorionic villi during the third week greatly increases the surface area of the chorion for the exchange of oxygen, nutrients and other substances between the maternal and embryonic circulations (**Fig. 6.5**).

The stages in the development of the embryo are summarised in **Table 6.1**.

Period of organogenesis (4–8 weeks)

The **embryonic period**, in which all major organs and systems of the body form from the three germ layers, is the period between weeks 4 and 8 of gestation (**Fig. 6.6**). At the beginning of week 4, folding of the embryo in the median and horizontal planes converts the flat, trilaminar, embryonic disc into a C-shaped, cylindrical embryo. The formation of head fold, caudal fold and lateral folds is a continuous sequence of events that results in the

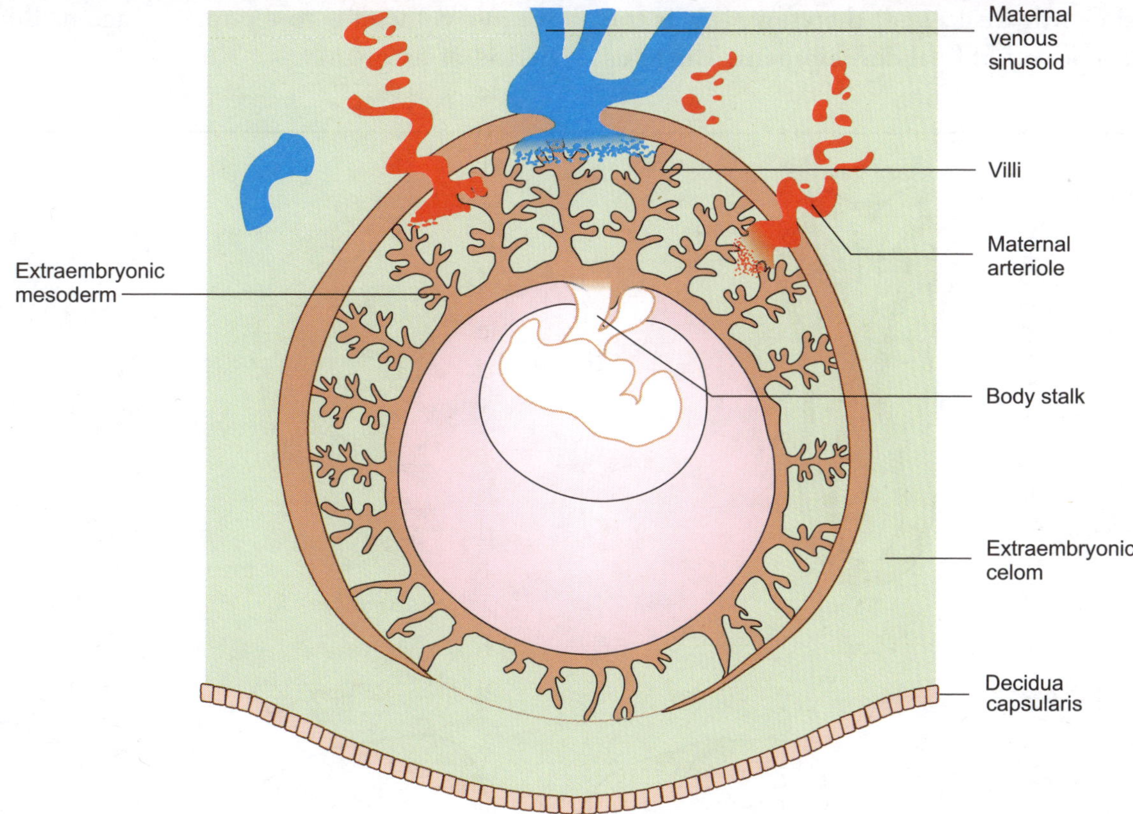

Fig. 6.5 Development of villi.

formation of a constriction between the embryo and the yolk sac. During the folding, a part of the yolk sac is incorporated into the embryo, leading to the formation of the gut. As the head region folds ventrally, part of the endodermal layer is incorporated into the developing embryonic head as the foregut. Folding of the head region results in the formation of the oropharyngeal membrane, the heart being carried ventrally and the brain becoming the most cranial part of the embryo. As the caudal eminence folds ventrally, part of the endodermal layer is incorporated into the caudal end of the embryo as the hindgut. The terminal part of the hindgut expands to form the cloaca. Folding of the caudal region results in the cloacal membrane, allantois and the connecting stalk being carried to the ventral surface of the embryo. Folding of the embryo in the horizontal plane incorporates part of the endoderm into the embryo as the midgut.

Table 6.1 Stages in the development of the embryo

Age (days)	Developmental event in embryo
5 days	Maturation of blastocyst
5 days	Loss of zona pellucida from blastocyst
6 days	Attachment of blastocyst to uterine epithelium
6–7 days	Epithelial penetration
7 ½–9 days	Trophoblastic plate formation and invasion of uterine stroma by blastocyst
9–11 days	Lacuna formation along with erosion of spiral arteries in the endometrium
12–13 days	Primary villus formation
13–15 days	Secondary placental villi, secondary yolk sac
16–18 days	Branching and anchoring villus formation
18–22 days	Tertiary villus formation

The external appearance of the embryo is greatly affected by the formation of the brain, heart, liver, somites, limbs, ears, nose and eyes. As these structures develop, the appearance of the embryo changes so that it has unquestionably human characteristics by the end of the eighth week. **Most essential external and internal structures are formed between the**

fourth and eighth weeks and, therefore, this is the most critical period of fetal development. The fetus is most vulnerable to teratogenic agents during this period of pregnancy.

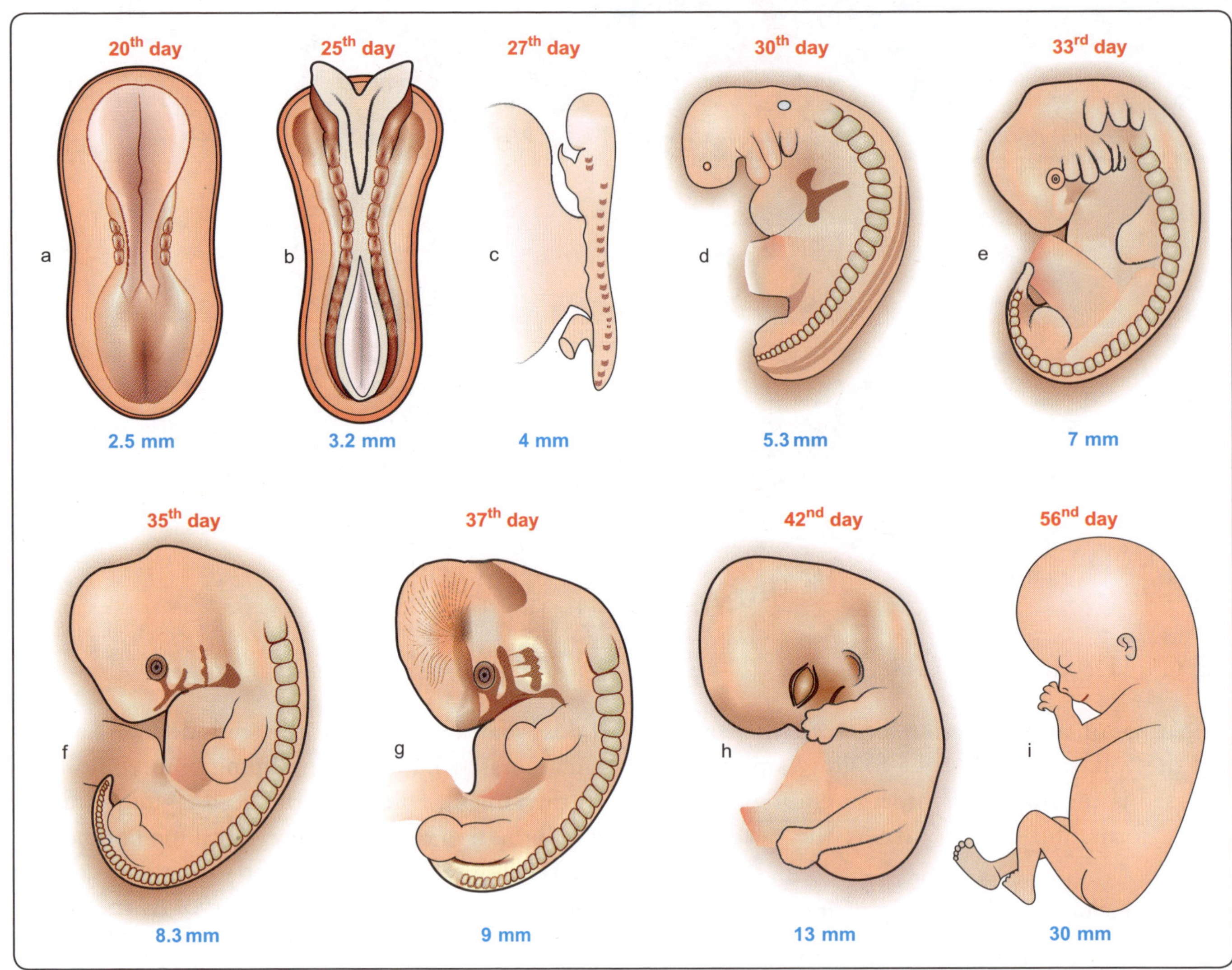

Fig. 6.6 Development of the embryo post-fertilisation. The crown–rump length is given in mm.
a: Dorsal view at 20 days shows 3–4 somites, neural plate, neural grooves and neural folds b: Dorsal view at 25 days shows 17–20 somites and fusion of the neural fold c: Sagittal view at 27 days shows 23–26 somites, head and tail, cardiac bulge, yolk sac and connecting stalk d: Lateral view at 30 days shows 32–35 somites, pharyngeal arches, lens and otic placodes, cardiac bulge, arterial arches and connecting stalk e: Lateral view at 33 days shows 36–38 somites, optic and otic vesicles, pharyngeal arches and four limb buds (paddle-shaped) f: Lateral view at 35 days shows 37–39 somites, optic and otic vesicles and well-developed limb buds g: Lateral view at 37 days shows 40–42 somites, optic and otic vesicles, arterial arches and the beginning of the ossification of skull bones h: Lateral view at 42 days shows well-formed eyes, external ear still in lower neck region and large head compared to the rest of the body i: Lateral view of embryo at 56 days, which has unquestionably human characteristics.

KEY POINTS

- The FSH influences the development of graafian follicles in the ovary. With a sudden surge in LH, one predetermined follicle develops to its full potential and ruptures, resulting in ovulation, 14 days before the first day of the next menstrual period.
- The ovum undergoes first meiotic division, with a reduction in chromosomal number to half. This is followed by the appearance of the secondary oocyte and the first polar body. The ovum is ready for fertilisation. Its effective lifespan is 36 hours.
- At the time of ovulation, the cervical mucus is thin and copious, and facilitates the passage of sperms through the cervical canal.
- Fertilisation is the process by which the pronuclei of the male and female gametes fuse. This fusion occurs in the ampullary part of the fallopian tube.
- The results of fertilisation are: restoration of the normal diploid number of chromosomes, completion of the second meiotic division, determination of the sex of the fetus and initiation of cleavage.
- By the end of week 1, the blastocyst is implanted in the superficial layer of the endometrium.
- At week 2, the amniotic cavity appears. The inner cell mass differentiates into a bilaminar embryonic disc.
- The most characteristic event in week 3 is gastrulation, which establishes all the three germ layers. The formation of the chorionic villi is completed.
- By eight weeks, the embryo assumes a human form.

QUESTIONS

Select the single most appropriate answer:

1. The most important event resulting in implantation of the fertilised ovum is
   a. formation of deciduas c. disintegration of zona pellucida
   b. formation of blastocyst d. cleavage
2. The oocyte completes its second meiotic division
   a. before ovulation
   b. at the time of ovulation
   c. immediately after penetration of spermatozoa
   d. at puberty
3. Fertilisation results in all of the following *except*
   a. restoration of haploid number of chromosomes
   b. determination of sex
   c. initiation of cleavage
   d. completion of second meiotic division of secondary oocyte
4. The corpus luteum of pregnancy is active till
   a. week 6 to 10 c. week 16 to 18
   b. week 12 to 14 d. week 20 to 22
5. The average lifespan of the ovum is
   a. 12 hours c. 36 hours
   b. 24 hours d. 48 hours
6. The cells surrounding the oocyte in a mature graafian follicle are known as
   a. theca interna
   b. corona radiata
   c. granulosa cells
   d. cumulus oophorus
7. The term embryo is used for the developing individual during the first
   a. 4 weeks c. 12 weeks
   b. 8 weeks d. 16 weeks
8. Which of the following is the most vulnerable period in fetal development?
   a. week 18 to 20 c. week 10 to 12
   b. week 14 to 16 d. week 6 to 8
9. The primordial germ cells are derived from the
   a. genital ridge c. allantois
   b. yolk sac d. celomic epithelium
10. Implantation of the fertilised ovum usually occurs on which day after ovulation?
    a. 3rd day c. 7th day
    b. 5th day d. 9th day

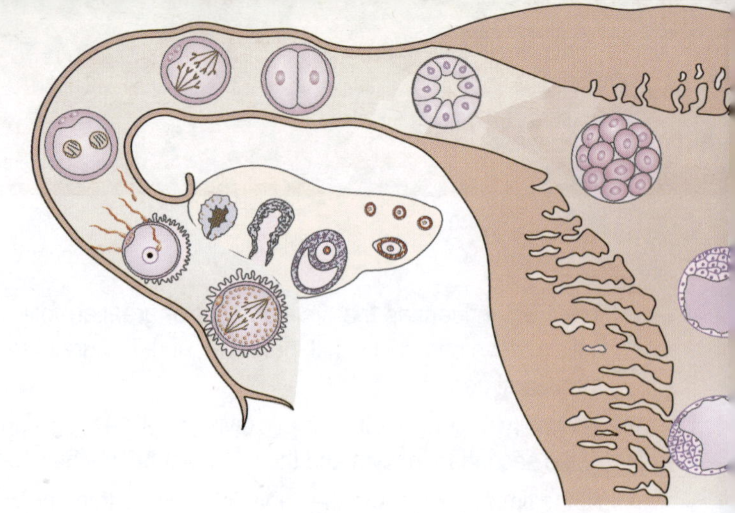

7

Development of the Fetus and Placenta

Sudha Rao

LEARNING OBJECTIVES

At the end of this chapter, the reader should be able to:

- explain the important aspects of the development of the fetus
- list the relevant stages in the development of the placenta
- describe the function of the 'fetoplacental unit'
- explain the clinical implications of abnormalities in fetal and placental development
- describe normal fetal circulation
- list the changes in fetal circulation that take place at birth

Introduction

From the third month of gestation till birth, the embryo is called the **fetus**. In the initial period of fetal development, differentiation of various organ systems takes place; in the latter period, mainly growth takes place. Organogenesis is complete by the end of the fourth month; thereafter the functional capacity is acquired and refined. Adverse influences in the early period will affect structural development and, in the later period, will cause abnormalities like growth restriction. Simultaneously, the placenta also grows and is responsible for the transfer of nutrition from the mother to the fetus and exchange of gases and clearance of excretory products from the fetus through the mother.

Development of the Fetus

Third month

- The length of the fetal head is half its entire length (crown–rump length or CRL).
- Face is broad, eyes are widely separated, ears are low-set and eyelids are fused until the sixth lunar month.
- Nails appear on the digits.
- Physiological umbilical hernia is reduced because of regression in the volume of the liver and kidneys and expansion of the abdominal cavity.

Fourth month

- Lanugo hair (primary) appears over the body surface.
- Eyes move further forward and medially.
- External ears shift position from the upper part of the neck to the side of the head.
- Male and female external genitalia are differentiated.

Fifth month

- Sebaceous glands become active; the secretion of sebum mixed with the desquamated epidermal cells forms a cheesy covering of the skin known as vernix caseosa which prevents maceration of the skin by the amniotic fluid.
- The mother experiences fetal movements known as 'quickening'.

Sixth month

- The skin is wrinkled due to the lack of deposition of subcutaneous fat.
- Eyelids are open and eyebrows are well developed.

Seventh month

- Growth of hair over the scalp, eyebrows and eyelashes is discernible.
- Pupillary membrane disappears.
- The body assumes a rounded contour due to the deposition of subcutaneous fat.
- Fetal lungs mature due to the development of rudimentary alveoli in a mesh of pulmonary capillaries and the appearance of surfactant from type II pneumocytes. Hence, the seventh month is called the **viable age of the fetus**.

Eighth to tenth month

- There is progressive loss of lanugo hair.
- Growth in length of the lower limbs is almost similar to that of the upper limbs at the time of birth.
- The thoracic cage increases in circumference and the infra-umbilical part of the abdominal wall shows a relative increase in surface area.
- A full-term fetus at the tenth lunar month has the umbilicus at the centre of the abdominal wall and the testes in the scrotum. The epiphyseal centre at the lower end of the femur appears.

Development of the Placenta

The fetus obtains oxygen, amino acids, minerals and vitamins from the mother and expels carbon dioxide and metabolic end products into maternal circulation. The decidua basalis and the chorion frondosum form a functional union between the mother and the fetus; it is called the **placenta**. At term, the placenta occupies 25%–30% of the endometrial surface of the uterus.

Placentation

The outer cell mass of trophoblast differentiates into a layer of multinucleated syncytiotrophoblast and an inner layer of mononucleated cytotrophoblast. Later, intercommunicating small lacunae appear in the syncytium and coalesce to form the intervillous space. Due to erosion of the endometrial vessels by the syncytium, the lacunae are filled with maternal blood and are incompletely separated by the trabeculae of the syncytium. The cytotrophoblast proliferates and extends into the trabeculae and forms the **villous stem**. The stems are invaded by the extraembryonic mesoderm and, later, blood vessels are formed. These vessels establish communication with the vitelline vessels, vessels of yolk sac and vessels of the chorionic mesenchyme. The free ends of the villous stem, which are covered only with cytotrophoblast, proliferate and pass through the thin syncytium; they further extend and fuse with a similar extension of the neighbouring villous stems, thus forming the cytotrophoblastic shell. This shell divides the syncytium into a peripheral layer that is applied to the decidua basalis and an inner layer of syncytium applied to the intervillous space. The peripheral layer degenerates, and at delivery, a cleavage in this zone leads to separation of the placenta. Initially, villi develop all over the chorionic sac. At the embryonic pole, the villi arborise extensively and form the chorion frondosum. In the remaining areas, the villi degenerate, leaving a smooth **chorion leve**. The chorion frondosum forms the fetal part of the definitive placenta and formation is completed by day 70.

Primitive blood vessels: By day 20, primitive blood vessels and blood cells are formed in the tertiary villi, making them more erectile and able to float more freely in the intervillous spaces, so nutrients may be exchanged.

Intervillous space: The endometrial spiral arteries open at intervals through the basal plate into the intervillous space. They dilate progressively, resulting in a considerable fall in pressure as the blood runs proximo-distally, so that it reaches the intervillous space at reduced pressure.

The blood bathes the villi, facilitating its transfer across the placental barrier. Even though there is very little difference between the arterial and venous blood pressure in the intervillous space, this difference is adequate to maintain the streams and prevent their mixing. The venous blood leaves the intervillous space through veins, which are distributed at intervals over the entire basal plate (**Fig. 7.1**).

Fetal vascular pattern: The umbilical arteries run in the chorionic plate and divide progressively into branches. Some branches enter into the villous stem and further divide into secondary and tertiary branches. The tertiary branches break up as capillaries in the terminal villi. The network of veins drains into the main vein of the villus through a series of venules. This complex system of fetal vessels in the placenta is meant for optimal rate of blood flow and for adequate exchange of gases, nutrients and waste products between the mother and the fetus.

Placental barrier: The capillary plexus in the villi is so arranged that normally, fetal blood is separated from maternal blood by the **placental barrier**, which is formed by syncytiotrophoblast, cytotrophoblast, the basement membrane of the cytotrophoblast, mesoderm, endothelium and the basement membrane of the fetal blood vessels.

The barrier becomes progressively thinner due to the loss of cytotrophoblast and the mesoderm. The syncytium also thins and allows for rapid and easy exchange to meet the demands of the growing fetus. With ageing of the placenta, deposition of calcium occurs within the vasculature of the villi and foci of fibrin are deposited on the surface of many villi.

Infarcts: The cause of fibrin deposition on the surface of the villi has not been established; however, larger deposits of fibrin may interfere with intervillous circulation. Any villus within the area of the fibrin deposit loses contact with maternal blood and dies, thus forming an infarct.

Clinical Aspects of the Placenta

Normal placenta: At term, the placenta is a flat, disc-shaped structure, weighing about 500 g. Viewed from the fetal surface, the umbilical cord is attached near the centre and the branching umbilical vessels are seen through the amnion. The maternal surface is covered with decidua and is divided into two lobes. Each lobe contains 15–20 maternal cotyledons, separated by the placental septa. Each lobe contains a number of anchoring villi and their branches. One such villus and its branches constitutes a functional fetal cotyledon; the rate of blood flow is 3–9 ml/min. A fully formed placenta has 60–100 functional fetal cotyledons (**Fig. 7.2**).

Maternal blood flow through the entire placenta has been estimated to rise from 300 ml/min at 20 weeks to 600 ml/minute at 40 weeks. The surface area of the villi has been calculated to be 11 m^2; it provides fetomaternal exchange of nutrients and gases.

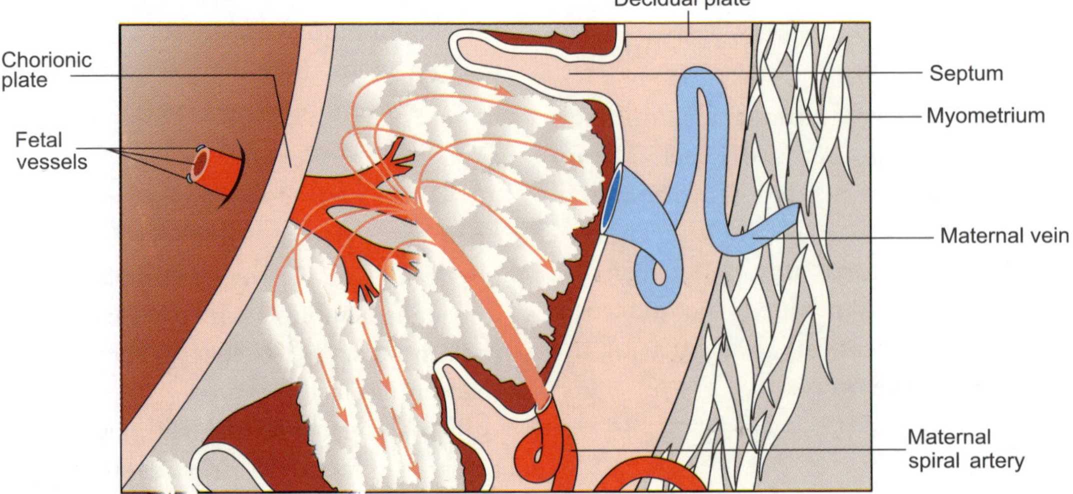

Fig. 7.1 Placental circulation.

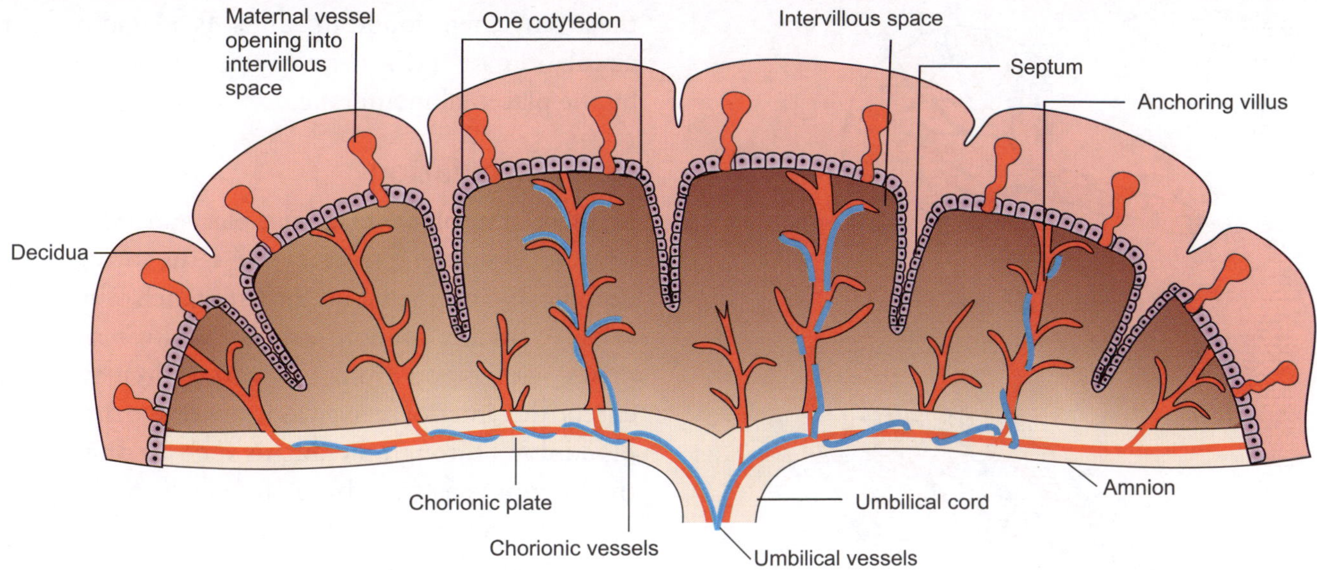

Fig. 7.2 Placental structure.

Gross abnormalities of the placenta

Battledore placenta: Normally, the umbilical cord is centrally inserted into the substance of the placenta. If the umbilical cord is inserted in the margin of the placenta, it is called battledore placenta (**Fig. 7.3a**).

Velamentous insertion: The fetal blood vessels travel through the umbilical cord and branch on the fetal surface of the placenta. Occasionally, the vessels branch before the cord inserts into the placenta. There is an increased risk of rupture of fetal vessels in such cases (**Fig. 7.3b**).

Placenta succenturiata: Sometimes, there may be one or more lobes found to be separate from the main placenta. The blood supply to these accessory lobes will arise from the main placental vessels. The clinical risk of this abnormality of placenta is that the accessory lobes may be retained in the uterus after delivery and may be missed. This may lead to delayed postpartum bleeding (**Fig. 7.3c**).

Placenta previa: The placenta is normally attached to the uterus in the upper segment. If the placenta is implanted partly or fully in the lower uterine segment, it is called placenta previa.

Placenta accreta, increta and percreta: Sometimes the deciduas basalis is extremely thin, deficient or absent. When the placental villi approach the myometrium, they may adhere to the myometrium (placenta accreta), invade the myometrium (placenta increta) or penetrate the serosal surface of the uterus (placenta percreta). Such placental tissue fails to separate during labour and will be retained.

Placenta extrachorialis: The chorionic plate in which villi arise is smaller than the basal plate. The transition from the smooth chorion to the villous chorion takes place not at the edge of the placenta but well within. The non-villous, membranous chorion contains the amnion and fibrin. If the transitional zone contains a ring of flat membrane, the placenta is classified as **circummarginate**. In the **circumvallate** type, the marginal ring is plicated with a raised or folded edge (**Fig. 7.3d**). The extrachorial placenta is associated with abortion, antepartum hemorrhage and premature onset of labour.

Placenta membranacea: This type of placenta is extensive and membranous. It envelops almost the entire gestational sac. Most of its external surface is covered with chorionic villi. Clinically, this is associated with premature labour, intrauterine growth restriction and postpartum hemorrhage.

Circulation Before and After Birth

The structure of the heart and the pattern of the blood vessels of fetal circulation are largely similar to

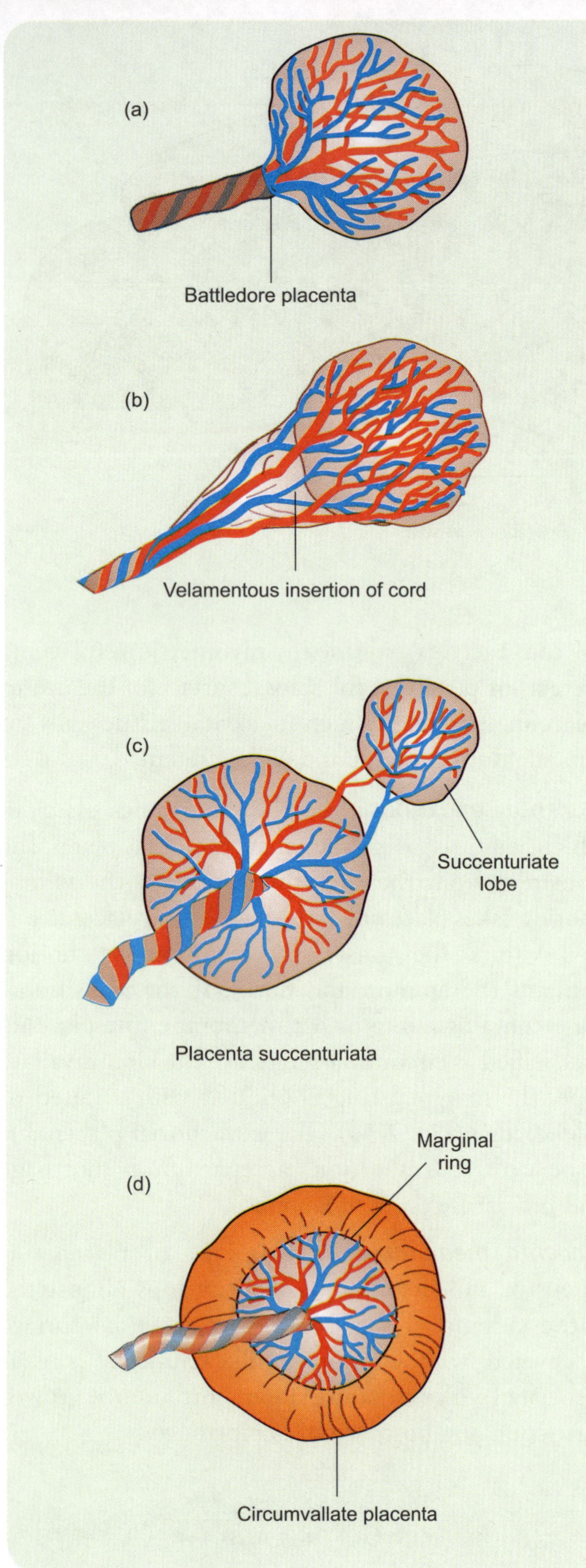

Fig. 7.3 Gross abnormalities of the placenta.

the arrangement found in adults. Fetal and maternal circulation are in intimate contact but are separated by the placental membrane.

Fetal circulation

In utero, the blood from the placenta (about 80% oxygen saturation) enters the fetus through the umbilical vein which joins the left branch of the portal vein. A smaller amount enters the liver sinusoids, mixes with blood from the portal circulation and enters the inferior vena cava; a greater amount of blood flows through the ductus venosus directly into the inferior vena cava, bypassing the liver.

The oxygenated blood (it is also rich in nutrients) reaches the right atrium through the interior vena cava; it is directed by the valve of the inferior vena cava towards the foramen ovale. Here it is divided into two by the lower edge of the septum secundum. Most of the blood passes through the foramen ovale into the left atrium.

In the left atrium, oxygenated blood mixes with a small amount of desaturated blood returning from the lungs. The blood then enters the left ventricle and the ascending aorta. The coronary arteries, myocardium, carotid arteries and the brain are supplied with well-oxygenated blood. Desaturated blood from the superior vena cava flows through the right ventricle into the pulmonary trunk. During fetal life, resistance in the pulmonary vessels is high, so that most of this blood passes directly through the **ductus arteriosus** into the descending aorta. After coursing through the descending aorta, blood flows towards the placenta through the two umbilical arteries. The oxygen saturation in the umbilical arteries is approximately 58% (**Fig.** 7.4).

Circulatory changes at birth

Changes in the circulatory system at birth are due to cessation of placental flow, the beginning of respiration and a fall in the infant's ambient temperature. Neural, chemical, thermal and mechanical stimuli cause the newborn to gasp and inflate its lungs for the first time. The lungs change from a solid to an expanded state, as air fills the bronchial tree and the alveoli. At birth, after the umbilical cord is tied,

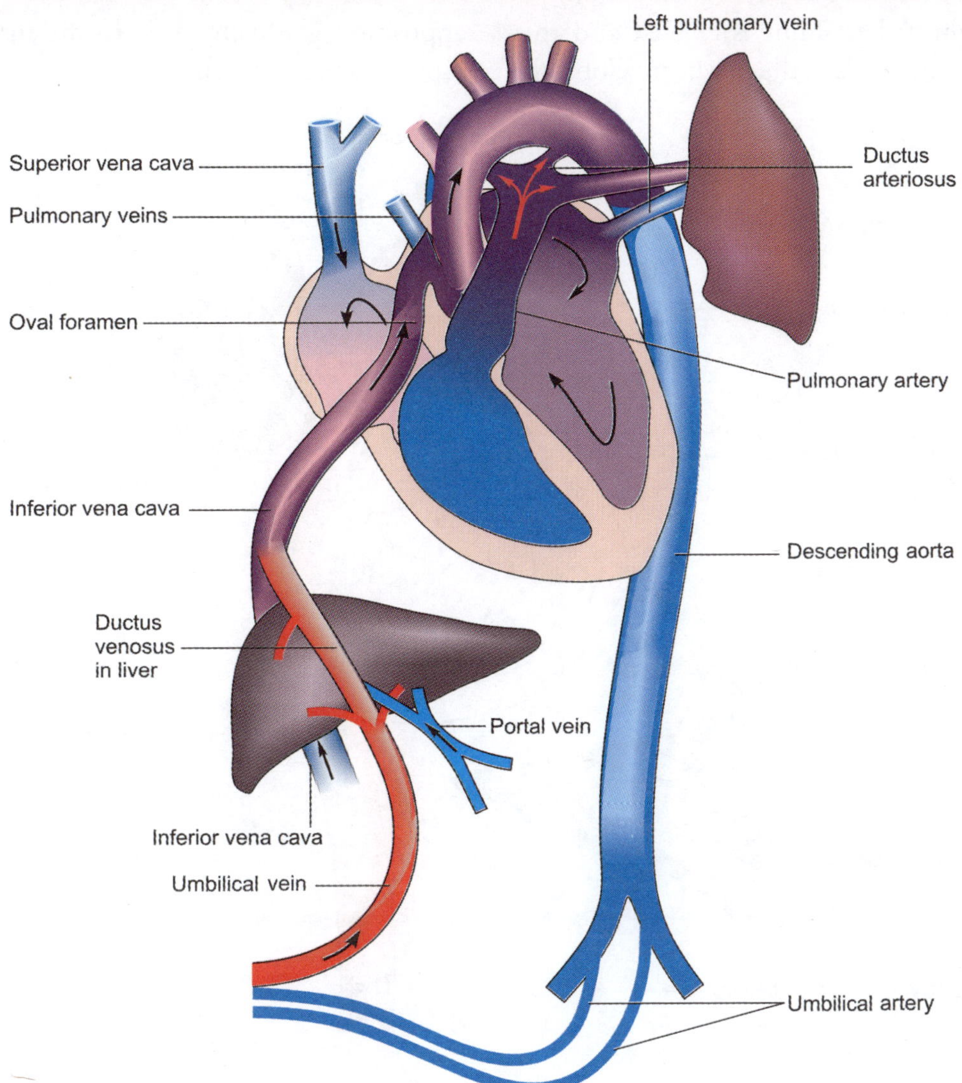

Fig. 7.4 Fetal circulation.

changes in circulation do not occur immediately. Some changes occur with the first breath and others take a few hours to days (**Fig. 7.5**).

When the smooth muscle in the walls of the umbilical arteries contract, the arteries close. The contraction is probably caused by mechanical stimuli, change in temperature and in oxygen tension. The arteries close a few minutes after birth and prevent the loss of infant blood. Although the actual obliteration of the lumen by fibrous proliferation may take 2–3 months, the distal parts of the umbilical arteries form the umbilical ligaments, and the proximal parts remain open as the superior vesical arteries.

The lumen of the umbilical vein and the ductus venosus close shortly after the umbilical arteries close. Hence, blood from the placenta may continue to flow into the newborn for some time after birth. The umbilical vein forms the ligamentum teres, and the ductus venosus forms the ligamentum venosum.

Closure of the ductus arteriosus is due to the contraction of its muscular wall after birth; it is mediated by bradykinin**,** a substance released from the lungs during initial inflation. Complete anatomical obliteration occurs at the end of three months, due to proliferation of the intima. Closure of the foramen ovale is caused by increased pressure in the left atrium, combined with a decrease in pressure on the right side.

The first breath presses the septum primum against the septum secundum. During the first days of life, however, this closure is reversible. When the baby cries, a right-to-left shunt is created and this accounts for cyanotic spells in the newborn. Constant apposition gradually leads to the fusion of the two septa in about an year.

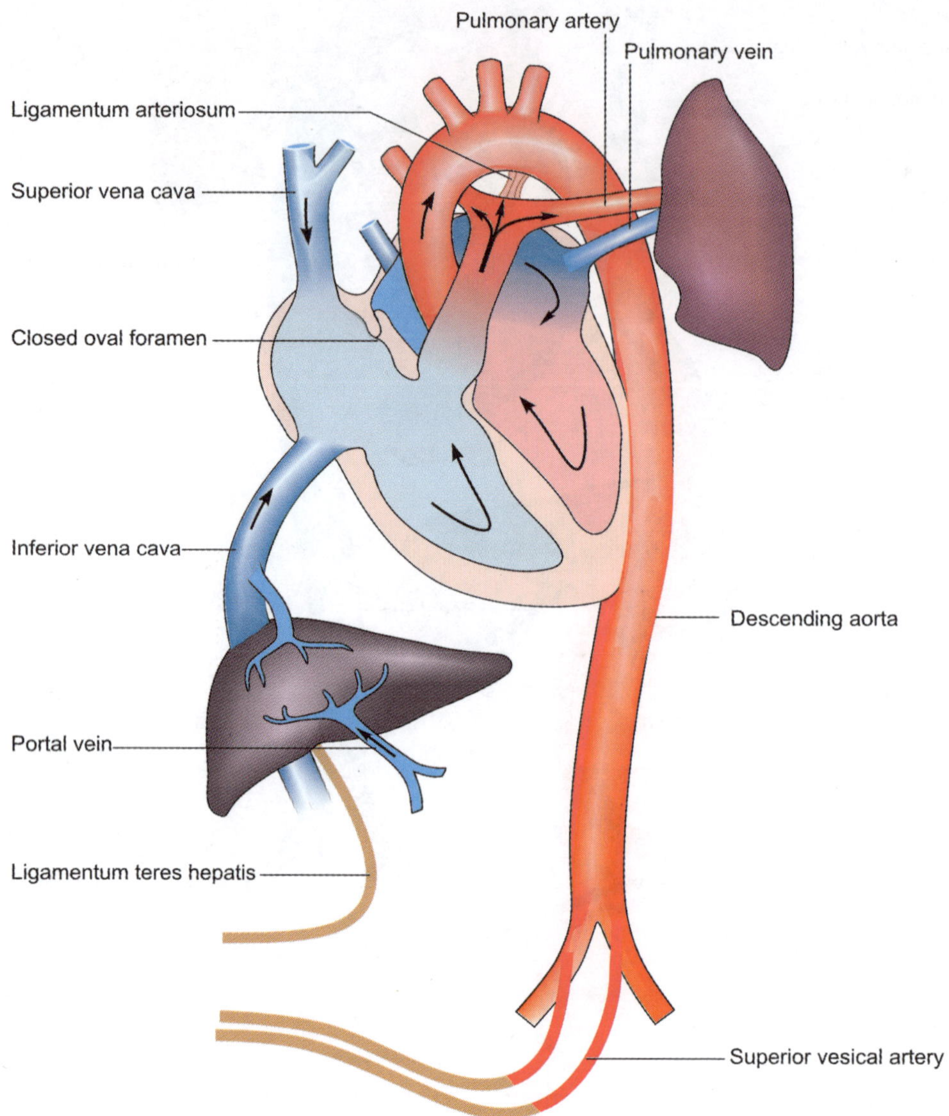

Fig. 7.5 Circulatory changes at birth.

KEY POINTS

- Organogenesis is completed by the fourth month and, thereafter, the organs begin to acquire functional capacity.
  - i. By the end of the month, lanugo hair is present and external genitalia are differentiated.
  - ii. By the end of the fifth month, the fetal body is covered with vernix caseosa. Fetal movements are felt by the mother.
  - iii. By the end of the seventh month, scalp hair appears and the lungs mature.
  - iv. From months 8 to 10, there is progressive loss of lanugo hair, the thoracic cage increases in circumference, the umbilicus is at the centre of the abdomen, the testes are in the scrotum and the epiphyseal centre appears at the lower end of the femur.
- The placenta is composed of about 60–100 functional lobules formed by the villous stem and its branches. It is divided by septae into 15–20 cotyledons.
- The endometrial spiral arteries open at intervals through the basal plate into the intervillous space. Blood flow through the placenta is 300 ml/minute at 20 weeks and 600 ml/minute at 40 weeks.
- At term, the placenta weighs 500 g. Near the centre on the fetal surface is the attachment of the umbilical cord; branches of umbilical vessels are visible.
- Abnormal placentation is associated with adverse pregnancy outcome for the mother and the fetus.
- In utero blood saturated with oxygen and nutrients enters the fetus through the umbilical vein. A greater amount of blood enters through the ductus venosus into the inferior vena cava. Blood rich in oxygen and nutrients passes into the left atrium through the foramen ovale.
- The resistance in the lungs being high, the blood reaches the descending aorta through the ductus arteriosus and further along the descending aorta to reach the placenta.
- Changes in fetal circulation at birth are caused by cessation of blood flow in the placenta, beginning of respiration and fall in the infant's ambient temperature.
- The umbilical arteries, veins, ductus arteriosus, ductus venosus and foramen ovale close after birth.

QUESTIONS

Select the single most appropriate answer:

1. The placental membrane is made up of all of the following *except*
   a. syncytiotrophoblast
   b. cytotrophoblast
   c. mesothelium of blood vessels
   d. connective tissue
2. Which of the following is true about the notochord?
   a. it gives rise to the spinal cord
   b. it persists as the vertebral column
   c. it degenerates
   d. it persists as the nucleus pulposus
3. Primitive streak gives rise to
   a. extraembryonic mesoderm
   b. intraembryonic mesoderm
   c. notochordal plate
   d. procaudal plate
4. Chorionic villus that has a core of syncytiotrophoblast, cytotrophoblast, mesoderm and blood vessels is called
   a. primary villus
   b. secondary villus
   c. tertiary villus
   d. anchoring villus
5. Neural crest cells give rise to
   a. melanocyte
   b. craniofacial skeleton
   c. adrenal medulla
   d. dorsal root ganglia
6. With advancing pregnancy, all of the following changes occur in the placenta *except*
   a. decrease in fibrous tissue in the core of villi
   b. thickening of basement membrane in fetal capillaries
   c. deposition of calcium
   d. obliteration in the small capillaries of the villi

7. The placental barrier is formed by all of the following *except*
   a. syncytiotrophoblast c. hypoblast
   b. cytotrophoblast d. connective tissue
8. All of the following statements are correct about ductus arteriosus *except*
   a. it connects the pulmonary artery to the aorta
   b. functional closure occurs one week after birth
   c. complete obliteration results in ligamentum arteriosus
   d. it develops from the left 6th artery
9. From the time of birth up to puberty, the number of oogonia
   a. remains constant c. increases marginally
   b. decreases d. increases significantly
10. When the placental villi invade the myometrium, the placenta is termed
    a. placenta accreta
    b. placenta increta
    c. placenta percreta
    d. placenta extrachorialis

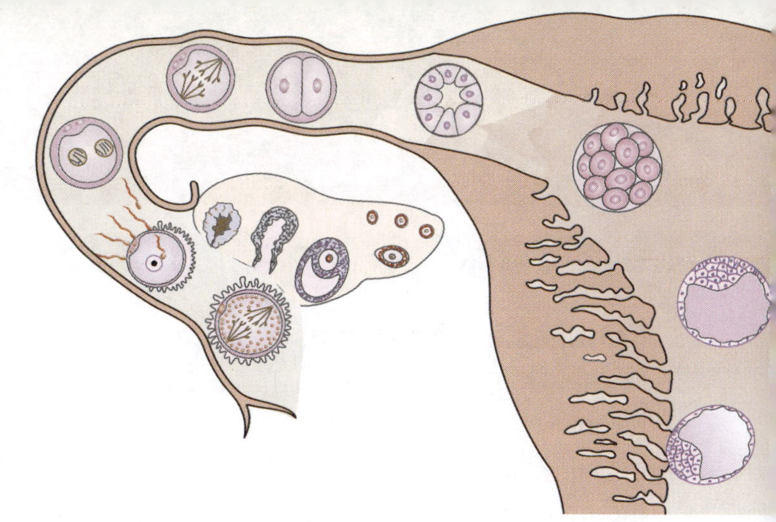

8

Maternal Changes in Pregnancy

Lakshmi Seshadri

LEARNING OBJECTIVES

At the end of this chapter, the reader should be able to:

- describe the salient anatomic, physiological and other changes during pregnancy
- appreciate the implications of these changes
- describe how an exaggeration of these changes can lead to complications
- enumerate the reasons why some of these changes can be interpreted as abnormal
- recapitulate how these changes affect the clinical course of the diseases complicating pregnancy
- recognise any deviation from normal

Introduction

Extensive anatomic, physiological and biochemical changes occur in the mother during pregnancy. These are intended to prepare the mother to meet the demands of pregnancy, labour and puerperium and to protect the fetus. Many of the changes are brought about by the pregnancy hormones. All the organ systems return to the prepregnancy state after delivery and lactation. The process takes about six weeks. Some of these changes would be considered abnormal in the nonpregnant state and may be interpreted as disease if one is not aware of these changes. Knowledge and understanding of these is, therefore, essential for the management of normal pregnancy and for recognising an abnormality.

Maternal characteristics that affect adaptation

The following important maternal characteristics influence the adaptation of the mother during pregnancy:

Gravidity: The physiological changes are more pronounced in the first pregnancy, as compared to subsequent ones.

Maternal age: Teenage mothers are less likely to adapt anatomically. Their pelvis is less capacious; therefore, cephalopelvic disproportion is common. Older women may have underlying diseases like diabetes and hypertension, which interfere with adaptation.

Medical conditions: Preexisting diabetes, hypertension and connective tissue disorders can affect adaptation.

Social class: Teenage pregnancies, grand multiparity, malnutrition, anemia and heavy physical work in women of a lower socioeconomic status can interfere with adaptation.

Ethnic variations: Due to variations in dietary habits, susceptibility to various diseases and basic physiological differences, different ethnic groups show some variation in adaptation.

Number of fetuses: The changes in organ systems are different in multifetal pregnancies.

Changes in the Genital Tract

Changes in the uterus

Major changes take place in the genital tract during pregnancy.

Changes in size and shape: In the prepregnant state, the uterus is a pear-shaped organ, weighing about 100 g and measures 8 × 5 × 2.5 cm. Rapid growth during pregnancy is due to hyperplasia and hypertrophy of the smooth muscle cells. By term, the uterus weighs 1,000 g. The shape of the uterus changes with advancing pregnancy, from pear-shaped to spherical at 20 weeks and elongates towards term, becoming longitudinally oval.

Lower segment: It develops from the isthmus and is about 3–4 cm wide by term. The difference between the two segments becomes more obvious as pregnancy advances. The junction between the two segments is at the level of the pubic symphysis and is marked by the level at which the peritoneum becomes loosely attached to the anterior uterine wall.

Blood flow: Blood flow to the uterus and cervix increase steadily to 500 ml/minute, which is five times more than in the nonpregnant state. Uterine vessels enlarge gradually and become tortuous.

Myometrium: It is arranged in three layers. The outer longitudinal layer is thin and passes from the fundus to the cervix. The middle layer is thick and consists of crisscrossing fibres. The blood vessels to the placenta pass through this layer; contraction of this layer leads to progressive expulsion of the fetus, and, in the third stage, to the closure of vessels and hemostasis. The inner layer is thin and circular, and forms sphincters around the opening of the fallopian tubes and cervix.

Uterine activity: Spontaneous contractions, called Braxton Hicks contractions, begin at around 10 weeks and continue till term. This uterine activity facilitates the development of the lower segment and softens the cervix.

Changes in the cervix

The cervix undergoes changes in pregnancy. The isthmus (the lower part of the uterus) softens; the fundus and cervix are firm. This softening and compressibility of the lower segment is described as the **Hegar sign**. The endocervical epithelium proliferates and gives rise to the ectropion. A lot of mucus is also produced and a thick plug of mucus forms in the cervical canal. This is expelled at onset of labour.

Changes in the vagina and vulva

There is increased vascularity and bluish discolouration, described as the **Chadwick sign**. Increase in glycogen-containing cells results in lowering of the pH due to increase in lactic acid. This offers protection from infection. The vulva becomes soft and varicosities may develop.

Changes in the ovary

The ovaries enlarge and become vascular, and the corpus luteum continues to grow till 7–8 weeks and begins to degenerate at 12 weeks.

Changes in the Breasts

Breast changes are more pronounced in primigravida. Estrogen and progesterone are responsible for the changes and cause hypertrophy and hyperplasia of ductal and glandular tissue. The breast enlarges from the first trimester and may become painful and tender. There is increased pigmentation of the nipples and areolae and Montgomery's tubercles become prominent. The nipples also enlarge. Secretion of colostrum starts from 12 weeks. Secondary areola forms by the fourth month. In the puerperium, milk secretion and letdown are controlled by prolactin and oxytocin.

Changes in Body Water Balance and Weight Gain

Changes in water balance affect all body systems. In pregnancy, total body water increases by about 8.5 l. Retention occurs mainly in the extracellular compartment, both in its intravascular and interstitial components. The retention of water is secondary to the retention of sodium mediated by the high levels of steroid hormones secreted during pregnancy.

Weight gain is usually 9–11 kg. This is mainly due to changes in maternal body water, fat, amniotic fluid, placenta and breasts besides the growing fetus. The average weight gain is about 0.5 kg per week in the second half of pregnancy. In the first trimester, women may lose about 2–3 kg due to a distaste for food and nausea and vomiting.

Metabolic Changes

Energy requirement

The mother and growing fetus require extra energy during pregnancy. The total requirement varies between individuals. It increases gradually from the end of the first trimester. There is little change till 10 weeks; requirement increases by 50–100 kcal/day till 36 weeks to 200–300 kcal/day in the last four weeks.

Carbohydrate metabolism

Pregnancy is a diabetogenic state. In the first trimester, the fasting plasma glucose concentration falls and the increase in blood glucose following a glucose load is marginal. Glycogen synthesis, storage, fat deposition and transport of amino acids into cells begin. By midpregnancy, insulin resistance sets in and plasma glucose concentrations rise. The response to the glucose load is slower but higher and lasts longer. The return to normal is delayed. This elevated plasma glucose is utilised as the primary source of energy by the fetus. Fasting glucose levels, however, remain low since the fetus utilises glucose continuously. Maternal utilisation of glucose is reduced, leading to glycogenolysis and gluconeogenesis. The mother uses fatty acids for energy. As a consequence, pregnant mothers develop ketosis rapidly, especially when energy requirements go up as in exercise, labour or hyperemesis.

The changes are attributed to estrogen, progesterone, cortisol and, to a large extent, human placental lactogen (hPL). Increase in insulin resistance, which becomes manifest at weeks 18–20 is concurrent with rising levels of hPL, indicating that this may be the main contributor.

Amino acid and fat metabolism

Amino acids are required by both the mother and the fetus for growth and energy. The level of amino acids, especially alanine, falls in pregnancy due to placental transfer and gluconeogenesis by the mother. Triglycerides, fatty acids, LDL cholesterol and HDL cholesterol increase. Fat is used as a source of energy by the mother.

The diagnosis of gestational diabetes should be with the prolonged glucose tolerance test (GTT). It should be performed at weeks 24–26, after the hPL levels rise. Diabetics require more insulin in pregnancy. One should watch out for ketosis during labour and in women who have been vomiting, as it occurs quite rapidly.

Changes in the Cardiovascular System

Anatomical changes

As the pregnant uterus enlarges, the diaphragm is pushed up; the heart is displaced upwards and laterally to the left with rotation in its long axis. The apex beat is, therefore, shifted upwards and to the left. The cardiac muscle hypertrophies, the chambers dilate and the heart size increases slightly. There can be functional hemic systolic murmurs of grade I or grade II intensity in the tricuspid and aortic areas. There is splitting of the first heart sound, and a third heart sound may also be heard. The ECG shows left axis deviation and ST depression.

Physiological changes

Peripheral resistance: It falls due to dilatation of the peripheral vessels by progesterone. The increased distensibility of veins along with pressure by the gravid uterus can result in varicose veins of the legs and vulva and hemorrhoids. Venous return decreases with peripheral pooling, which along with pressure by the gravid uterus on the great vessels, may lead to edema of the feet.

Cardiac output: It increases by 30%–50%, the increase beginning by about 10 weeks and reaching a peak at weeks 24–26. This is a combined effect of increase in stroke volume and heart rate (**Fig. 8.1**). In the supine position, the pressure of the gravid uterus on the inferior vena cava leads to reduction in venous return and hence cardiac output, leading to supine hypotension. These changes are seen in the third trimester and during labour. Renal and placental blood flow are also affected in the supine position. In labour, with pain and associated catecholamine release, the heart rate increases further. The pumping of blood from the uterus during the contractions increases venous return and cardiac output.

Blood pressure: There is no change in systolic blood pressure; diastolic pressure falls by 10–15 mm Hg in the second trimester due to a decrease in peripheral resistance and returns to normal by the third trimester. This should be borne in mind when diagnosing pregnancy-induced hypertension in the third trimester.

Diagnosis of valvular disease has to be made with caution, keeping in mind the shifting of the apex beat and ECG changes in pregnancy. Murmurs of intensity higher than grade III, those that are associated with thrill and diastolic murmurs are diagnostic of cardiac disease.

The increase in blood volume, cardiac output and heart rate can adversely affect women with valvular disease, leading to pulmonary edema and congestive cardiac failure. These risks are further increased in labour.

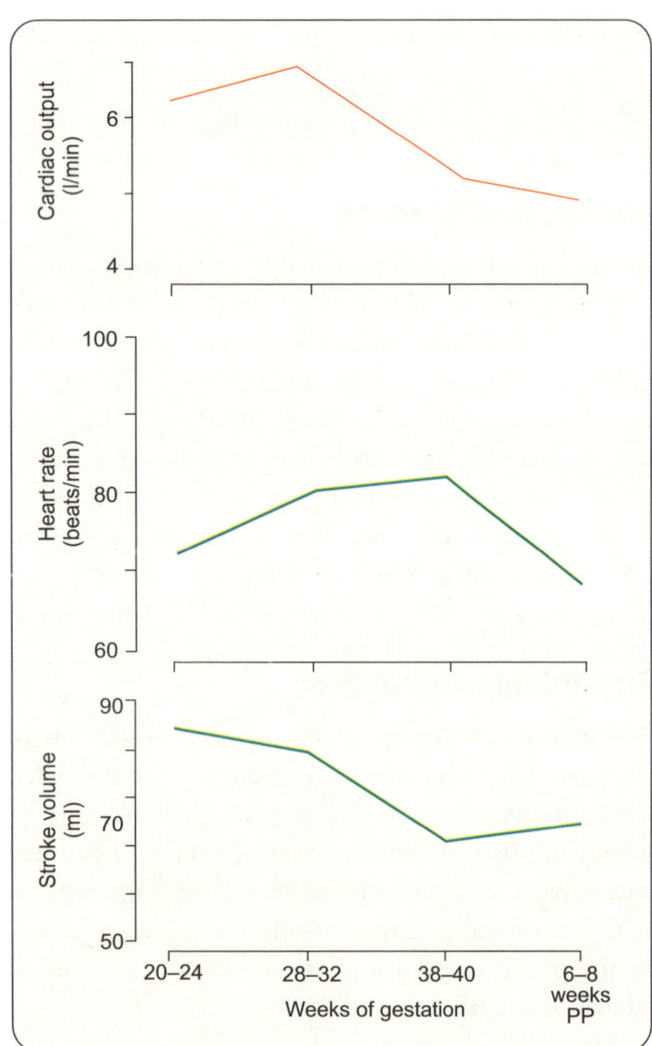

Fig. 8.1 Cardiac output.

Hematological Changes

The following important hematological changes occur during pregnancy:

Blood volume: It increases by 40%–50%. It starts in the first trimester and reaches a peak by weeks 32–34. Plasma volume increases by 50% and red cell volume by 30%, leading to 'physiological hemodilution' (**Fig. 8.2**). The increase in blood volume is meant for extra blood flow to the uterus, placenta and kidneys and to compensate for blood loss at delivery.

Blood cells: The need for iron increases since it is used up for producing extra maternal and fetal hemoglobin and placenta. If iron intake is inadequate, the iron stores may become depleted. White cell count increases from 12,000/µl to 16,000/µl. Neutrophils increase but other white cells and platelets are unaltered.

Coagulation factors: These also increase and hence pregnancy is considered a hypercoagulable state. Plasma levels of fibrinogen and factors VII, VIII, IX and X increase. Fibrinolysis is reduced. Erythrocyte sedimentation rate (ESR) increases due to increase in plasma globulin and fibrinogen.

Iron supplementation is required for most women in the developing countries and iron-deficient women in the developed world. White cell count and ESR cannot be used to diagnose infection in pregnancy.

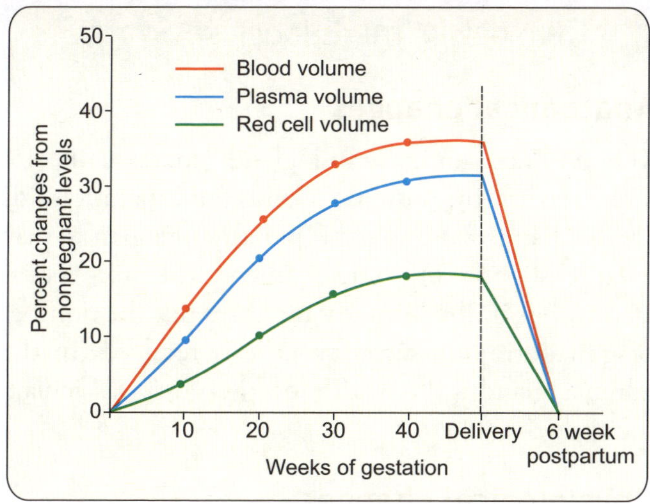

Fig. 8.2 Blood volume.

Normal blood loss in labour is tolerated well and signs of hypovolemia will not be manifest till a large volume of blood (1,000 ml) is lost. Due to the increase in coagulation factors and decrease in fibrinolysis, disseminated coagulation occurs easily.

Changes in the Respiratory System

Anatomical changes

As the uterus enlarges, the diaphragm is pushed up by as much as 4 cm, and the rib cage widens and is displaced upwards. There is mucosal congestion of the entire respiratory tract.

Physiological changes

Tidal volume and inspiratory capacity increase while functional residual capacity and residual volume decrease. These are due to relaxation of the musculature of the airways. With advancing pregnancy, there is increase in minute ventilatory volume and minute oxygen uptake. The threshold of the respiratory centre is reduced, probably as an effect of progesterone, and results in a reduction in maternal pCO_2. There is physiological dyspnea.

These changes have implications during anesthesia. Increased oxygen consumption and decreased reserve leads to a rapid fall in arterial oxygen. Diseases of the respiratory tract may be more serious during pregnancy.

Changes in the Urinary System

Anatomical changes

In early pregnancy, while the uterus is still a pelvic organ, there is pressure on the bladder by the enlarging uterus causing frequency and urgency. This is relieved in the second trimester. In the last weeks of pregnancy, the pressure of the fetal head on the lower pole of the uterus may again cause these symptoms. In labour, the fetal head can compress the bladder and urethra against the pubic bone and cause urinary retention. Prolonged pressure can lead to edema of the base of the bladder and voiding difficulties in the puerperium.

The kidneys increase in size and weight. The renal pelvis is dilated. The ureters dilate and become more tortuous. The changes are limited to the part of the ureters above the pelvic brim. Relaxation of smooth muscles due to progesterone and the pressure of the enlarging uterus are responsible for these changes. These are more on the right side due to dextrorotation of the uterus. Bladder tone decreases and bladder capacity increases. The bladder supports relax.

Physiological changes

The glomerular filtration rate (GFR) increases by 50% and renal plasma flow by 25%–50%. These are altered by posture, being more in the lateral position when the pressure of the uterus on the aorta and vena cava is relieved. With the increase in GFR, creatinine clearance increases. The renal threshold for glucose decreases and reabsorption of various substances like glucose, amino acids and uric acid by renal tubules also reduces. This results in glycosuria, mild proteinuria (<300 mg in 24 hours) and fall in blood levels of amino acids and uric acid.

There is an increase in the renin–angiotensin II and prostacyclin levels. These regulate efferent arteriolar resistance and glomerular filtration. Systemic vascular sensitivity to renin–angiotensin II is an reduced. There is an increase in total body water, leading to a fall in plasma osmolality. There is retention of sodium.

Anatomical changes lead to urinary frequency in the first trimester due to the pressure of the pregnant uterus on the bladder. Urinary infections are common due to ureteric and renal pelvic dilatation and stasis. Relaxation of the bladder supports can cause stress incontinence. Renal glycosuria should not be interpreted as diabetes.

Changes in the Gastrointestinal System

Anatomical changes

The enlarging uterus displaces the stomach and intestines upwards. The intragastric pressure changes and the angle at the gastroesophageal junction is altered. The appendix is displaced superiorly and reaches the right flank.

Gums become hypertrophic, hyperemic and may bleed; this is commonly known as **gingival hypertrophy of pregnancy**.

Physiological changes

Secretion by the salivary glands increases in the first trimester. With increasing progesterone levels, production of motilin decreases. Therefore, motility of the entire gastrointestinal tract is reduced. The sphincters relax. These changes lead to increased emptying time and transit time of food through the gastrointestinal tract. These result in gastroesophageal reflux or 'heart burn' worsening in the later part of pregnancy. Increased reabsorption of fluid due to increase in transit time in the bowel leads to constipation.

No anatomical or histological changes are seen in the liver. But plasma globulin and fibrinogen levels increase. Increase in hormone-binding globulins leads to reduction in the levels of free hormones. Transaminases are unaltered but alkaline phosphatase levels increase. A major part of this rise is due to secretion by the placenta. Gall bladder emptying is slow and causes cholestasis.

Increased gastric stasis can lead to aspiration of gastric contents during anesthesia. Aspiration of acid gastric contents can lead to Mendelson syndrome and maternal mortality.

A diagnosis of appendicitis can be difficult since the organ is displaced. Cholestasis can, in some women, be recurrent and associated with pruritus, and is known as **recurrent cholestasis of pregnancy**.

Changes in the Endocrine System

Anatomical changes

The pituitary and thyroid glands increase in size and weight; the adrenal glands and parathyroids are unchanged though the parathyroid glands may enlarge slightly in some women. The number of lactotrophs in the pituitary increases but the number of gonadotrophin-secreting cells is reduced. In the adrenal glands, the width of the zona fasciculata increases.

Physiological changes

The trophoblastic cells of the placenta synthesise several hormones from early gestation. They begin to secrete human chorionic gonadotrophin (hCG) seven days after conception. The levels increase rapidly following implantation to reach a peak at 60–70 days (**Fig. 8.3**). The detection of hCG is used for the diagnosis of pregnancy. Other steroid and protein hormones like progesterone, estradiol, estriol, adrenocorticotropic hormone, hPL and renin are also secreted in large quantities. The estrogens enhance hepatic synthesis of binding globulins and this, in turn, leads to increased circulating levels of bound hormones but not necessarily free hormones. Human placental lactogen and other steroid hormones are responsible for the development of gestational diabetes in susceptible women.

The secretion of anterior pituitary hormones is unchanged or reduced. Prolactin levels rise from early pregnancy and can be 20 times higher than in the nonpregnant state.

Renal clearance of iodide doubleds due to the increase in GFR but the thyroid gland compensates by increasing the uptake of iodine. This results in increase in size of the gland and in frank goitre if the mother's diet is iodine-deficient. Free plasma triiodothyronine (T3) and thyroxine (T4) levels remain normal but the levels of the bound fraction increase due to an increase in the binding globulin. The mother, however, remains euthyroid.

The long-acting thyroid stimulator, T4, iodide and the thyrotrophin-releasing hormone cross the placenta. Elevated levels of these when the mother

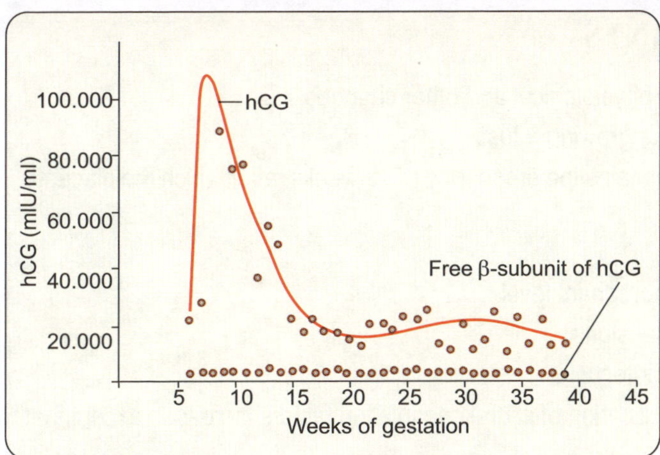

Fig. 8.3 Levels of hCG in pregnancy.

is hypo or hyperthyroid can, therefore, affect the fetus.

Plasma cortisol and other corticosteroids increase from week 12 onwards but progesterone has an antiglucocorticoid effect and occupies the receptors. The placental enzymes metabolise the excess corticoids and prevent a rise in fetal circulating levels.

The renin–angiotensin system undergoes changes resulting in elevated levels of plasma renin, angiotensinogen II and angiotensin II.

Implications: Increase in the size of the thyroid gland can be misdiagnosed as pathological goitre.

The mood swings and altered behaviour in pregnancy are due to endocrine changes. Progesterone increase leads to dyspnea, altered gut motility and several changes in other systems. Elevated corticosteroid levels may explain the euphoria and 'blues' experienced by some women especially after childbirth. Placental hormones cause altered glucose metabolism and gestational diabetes. Interpretation of the results of hormone levels can be difficult unless the changes in binding globulin levels are kept in mind. Most hormones cross the placenta and can affect the fetus if the levels are abnormal. Fetal maturation, onset of labour and several other events are hormone-dependent. Therefore, the endocrine system, along with the placental hormones, plays a key role in pregnancy, labour and lactation.

Changes in the Skin

Pigmentation is common, especially on the face and abdomen. This is more obvious on the cheeks and nose over a butterfly-shaped area and is referred to as **chloasma gravidarum**. Linea nigra is the linear pigmentation below the umbilicus in the midline and is characteristic of pregnancy. Striae occur on the lower abdomen, flanks, inner thighs and breasts and are caused by increased levels of corticosteroids and stretching, with resultant rupture of the elastic fibres in the dermis. Palmar erythema and spider nevi are common, due to increased estrogen levels.

Changes in the Musculoskeletal System

There is relaxation of connective tissue due to biochemical changes. The laxity of intervertebral joints and lordosis of pregnancy cause a shift in the centre of gravity and may cause backache. The pubic symphysis becomes lax and can cause pain. Late in pregnancy, the gait of the woman is described as 'waddling'.

KEY POINTS

- During pregnancy, a woman undergoes profound anatomical, physiological and other changes.
- The weight of the uterus increases tenfold to accommodate the growing fetus.
- The corpus luteum in the ovary secretes progesterone and maintains the pregnancy till 12 weeks, after which the placenta takes over.
- Total weight gain during pregnancy is 9–11 kg.
- The blood volume increases near term by 50% above the nonpregnant level.
- The physiological cardiovascular changes may mimic abnormal signs.
- Changes in the urinary tract predispose the woman to urinary infection.
- Pregnancy is essentially a hypercoagulable state as the concentration of all the coagulation factors increases except that of factors XI and XIII.
- Dyspnea of pregnancy occurs due to increased oxygen consumption and decreased reserve.
- Pregnancy is essentially diabetogenic; diabetes may be unmasked for the first time during pregnancy.
- The plasma levels of free T3 and T4 remain normal, but the level of the bound fraction increases due to an increase in binding globulin. The pregnant woman remains euthyroid.
- There is an increase in glomerular filtration rate and a lowering of the renal threshold.
- The motility of the intestinal tract is reduced and gastric emptying is delayed as a result of raised progesterone levels.

QUESTIONS

Select the single most appropriate answer:

1. The uterus in the prepregnant state weighs 100 g. Its weight increases rapidly through pregnancy to weigh on an average
   a. 500 g b. 1,000 g c. 1,500 g d. 2,000 g
2. By term pregnancy, the blood flow to the uterus increases to
   a. 900 ml/min c. 500 ml/min
   b. 700 ml/min d. 300 ml/min
3. Spontaneous uterine contractions known as Braxton Hicks contractions begin by
   a. 10 weeks c. 18 weeks
   b. 14 weeks d. 22 weeks
4. Hegar sign is due to
   a. uterine enlargement
   b. softening of the cervix
   c. compressibility of the isthmus
   d. increased vascularity of the genital tract
5. During pregnancy, the average increase in total body water is
   a. 4.5 litres b. 6.5 litres c. 8.5 litres d. 10.5 litres
6. The main contributor to increased insulin resistance during pregnancy is
   a. progesterone c. cortisol
   b. hPL d. estrogen
7. During pregnancy, the blood volume begins to rise by
   a. 8 weeks c. 12 weeks
   b. 10 weeks d. 14 weeks

In the following questions, there are two statements. Select the appropriate answer using the following key:

a. if both statements are true and causally related
b. if both statements are true but not causally related
c. if the first statement is true and the second is false
d. if the first statement is false and the second is true
e. if both statements are false

8. Pregnancy is a state of glucose intolerance *because* Insulin resistance increases during pregnancy.
9. A pregnant mother under stress is prone to developing ketosis *because*

   A pregnant mother predominantly utilises glucose for energy.
10. In the second trimester, the diastolic blood pressure remains unchanged *because*

    In the second trimester there is more pronounced peripheral vasodilatation.

Select the appropriate answer using the following key:

a. if only responses 1, 2 and 3 are correct
b. if only 1 and 3 are correct
c. if only 2 and 4 are correct
d. if only 4 is correct
e. if all are correct

11. During pregnancy, the following changes are noted in the respiratory physiology
    1. tidal volume is increased
    2. functional residual capacity is decreased
    3. inspiratory capacity is increased
    4. residual volume is increased

12. What functional changes occur in the renal system during pregnancy?
    1. increase in GFR
    2. decrease in plasma flow
    3. decrease in renal threshold to glucose
    4. decrease in creatinine clearance

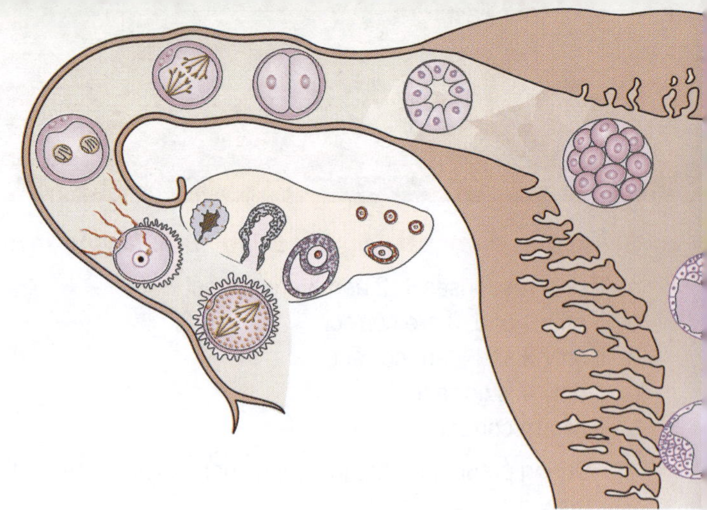

9

Diagnosis of Pregnancy

Kapila Bharucha

LEARNING OBJECTIVES

At the end of this chapter, the reader should be able to:

- appreciate the need for the early diagnosis of pregnancy
- list the symptoms suggestive of pregnancy
- enumerate the signs of pregnancy
- list the investigations that help confirm pregnancy
- list the differential diagnosis of pregnancy

Introduction

Whenever a woman in the reproductive age group, who earlier had regular menstruation, presents with amenorrhea, one should first think of pregnancy. Pregnancy is a physiological condition but its correct diagnosis is essential. The diagnosis has far-reaching psychosocial consequences to the woman. Any health care provider, when consulted by a woman in the reproductive age group, should always know if the woman is pregnant, so that any interventions that may harm the fetus can be avoided. It is prudent to remember that many symptoms of pregnancy may be seen in other diseases and failure to diagnose pregnancy may lead to wrong diagnosis and incorrect treatment. The diagnosis of pregnancy has traditionally been based on history and examination findings; however, currently, urine tests to detect the presence of human chorionic gonadotrophin and ultrasonography are used to confirm pregnancy.

Symptoms of Pregnancy

The following symptoms in a woman of reproductive age should make one suspect pregnancy: amenorrhea, nausea, vomiting, frequency of micturition and fatigue. They point to presumptive evidence of pregnancy.

First trimester

Amenorrhea: Sudden cessation of menstrual cycles in a woman of reproductive age, who earlier had regular menstruation, is highly suggestive of pregnancy. A woman will suspect pregnancy whenever she misses her periods: the suspicion is even greater when a second period is missed. Amenorrhea is a reliable indicator of pregnancy. Rarely, a woman may continue to menstruate till the completion of 12 weeks of gestation. Also, conception may occur in the absence of previous menstruation. For example, pregnancy can take place during lactational amenorrhea. Cessation of menstruation may also be a manifestation of other diseases like polycystic ovarian syndrome (PCOS) and genital tuberculosis.

Nausea and vomiting: Many women may complain of nausea with or without vomiting. It is also known as morning sickness as the symptoms begin in the morning but may continue through the day. Nausea and vomiting can be very disturbing as the woman would be unable to eat or drink. The symptoms characteristically occur in early pregnancy and are resolved by the end of the first trimester. They may occasionally persist in the second trimester, especially if the woman has a multiple pregnancy. The symptoms are attributed to high levels of hCG, but no definite cause has been established.

Disturbances in the digestive system associated with nausea and vomiting, like gastritis, are common throughout pregnancy; the cause should be detected and appropriate treatment instituted.

Disturbances in micturition: The enlarging gravid uterus in early pregnancy exerts pressure on the base of the bladder causing frequent micturition. The frequency diminishes as pregnancy advances, but may reappear at the end of pregnancy, when the fetal head enters the pelvis.

Fatigue: Some women complain of tiredness in early pregnancy. The symptoms are only presumptive of pregnancy, and diagnosis will be based on clinical signs or laboratory tests.

Pain in the breasts: Some women may complain of pain in the breasts.

Second trimester

Amenorrhea persists. The woman is relieved of nausea and vomiting by 14 weeks of gestation. Disturbances in micturition disappear as the uterus becomes an abdominal organ.

Abdominal enlargement: This is perceived once the uterus is larger than 14 weeks. It is confined to the lower abdomen in the second trimester.

Perception of fetal movements: A woman is likely to perceive fetal movements between 18 and 20 weeks of gestation. In a multigravida, the fetal movements are felt between 16 and 18 weeks, and about two weeks later in a primigravida. The movements are described as 'fluttering' in the abdomen. As pregnancy advances, they become more obvious. In case the woman remembers the first day she recognised the movements (known as 'quickening'), the information may be useful in calculating the period of gestation.

Tightening of the abdomen: Women become aware of a feeling of tightening of the uterus. This is due to painless uterine contractions, known as Braxton Hicks contractions, which are infrequent till the last one or two weeks.

Third trimester

Amenorrhea: It continues and enlargement of the abdomen is progressive.

Other symptoms: The pregnant woman is likely to complain of breathlessness, pedal edema and difficulty in walking, and palpitation.

Fetal movements: These become more pronounced and sometimes may cause discomfort.

Lightening: Towards term, the woman experiences a sudden relief as the head enters the pelvis.

Frequency of micturition: It increases when the fetal head enters the pelvis, towards term.

Signs of Pregnancy

Most of the signs of pregnancy are probable evidence of pregnancy.

First trimester

Breasts: With advancing pregnancy, the breasts enlarge and become heavy; the nipple and areola become darker; the pigmentation around the areola gives rise to 'secondary areola'. These changes may be seen at 6–8 weeks and are more marked in a primigravida. Montgomery's tubercles become more prominent in the primary areola. Colostrum or milk-like secretion can be expressed from the breasts.

Vagina: On speculum examination, the vaginal mucosa appears dark-blue or purple and is known as the Chadwick or **Jacquemier sign**. It is not specific to pregnancy and may be seen in disorders associated with pelvic congestion.

Cervix: This is also dark blue and feels soft and is known as the **Goodell sign**.

Uterus: The uterus softens and enlarges to accommodate the growing fetus. Between 6 and 8 weeks of gestation, the products of conception are lodged in the upper segment and the isthmus is extremely soft and compressible. On bimanual examination, the lower part is easily compressed between the fingers, with the cervix below and the globular upper part above. This finding is referred to as the **Hegar sign**; it disappears once the products of conception occupy the entire uterus (**Fig. 9.1**). As pregnancy advances, the original pyriform shape of the uterus becomes globular, from the size of an egg at six weeks to a cricket ball at eight weeks and that of the fetal head at 12 weeks. In the case of asymmetrical implantation, the consistency of the two halves of the uterus may be different, giving the impression of an extrauterine mass (**Piskacek sign**). Because of increased vascularity, the pulsations of vessels are felt in the fornices; this is known as the **Osiander sign**.

Second trimester

Breasts: The changes seen in the first trimester continue.

Skin changes: The pigmentation becomes more intense as pregnancy progresses. Butterfly-like pigmentation appears around the cheeks (known as **chloasma**); pigmentation of the armpits and breasts occurs and linea nigra, a dark line in the midline of the abdomen, is seen. Stretch marks, called **striae gravidarum**, appear on the lower abdomen and flanks.

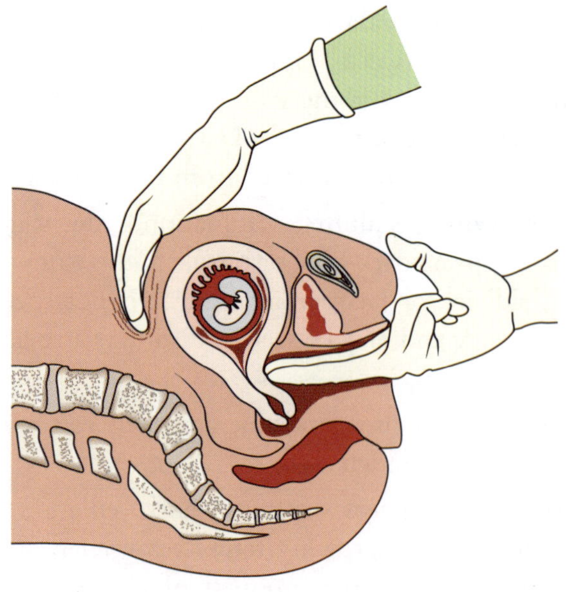

Fig. 9.1 Hegar sign.

Abdomen: The enlarging uterus rises out of the pelvic cavity, distending the abdomen progressively till term. The uterus is palpable abdominally after 12 weeks. It reaches the umbilicus by 24 weeks of gestation and is at the junction of the lower third and upper two-thirds of the distance between the umbilicus and the xiphisternum at 28 weeks.

Braxton Hicks contractions: Palpable uterine contractions occur in a pregnant uterus. They start in early pregnancy, are painless and come on at irregular intervals. Their presence helps to confirm an intrauterine pregnancy. Towards the end of pregnancy, the contractions increase both in frequency and intensity.

Ballottement: In this trimester, the volume of amniotic fluid is greater compared to that of the fetus. Around 20 weeks, tapping the uterus between the palpating hands reveals the feeling of ballottement. This sign is called **external ballottement**.

At about 16 weeks, on vaginal examination, when the fetus is pushed up, it returns and hits the examining fingers with a thud. This sign is known as **internal ballottement**.

Fetal movements: The examining hand can appreciate active fetal movements after about 20 weeks. Initially felt as a flutter, the movements become more intense as pregnancy advances.

Fetal heart sounds: These are audible with a stethoscope or a fetoscope from 18 to 20 weeks of gestation. The fetal heart rate at this time of pregnancy is 120–160 per minute and is heard as the 'ticking' of a watch. It is important to count the rate to ensure that it is different from the maternal pulse. The Doppler machine can detect the fetal heart tones as early as week 12 of gestation, but more regularly after week 14.

Third trimester

Breasts: The enlargement progresses and the likelihood of secretion from the nipples increases.

Uterine enlargement: The uterus continues to increase to reach the xiphisternum by 36 weeks, and then descends to the costal margin with fullness of the flanks, as the volume of liquor decreases and the head enters the pelvis.

Fetal parts: The fetal parts like the head and back are identified more distinctly and definitely by the examiner as pregnancy advances.

Fetal heart sounds: These are heard well. One is less likely to mistake uterine soufflé for fetal heart sounds.

Diagnostic Tests for Confirmation of Pregnancy

Advances in diagnostic techniques have contributed not only to the early diagnosis of pregnancy, but also that of abnormal conditions like hydatidiform mole and ectopic pregnancy.

Immunological tests for pregnancy

The immunological tests for pregnancy are based on the principle that the β subunit of hCG produced by the cytotrophoblast in early pregnancy is detectable in maternal serum/urine 8–10 days after conception. The tests currently available can detect 1–2 mIU/ml in serum within 10 days of conception.

Indirect or agglutination inhibition test: When the pregnant woman's urine containing hCG is treated with anti-hCG antibody, the antibody is neutralised. Subsequently, when latex coated with hCG is added, there is no agglutination, indicating pregnancy. If there is no pregnancy, there is no hCG in the urine and the antibody, unneutralised, agglutinates the latex with hCG. This test is rapid, can detect 15–25 mIU/ml of hCG and becomes positive two days after the missed period.

Direct or agglutination test: In this test, latex particles coated with anti-hCG monoclonal antibodies are mixed with the urine to be tested. If it contains hCG, agglutination is seen. This test is similar to the indirect test in its sensitivity and time of detection of hCG.

Radioimmunoassay (RIA): The test uses radiolabelled hCG antibodies to detect the β-subunit of hCG up to 2 mIU/ml in serum. It is positive three days before the missed period.

Enzyme-linked immunosorbent assay (ELISA): It is based on one monoclonal antibody for hCG and another for alkaline phosphatase. The two antibodies sandwich the hCG; it shows colour changes after binding. It is a very sensitive test (1–2 mIU/ml of serum) and can detect pregnancy five days before the missed period. It takes 3–4 hours to perform the test.

Immunoradiometric assay (IRMA): The assay uses the sandwich principle to detect the hCG antigen in serum, is rapid and can detect as low as 0.05 mIU/ml of hCG. The test is positive within eight days of conception.

Ultrasonography

First trimester: Transvaginal sonography (TVS) is the most accurate method for confirming an intrauterine pregnancy and assessing the gestational age early in the first trimester. Ultrasonography is not used to diagnose pregnancy unless there is clinical suspicion of pregnancy or the woman presents with vaginal bleeding or abdominal pain early in gestation.

The earliest structure identified by TVS is the gestational sac, by 4–5 weeks. The gestation sac grows at 1 mm/day in early gestation. By 5–6 weeks, the **double decidual sign** can be seen, which is the gestational sac surrounded by the thick decidua. The yolk sac appears as a small sphere with a hypoechoic centre and is located within the gestational sac around 4–5 weeks. The fetal pole is a linear hyperechoic structure first seen at 5–6 weeks of pregnancy and grows at a rate of 1 mm/day (**Fig. 9.2**). Cardiac activity can be identified by six weeks.

Besides the diagnosis of early pregnancy, ultrasonography is useful for identifying conditions

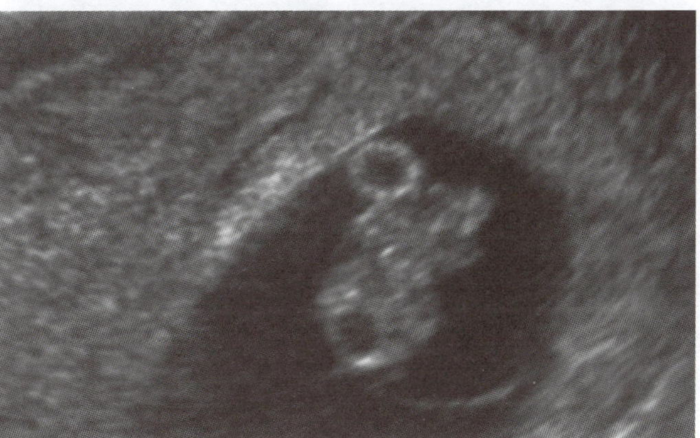

Fig. 9.2 Ultrasound picture of six weeks pregnancy.

like multiple pregnancy and ectopic pregnancy when used along with quantitative hCG levels.

Second and third trimesters: Sonography may be required for the diagnosis of pregnancy in the first trimester. In subsequent trimesters, it is useful in complicated pregnancies where clinical detection is difficult.

Routine obstetric sonography is recommended to ascertain the location of the placenta, amount of amniotic fluid and state of the internal cervical os. Apart from this, it is used to detect fetal abnormalities.

An ultrasound scan between 8 and 16 weeks of gestation can help date the pregnancy.

Table 9.1 summarises the clinical and laboratory criteria for the diagnosis of pregnancy.

Differential diagnosis of pregnancy

Pregnancy may be mistaken for abdominopelvic swellings, such as those of the bladder, uterine fibroids and ovarian cysts, and should always be ruled out in a young woman.

Distended bladder: A distended bladder may be mistaken for any abdominopelvic swelling, including pregnancy, and it is essential to ensure that the bladder is empty before examining a woman.

Uterine fibroid: A symmetrically enlarged uterus with a submucosal fibroid can simulate pregnancy. Amenorrhea is not a symptom of fibroid unless pregnancy is coexisting and the fibroids are usually firm in consistency. It can sometimes be difficult to diagnose pregnancy in a uterus with multiple fibroids, and a urine pregnancy test and ultrasound scans must be done to rule out pregnancy. In later pregnancy, a fibroid in the pelvis may be mistaken for the fetal head on vaginal examination.

Ovarian cysts: These are not associated with amenorrhea. Generally on bimanual palpation, the

Table 9.1 Symptoms, signs and laboratory tests for the diagnosis of pregnancy

Period of gestation	Symptoms	Signs	Laboratory tests
4 to 5 weeks	Occasional nausea and vomiting		Raised serum β hCG levels, urine pregnancy test positive TVS: Gestational sac
6 to 8 weeks	Amenorrhea, nausea and increased frequency of micturition	Hyperpigmentation of nipple and areola Bluish-purple discolouration of cervix and vagina Hegar sign positive	Double decidual sign, yolk sac appears Fetal pole with cardiac activity
9 to 12 weeks	Amenorrhea, nausea and vomiting	Uterus is palpable just above symphysis pubis	
Second trimester	'Quickening' felt around 18–20 weeks; Braxton Hicks contractions	Growth of breasts continues Fetal parts felt and fetal heart sounds heard External and internal ballottement elicited	Not necessary for diagnosis Useful to determine fetal and placental anatomy Done to detect any abnormalities of fetus, placenta or liquor
Third trimester	Breast secretion may appear	Uterus reaches the xiphisternum at 36 weeks and then comes down as the head descends in the pelvis Fetal head, neck and back identified Fetal heart sounds heard distinctly	Same as above

uterus can be felt separately from the ovarian cyst. Further, the absence of fetal parts and a negative pregnancy test is suggestive of an ovarian cyst. Ultrasound examination will confirm the cyst.

Pseudocyesis

Pseudocyesis is a psychological disorder in which the patient fantasises that she is pregnant. It is usually seen in elderly women undergoing treatment for infertility. The patient has amenorrhea, morning sickness and, breast tenderness and perceives fetal movements. Even the abdomen may appear distended, fetal parts cannot be felt and the fetal heart cannot be heard. A pregnancy test and ultrasound examination may be performed to convince the patient.

KEY POINTS

- It is very important to make an accurate diagnosis of pregnancy, as it can have far-reaching emotional and social consequences.
- Symptoms like amenorrhea, nausea and vomiting are presumptive of pregnancy.
- The probable signs are changes in the breasts, skin, vagina and uterine enlargement.
- Palpation of fetal parts and the presence of fetal heart sounds are definitive signs of pregnancy.
- Detection of hCG in the urine or raised levels in the serum are useful tests to confirm pregnancy in the first trimester.
- Sonography can confirm pregnancy by five weeks of gestation.

QUESTIONS

Select the single most appropriate answer:

1. Nausea and vomiting usually disappear by
   a. 8 weeks
   b. 12 weeks
   c. 16 weeks
   d. 20 weeks
2. Which of the following is *not* presumptive of pregnancy?
   a. vomiting
   b. increased frequency of micturition
   c. pain in the breasts
   d. auscultation of fetal heart sounds
3. A multigravida perceives fetal movements by
   a. 12 weeks
   b. 16 weeks
   c. 20 weeks
   d. 24 weeks
4. During pregnancy, due to increased vascularity, pulsations of vessels are felt in the fornices; this is known as
   a. Chadwick sign
   b. Jacquemier sign
   c. Osiander sign
   d. Goodell sign
5. By 28 weeks of gestation, the fundus of the uterus is
   a. midway between the umbilicus and the xiphisternum
   b. at one-third the distance between the umbilicus and the xiphisternum
   c. just above the level of the umbilicus
   d. at two-thirds the distance between the umbilicus and the xiphisternum
6. External ballottement can be elicited by what period of gestation?
   a. 8 weeks
   b. 12 weeks
   c. 16 weeks
   d. 20 weeks
7. With the immunological tests currently available, pregnancy can be detected
   a. 4 days after conception
   b. 6 days after conception
   c. 8 days after conception
   d. 10 days after conception

Select the appropriate answer using the following key:

a. if only responses 1, 2 and 3 are correct
b. if only 1 and 3 are correct
c. if only 2 and 4 are correct
d. if only 4 is correct
e. if all are correct

8. What are the definitive signs of pregnancy?
   1. striae gravidarum
   2. palpation of fetal parts
   3. uterine enlargement
   4. presence of fetal heart sounds
9. On transvaginal ultrasonography at 4 to 5 weeks of pregnancy, the following may be seen
   1. yolk sac
   2. cardiac pulsation
   3. gestational sac
   4. embryonic movements
10. Transvaginal sonography in early pregnancy is useful in the diagnosis of
    1. intrauterine pregnancy
    2. hydatidiform mole
    3. multiple pregnancy
    4. ectopic pregnancy

10

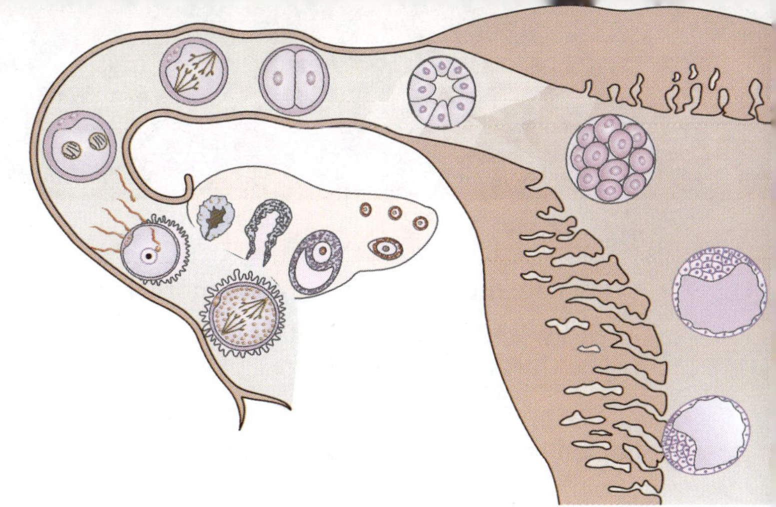

Antenatal Care

Asha Oumachigui

LEARNING OBJECTIVES

At the end of this chapter, the reader should be able to:

- define antenatal care
- appreciate the status of antenatal care in India
- enumerate the components of antenatal care
- assess the duration of gestation
- monitor the health of the mother and the fetus
- impart comprehensive care according to national guidelines
- appreciate any deviation from normal
- manage minor ailments
- refer the pregnant mother appropriately for further care or for delivery

Introduction

Antenatal care (ANC) started as a social service for unmarried mothers in Paris at the end of the eighteenth century. It was in 1901 that a paper by Ballantyne, *A Plea for a Pro-Maternity Hospital,* secured one antenatal bed in the Edinburgh Royal Maternity Hospital. Subsequently, antenatal clinics were set up in England, Wales and Australia. Antenatal care as we know it today emerged in the 1960s. India took the first steps to strengthen maternal and child health services in the first two Five-Year Plans (1951–1956 and 1956–1961). Advances in medical sciences in general and technology in particular have made ANC medically and scientifically effective, documented by a drop both in maternal and infant mortality and morbidity.

The ANC programme is a systematic health care programme for a pregnant mother that involves a coordinated approach to medical, social and psychological management; it should ideally begin before conception and continue till delivery so that the outcome of a healthy mother and a healthy baby are achieved at the end. However, most mothers consult a health professional only when they suspect or know that they are pregnant. The recommended number of antenatal visits is 14, but it is likely to vary depending on the complications detected. It must be remembered that social and economic factors may make it difficult for the mothers to follow a 'strict' schedule of antenatal visits, and some flexibility is required without compromising on the essential care. The Ministry of Health and Family Welfare (MOHFW), Government of India in 1997 advocated at least three visits. The National Family Health Survey II (NFHS II) 1998–99, revealed that only 44% of mothers had three or more visits. There is certainly a need to improve the implementation of ANC in order to improve both maternal and perinatal outcome.

The overall goals of ANC are:

- evaluate the health status of the mother and fetus
- monitor the progress of pregnancy
- plan further obstetrical care.

These goals are best achieved through implementation of the components of ANC.

Components of Antenatal Care

The components of antenatal care are:

- preconceptional counselling
- diagnosis of pregnancy
- assessment of duration of pregnancy
- monitoring the progress of pregnancy
- advice about immunisation, drug intake, breastfeeding and contraception
- screening for infections and cervical cancer.

The information obtained from history, physical examination and investigations is noted in antenatal records systematically and should be easily accessible for decision-making later in pregnancy.

Preconceptional counselling

Preconceptional counselling is preventive medicine par excellence. A host of factors like the mother's age, parity, occupation, socioeconomic status, lifestyle, heredity, addictions, medical disorders and environment influence the outcome of pregnancy. The mother-to-be could be cautioned or educated about many factors that gain importance in pregnancy. For example, if a mother is suffering from diabetes mellitus and if it is uncontrolled, it affects her and the baby adversely; some oral hypoglycemic agents could be teratogenic. Supplementation of 400 μg of folic acid in the preconceptional period has been documented to reduce the incidence of neural tube defects in the child. Thorough history-taking, clinical examination and appropriate investigations can alert the doctor to many of these factors. Preconceptional counsellors can then help the mother modify or eliminate some of these factors by proper counselling. The best time to counsel is when a woman consults a physician for missed periods and the pregnancy test is negative.

Diagnosis of pregnancy

Pregnancy is suspected when a woman in the reproductive age group has amenorrhea. Often, associated symptoms like morning sickness may be elicited. Clinical examination will detect pregnancy with reasonable certainty. When in doubt, urine pregnancy test or ultrasound may be done (see Chapter 9).

Assessment of the period of gestation

The normal duration of pregnancy is 280 days, as calculated from the first day of the last menstmal period (LMP). It is customary to calculate the expected date of delivery (EDD) by adding seven days to the first day of the LMP and by going back three months (alternatively, going forward nine months and adding seven days). For instance, if the LMP is March 12, 2010, the EDD will be December 19, 2010. This is known as **Naegele's rule** and it presumes that the menstrual cycle is of 28 days' duration. Sometimes a woman may have longer menstrual cycles (say 40 days), in which case one needs to add 12 days to the calculated EDD. Now, if the LMP was on March 12 and the woman had cycles of 40 days, her revised EDD would be December 31. It is therefore imperative not only to ask for the date of LMP, but also to ascertain the duration of menstrual cycles, if necessary by finding out the date of the menstrual period prior to the LMP, expressed as last to last menstrual period (LLMP).

The findings of the clinical examination or ultrasonogram performed in early pregnancy are the most accurate for the assessment of the period of gestation (POG).

History

The principles of history-taking in obstetrics are the same as in other branches of medicine. The information must be gathered meticulously, with the doctor listening to what the mother has to say. Towards this objective, she should be made to relax so as to create an environment conducive to gathering the necessary information.

Background information: The pregnant mother's name and address must be noted carefully. It is important to make a note of her age, occupation, socioeconomic status, education, religion and race. The pregnant mother's economic and literacy status influence her health-seeking behaviour. Women from the lower socioeconomic strata are more likely to suffer from malnutrition and communicable diseases like tuberculosis and parasitic infections. The mother's occupation can influence her and her fetus to a variable extent. For example, occupations requiring long hours of standing can predispose her to varicose veins and preterm labour.

Obstetric index: It is customary to note the number of pregnancies the woman has had and the POG at which they ended. The term **gravida** refers to a pregnant woman and the number of times she has been pregnant earlier. For example, fifth gravida is one who had four pregnancies in the past and is pregnant for the fifth time. **Parity** refers to the number of pregnancies that ended after the period of viability (28 weeks for India and 20 weeks according to the World Health Organization). A woman who had two deliveries and an abortion, and is pregnant for the fourth time and has two live children, will be a gravida 4, para 2, abortion 1 and live 2. Multiple pregnancies beyond viability increase the parity by 1 irrespective of the number of fetuses carried in such a pregnancy. While ectopic pregnancy will add to the gravidity, it does not increase the parity.

Presenting symptoms: A careful note must be made about the presenting symptoms: some of these are specific to each trimester. In early pregnancy, the mother may present with vomiting. Later on, she is likely to consult for swelling of the feet, breathlessness or headache/giddiness; bleeding per vaginum could occur at any time. It is important to elicit information about the medication being taken and details of the ANC received so far.

Menstrual history: This should be noted very carefully, as indicated above.

Marital history: Ask about the duration of marriage and whether the marriage is consanguineous (and, if yes, the degree of consanguinity). If there has been a long gap since the time of marriage, note whether the postponement was by use of contraceptives; if not, ask if any treatment was taken for infertility and record it.

Obstetric history: This should be recorded meticulously with reference to the year of pregnancy, outcome of the pregnancy, type of health facility where she delivered, her health during pregnancy and the ANC she received. It is necessary to find out about the type of delivery, indication for intervention if delivery was not normal, complications during puerperium and the status of the child at birth and at present. Enquire gently whether intrauterine fetal death or intrapartum fetal death occurred. Similarly, enquire about abortions, the POG at which pregnancy terminated, and whether it was spontaneous or otherwise. Spontaneous abortions in the first 12–14 weeks are attributed to genetic or endocrine causes. Those occurring after 14 weeks are due to anomalies like bicornuate uterus or incompetent os. In case the pregnancy was terminated deliberately, it is necessary to find out the method of termination, medical or surgical. **Any obstetrical complication in the past can adversely influence the outcome of the current pregnancy.** Details of breastfeeding and contraceptive use should be noted.

Medical and surgical history: Information about any medical or surgical illness and the treatment used need to be noted. Diabetes, hypertension, cardiac disease, asthma or epilepsy are examples of diseases which may be affected by pregnancy or may have an effect on pregnancy.

Family history: This is taken as in any branch of medicine. However, particular attention must be paid to a history of preeclampsia/eclampsia in the mother or sister, diabetes mellitus, hypertension or any twinning/congenital anomalies.

Psychosocial history: A pregnant woman and her fetus can be affected adversely if she is suffering from psychosocial problems. Addiction to tobacco, alcohol and hard drugs is associated with fetal growth restriction and other undesirable outcome in the newborn. Domestic violence and violence against adolescent and adult women adversely affect the health of the mother and her unborn child. It has also been documented that a significant number of pregnant women are subjected to domestic violence; this aspect should be considered and specifically enquired into.

Physical examination

General and systemic examination: At the first visit, the pregnant woman must be examined thoroughly. In the general examination, make particular note of the height, weight, blood pressure, pallor, oral hygiene, varicose veins, edema of the feet and any evidence of a thyroid disorder. The respiratory, cardiovascular and skeletal systems must be examined. While examining the breasts, one must look for changes suggestive of pregnancy, cracked and retracted/flat nipples and any lumps.

Obstetrical examination: After explaining to the woman and obtaining her consent, an abdominal examination is performed to detect the presence of any scar, organomegaly, tumours, ascitis or hernia.

Obstetrical palpation: This consists of abdominal palpation and its main objectives are discussed below:

- Assess the period of gestation. The uterus can be palpated just above the symphysis pubis at 12 weeks of gestation. The distance between the symphysis pubis and the umbilicus is divided into three parts, marking 16, 20 and 24 weeks. The distance between the umbilicus and the xiphisternum is divided into three parts, marking 28, 32 and 36 weeks. At term, the fundus comes down to the level of the costal margin and there is fullness in the flanks (**Fig. 10.1**). The distance between the symphysis pubis and the fundal height, termed symphysiofundal height (SFH), measured in centimetres, corresponds approximately to the POG in weeks between 18 and 30 weeks. While measuring the SFH serially, it is best to mark this parameter on a gravidogram; if the SFH is close to or below the 50th percentile curve, the mother is suspected to have intrauterine growth restriction (IUGR). If it is close to or beyond the 90th percentile, one must think of macrosomia or multiple pregnancy (**Fig. 10.2**). In both situations, the mother is referred to a specialist for consultation.

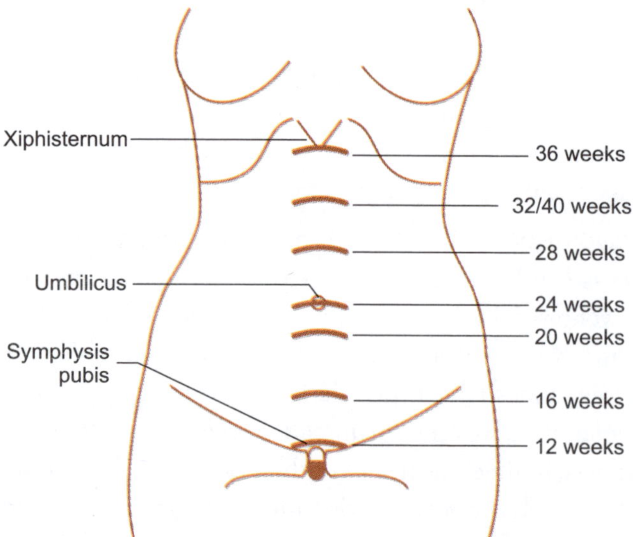

Fig. 10.1 Fundal height at different periods of gestation.

- Detect the lie of the fetus. This is the relation of the long axis of the fetus to the long axis of the mother. The lie is said to be longitudinal if both are parallel to each other.
- Ascertain the attitude. It refers to the relationship of the fetal parts to one another. The fetus is normally in a state of universal flexion.
- Detect the presentation which is the part occupying the lower pole of the uterus.
- Position. This is the relationship of a fixed point on the presenting part, known as the denominator, to fixed points on the maternal pelvis.
- Assess the level of fetal presenting part in relation to the pelvic brim. The head is said to be engaged if the biparietal diameter has crossed the pelvic brim.
- Evaluate fetal wellbeing. This is ascertained by fetal growth as noted by a progressive increase in fundal height and by listening to fetal heart sounds.

The technique of palpation is described in Chapter 23.

Speculum examination: Next, the vulva and the perineum are inspected for the presence of any lesions. A speculum lubricated with warm water is used to view the cervix and the vagina. A bluish discolouration is characteristic, but not diagnostic, of pregnancy. One must look for yellow frothy discharge suggestive of trichomonal vaginitis or curdy white discharge characteristic of candidiasis. If there is no infection, a pap smear is taken in order to identify cytological abnormalities. In India, the prevalence of cervical cancer is high and, therefore, this opportunity for screening should not be missed.

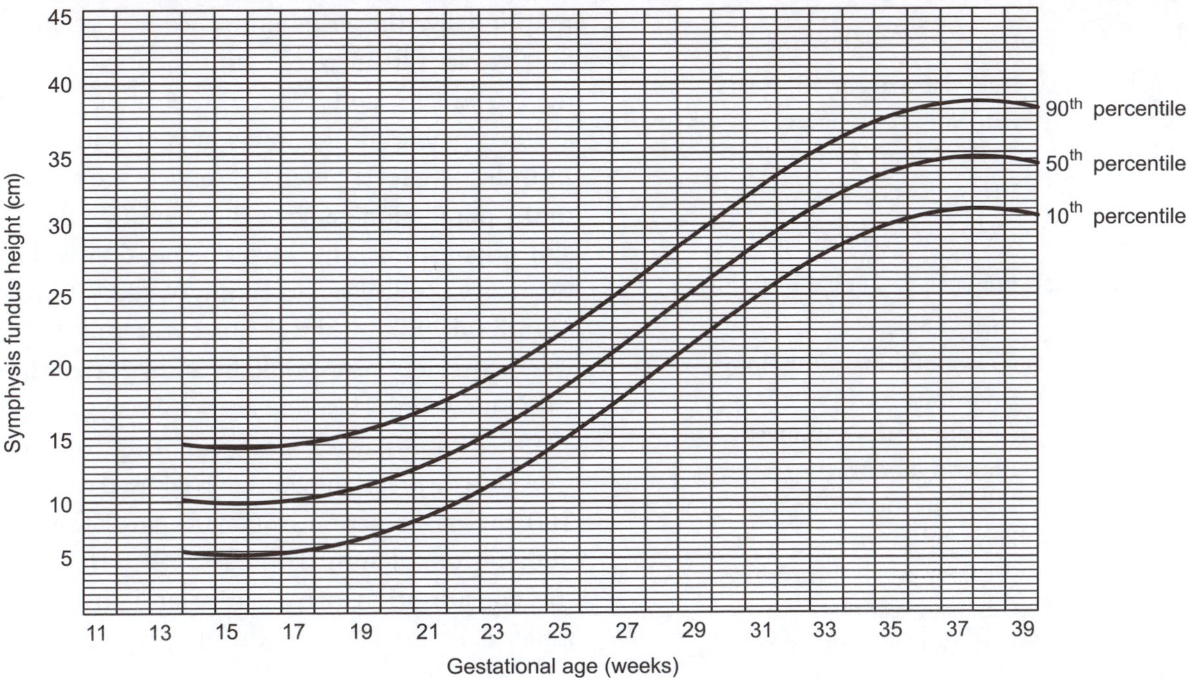

Fig. 10.2 Gravidogram: Maternal symphysis–fundus growth chart.

Bimanual examination: The speculum is removed and bimanual examination is performed, particularly to check the consistency, length and position of the cervix. One must also note the direction, consistency and size of the uterus. In early pregnancy, uterine enlargement corresponds fairly accurately with the period of gestation.

Laboratory investigations

The essential investigations are:

- hemoglobin to assess the degree of anemia
- urine for sugar and albumin
- VDRL for the detection of syphilis
- blood grouping and rhesus typing.

Even though syphilis is now uncommon, because it has a devastating effect on pregnancy and yet is easily treatable, VDRL a routine investigation. There are definite advantages in testing pregnant mothers for hepatitis B and HIV infections. The mother should be informed about the benefits of testing and counselled voluntary testing is recommended for HIV. Other laboratory tests should be requested only when complications are anticipated or detected.

Ultrasonography (USG)

A first trimester USG helps date the pregnancy accurately and to exclude conditions like ectopic pregnancy or hydatidiform mole. In the second trimester, it is less reliable for dating, but is useful for excluding malformations. Routine USG for every pregnant woman is not practical in many situations, but, where possible, may be done in the second trimester. Otherwise, USG may be used depending on the clinical need.

High-risk Pregnancies

In an attempt to improve the effectiveness of ANC, a **'risk approach'** has been adopted to try and use the resources optimally. A woman can be formally evaluated against a checklist of risk factors. Whenever these risk factors are present, they are likely to influence obstetric decision-making and the outcome of the pregnancy.

The presence of one or more of these factors must be considered as a risk to the pregnant mother and her unborn child (**Table 10.1**).

Table 10.1 Risk factors in pregnancy

1. Maternal characteristics	Age <18 years or >35 years Addiction to tobacco, alcohol, hard drugs Below poverty line
2. LMP details	LMP uncertain
3. Vaginal bleeding	Presence of vaginal bleeding
4. Obstetric history	Parity ≥5 Congenital malformation Abortions (spontaneous or induced) Preterm labour IUGR or macrosomia Perinatal death Previous cervical suture Cesarean section Hypertension/eclampsia Third-stage complications
5. Medical/ surgical history	Surgery to genital tract Diabetes mellitus, cardiac/renal disease, thromboembolism Epilepsy Heart disease Bronchial asthma Tuberculosis
6. Family history	Diabetes mellitus Hypertension, preeclampsia/ eclampsia in mother/sister Multiple pregnancy Congenital anomalies
7. Examination on first visit	Maternal weight ≥85 kg or ≤45 kg Maternal height ≤140 cm BMI <18.5 or >30 Blood pressure ≥140/90 mm Hg Detection of cardiac murmur Uterus not corresponding to POG Gynecological disorder Moderate to severe anemia

OCP = oral contraceptive pills; IUGR = intrauterine growth restriction

Follow-up visits

The subsequent visit is scheduled according to the POG and the presence of any complications. If all the parameters are within normal limits, traditionally, the visits are scheduled at intervals of four weeks till 28 weeks, and then every two weeks till 36 weeks and weekly thereafter. Fewer visits are acceptable if the pregnancy is uncomplicated. In India, wherever antenatal services are not accessible to the population (such as those residing in rural areas and urban slums), the recommendation is three visits (Ministry of Health and Family Welfare, Government of India, 1997). Ideally, the first visit must be at 12–16 weeks; the next visit should be at the end of the second trimester and the last one after 36 weeks.

Once the nausea and vomiting of pregnancy subside, the pregnant woman is advised to supplement 100 mg of elemental iron, 500 µg of folic acid and 500 mg of calcium daily. The MOHFW advocates the consumption of one iron and folic acid (IFA) tablet daily for 100 days during pregnancy.

Recommended Measures for ANC

- **At each visit**: The mother should be asked if she has any complaints like bleeding/discharge per vaginum or abdominal pain. It is important to record the weight, blood pressure, edema of the feet, urine for sugar and protein, hemoglobin (at first visit and 34 weeks), fundal height and fetal heart sounds.

  The average weight gain from the second trimester should be 300–500 g per week. An increase of less than 300 g points to conditions like IUGR and maternal malnutrition. Excessive gain of 1,000 g per week must alert the doctor to the possibility of preeclampsia, multiple pregnancy and fetal macrosomia.

  If the blood pressure is ≥140/90 mm Hg recorded on two occasions six hours apart after 20 weeks of gestation, a diagnosis of pregnancy-induced hypertension is made.

  In recent years it is recommended that all pregnant women, irrespective of their age, should be screened for trisomy. This screening includes the measurement of nuchal translucency, estimation of maternal serum hCG and pregnancy-associated placental proteins (PAPP-A), between 11 and 14 weeks of gestation.

During the second trimester, a triple test is done with maternal serum alpha fetoprotein (MSAFP), unconjugated estriol and hCG. The quadruple test includes the estimation of inhibin in addition to the above. A large number of soft markers by ultrasound examination have also been identified to detect trisomy.

- **At 18–20 weeks**: An ultrasound examination is advocated to screen for congenital anomalies. Other screening tests are done only if indicated.
- **At 24–28 weeks**: Screening for gestational diabetes.
- **After 36 weeks**: Fetal presentation is evaluated.
- The pregnant mother should be advised about nutrition and drugs (see Chapters 11 and 12).

If the mother's hemoglobin is 11 g/dl, and she is well nourished, she can take 100 mg of elemental iron, 500 µg of folic acid and 500 mg of calcium as supplement. The MOHFW advocates 100 tablets of iron and folic acid (IFA) during pregnancy.

- **Breastfeeding:** Advice should be given for the correction of retracted or flat nipples, and the benefits of breastfeeding should be explained. Early preparation of the mother for lactation helps in establishing successful breastfeeding.
- **Contraception:** A dialogue regarding contraception should be started to bring about awareness of the various methods available.
- **Immunisation against tetanus:** In India, an important cause of neonatal mortality is tetanus, as most deliveries take place at home under unhygienic conditions. According to the National Immunisation Schedule, every pregnant mother must be administered an injection of tetanus toxoid 0.5 ml intramuscularly around 20 weeks of gestation; a second dose is given 4–6 weeks later. However, the second dose must be given at least four weeks before the delivery to ensure protection to the newborn. A booster dose is recommended every five years; if two doses have been received in the previous five years, a single booster dose is recommended.
- **Monitoring the progress of pregnancy:** At each follow-up visit, measures are taken to assess the wellbeing of the mother and her fetus. Information is obtained about the mother and fetus from history and examination.

In the mother

- **Symptoms:** Headache, visual disturbance, edema not relieved by rest, abdominal pain, bleeding/watery discharge per vaginum, nausea/vomiting or dysuria
- **Weight gain:** Ideally, this should be 300–500 g per week. Note if it is inadequate or excessive.
- **Blood pressure:** Actual and extent of change
- **Height in centimetres from symphysis pubis to uterine fundus:** The serial measurements plotted on a gravidogram help detect IUGR and macrosomia.
- **Vaginal examination:** This is useful in late pregnancy (38 weeks) to confirm the presenting part and to assess the consistency, effacement and dilatation of the cervix and clinical estimation of the pelvic configuration and capacity.

In the fetus

- fetal heart rate
- fetal activity, also noted by the mother
- size, appropriate or inappropriate for the period of gestation
- amount of amniotic fluid
- presenting part.

Plan for Delivery

This is dictated by the risk factors present or by those that arise during pregnancy. The decision should be made with reference to the following points:

- the POG at which pregnancy should be terminated
- the method of termination
- the type of health facility where the delivery should take place.

Therefore, during the ANC, one needs to be vigilant and refer the pregnant mother to a carefully selected health facility. A pragmatic approach is to consider the following categories of mothers for delivery at primary health centres or at home:

- absence of medical/surgical disorders
- normal obstetric history
- age over 18 years and below 35 years
- gravidity second to fourth

- normal fetal growth
- normal fetopelvic relation (vertex presentation).

It is imperative that a skilled attendant be present at delivery. This is a guideline issued by the MOHFW and should be implemented in totality.

Advice During Pregnancy

Pregnant mothers have concerns regarding issues that they may not worry about in the nonpregnant state. These are:

Nutrition: A mother whose pregnancy is normal should be advised to eat whatever she wants in the quantity she wants. However, one must ensure that she takes enough proteins and food rich in iron and calcium (see Chapter 11).

Rest: The mother must rest for at least two hours during the day, apart from her night time sleep of at least six hours.

Clothing and footwear: She must be advised to wear loose comfortable cotton clothing. She must be advised against using footwear with high heels.

Drugs: Vitamins, analgesics and antipyretics are the most common drugs a pregnant women is likely to consume. Should there be a need to take other medication, one must select a drug that is relatively safe for the fetus (see Chapter 12).

Addictions: These must be enquired into. The most common addiction is to tobacco, either in the form of smoking, chewing or snuff. Tobacco can lead to fetal growth restriction and it is best to stop it or reduce it considerably. The pregnant mother must be advised against the use of alcohol and hard drugs as they are harmful to both the mother and her fetus in many ways.

Travel: It is best avoided in early pregnancy and close to term. A woman with a history of previous obstetric mishaps and complications in the current pregnancy, like hemorrhage or fetal growth restriction, should be advised not to travel. Air travel is safe since aircraft cabins are pressurised.

Physical activity: This is not restricted unless there is a history of spontaneous abortion or preterm delivery and complications in the present pregnancy.

Coitus: It should be avoided whenever there is a threat of abortion or preterm delivery. In healthy pregnant women, sexual intercourse is perfectly acceptable except in the last four weeks of pregnancy.

Minor Complaints During Pregnancy

Nausea and vomiting: These are common complaints during early pregnancy. Proper dietary advice and reassurance are effective, but in some cases antiemetics are necessary (see Chapter 38).

Heartburn: It is due to the reflux of gastric contents into the esophagus. The pregnant woman should be advised to take small, frequent meals and avoid lying flat immediately after a meal. Antacids are prescribed if there is no relief.

Constipation: It occurs because of high levels of progesterone, which slows down the transit time and pressure of the enlarged uterus. The pregnant woman should be advised to take plenty of fluids, fruits and vegetables and daily exercise. If necessary, mild laxatives and stool softeners may be prescribed. These measures will prevent the occurrence of anal fissures and worsening of hemorrhoids.

Pica: It refers to is the craving of pregnant women for specific kinds of food. Most of them seem to have a craving for pickles, but a few may consume an excess of starch, leading to iron deficiency anemia.

Ptyalism: It means excessive salivation among pregnant women. No definite reason has been attributed; it may be stimulated by the consumption of starch. The mother should be reassured if it is bothersome.

Backache: It is experienced by more than 50% of women during pregnancy. It is caused by relaxation of the ligaments and lordosis. A pillow to support the back, advising the woman to squat into the sitting position instead of bending the back to pick up something, will help. She must be advised regarding correct posture and proper footwear. Local heat and analgesics may be advised when the pain is not relieved by other measures. However, if backache is persistent or there is a definite tenderness at any vertebral level, the woman must be referred to an orthopedic surgeon for further management.

Headache: It is a common complaint; if it persists in spite of symptomatic treatment, other causes like refractive errors of the eye must be looked for. Later in pregnancy, headache is attributable to hypertensive disorders of pregnancy and is associated with severe preeclampsia and eclampsia.

Fatigue: It is more common in early pregnancy. The pregnant woman tends to feel sleepy; this is due to the effect of progesterone. It is often due to anemia, vomiting in early pregnancy and mechanical factors.

Varicosities of the lower limbs: These may manifest during pregnancy; they could worsen if already present. The symptoms may vary from mild to severe discomfort following long hours of standing. Treatment consists of rest, elevation of legs and elastic stockings. Surgical treatment is not advised during pregnancy.

Leukorrhea: Pregnant women often complain of white discharge. It is mainly caused by the increased secretion of mucus from the cervical and vaginal transudation due to increased levels of estrogen. It is usually not pathological and the woman needs to be reassured.

If the discharge is greenish yellow, one should suspect trichomonal vaginitis. If the discharge has a fishy odour, it is due to bacterial vaginosis. These infections must be treated with metronidazole only if the women are symptomatic. One must be very cautious in using the drug in the first trimester. White discharge could be due to candidiasis. It is useful to prescribe clotrimazole as vaginal pessaries or cream.

KEY POINTS

- Antenatal care is a comprehensive, systematic, health care programme for pregnant mothers.
- Preconception care improves both maternal and fetal outcome.
- Efforts must be made to identify obstetric, medical and psychosocial complications.
- The recommendations of Ministry of Health and Family Welfare (Government of India) are: three antenatal visits, iron and folic acid prophylaxis, administration of tetanus toxoid and measures for early detection of preeclampsia.
- Women with no risk factors, second to fourth gravida, and with normal fetopelvic relation may be selected for delivery at home or at a primary health centre.
- Women must be counselled regarding issues like nutrition and drugs, and treated for minor common complaints associated with pregnancy.

QUESTIONS

Select the single most appropriate answer:

1. The minimum number of antenatal visits recommended by the Government of India (1997) is
   a. 3 b. 5 c. 7 d. 9
2. Which of the following has the maximum influence on the health-seeking behaviour of a pregnant woman?
   a. socioeconomic status c. proximity to health facility
   b. literacy d. advice given by neighbour
3. Which of the following information in family history has no relevance to the woman's current pregnancy?
   a. hypertension c. mitral stenosis
   b. diabetes mellitus d. multiple pregnancy
4. What is the best time to ask a woman to start taking folic acid supplements to reduce the risk of neural tube defects?
   a. second half of menstrual cycle
   b. when she consults for a missed period
   c. when pregnancy is confirmed
   d. once she plans a pregnancy
5. The gravidogram is a simple tool to alert the obstetrician to all of the following *except*
   a. fetal growth restriction
   b. occipitoposterior position

c. macrosomia
d. multiple pregnancy

In the following questions there are two statements. Select the appropriate answer using the following key:

a. if both statements are true and causally related
b. if both statements are true but not causally related
c. if first statement is true and the second is false
d. if first statement is false and the second is true
e. if both statements are false

6. Information obtained regarding obstetric history is important *because*

   Information obtained regarding obstetric history determines the management of the present pregnancy.

7. During pregnancy, examination of the breasts is not necessary *because*

   During pregnancy the incidence of breast cancer is very low.

8. It is unsafe for an adolescent girl to become pregnant *because*

   An adolescent girl is not likely to suffer from anemia.

Select the appropriate answer using the following key:

a. if only responses 1, 2 and 3 are correct
b. if only 1 and 3 are correct
c. if only 2 and 4 are correct
d. if only 4 is correct
e. if all are correct

9. In pregnant women
   1. VDRL test should be done routinely
   2. syphilis is uncommon
   3. syphilis is easily treatable
   4. syphilis has no significant ill effect

10. A pregnant woman is said to be at high risk if
    1. her BMI is 21
    2. her height is 150 cm
    3. her parity is 4
    4. she is below the poverty line

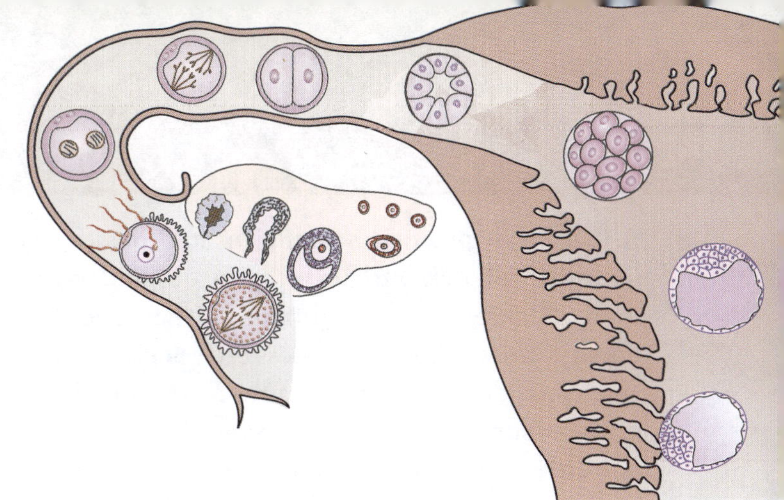

11

Nutrition in Pregnancy

Prema Ramachandran

LEARNING OBJECTIVES

At the end of this chapter, the reader should be able to:

- appreciate the need for focus on nutrition during pregnancy
- define the recommended dietary allowances (RDA) during pregnancy and lactation
- describe the dietary intake for pregnant and lactating women in India
- describe the effect of maternal nutrition on the course and outcome of pregnancy
- list the causes for the deterioration of maternal nutrition during pregnancy and lactation
- describe the interventions used to prevent, detect and combat undernutrition, micronutrient deficiencies and obesity during pregnancy and lactation
- describe how to assess each person carefully and give appropriate advice

Introduction

From time immemorial it has been recognised that the nutrition of pregnant and lactating women is immensely important. The ill-effects of maternal macro- and micronutrient deficiency affect the mother as well as the offspring. Macronutrients are those like carbohydrates, proteins and fats that the body uses in relatively large amounts, whereas micronutirents like vitamins and minerals are used in smaller amounts.

Research studies carried out in the last five decades have helped to define the nutritional requirements of both macro- and micronutrients during pregnancy and lactation. Epidemiological studies from India and other developing countries documented the magnitude and adverse consequences on the mother-child dyad of:

- chronic energy deficiency (CED)
- anemia due to iron and folate deficiency and
- iodine deficiency disorders in pregnancy.

Accordingly, during antenatal care, stress has been laid on early detection and effective intervention for minimising maternal undernutrition with reference to both macro- and micro-nutrients. While undernutrition continues to be a major problem as in the earlier decades, the 1990s have witnessed a progressive rise in obesity and diabetes mellitus among women of the reproductive age due to overnutrition.

Undernutrition and micronutrient deficiencies increase susceptibility to infections; infections aggravate nutritional deficiencies. With the advent of the HIV epidemic in India, it is inevitable that over the next decade there will be an increase in the severe undernutrition associated with HIV infection in pregnancy and the adverse impact of maternal HIV infection on the fetus. On the other hand, obesity and diabetes are also associated with some adverse pregnancy outcomes.

Currently, practising physicians and obstetricians in India will have to prevent, detect and combat undernutrition, micronutrient deficiencies and obesity. They will have to assess each person carefully and provide appropriate advice regarding diet, nutrient supplements and exercise; they have to pay due attention to infection and contraception in order to improve the health and nutritional status of the mother and her child.

Recommended Dietary Allowance

The recommended dietary allowance (RDA) is based on an assessment of nutrient requirements estimated in apparently healthy individuals. Energy requirement is defined as the amount that will balance the energy expenditure of the individual (as determined by body size and composition and level of physical activity) consistent with long-term good health. This intake will allow for the maintenance of physical activity which is economically necessary and socially desirable. Both lower and higher energy intakes are associated with health hazards. For all other nutrients, the RDA is based on mean +2SD value of a group of persons, because with this allowance, over 97% of the persons in the group would obtain their requirements. If they consume a balanced diet, all the nutrient requirements will be met if the energy needs are met.

RDA in pregnancy

The ideal situation is for a woman to enter pregnancy with normal weight and good nutritional status. The dietary intake during pregnancy must provide the energy that will ensure the delivery of a full-term healthy baby with appropriate body composition. Good nutritional intake will also be consistent with long-term good health and wellbeing as well as sufficient energy stores required during lactation and beyond.

The energy requirement for pregnancy in well-nourished women was calculated based on the following assumptions:

- The gestational weight gain of 12 kg is associated with the optimal outcome of pregnancy;
- During pregnancy, extra energy is needed for:
  i. growth of the fetus, placenta and various maternal tissues such as the uterus, breast and fat stores
  ii. changes in maternal metabolism and
  iiii. increase in physical effort at rest and during physical activity.

The total energy requirement during pregnancy is not equally distributed throughout pregnancy; additional daily energy requirement in the first, second and third trimesters were computed to be 85, 285 and 475 kcal, respectively.

RDA in lactation

The energy cost of lactation has two components: the energy content of the milk secreted and the energy required for producing milk. Well-nourished women can derive part of this additional requirement from body fat stores accumulated during pregnancy. Well-nourished women should have an additional 550 kcal per day and those with insufficient gestational weight gain, an additional 675 kcal/day during the first six months of lactation.

RDA for Indians

An expert committee constituted in 1988 by the Indian Council for Medical Research (ICMR) recommended an additional intake of 300 kcal during the second and third trimesters of pregnancy, 550 kcal during the first six months of lactation and 400 kcal during 7–12 months of lactation. The recommendations for a woman weighing 50 kg who does moderate work are given in **Table 11.1**.

Nutritional Status and Outcome of Pregnancy in India

Maternal weight (prepregnancy weight plus weight gain) is the most significant predictor of low birth weight (LBW) and intrauterine growth restriction (IUGR). The relation of maternal BMI and prevalence of LBW is shown in **Fig. 11.1**. Low prepregnancy weight and BMI, and poor weight gain between 20 and 28 weeks of gestation were moderate predictors

Table 11.1 Recommended dietary allowances

Status	Energy kcal/day	Protein g/day	Fat g/day	Calcium mg/day	Iron mg/day	Vit. A µg/day	Vit. C mg/day	Folic acid µg/day	Vit. B_{12} µg/day
Nonpregnant	2200	50	20	400	30	600	40	100	1
Pregnant	2500	100	30	1000	38	600	40	400	1
Lactating	2750	75	45	1000	30	950	80	150	1.5

of preterm delivery, and low maternal height (for example 146 cm compared with 160 cm) was a moderate predictor of cesarean delivery. Women with short stature, especially in developing countries with inadequate health care systems and high prevalence of impaired growth during childhood, are also at high risk of LBW. These women are also prone to preterm delivery and a number of obstetric complications during labour and puerperium.

Course and outcome of pregnancy in well-nourished women

Epidemiological data from India show that well-nourished women may be subsisting on a wide range (1,500 and 2,500 kcal/day) of dietary intakes. There is no increase in dietary intake during pregnancy in women who 'eat to appetite'. This practice was not associated with any adverse effect on pregnancy outcome, like birth weight or maternal nutritional status during pregnancy. Increasing parity had no detrimental effect on the nutritional status provided the inter-pregnancy interval was more than two years. Other studies suggested that increased dietary intake during pregnancy and lactation might, in fact, lead to obesity in pregnant women.

Women from the upper income group consume 2,000 and 2,500 kcal per day during pregnancy. In this group, pregnant women do not perform hard physical labour; in fact their routine work activity is reduced during pregnancy. Their prepregnancy weight is 45–55 kg and the mean pregnancy weight gain is about 11 kg. The mean birth weight of infants is 3.1 kg.

Table 11.2 compares the birth weight in relation to various factors among women from different socioeconomic strata.

Course and outcome of pregnancy in undernourished urban women

The dietary intake of the urban low-income group varies between 1200 and 1800 kcal during pregnancy. Pregnant women continue to do their household and other activities, and remain moderately active throughout pregnancy. Some women may be engaged in heavy physical work. The women in the lower socioeconomic group weigh on an average 44 kg prior to pregnancy and gain 6 kg during pregnancy. The mean birth weight of infants is 2.7 kg. There is no obvious deterioration in the maternal nutritional status during pregnancy or following repeated pregnancies provided the inter-birth interval is longer than two years.

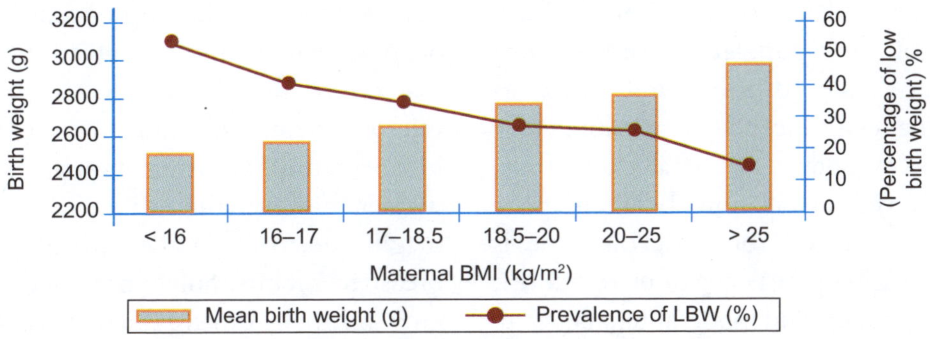

Fig. 11.1 Birth weight in relation to maternal BMI. ***Source:*** Tenth Five-year Plan, GOI 2002.

Table 11.2 Birth weight and socioeconomic status

Income level	Poor	Middle	High
Age (years)	24.1	24.3	27.8
Parity	2.41	1.96	1.61
Height (cm)	151.5	154.2	156.3
Weight (kg)	45.7	49.9	56.2
Weight gain (kg)	6	8	11
Hb (g/dl)	10.9	11.1	12.4
Birth weight (kg)	2.70	2.90	3.13

Source: Prema Ramachandran. 1989. Nutrition in pregnancy. In C Gopalan and S Kaur (eds), *Women and Nutrition in India*. Special Publication No. 5. Nutrition Foundation of India, New Delhi.

Course and outcome of pregnancy in undernourished rural women

In rural India, the dietary intake of women from the low income group is essentially similar to that of urban women. However, rural women spend more energy in daily household chores. These women gain about 5 kg during pregnancy and the mean birth weight of their infants is 2.7 kg. There is no significant deterioration in the maternal nutritional status during pregnancy and after repeated pregnancies, provided the inter-birth interval is longer than two years.

Maternal undernutrition and outcome of pregnancy

It has been computed that fetal wastage—abortion, intrauterine death and stillbirth—occurs in about 20% of conceptions in the poorer segments of the population. Perinatal mortality varies between 50 and 70 per thousand live births. Women from these segments of the population suffer from several pregnancy-associated problems such as anemia and pregnancy-induced hypertension. Very few of them seek or obtain antenatal care. Thus, part of the observed association between poor maternal nutrition and poor obstetric outcome is attributable to the higher prevalence of maternal risk factors during pregnancy and poor antenatal care. Combining adequate antenatal care with effective food supplementation programmes is likely to result in a substantial improvement in the outcome of pregnancy in undernourished communities.

Dietary Intake and Nutritional Status of Lactating Women

The importance of breastfeeding in infant nutrition and survival has long been recognised. The recognition that lactation may have a profound effect on maternal nutrition and fertility is of more recent origin. Maternal nutrition may affect lactation and lactation may have some effect on maternal nutrition and return to fertility. Conception during lactation or the use of contraceptives may have an effect on lactation and maternal nutritional status.

Effect of lactation on maternal nutrition

Successful prolonged breastfeeding for 18–24 months is the traditional practice among the poorer segments of the population in India. The recognition of the importance of breastfeeding in infant survival, growth and nutrition in this population has resulted in sustained efforts to protect and strengthen the existing practice. Lactation involves considerable nutrient expenditure for the mother; the estimated calorie expenditure is 400–700 kcal/day.

Effect of maternal nutrition on lactation

Available data from India shows that mild and moderate maternal undernutrition does not have any adverse effect on the duration of lactation, quantity of milk secreted and composition of milk regarding macronutrients. In undernourished women with micronutrient deficiency, the micronutrient content in breast milk is lower than that of well-nourished women; however, these differences are not of sufficient magnitude to affect the nutritional status of solely breastfed infants. Solely breastfed infants thrive and grow normally during the first six months of life and have lower morbidity rates than infants who receive milk other than breast milk.

Factors Associated with Deterioration in Maternal Nutritional Status

Studies carried out in India during the 1980s have defined some of the situations where, inspite of preventive measures, the nutritional status of women deteriorates during pregnancy and lactation. These situations include:

- drought—when there is a further reduction in the dietary intake below the habitual level
- food-for-work programmes—increase in physical activity above the habitual level
- drought relief through food-for-work programme —where physical activity increases markedly
- pregnancy in an adolescent girl
- pregnancy in lactating women
- pregnancy within two years of the last delivery
- infections during pregnancy.

Health care includes efforts to prevent, detect and manage all these situations. Adequate food supplementation is the key to preventing deterioration in nutritional status.

The Integrated Child Development Services (ICDS) programme envisaged that pregnant and lactating women should receive food supplements containing 500 kcal and 20 g of protein. Available data from the Department of Women and Child Development showed that:

- coverage was low (<15%).
- quality and quantity of food was variable.
- continuous access throughout pregnancy was rare.
- food often acted as a substitute and not as an addition to home food.

The Tenth Five-year Plan recommended that all pregnant women should be weighed and those who are undernourished (<40kg) should get targeted food supplements and good antenatal care.

Obesity: The emerging problem

Over the last three decades, there have been substantial changes in socioeconomic status among some segments of the population. This has led to some increase in the dietary intake of men and women, especially from the rural and urban affluent segments. Ready availability and easy access to energy-rich fast foods like ice creams at affordable prices have resulted in increased energy consumption. Improved access to piped water supply, cooking gas and labour-saving appliances has resulted in a substantial reduction in energy expenditure in women. Data from the National Family Health Survey-3 (2005–2006) indicates that though undernutrition continues be a major problem among women, overnutrition is emerging as a public health problem (**Fig. 11.2**).

In the current decade it is, therefore, essential that those dealing with pregnant and lactating women who are well nourished, modify their advice regarding diet during pregnancy and lactation suitably. A careful watch should be kept for undue weight gain and appropriate corrective steps initiated, if not during pregnancy at least during the lactation period, so that these women do not become overweight and incur subsequent long-term health hazards.

Micronutrient Deficiencies

Anemia in pregnancy

India has the dubious distinction of being one of the countries with the highest prevalence of anemia in the general population and in pregnant women (**Fig. 11.3**). This is mainly due to low dietary intake, poor bioavailability of iron from the Indian diet and poor intake of folic acid. Anemia antedates pregnancy, becomes aggravated during pregnancy and gets perpetuated by blood loss during labour. Anemia continues to be responsible for the majority of perinatal and maternal morbidity and mortality.

Realising the magnitude of the problem, obstetricians made screening and effective management of anemia an essential component of antenatal care. In 1972, the National Anemia Prophylaxis Programme for distributing iron and folic acid was started to reduce the prevalence of anemia during pregnancy. In the Tenth Five-year Plan, the following goals were set to reduce anemia:

- universal screening of pregnant women for anemia and appropriate treatment

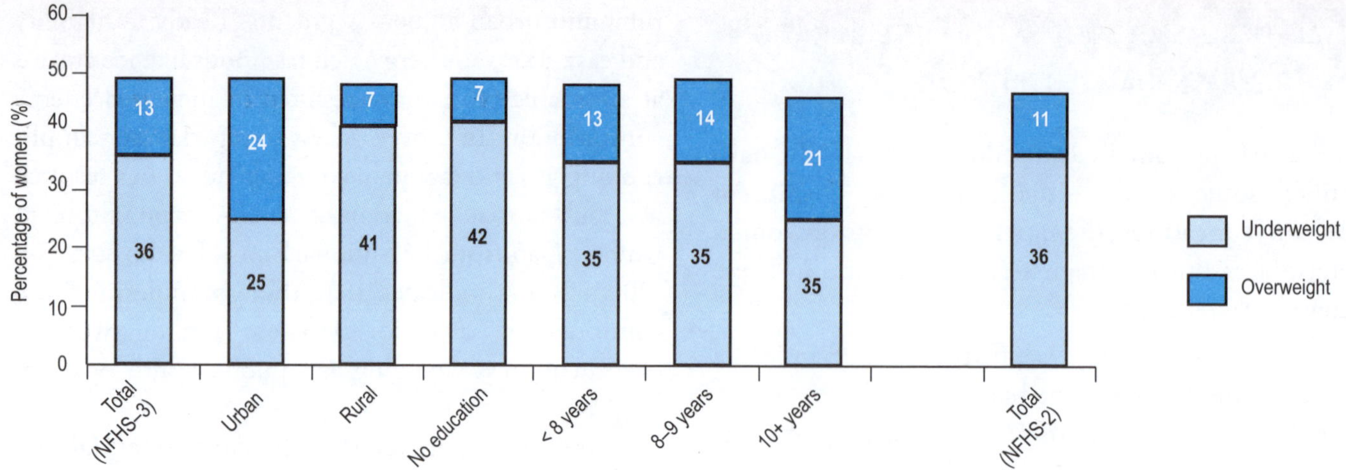

Fig. 11.2 Malnutrition in women by residence and education. *Source:* NFHS–3, 2006.

- reducing the prevalence of anemia by 25% in pregnant and lactating women
- reducing moderate and severe anemia by 50%.

In spite of several programmes being in place for the control of anemia, 56% of married women and 59% of pregnant women continue to be anemic, as noted by the NFHS-3 (2005–2006).

Vitamin A deficiency in pregnancy and lactation

It has been estimated that 1%–5% of all pregnant women show symptoms and signs of vitamin A deficiency. Subclinical deficiency may be more widespread but remains undetected. Unlike anemia, vitamin A deficiency in pregnancy is not associated with any major health problem or adverse obstetric outcome. With improved antenatal coverage, it will be possible for women with this deficiency to be identified by the ANM and 10,000 IU of vitamin A administered daily for the next four weeks.

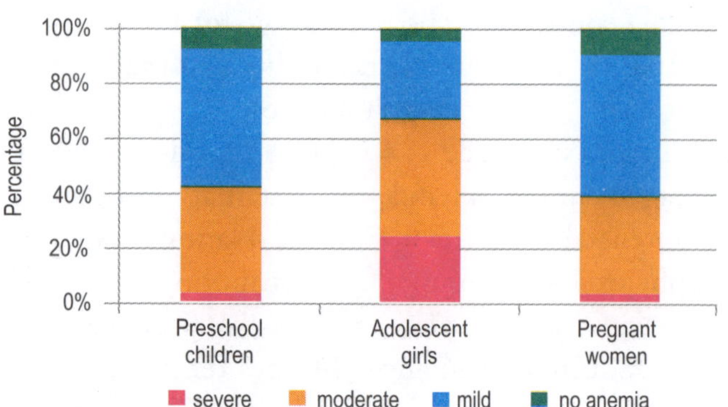

Fig. 11.3 Prevalence of anemia. *Source:* DLHS 2004

Vitamin B complex deficiency

Biochemical evidence of vitamin B complex deficiency is fairly widespread among pregnant women from the poorer segments of the population. Prevalence of clinical signs of B complex deficiency such as glossitis and angular stomatitis are higher in pregnant women. They respond readily to therapy. So far there is no clear-cut evidence of adverse consequences associated with vitamin B complex deficiency during pregnancy. Efforts to promote the cultivation and consumption of micronutrient-rich vegetables are the most appropriate strategy for improving vitamin B status during pregnancy. Women with clinical lesions require treatment with B complex vitamins.

Iodine deficiency disorders (IDD)

Iodine deficiency disorder is due to deficiency of iodine in water, soil and food and affects all socioeconomic groups living in defined geographic areas. An estimated 167 million people are at risk of IDD in India, of which 54 million have goitre and over 8 million have neurological handicaps. Goitre is the most well-recognised visible manifestation of iodine deficiency. However, the most damaging effect of the deficiency is on the unborn fetus. The association between maternal IDD and higher abortion rate, higher stillbirth, cretinism and infant mortality rate has been documented.

Vitamin D deficiency in pregnancy

In the first decades of the last century, osteomalacia due to vitamin D deficiency was reported in pregnant women who did not have adequate exposure to sunlight. With changes in lifestyle, subsequent studies showed that it was no longer a major public health problem. However, recent studies have shown that there is biochemical evidence of vitamin D deficiency, especially in winter, in women from the middle and upper income groups whose lifestyle reduces their exposure to sunlight.

KEY POINTS

- Chronic energy deficiency (CED) and micronutrient deficiencies precede pregnancy.
- Major factors responsible for undernutrition during pregnancy and lactation are low dietary intake, heavy manual work and, too early and too frequent pregnancies.
- Adverse effects of CED and micronutrient deficiencies on the mother–child dyad are partly due to deficiencies and partly due to poor antenatal care.
- Iron deficiency anemia during pregnancy is of great concern, and therefore a programme to detect and treat it forms an important component of antenatal care.
- Nutrition and health education for prevention of these deficiencies and early detection and appropriate management among adolescent girls is of paramount importance.
- Appropriate interventions are required to detect and correct not only undernutrition, but also obesity, likely to be encountered among women of the middle-to-high income groups.
- Infection–nutrition interaction can adversely influence maternal and fetal health.

QUESTIONS

Select the single most appropriate answer:

1. Which is the most common clinical manifestation of undernutrition during pregnancy?
   a. infection
   b. anemia
   c. BMI <18.5
   d. Low birth weight babies
2. For a pregnant woman, the daily caloric requirements according to the recommended dietary allowances is
   a. 2,100 kcal
   b. 2,300 kcal
   c. 2,500 kcal
   d. 2,700 kcal
3. Regarding nutrition in women, which of the following statements is true?
   a. obesity is increasing.
   b. there is a decline in undernutrition.
   c. on an average, 20% of pregnant women are anemic.
   d. moderate undernutrition affects lactation adversely.
4. The recommended dietary allowance of calcium for a pregnant woman is
   a. 400 mg/day
   b. 600 mg/day
   c. 800 mg/day
   d. 1,000 mg/day
5. What is the recommended dietary allowance of folic acid for a nonpregnant woman?
   a. 100 µg/day
   b. 200 µg/day
   c. 300 µg/day
   d. 400 µg/day

In the following questions, there are two statements. Select the appropriate answer using the following key:

a. if both statements are true and causally related
b. if both statements are true but not causally related
c. if the first statement is true and the second is false
d. if the first statement is false and the second is true
e. if both statements are false

6. Increasing parity has an adverse nutritional effect on pregnant women *because*

   Increasing parity is associated with women who are already malnourished.
7. Women of a lower socioeconomic status gain 11 kg during pregnancy *because*

   Women of a lower socioeconomic status perform hard labour.
8. Vitamin A deficiency is not associated with adverse obstetric outcome *because*

   Symptoms due to Vitamin A deficiency are noted in 1%–5% of women.

Select the appropriate answer using the following key:

a. if only responses 1, 2 and 3 are correct
b. if only 1 and 3 are correct
c. if only 2 and 4 are correct
d. if only 4 is correct
e. if all are correct

9. The nutritional status of women may continue to deteriorate despite preventive measures in which of the following situations?
   1. adolescent pregnant girls
   2. pregnancy during lactation
   3. infections during pregnancy
   4. in drought conditions
10. Obesity among pregnant women may be attributed to
    1. decrease in physical activity
    2. alteration in preference for certain foods
    3. overweight status in the nonpregnant state
    4. increased requirement of calories

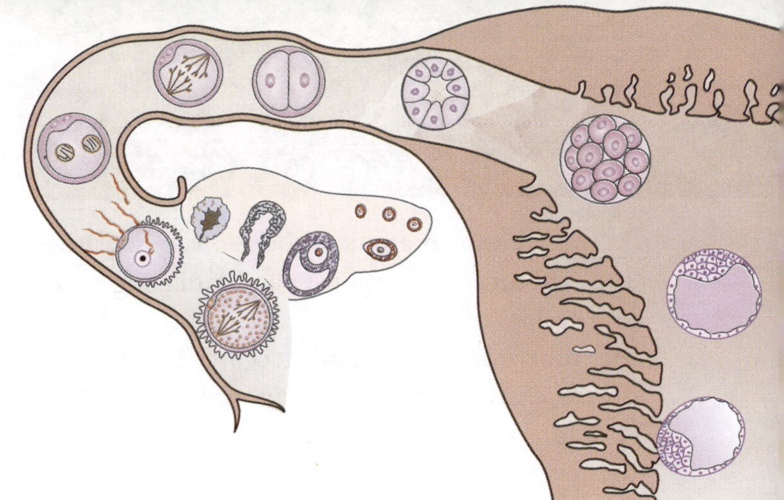

12

Drugs in Pregnancy

CH Shashindran

LEARNING OBJECTIVES

At the end of this chapter, the reader should be able to:

- appreciate the need for caution while deciding on administering drugs during pregnancy or lactation
- list the pharmacokinetic principles governing the passage of drugs across the placenta
- enumerate the pharmacokinetic parameters that govern the passage of drugs into breast milk
- categorise drugs according to the FDA categorisation and based on the latest available evidence
- assess the risk–benefit ratio to the mother and the fetus/child and prescribe medications only if essential
- list some drugs which can be prescribed and those that should be avoided during pregnancy and lactation

Introduction

During pregnancy and lactation, caution has to be exercised while using drugs for therapy, since drugs administered to the mother can have effects on the fetus too. While there should be no hesitation to use drugs to save the pregnant woman's life, it may be necessary to choose different drugs during pregnancy or defer treatment with drugs for low-risk conditions and wait for a more appropriate period of pregnancy.

While deciding to administer drugs during pregnancy and lactation, the physician has to take into account several factors. The first and foremost is to decide whether the medication is essential—only if it is essential should medication be considered. Once the decision to administer a drug is taken, one has to consider two very important factors:

- Do the benefits justify the risks, both to the mother and the developing fetus or the breastfed neonate?
- The molecule which offers the maximum benefits with the least risks should be selected.

Placental transfer of drugs

Some drugs can harm the developing fetus. Some drugs administered just before delivery can produce an untoward effect in the neonate. Several factors influence the transfer and its extent. These include:

- lipid solubility
- extent of ionisation
- plasma protein binding
- molecular weight: water-soluble molecules, above molecular weight 600, traverse the placenta only sparingly, if at all.

The placenta has P-glycoprotein-gated channels which efflux many drugs, thereby reducing fetal exposure. However, it is important to remember that any molecule that gets into the maternal bloodstream and stays there long enough has a chance of reaching the fetus, though in very small amounts.

Drug effect and period of gestation

For any molecule to affect the structure and function of the developing fetus, exposure should occur at critical periods during gestation. These periods are:

- from fertilisation to implantation, termed the **preimplantation period**
- from the third week to the eighth week, termed the **embryonic period**
- from nine weeks to term, termed the **fetal period.**

The preimplantation period is a very sensitive one and exposure of the zygote to any damaging factor can lead to loss of the zygote. Exposure in weeks 3 to 8, the embryonic period, can affect organogenesis. Insult during critical periods of organogenesis can affect the structure and function of the organ. Exposure during the fetal period can affect the maturation of various organs. It can also affect the functional development of various systems.

Drugs for use in Pregnancy

Based on data from human and animal studies, the Food and Drug Administration (FDA) has categorised drugs in terms of maternal and fetal benefits and risks (**Table 12.1**). However, caution has to be exercised as many of these recommendations are based on case reports or limited animal studies, thus restricting the reliability of such evidence.

Table 12.1 FDA categories for drugs and medications in pregnant women

Category A Controlled studies in humans have demonstrated no fetal risks. There are a few category A drugs, such as multivitamins or prenatal vitamins, but not 'megavitamins'.
Category B Animal studies indicate no fetal risks, but there are no human studies; or adverse effects have been demonstrated in animals, but not in well-controlled human studies. Several classes of commonly used drugs, for example, penicillins belong to this category.
Category C There are not enough studies, either animal or human; or there are adverse fetal effects in animal studies but no available human data. Many drugs or medications commonly taken during pregnancy are in this category.
Category D There is evidence of fetal risk, but benefits are thought to outweigh these risks. Carbamazepine and phenytoin are examples.
Category X Proven fetal risks clearly outweigh any benefits. An example is the acne medication isotretinoin, which may cause multiple central nervous system, facial and cardiovascular anomalies.

Analgesics and antiinflammatory agents

Aspirin, paracetamol and ibuprofen are frequently used drugs. Aspirin may cause oligohydramnios, premature closure of ductus arteriosus and cardiac and pulmonary abnormalities; other NSAIDs too may have similar effects. Paracetamol is safe for use.

Antiemetics

No obvious teratogenic effects have been demonstrated with the use of doxylamine, pyridoxine, meclizine, cyclizine, phenothiazines and metoclopramide. Ondansetron is best avoided in early pregnancy.

Antimicrobials

Tetracycline exposure can lead to maldevelopment and staining of teeth and reversible retardation of fetal bone growth. Aminoglycosides are best avoided because of the possibility of ototoxicity in the fetus. Sulphonamides taken late in pregnancy can produce hemolysis and kernicterus in the infant. In those with glucose-6-phosphate dehydrogenase deficiency, these can precipitate hemolytic anemia. Quinolones have been found to produce irreversible arthropathy in animals and are best avoided.

The penicillin group of drugs, macrolides and cephalosporins are safe for use during pregnancy and lactation.

Anticonvulsants

There are a number of medications and substances strongly suspected of being teratogenic to humans. These include anticonvulsants such as carbamazepine, phenytoin, trimethadione and valproic acid. The mechanism is thought to be the generation of oxidative stress in fetal tissues. Frequent malformations with phenytoin include cleft lip and congenital abnormalities of the heart. Fetal exposure to valproic acid in the first trimester is associated with the development of spina bifida.

Antihypertensives

Angiotensin converting enzyme inhibitors (ACE inhibitors) have been associated with various fetal abnormalities such as renal tubular dysgenesis, pulmonary hypoplasia, hypocalvaris and growth restriction. Prolonged fetal hypotension, hypoperfusion and renal ischemia result in oligohydramnios. In many instances, these lead to fetal death.

Alpha methyl dopa, beta blockers and calcium channel blockers belong to category C, but are used for the effective control of pregnancy-induced hypertension.

Antidiabetics

Oral hypoglycemic drugs are not advised during pregnancy. Metformin has not been found to be associated with any risk, but these drugs may have an unpredictable effect and the safety of some of the newer drugs like thiazolidinediones is yet to be established. Insulin is considered best for the treatment of diabetes in pregnancy.

Diuretics

Diuretics are sometimes needed during pregnancy. Thiazides given in late pregnancy can cause neonatal thrombocytopenia and electrolyte imbalance.

Antiasthmatics

Most medications like terbutaline and aminophylline can be safely prescribed during pregnancy. There is insufficient evidence regarding the safety of chromoglycate. The use of steroids produces cleft lip and palate.

Anticoagulants

Coumarin exposure can produce fetal abnormalities during two stages of development. Exposure between weeks 6 and 9 results in embryopathy, characterised by nasal hypoplasia and stippling of the femoral and vertebral epiphyses. These are thought to be due to the effect of coumarins on proteins called osteocalcins which control calcification during the embryonic period. Exposure during the second and third trimesters leads to central nervous system abnormalities and abnormalities in the development of the eyes.

Retinoids

There are some unconfirmed reports that high doses of vitamin A can be teratogenic. Therefore, it is recommended that the intake of vitamin A during pregnancy should not exceed the recommended daily intake.

Isotretinoin: This isomer of vitamin A has the property of stimulating epithelial cell differentiation. It is used to treat cystic acne. Isotretinoin is one of the most powerful tetratogens if the exposure happens in the first trimester. Abnormalities involving the face, heart, thymus, cranium and central nervous system have been reported. Women in the reproductive age group taking isotretinoin should be protected against pregnancy by reliable means.

Etretinate: This isomer is recommended for use in psoriasis. Traces of this drug can be detected in the body for up to one year after discontinuation. Etretinate can produce abnormalities similar to those produced by isotretinoin. Its use in women in the reproductive age group should be avoided.

Hormones

Androgens, anabolic steroids and androgenic progestins: Exposure to these hormones or drugs between weeks 7 and 12 can lead to masculinisation of the female fetus or the development of ambiguous external genitalia. Exposure to androgens for prolonged periods during fetal life can lead to a more masculine orientation and aggressiveness.

Estrogens: Unlike androgens, most estrogens do not affect fetal development. However, diethylstilbestrol is an exception. Vaginal and cervical clear cell carcinoma may develop in a small number of women who were exposed during fetal life. When ingested early during pregnancy, it can affect normal development of the vagina, uterus and fallopian tubes. A male fetus exposed to estrogen may have a penis of reduced size and testicular hypoplasia.

Alcohol: Ethyl alcohol is a powerful teratogen and fetal exposure can lead to a number of abnormalities.

These include craniofacial maldevelopment, behavioural abnormalities, growth retardation, and cardiac and spinal defects.

Anticancer drugs

By general perception, these agents are believed to be teratogens and carcinogens; however, in practice they are rarely so.

Cyclophosphamide: When given during early pregnancy, this agent can cause the defective development of limbs and deformities of the hands and feet. Cleft palate has been reported. It is best to avoid alkylating agents during the first trimester.

Aminopterin and methotrexate: These agents interfere with folic acid metabolism. Fetal effects include defects in cranial bone development and facial deformities.

Thalidomide

This drug, which was withdrawn in the 1960s, has again been made available for the treatment of lepra reaction and some connective tissue disorders. This is a very powerful teratogen and its use in women in the reproductive age group should be avoided unless the woman is using reliable contraceptive measures.

Medication in Lactating Women

Most of the drugs present in plasma appear to be excreted in breast milk. However, the quantity excreted is too small to affect maternal drug levels. Some of these drugs can affect the suckling infant, and the child needs to be observed for the appearance of untoward effects. Some drugs have inherent toxicity; when taking these, mothers should avoid breastfeeding. In general, these include cytotoxic drugs, radiopharmaceuticals, immunosuppressants and retinoids. Moreover, drugs affecting lactation such as ergotamine, bromocriptine, androgens and estrogens should be avoided in the interests of the suckling infant.

Whenever a drug is prescribed to a lactating woman, the first question that comes to the prescriber's mind is whether it is excreted in breast milk. Understanding the pharmacokinetics of drugs and their relationship with breast milk can help physicians assess the risk. Note that drug metabolising and eliminating mechanisms are not fully developed in the newborn. This is especially so in premature infants, which makes them vulnerable to adverse effects.

Passage of drugs into breast milk

Most drugs pass from plasma to breast milk by passive diffusion. This diffusion is affected by the characteristics of the milk such as water, lipid and protein content and the pH. The properties of the drug such as protein binding, lipid solubility and pKa also determine the extent of plasma-to-milk transfer. Milk contains less protein and more lipids as compared to plasma. It is also a little more acidic. Hence, weakly basic drugs with strong lipophility tend to pass into breast milk.

It is arbitrarily believed that an infant dose equivalent to 10% or less of the maternal dose (on an mg/kg basis) is safe for most drugs. However, this figure has to be scaled down in the case of drugs which have inherent toxic potential, and substances used socially such as caffeine, nicotine and alcohol, whose dose range varies widely. It can be concluded that the science of predicting the safe dose for the suckling infant is, at best, inexact: it is best to search databases for specific evidence-based information. The package inserts of most of the drugs are unhelpful because of the manufacturers' fear of litigation.

The safety of some commonly prescribed drug groups in lactation is described below.

Anticonvulsants: Sodium valproate, clonazepam, phenytoin and carbamazepine are believed to be safe during lactation. However, the infant has to be monitored closely for signs and symptoms of sedation. Phenobarbitone and primidone are best avoided. Newer drugs such as lamotrigine and vigabatrin are also best avoided till enough evidence is available about their safety during lactation.

Antiinflammatory and analgesic agents: Paracetamol, ibuprofen, indomethacin, naproxen and codeine can be used safely. Aspirin is best avoided.

Antidepressants: Mothers suffering from postnatal depression may need to take antidepressants during lactation. Tricyclic antidepressants can be used with caution. The child will have to be monitored for sedation and anticholinergic side effects. Doxepin is best avoided. Selective serotonin reuptake inhibitors may be considered safe. However, more evidence is needed regarding their use.

Anticoagulants: Heparin is listed as safe. Warfarin excretion in breast milk is minimal, if at all, and is considered safe. Phenindione is contraindicated because of concerns about bleeding in the infant.

Antiinfective agents: Penicillins and cephalosporins are generally considered safe. However, all antimicrobials have the potential to alter bowel flora in the infant. This is especially so with broad-spectrum ones like third-generation cephalosporins. Macrolide antibiotics including roxithromycin are considered safe. Tetracyclines should be avoided because of the risk of staining teeth and of fetal bone growth inhibition. Sulphonamides are best avoided in infants with hyperbilirubinemia and in those with glucose-6-phosphate dehydrogenase deficiency. Quinolones should not be used because of the risk of damage to the developing cartilage. Metronidazole in usual doses is considered safe; breastfeeding is avoided when using high doses. Moreover, metronidazole renders a bitter taste to milk and babies may be reluctant to suckle. Milk may have to be expressed before breastfeeding so that the bitterness may be reduced. Anthelmintics such as mebendazole, praziquantel and pyrantel are considered safe. Acyclovir is considered safe.

Antihistamines: Chlorpheniramine and diphenhydramine which have been in use for many years are considered safe. However, the infants should be observed for restlessness and excessive irritability. The same applies for cough and cold remedies which contain antihistaminics with phenylpropanolamine. For want of evidence, newer non-sedating antihistaminics are best avoided.

In conclusion, it may be said that any drug present in the plasma of the mother has the potential to appear in the milk. In most cases it is present in very small quantities and may not affect the suckling infant. However, it is important for the prescribing physician to consider the possibility and effects of infant exposure and choose a drug which exposes the infant to minimal risk.

KEY POINTS

- Caution should be exercised while prescribing drugs during pregnancy and lactation.
- Drugs can cross the placenta and affect the fetus.
- The gestation period of pregnancy has a bearing on the drug effect.
- The benefit of the drug should be weighed against the risk before prescribing.
- Plasma level, lipid solubility, molecular weight, ionising extent and protein binding capacity of the drug will determine the placental transfer.
- Drugs are secreted in breast milk by passive diffusion.
- The concentration of drugs in breast milk is generally low.
- If the mother's need for a drug is paramount, the drug should be given to her.

QUESTIONS

Select the single most appropriate answer:

1. The anticonvulsant that is best avoided by breastfeeding mothers is
   a. phenobarbitone   c. sodium valproate
   b. phenytoin   d. carbamazepine
2. Breastfeeding should be avoided by the mother while she is taking
   a. heparin   c. warfarin
   b. phenindione   d. dicoumarol
3. All of the following drugs are contraindicated during lactation *except*
   a. ibuprofen   c. isotretinoin
   b. amiodarone   d. ergotamine
4. Drugs that tend to concentrate in breast milk are
   a. highly protein bound   c. weak bases
   b. of low lipid solubility   d. weak acids
5. The analgesic considered unsafe during lactation is
   a. codeine   c. methadone
   b. ibuprofen   d. aspirin
6. Phocomelia is a characteristic deformity produced due to prenatal exposure to
   a. methotrexate   c. tritretinoin
   b. thalidomide   d. cyclophosphamide
7. The antihypertensive agent contraindicated during pregnancy is
   a. methyldopa   c. captopril
   b. nifedipine   d. hydralazine
8. The drug of choice for the management of gestational diabetes mellitus is
   a. troglitazone   c. glipizide
   b. metformin   d. insulin
9. The antimicrobial contraindicated during pregnancy is
   a. cefaclor   c. ciprofloxacin
   b. erythromycin   d. ceftriaxone
10. For a pregnant woman allergic to beta lactam antibiotics, the drug of choice for the treatment of gonorrhea is
    a. ofloxacin   c. ceftriaxone
    b. doxycycline   d. spectinomycin

13

Imaging in Obstetrics

S Soundara Raghavan

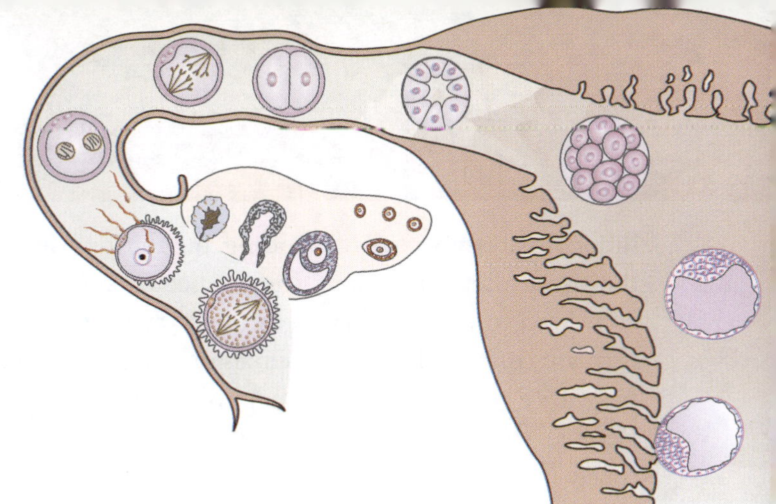

LEARNING OBJECTIVES

At the end of this chapter, the reader should be able to:

- describe the basic principles of how ultrasonography (USG) works
- appreciate the various applications of ultrasound in obstetric practice
- enumerate the conditions in early pregnancy where USG will be useful
- list the measurements that help in obstetric management
- explain how USG is used to date pregnancy
- appreciate the uses of USG in screening for malformations
- understand the principles of growth monitoring
- appreciate how USG helps in the assessment of fetal wellbeing
- understand the role of Doppler in obstetrics
- understand the role of computerised tomography (CT) scan and magnetic resonance imaging (MRI)
- understand the basics of interventional ultrasound

Introduction

Ultrasonography (USG) is one of the major discoveries that has revolutionised obstetric practice. Prior to this, radiography was used, and it had the obvious limitation of maternal and fetal exposure to radiation. Real-time imaging did not exist. The advantages of ultrasound are noninvasiveness and lack of evidence of harmful biological effects: these have led to the extensive use of ultrasound and its offshoot, Doppler, in obstetrics. Apart from diagnostic use, it is also used for therapeutic interventions. Computerised tomography (CT) and magnetic resonance imaging (MRI) are occasionally used, but are more expensive and less widely available.

In most developed countries, ultrasound is used routinely to screen pregnancies. Major uses currently are: confirming pregnancy, charting antenatal fetal growth, assessing fetal wellbeing and screening for congenital abnormalities. Doppler is used to view continuous waveforms of the fetal heart. Colour and spectral Doppler are useful for identifying fetal and placental vessels and for collecting information about placental function and fetal oxygen status.

Basics of ultrasound

Ultrasound equipment used in diagnostic practice uses high-frequency, low-intensity sound waves, produced by piezoelectric crystals which convert electrical energy to sound waves. These crystals are placed in the transducer and emit and receive sound waves. When the transducer is placed on the body, the waves are transmitted to the body through a gel, which prevents the presence of air between the transducer and the body, as air is a poor conductor of sound waves. The sound waves, which pass through the body, are differentially reflected, depending on the density of the tissue they encounter. These reflected signals are converted to electric charges in the crystals, which in turn are converted to visual signals on the screen. This provides a two-dimensional image of the human body. Because the array of crystals is triggered rapidly, the image is constantly updated and hence, movements in the body can be studied. The transducer can be moved over the body and a three-dimensional image can be created. The wavelength of most machines varies between 3 MHz and 7.5 MHz.

The quality of images obtained depends to some extent on the machine, and heavily on the skill of the operator.

Currently, there is no evidence that the use of ultrasound is harmful to the mother or the fetus. It has been routinely used in obstetrics for several decades and millions of pregnant women have undergone ultrasound examinations. However, ultrasound should not be considered totally noninvasive. It can cause bioeffects by generating heat. Some newer methods use more focused beams with higher intensity. Hence, while ultrasound may be safe, care should be taken to avoid unnecessary prolonged exposure, particularly to high-intensity waves, and frivolous indications should be avoided.

Applications of Obstetric Ultrasound

Ultrasound is commonly used for the following applications:

- diagnosis of pregnancy
- fetal biometry and dating of pregnancy
- evaluation of early pregnancy bleeding
- ectopic pregnancy
- diagnosis of multiple pregnancy
- anomaly screening
- fetal growth monitoring
- fetal weight estimation
- assessment of fetal wellbeing
- placental localisation and study of umbilical cord
- evaluation of liquor amnii
- interventional ultrasound.

Diagnosis of pregnancy

The intrauterine gestational sac can be identified as early as five weeks from the last menstrual period (**Fig. 13.1**), particularly by TVS. The embryo can be identified by six weeks with cardiac activity (**Fig. 13.2**). By the seventh week, embryonic movements may be appreciated. Occasionally, a pseudo-gestational sac may be seen and may confuse the issue; however, it can be definitively identified by its central location, irregular outline, absence of yolk sac, fetal pole and no increase in size.

Dating of pregnancy

Dating means assessing the gestational age: this is vital in obstetric management. Ultrasound is more accurate than clinical assessment with the last menstrual period, vaginal or abdominal examination. It must be remembered that a single assessment of gestational

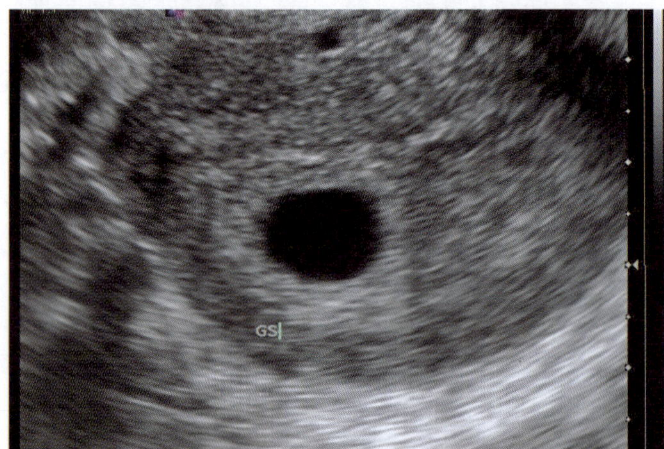

Fig. 13.1 Gestational sac at five weeks.

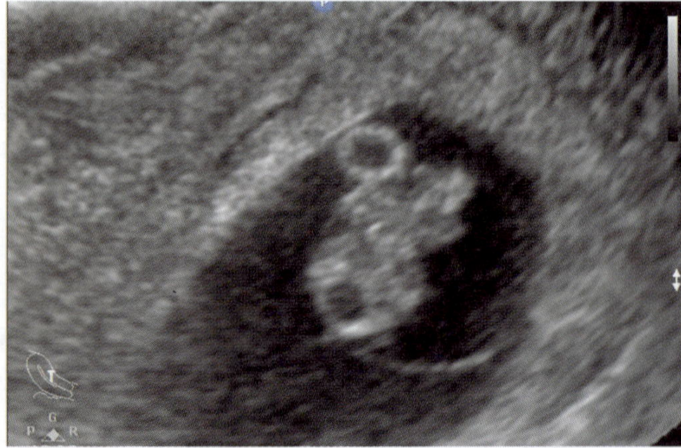

Fig. 13.2 Gestational sac with fetal echo.

age late in pregnancy is likely to have an error margin of ±2–3 weeks. The earlier the measurement is made, the more accurate is the assessment. Measurement of crown–rump length (CRL) in the first twelve weeks has an error margin of ±5 days (**Fig. 13.3**). A combination of the last menstrual period and a first trimester ultrasound is the most accurate and considered to be 'excellent dates'.

Biparietal diameter (BPD) (**Fig. 13.4**), head circumference (HC) (**Fig. 13.5**), abdominal circumference (AC) (**Fig. 13.6**) and femur length (FL) (**Fig. 13.7**) are the other measurements used to assess gestational age in the second and third trimesters. At 20 weeks, BPD has an error margin of ±1–2 weeks and in the third trimester, it increases to ±2–3 weeks. As the measurements are taken, the software of the equipment calculates the expected date of delivery (EDD) and the period of gestation.

Evaluation of early pregnancy bleeding

Ultrasound is invaluable in evaluating early pregnancy bleeding. Local lesions should be ruled out by clinical examination. Apart from these, the important conditions are abortion, molar pregnancy and ectopic gestation.

Abortion: In case of threatened abortion, ultrasound is the only way to ascertain the viability of the fetus in the first trimester and up to 20 weeks in the second trimester, which will determine the management. The presence of cardiac activity by

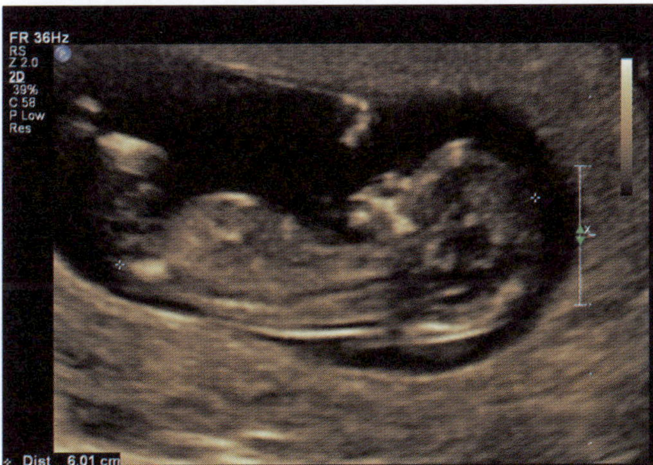

Fig. 13.3 Measurement of CRL.

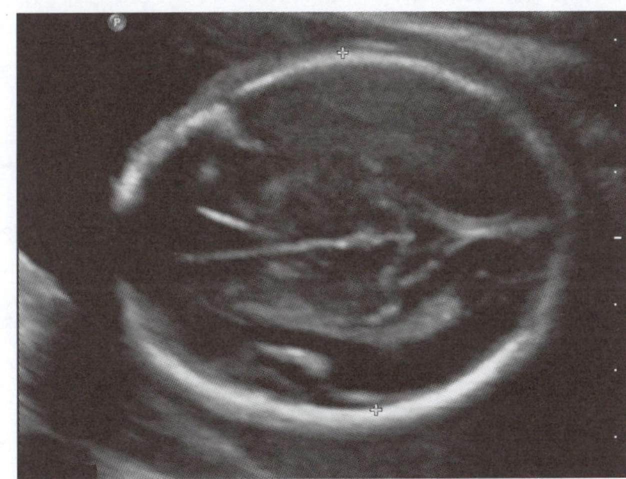

Fig. 13.4 Measurement of BPD.

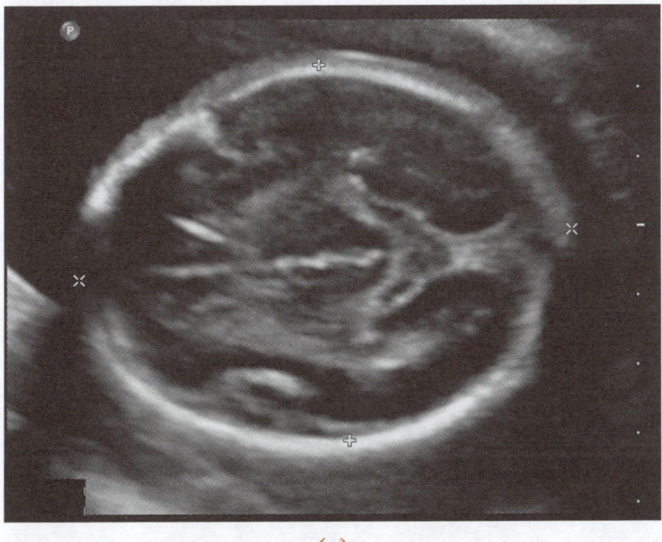

(a)

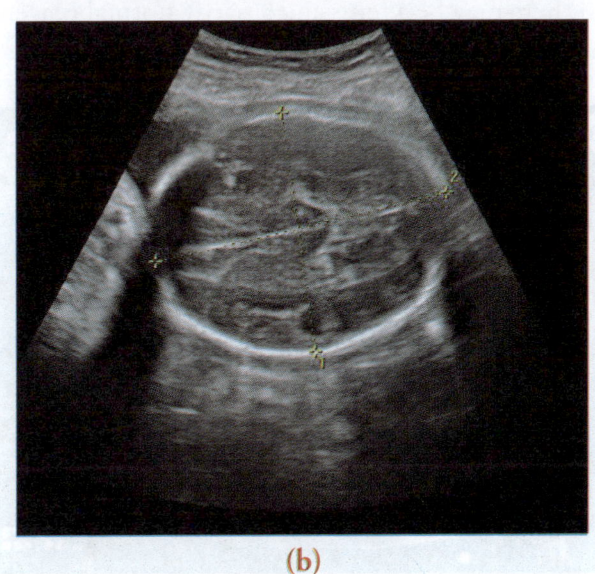

(b)

Fig. 13.5 Measurement of HC.

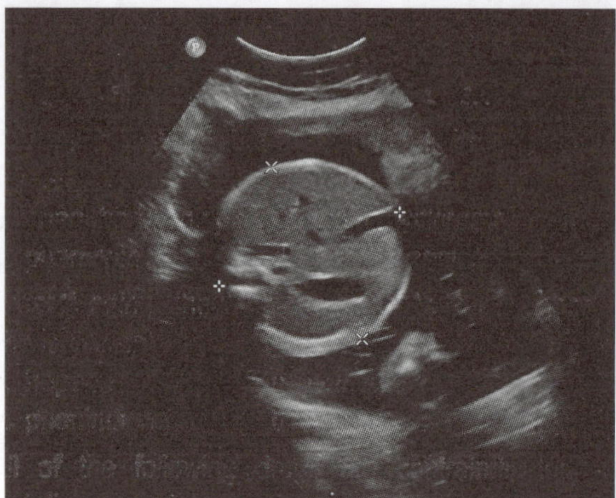

Fig. 13.6 Measurement of AC.

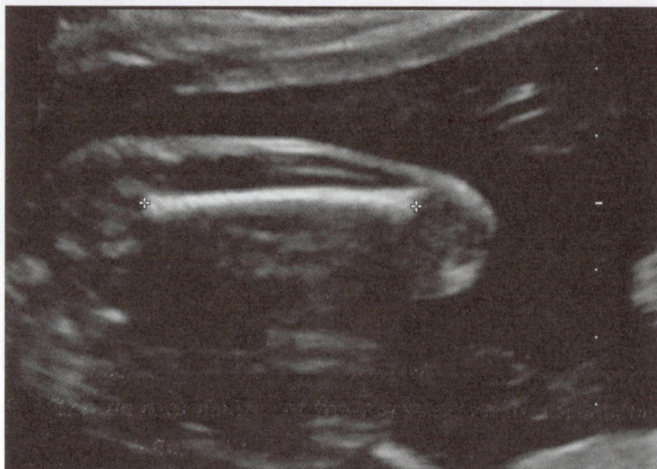

Fig. 13.7 Measurement of FL.

USG or demonstration of fetal heart by Doppler will suggest conservative management in the absence of major malformations.

Inevitable and incomplete abortions are often diagnosed clinically, and are emergencies; USG should be resorted to only in rare occasions. Sometimes, USG may be needed to confirm that the process of abortion is complete when the clinical picture is inconclusive.

Molar pregnancy: This can be diagnosed by the absence of the fetus in the complete variety, and the typical 'honeycomb' or 'snowstorm' appearance (**Fig. 13.8**). In cases of partial mole, the above appearance will be restricted to a part of the placenta and there may be a fetus and a partly normal placenta (**Fig. 13.9**).

Ectopic gestation: Ultrasound is a very important tool in the diagnosis of ectopic tubal gestation in the very early stages (before it ruptures) and helps in the planning and follow-up of medical management (when such management is necessary). Absence of intrauterine gestation in the presence of amenorrhea, pain, vaginal bleeding and a positive test for β-hCG strongly suggests an ectopic pregnancy. It may be possible to view the gestational sac with the fetus in the adnexal region (**Fig. 13.10**). In addition, measurement of the ectopic gestation (<3.5 cm) helps in selecting cases for medical management.

Multiple pregnancies

Ultrasound helps in diagnosing multiple pregnancy early, when two or more gestational sacs may be

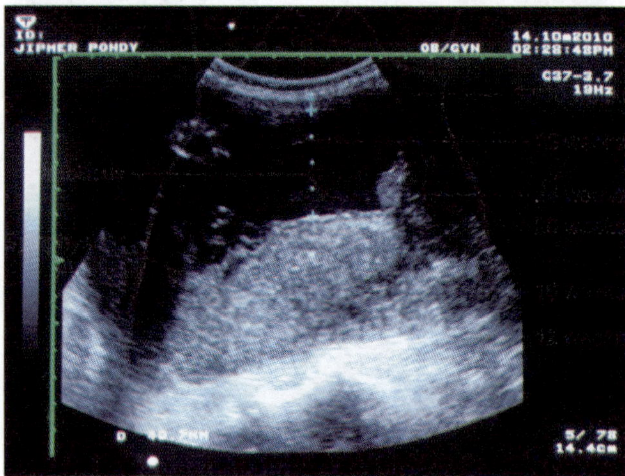

Fig. 13.8 Molar pregnancy.

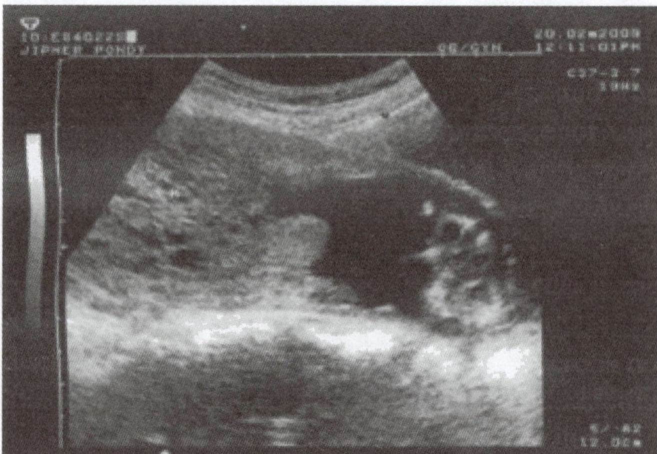

Fig. 13.9 Partial mole.

seen (**Fig. 13.11**). As the pregnancy advances, USG helps in diagnosing the zygosity by the number of amniotic cavities and placentae. Monoamniotic twins are monozygotic. Dizygotic twins are always dichorionic diamniotic. Some monozygotic twins may be dichorionic and diamniotic.

Ultrasound also helps in determining the lie of the fetuses, presence of disparity in growth, twin-to-twin transfusion, single fetal demise and placenta previa.

Anomaly screening

The best time to carry out an anatomical screening for malformations is at about 18–20 weeks, though such a scan can be done at any stage of pregnancy. Every organ should be examined: this usually takes 15–20 minutes. The overall detection rate will depend on the operator's skill and anatomical knowledge, but is generally around 80%. False positives are low.

Nuchal translucency (**Fig. 13.12**) is probably the earliest parameter which can be measured (at around 12 weeks). It should be remembered that it only helps in identifying a risk group and is not diagnostic. Gross structural abnormalities like anencephaly (**Fig. 13.13**) or encephalocele (**Fig. 13.14**) can be identified by TVS in the first trimester.

Abnormalities of the central nervous system and cardiac defects are the most common. A detailed study of the cranium, particularly of the ventricles and the cerebellum, must be carried out. The head circumference is large in hydrocephalus, but this occurs late in pregnancy. Hence, the diagnosis is based on enlarged ventricles. A small head circumference will point to microcephaly.

The vertebral column should be examined; both the anterior view and the clear, continuous skin margin must be looked for. Spina bifida (**Fig. 13.15**) and meningomyelocele (**Fig. 13.16**) can be diagnosed.

The face is better studied with 3D ultrasound, which may not be universally available. However, with the regular machine, the orbits, lips, nose and mandible can be reasonably assessed.

A four-chamber view of the fetal heart is obtained and the outflow tracts can be viewed. Doppler studies may be undertaken as indicated.

The abdomen is scanned, noting the cord insertion, diaphragm, liver, stomach, bowel, kidneys and

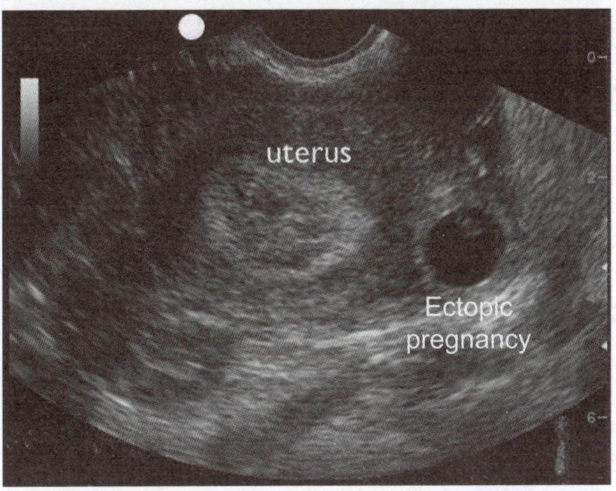

Fig. 13.10 Gestational sac with fetus in the adnexal region.

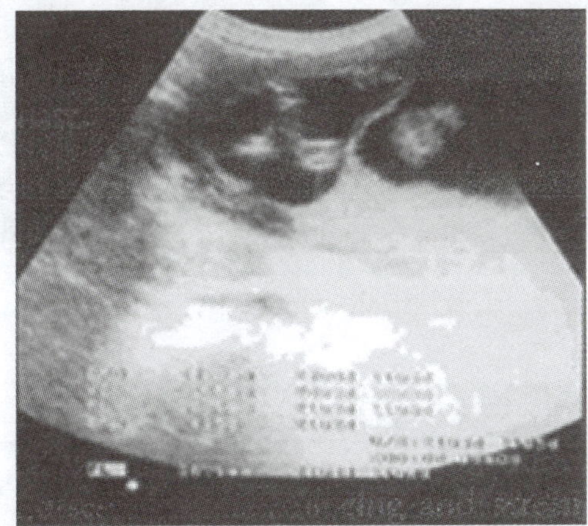

Fig. 13.11 Twin pregnancy.

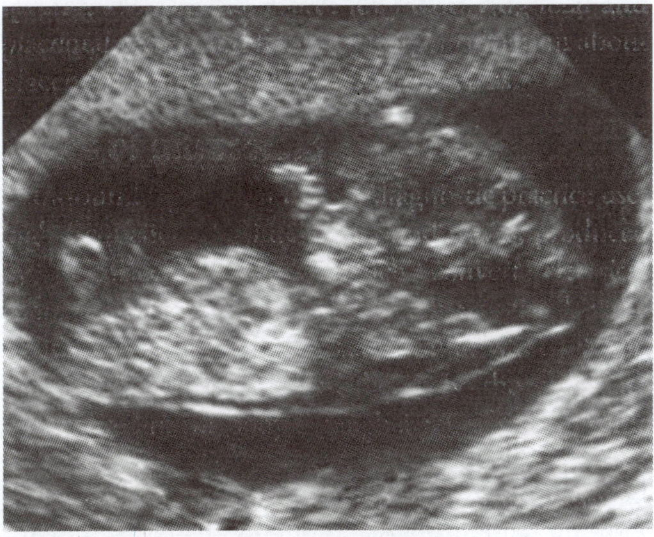

Fig. 13.12 Nuchal translucency.

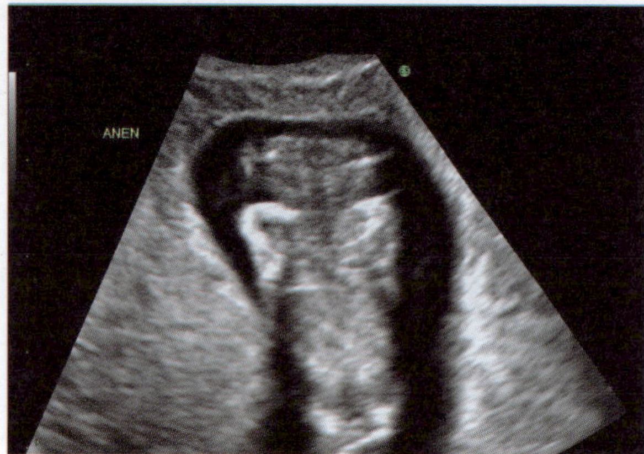

Fig. 13.13 Anencephaly.

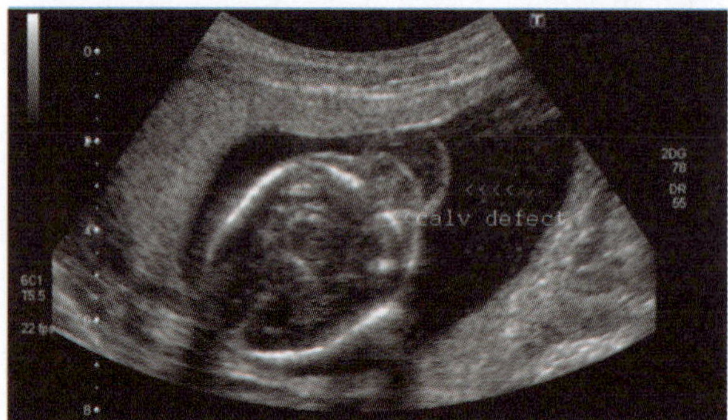

Fig. 13.14 Encephalocele.

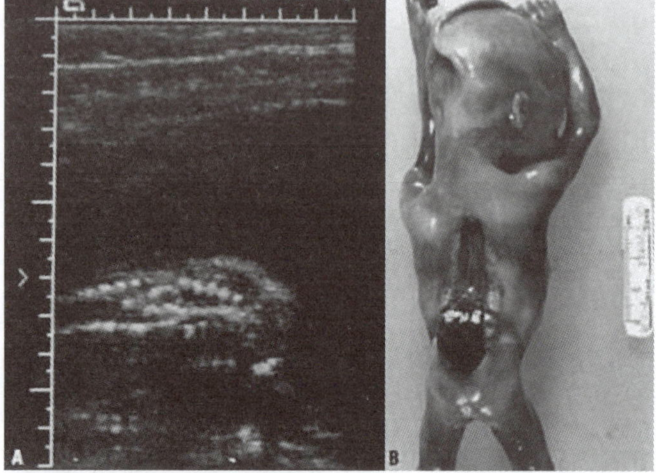

Fig. 13.15 Spina bifida.

urinary bladder. A small abdominal circumference may indicate triploidy, like trisomy 18.

The limbs are serially studied, one after the other, from the long bones to the digits. A small femur may indicate achondroplasia, though serial measurements should be performed to confirm the diagnosis.

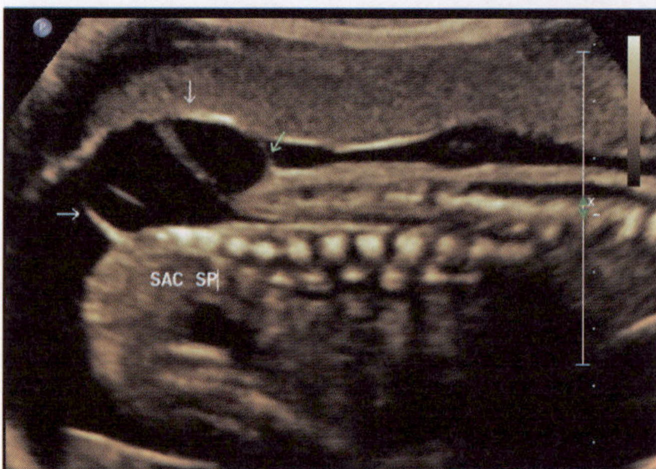

Fig. 13.16 Meningomyelocele.

Fetal growth assessment

Serial charting of fetal measurements like the BPD, HC, AC and FL will help to ascertain if fetal growth is appropriate. It will help to identify at an early stage the fetuses which are lagging behind in growth and will also distinguish between symmetrical and asymmetrical intrauterine growth restriction (IUGR). In the former, the ratio of HC to AC will be about 1, while in the latter it will be more than 1, since the head grows preferentially over the viscera due to a greater amount of blood flow being directed to the brain. In a diabetic pregnancy, the abdominal circumference will be larger, due to the effect of insulin on the liver and fat stores.

Fetal weight estimation

Estimation of fetal weight may be important in conditions like breech presentation and diabetic pregnancies since it will assist in deciding the mode of delivery. Abdominal circumference is the best predictor of fetal weight. Calculation of fetal weight using several parameters will reduce the error. Fetal weight can be predicted within 200 g of the actual weight. Fetal weight estimations tend to have higher margins of error when the fetus is too small or big.

Fetal wellbeing

Assessment of fetal biophysical profile (BPP) is currently the most commonly used method for assessing fetal wellbeing. Cardiotocography, along with sonological assessment of the fetal tone, movements, breathing movement and the amount of amniotic fluid form the components of BPP. In addition, Doppler study of the umbilical artery and detailed assessment of fetal arterial and venous circulation are undertaken (see Chapter 15).

Placental localisation and study of the umbilical cord

One of the clinical conditions where ultrasound is most useful is antepartum hemorrhage. Ultrasound provides a quick noninvasive method of identifying placenta previa (**Fig. 13.17**). In addition, placental morphology can also be studied. The placenta has a uniform texture in the second and early third trimesters. Towards the end of pregnancy, as well as in severe placental dysfunction, it may appear distinctly lobular with areas of calcification. The size of the placenta may be large in diabetic pregnancy as well as in Rh isoimmunisation.

Check for umbilical cord insertion into the fetal abdomen and also confirm the presence of three vessels in the cord. The presence of a single umbilical artery has been shown to be associated with a higher incidence of malformations. Diffuse swelling of the placenta and cord may be appreciated in hydrops fetalis.

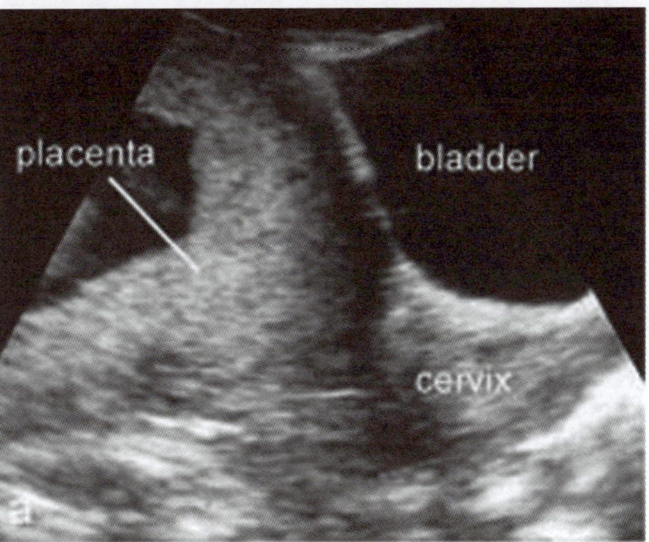

Fig. 13.17 Placenta previa.

Amniotic fluid assessment

The amount of liquor can be studied by calculating the amniotic fluid index (AFI), which is the total of measurements of largest vertical pockets of amniotic fluid measured in the four quadrants of the uterus. A single maximum vertical pocket (MVP) is also used by some (**Fig. 13.18**). An AFI of more than 25 or an MVP of more than 8 is said to be diagnostic of polyhydramnios. When the AFI is less than 5 or MVP is less than 2, the diagnosis of oligohydramnios is made.

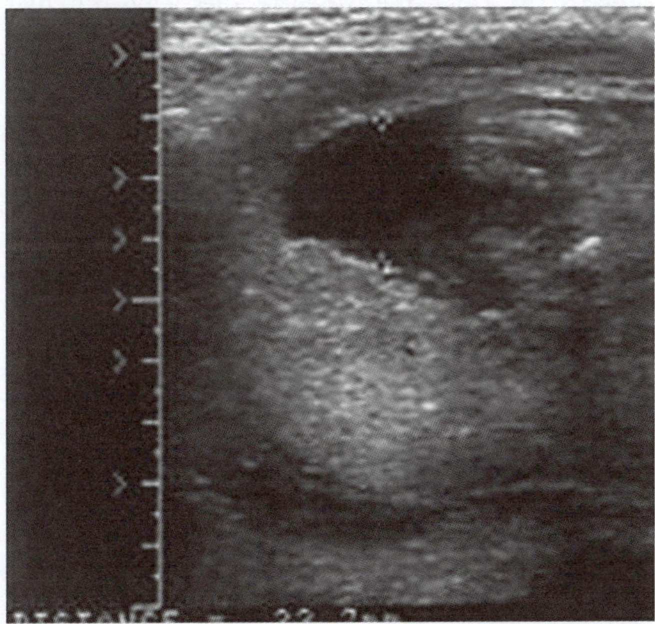

Fig. 13.18 Maximum vertical pocket.

Interventional ultrasound

In specialised centres, ultrasound is used for several diagnostic and therapeutic procedures like chorion villus sampling (CVS), amniocentesis (both diagnostic and therapeutic) and cordocentesis, where the umbilical cord is accessed for drawing fetal blood or for intrauterine fetal transfusion as in cases of Rh isoimmunisation. Other procedures such as fetal tissue biopsies, placement of coils in abnormal vessels or catheters in urinary obstruction are also carried out with the help of ultrasound.

Doppler in obstetrics

The Doppler principle involves the use of frequency shift, where the frequency of the transmitted and received waves differs when the wave encounters a moving medium like blood in a vessel. If the blood moves towards the beam, the reflected wave has a higher frequency than the transmitted one. Conversely, the frequency reduces if the blood is moving away from the beam. The equipment can show the blood vessels as a colour map: this is called **colour Doppler.** Blood flowing towards the transducer is red and that flowing away, blue. The velocity and resistance to flow can be quantitatively documented. High diastolic flow in the placental and fetal vessels indicates low resistance and high perfusion. A ratio of the systolic to diastolic flow is calculated: the higher the index, the more the resistance. Moreover, the appearance of a diastolic notch in uterine artery blood flow indicates resistance in spiral arterioles (**Fig. 13.19**). This is due to the arterioles being muscular and noncompliant because of poor penetration of these vessels by the trophoblast. The appearance of the diastolic notch has been shown to have a correlation with the occurrence of preeclampsia. Doppler studies are invaluable, particularly in assessing fetal status in intrauterine growth restriction.

Computerised tomography (CT)

The radiation hazard is much less with CT scan than with routine radiography. The possible hazards of radiation and the utility of ultrasound have limited the use of CT scan in obstetrics to general indications.

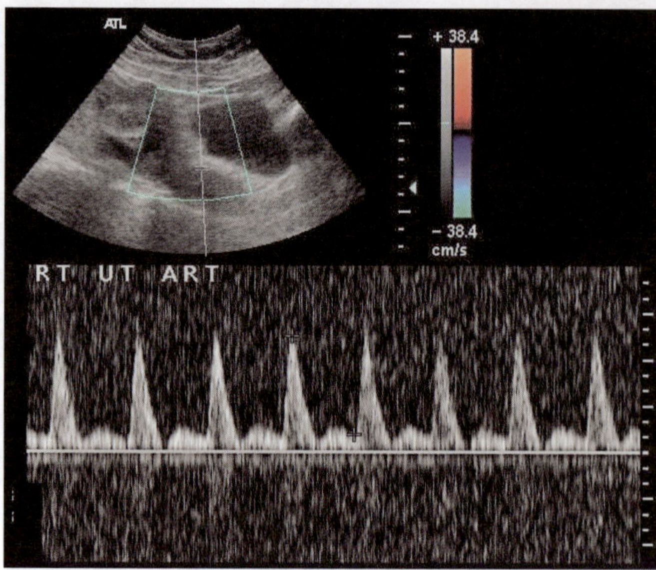

Fig. 13.19 Diastolic notch.

If CT scan is warranted for a maternal condition, it may be used.

Magnetic resonance imaging (MRI)

MRI is sometimes used to study the maternal pelvis and its fetal relationship, particularly in breech presentation, and in some centres in rare cases for intrapartum assessment. It is radiation-free. It may also be used to study fetal structural abnormalities. Contraindications for its use are the presence of cardiac pacemakers or other implants. It is an expensive method and is not widely available.

KEY POINTS

- Ultrasound is the most commonly used imaging modality in obstetrics.
- It can diagnose pregnancy as early as five weeks after a missed period.
- It is most useful in the management of early pregnancy disorders like abortion and ectopic pregnancy.
- Screening for fetal malformations is advocated between 18 and 20 weeks of pregnancy.
- It is used primarily to evaluate gestational age, fetal growth and wellbeing.
- It is a noninvasive method of detecting the cause of antepartum hemorrhage.
- Doppler ultrasound is used to study blood flow in fetuses with compromised uteroplacental function.

QUESTIONS

Select the single most appropriate answer:

1. Obstetric ultrasound is useful for all of the following *except*
   a. confirmation of pregnancy
   b. dating of pregnancy
   c. evaluation of pelvis
   d. assessment of fetal wellbeing
2. Ultrasound is extensively used in obstetric practice because it is
   a. technically easy
   b. universally available
   c. very cheap
   d. has no adverse biological effect
3. Gel is used while performing an ultrasound because it
   a. prevents air interface between the probe and body
   b. produces thermocoupling
   c. permits good conduction of electromagnetic waves
   d. prevents damage to tissues by attenuating the waves
4. Unnecessary prolonged ultrasound examination should be avoided because
   a. it is expensive
   b. expertise is not available
   c. to avoid any unknown biological harmful effect
   d. supine position during pregnancy predisposes to hypotension
5. The best measurement for dating of pregnancy in the first trimester is
   a. biparietal diameter
   b. crown–rump length
   c. abdominal circumference
   d. head circumference
6. The earliest time after the last menstrual period when pregnancy can be diagnosed by ultrasound is
   a. 8 weeks
   b. 7 weeks
   c. 6 weeks
   d. 5 weeks
7. Ultrasound is most helpful in the management of threatened abortion because it
   a. helps to assess cervical status
   b. can predict expulsion of products
   c. helps confirm that the fetus is alive
   d. detects minor placental hemorrhage
8. The best time to screen for anomaly during pregnancy is
   a. weeks 10–12
   b. weeks 14–16
   c. weeks 18–20
   d. weeks 22–24
9. Normal amniotic fluid volume reasonably excludes
   a. neural tube defects
   b. renal defects
   c. gastrointestinal malformations
   d. cardiac defects
10. Polyhydramnios is diagnosed if
    a. MVP is more than 5
    b. AFI is more than 15
    c. the examiner subjectively feels there is more liquor
    d. MVP is more than 8

14

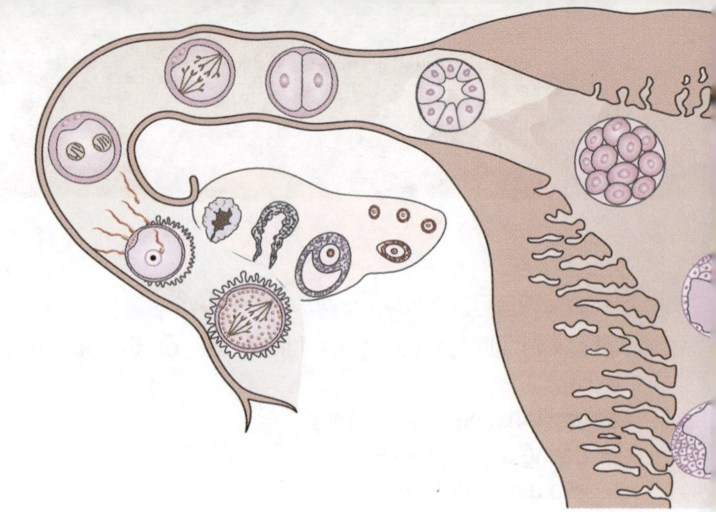

Screening and Prenatal Diagnosis of Fetal Anomalies

Lavanya Rai

LEARNING OBJECTIVES

At the end of this chapter, the reader should be able to:

- define prenatal diagnosis
- list the indications for prenatal diagnosis
- enumerate the types of and indications for prenatal diagnostic tests
- select imaging and biochemical screening tests for the first and second trimesters
- list the advantages and disadvantages of invasive prenatal diagnostic tests
- select the tests for the prenatal diagnosis of common anomalies
- explain the basis of investigations for genetic disorders
- list the salient features of the Prenatal Diagnostic Technique (PNDT) Act

Introduction

Though most women deliver healthy babies, about 3% of pregnant women have babies with anomalies. Congenital fetal anomalies not only increase the perinatal mortality but also cause significant morbidity. **Prenatal diagnosis is the diagnosis of a disease or condition in a fetus or embryo before it is born.** The majority of these fetal anomalies occur in a 'low-risk' population: women who have no known predisposition to such anomalies. The objective of prenatal diagnosis is to reduce birth incidence of fetal anomalies. Screening of all pregnant women will identify those who require further diagnostic tests to check for specific anomalies. Prenatal diagnosis can be performed by various invasive and noninvasive techniques.

Recommendations for prenatal diagnosis

The majority of fetal malformations occur sporadically in 'low-risk' pregnancies. Therefore, routine ultrasound and biochemical screening is recommended for the general obstetric population. Specific prenatal tests are required in the following circumstances:

- previous child with malformation or chromosomal abnormality
- parents with an anomaly
- mother on drugs like anticonvulsants, lithium or other teratogens
- history of rubella, toxoplasmosis during pregnancy
- women with a history of recurrent abortions, fetal or neonatal deaths

- known diabetic mothers or those with phenylketonuria
- genetic disorders in families
- older age couples
- ultrasound detected anomaly
- presence of clinical markers such as oligoamnios, polyhydramnios, growth restriction or malpresentations.

Types of Tests

There are two types of tests for prenatal diagnosis: **screening** and **diagnostic**. A **screening test** identifies women who require further diagnostic tests. An ideal prenatal screening test should be reliable, cost-effective, have a low false positive rate with good sensitivity and should be applicable in early gestation. Appropriate **diagnostic tests** should be available after the screening test that identifies the 'at risk' pregnancy (**Fig. 14.1**). The diagnostic tests are generally invasive and, therefore, there is a small risk of pregnancy loss.

Noninvasive Tests: Screening Tests

First trimester

There are two tests in the first trimester and both are used for Down syndrome (trisomy 21) screening.

- USG screening for nuchal translucency (NT) thickness
- Estimating serum levels of hCG and pregnancy-associated plasma protein A (PAPP-A); high β-hCG with low serum PAPP-A is considered screen positive for Down syndrome (**Table 14.1**).

Ultrasound done between weeks 10 and 14 for dating pregnancy should also be used for NT screening. Nuchal translucency (NT) is a fluid-filled space in the posterior nuchal area. A thickness of more than 3 mm is significant and is indicative of Down syndrome. A combination of biochemical and NT screening detects almost 90% of cases of Down syndrome. The absence of nasal bone is also a USG marker detectable between weeks 11 and 14. The diagnostic test at this stage of pregnancy is karyotype by CVS. Fetuses with abnormal NT and a normal karyotype are at risk of cardiac defects and major genetic syndromes. Fetal echocardiography and a detailed scan at a later stage are therefore mandatory.

Second trimester

Biochemical screening involves maternal serum alpha fetoprotein (MSAFP), triple or quadruple tests.

MSAFP screening is done between weeks 16 and 20 to detect neural tube defects (NTD) and other structural malformations. It is elevated in these malformations while it is low in chromosomal

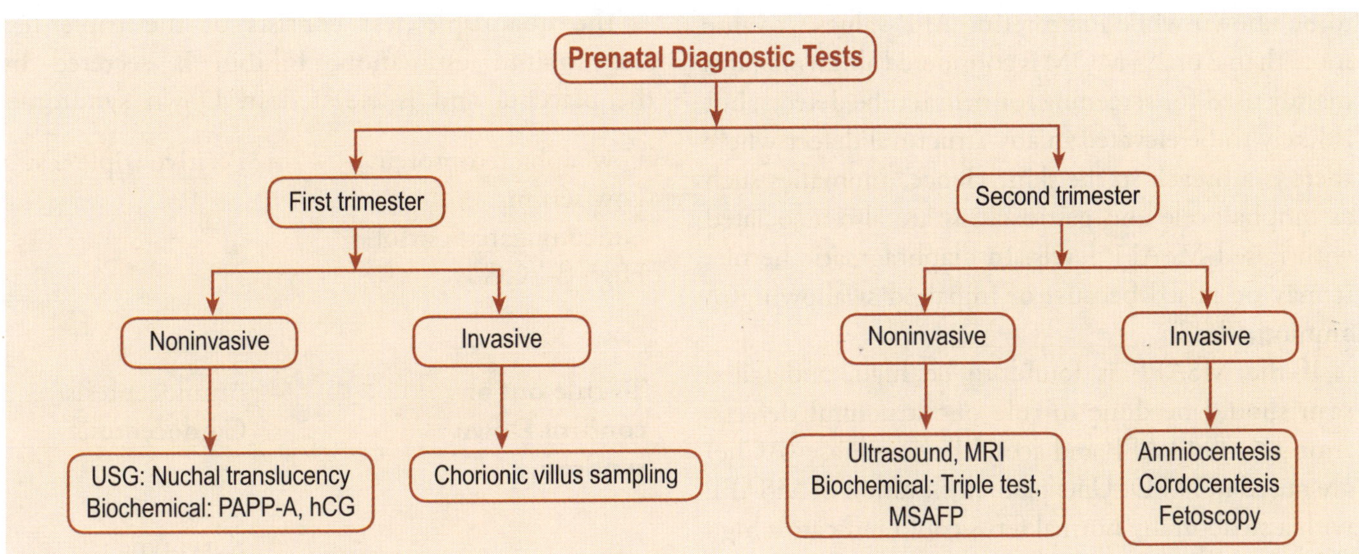

Fig. 14.1 Various types of prenatal diagnostic tests.

Table 14.1 Down syndrome screening tests

Method	Gestational week	Result	Detection rate
First trimester			
USG			
Nuchal translucency	10–13	>3 mm	60%–69%
Biochemical			
PAPP-A	8–13	Low	42%
Free β-hCG	8–13	High	25%
Combined tests (NT + Biochemical)			85%
Second trimester			
Triple Test AFP+ hCG + estriol	16–18	Low AFP, high hCG, low unconjugated estriol	69%
Quadruple Test Triple test + inhibin		High inhibin	76%
Integrated test NT + PAPP-A + Quadruple test	10–13 + 16–18	Positive combined and quadruple test	94%

abnormalities. Alpha fetoprotein (AFP) is produced by the yolk sac early in pregnancy and in the fetal liver later. It crosses over to the maternal circulation through the placenta and membranes. Fetal urine adds to the levels in the amniotic fluid. During pregnancy, maternal AFP rises while in non-pregnant women it is found to be very low. It is expressed in multiple of median (MOM), though it is measured in ng/ml. MSAFP increases by 15% with every week of gestation. Therefore, the exact gestational age has to be known while interpreting AFP values. A value more than 2 or 2.5 MOM is considered abnormal. It is mainly used for screening for neural tube defects, but is likely to be elevated in any structural defect where there is a breach in the skin. Hence, anomalies such as omphalocele and gastroschisis are also associated with raised MSAFP levels. In diaphragmatic hernia, it may be raised because of impaired swallowing of amniotic fluid.

If the MSAFP is found to be high, a detailed scan should be done to rule out structural defects. Amniotic fluid AFP and acetylcholinesterase (AChe) are raised in NTD. Unexplained elevation of MSAFP with a structurally normal fetus could indicate a high risk of perinatal complications. MSAFP is believed to be a marker of a diseased placenta.

Triple test is the most widely used biochemical screening test for Down syndrome (**Fig. 14.2**). Serum analytes altered by aneuploidy are hCG, AFP and estriol. These three substances are independent variables; therefore, their values can be combined and used along with maternal age to calculate the risk of Down syndrome. A risk threshold of about 1:270 is taken as the cut-off, indicating that a karyotype should be done. If values of all three are low, it may be indicative of trisomy 18.

The quadruple test consists of the triple test and inhibin estimation. Inhibin is secreted by the placenta and is elevated in Down syndrome.

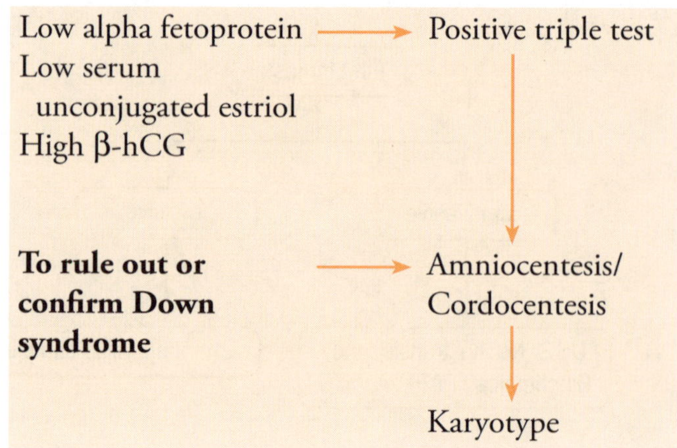

Fig. 14.2 Down syndrome: Diagnosis.

Table 14.1 lists the different tests used for screening for Down syndrome.

When both the first and second trimester screening is combined, the test is called the two-stage integrated test. This test not only increases the detection rate but also allows sufficient time for parents to understand and accept the positive results.

Ultrasonography

Ultrasonography is indispensable to prenatal diagnosis. All invasive tests are done under ultrasound guidance. Besides prenatal diagnosis, USG can evaluate fetal growth, gestational age and fetal wellbeing.

- A first trimester booking scan is used for dating and NT. Gross anomalies such as anencephaly, conjoint twins and limb anomalies such as sirenomelia may be detectable by 12 weeks.
- Detailed scan or target-oriented scan is generally done at 18–20 weeks. At this stage of pregnancy, liquor is adequate and it is easy to visualise the whole body of the fetus and the majority of the anomalies are detectable.

In addition to the above, anomalies should always be looked for while checking for growth or biophysical profile in the third trimester. Anomalies such as hydrocephalus, hydronephrosis and gastrointestinal tract obstructions may only be evident late in pregnancy. **Table 14.2** depicts the systematic anatomical survey and some common anomalies.

Genetic sonogram: This is a targeted examination for fetal aneuploidy. Chromosomal disorders such as trisomy 21, 13 and 18 have a pattern of malformations, abnormal biometry and subtle markers which can be diagnosed on ultrasound.

Fetal echocardiography: Using ultrasound and duplex or colour Doppler, details of fetal structural cardiac defects and rhythm disturbances can be diagnosed in the second trimester. Fetal echocardiography is essential when there is a previous child with a cardiac anomaly, the mother is on anticonvulsants, or lithium therapy or has been exposed to other teratogens. Maternal diseases such as diabetes, phenylketonuria and rubella in early pregnancy are other indications for fetal echocardiography.

Three-dimensional ultrasound: It is an advanced, high-quality ultrasound that can enhance diagnostic capability over standard 2D ultrasound. The 3D ultrasound is useful in the evaluation of facial, limb and CNS anomalies. Sensitivity of ultrasound to such anomalies varies from 40% to 85%, depending on the skill, resolution of the machine and gestational age. Abnormal fetal position, thick maternal abdominal

Table 14.2 Ultrasound checklist and common anomalies

Anatomical site	Check	Anomaly
Head	Size, shape, configuration Atria of lateral ventricles Posterior fossa	Anencephaly, hydrocephalus
Face	Profile and 'face on' views	Cleft lip
Neck	Masses	Cystic hygromas
Spine	Longitudinal and transverse sections	Spina bifida
Chest	Four-chamber view and cardiac outflow tracts Pleural cavity, diaphragm	Cardiac defects, pleural effusion Diaphragmatic hernia
Trunk	Cord insertion in fetal abdomen Stomach bubble, liver, kidneys, bladder	Abdominal wall defects: omphalocele, gastroschisis Renal anomalies: agenesis, hydronephrosis GI tract: obstruction
Limbs	Upper and lower; right and left; hands, feet, long bone lengths	Skeletal dysplasias
Others	Cord vessels, external genitalia	Nonimmune hydrops, single umbilical artery

wall and oligohydramnios limit the visualisation of the fetus.

Magnetic resonance imaging

An MRI is very useful in certain situations where the USG is not helpful, such as oligohydramnios. MRI use is limited to the second and third trimesters. It is not used in the first trimester because its teratogenicity is not known. It is useful in the diagnosis of CNS anomalies, fetal tumours and posterior placenta previa. The disadvantages are that it is expensive, not easily available and fetal movements impair the images.

Invasive Tests

All the tests carry a risk of pregnancy loss by spontaneous abortion or preterm labour. Hence, it is important to counsel and obtain informed consent before carrying out invasive tests.

Chorionic villus sampling

This is an invasive diagnostic test performed in the first trimester (**Fig. 14.3**). It is done at 10–12 weeks on an outpatient basis. Under ultrasound guidance, the villi are aspirated from the chorion frondosum either transcervically or transabdominally. CVS should be avoided before 9 weeks because it can cause ischemic effects on the fetus, resulting in limb reduction effects. The transcervical route has more risk of infection and abortion. Transabdominal CVS, also called placental biopsy, can be performed at any period of gestation as an alternative to fetal blood sampling and amniocentesis.

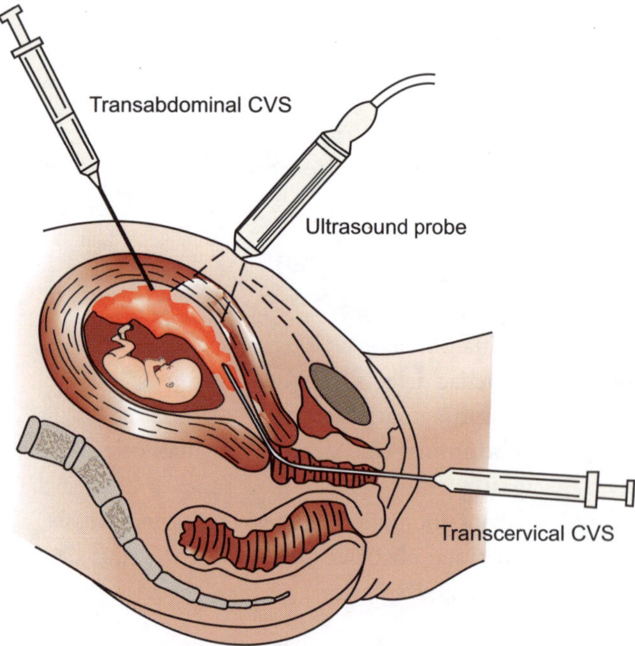

Fig. 14.3 Chorionic villus sampling.

Amniocentesis

This is the most commonly performed invasive procedure for prenatal diagnosis (**Fig. 14.4**). About 10–15 ml of amniotic fluid is aspirated under USG guidance between 15–20 weeks under local anesthesia. The cells and the fluid can be used for diagnosis. As the cells in the amniotic fluid are not actively dividing, they need to be cultured and thus the results take 2–3 weeks. However, using fluorescent in situ hybridisation (FISH) (a recent technology) these cells can be used for rapid

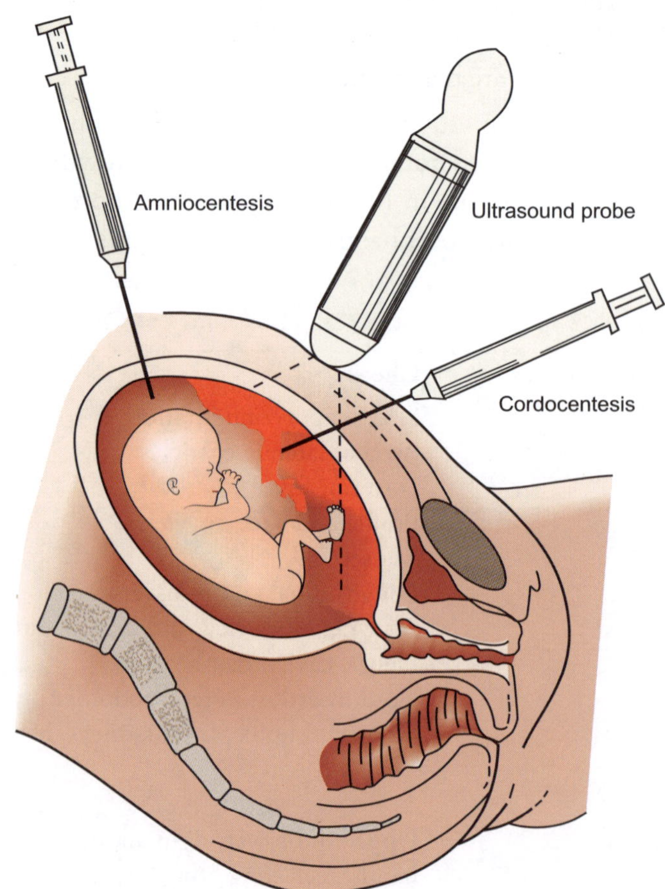

Fig. 14.4 Amniocentesis and cordocentesis.

diagnosis. Unlike CVS, the fibroblasts obtained in amniocentesis truly represent the fetus as they are shed from fetal skin. Supernatant fluid can be used for the estimation of enzymes like acetyl cholinesterase, 17-α hydroxyprogesterone and alpha fetoprotein.

Amniocentesis in the third trimester can help assess lung maturity or the severity of hemolysis in Rh isoimmunised pregnancies. Amnioreduction has a therapeutic role in polyhydramnios and the management of twin-to-twin transfusion. Amniocentesis is associated with talipes equinovarus and fetal loss in the first trimester, and vaginal spotting, fluid leakage and chorioamnionitis in the second trimester.

Fetal blood sampling

This procedure is also known as **cordocentesis** or **percutaneous umbilical cord blood sampling (PUBS)**. Occasionally, when the cord is inaccessible, fetal blood may be taken from the fetal intrahepatic vein or fetal heart. This is done after 18–20 weeks. Besides diagnosis, this procedure is used for intrauterine transfusion in fetal anemia. Cordocentesis gives a quicker chromosomal report than CVS or amniocentesis (**Fig. 14.4**). It is also useful when the mother presents late in gestation or when amniocentesis fails. Nongenetic indications of cordocentesis include evaluation of fetal anemia, thrombocytopenia and fetal infections. Cord hematoma, bradycardia and chorioamnionitis are some complications of the procedure which may lead to pregnancy loss.

Fetoscopy

This procedure is used for visualising the fetus in the second trimester. A fine calibre endoscope is introduced into the uterine cavity through the abdomen and the fetus is visualised directly. However, it only provides a limited view of a small portion of the fetus. It is useful for the diagnosis of the following conditions:

- inherited skin disorders
- subtle cleft lips
- for laser coagulation of placental vessels in twin-to-twin transfusion syndrome (TTS)
- skin biopsy.

Fetoscopy has an associated risk of 3%–5% of miscarriage, and is rarely performed today. There is a similar technique in the first trimester to visualise the fetus, known as embryoscopy.

Fetal tissue biopsy

This is done for the direct analysis of fetal tissue. Biopsy material is obtained under ultrasound guidance or fetoscopy. Liver biopsy has been used for the diagnosis of some storage disorders and inborn errors of metabolism. Skin biopsies are occasionally done to diagnose certain conditions like epidermolysis bullosa. Muscle biopsy may help when the genetic test is inconclusive, as in muscular dystrophy. Fetal tissue heals well after biopsy.

Fluid aspiration

Urine can be aspirated from the bladder for renal function assessment. Chylothorax is diagnosed by aspirating pleural effusion.

All invasive tests are done as outpatient procedures with aseptic precautions, after informed consent. Antibiotics may be given if required. Anti-D immunisation should be given for Rh-negative mothers.

Recurrence Risk of Common Anomalies

The two most common congenital disorders for which screening is done are neural tube defects and Down syndrome.

Neural tube defects

These are congenital structural abnormalities of the brain and vertebral column and are the commonest reported anomalies in India; the incidence varies from 6 to 11.4 per thousand births. The two most common types of lesions are anencephaly and spina bifida.

Neural tube defects occur because there is a failure in closure of the neural tube (it usually closes between 26 and 28 days of conception). When the cranial end fails to close, the result is anencephaly; distal end failure results in spina bifida. Both anencephaly and spina bifida are common and coexist in about 20% of cases.

MSAFP evaluation is an effective screening test for NTDs and should be offered to all pregnant women. However, ultrasound is considered superior to biochemical screening as it gives detailed information regarding the type, site and size of the defect which would help in assessing the prognosis. Ultrasound is used as both screening and as a diagnostic test wherever MSAFP is not available.

- **Anencephaly** was the first anomaly to be diagnosed by ultrasound. It is characterised by the absence of cranial vault and cerebral hemispheres. It is a lethal anomaly incompatible with life, and can be diagnosed at weeks 10–12 by TVS. If TAS is used, it is detectable after 14 weeks (the diagnosis is thus delayed by two weeks) (**Fig. 14.5**).
- **Spina bifida** is a midline defect of the vertebrae resulting in exposure of the neural canal (**Fig. 14.6**). It is most commonly seen in the lumbosacral area and is associated with incontinence and paralysis. In open spina bifida, very often the herniating neural tissue is contained in a sac; this is called **meningomyelocele**. It may be associated with other malformations like hydrocephalus and club feet.

It can be diagnosed by the second trimester scan and pregnancy can be terminated. If spina bifida is diagnosed in the third trimester, a conservative approach is adopted and surgery can be tried after delivery. Many babies who survive have disability. Only 10% may survive without any problem.

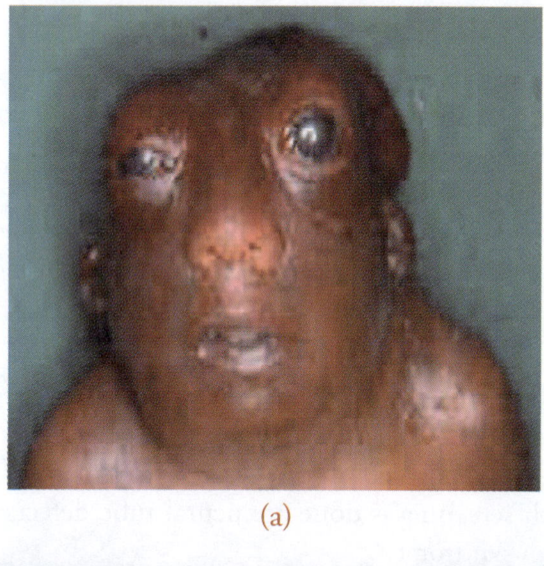

(a)

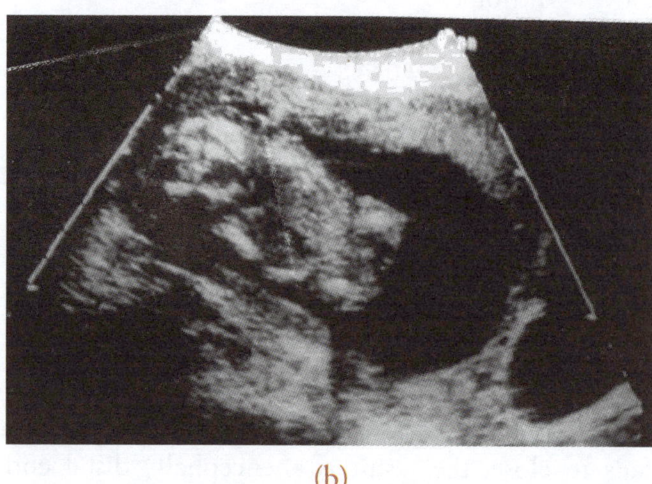

(b)

Fig. 14.5 Anencephaly a: Late second trimester b: USG at 15 weeks' gestation.

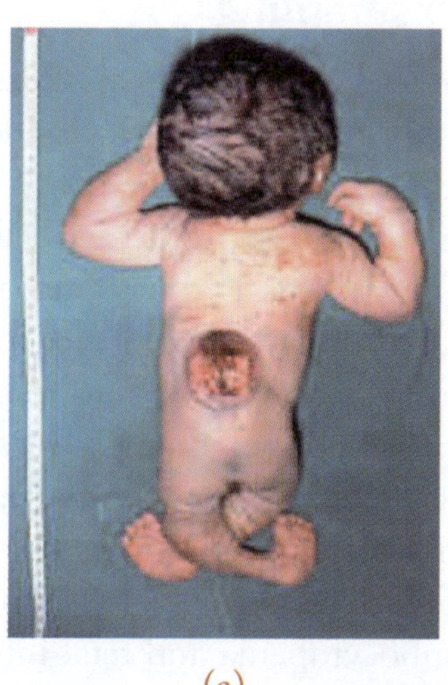

(a)

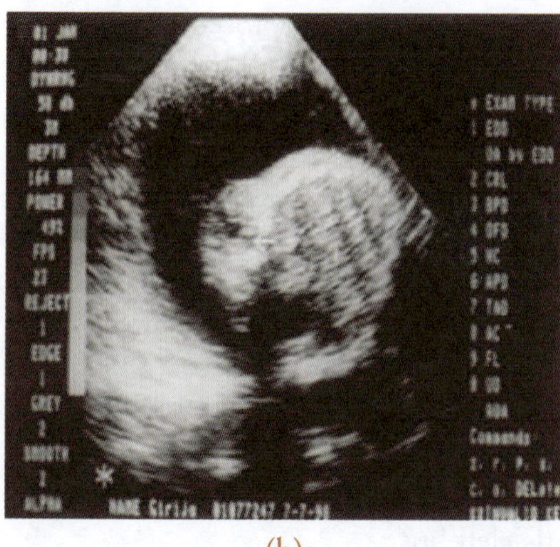

(b)

Fig 14.6 Spina bifida a: Lumbosacral spina bifida b: Transverse section of thoracic spina bifida.

USG findings can be grouped as direct and indirect signs. Though diagnosis should be based on direct signs, the indirect ones have improved the sensitivity and accuracy of diagnosis.

Direct signs:

Defect in the spine, seen in both transverse and longitudinal sections
Presence of meningocele sac
Splaying of spine in the coronal section
Abnormal curvature of the spine

Indirect signs:

Lemon sign: scalloping of forehead
Banana sign: cerebellum is shaped like a banana
Club foot
Polyhydramnios

- In **encephalocele** there is a defect in the skull with protrusion of neural tissue (**Fig. 14.7**). Though it is most often an isolated anomaly, it can be a part of a genetic syndrome called Meckel syndrome; associated polydactyly and polycystic kidneys are seen.

Prevention and counselling: Recurrence risk is 3%–5% after one pregnancy, 6%–8% after two affected babies and about 25% after three affected children. Since it is a multifactorial disorder, it is better to delay the next pregnancy by at least six months to one year. When pregnancy is contemplated, periconceptional folic acid 5 mg/day should be given. Ideally it must be started three months prior to conception and continued till the end of the first trimester to reduce the risk of recurrence.

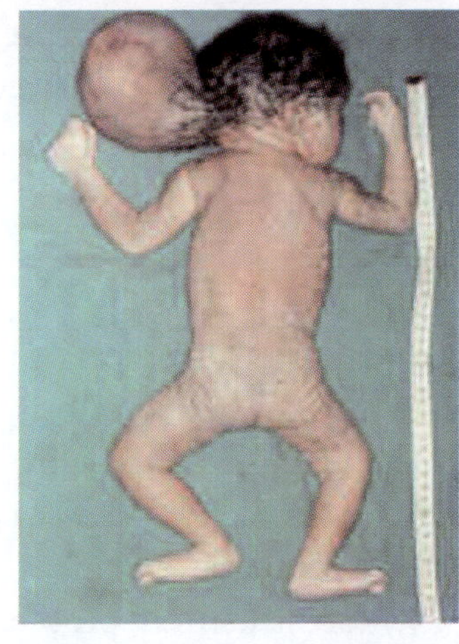

(a)

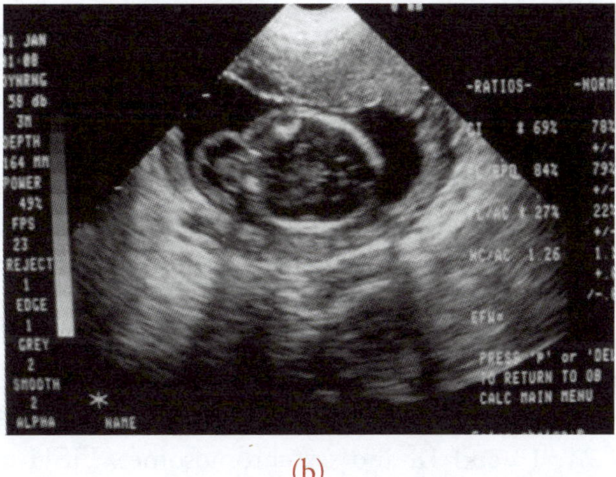

(b)

Fig. 14.7 Encephalocele a: Third trimester
b: Ultrasound picture of encephalocele (early second trimester).

Down syndrome

This syndrome occurs when either the whole or a segment of the long arm of chromosome 21 is present in three copies instead of two. Among all the trisomies, screening for Down syndrome is useful because this fetus usually survives with mental and physical disabilities. Trisomy 13 and 18 are generally lethal and are easily detectable by ultrasound because of the associated multiple anomalies. Sonographic findings in Down syndrome are more subtle and less conspicuous.

The association of Down syndrome with advanced maternal age is well known. However if screening is based on age alone, it will detect only 20% of Down syndrome cases because 80% of the cases are born to mothers below the age of 35 years.

The incidence of Down syndrome is 1 in 700–800 births. Overall, the mother contributes the extra chromosome in 80% of cases and the father in 20%. Affected children have a characteristic facial appearance, mental retardation and may die young. They are prone to develop congenital heart disease and acute leukemia. The risk of Down syndrome increases with age: it is 1:300 at 35 years, 1:100 at 40 and 1:20 at age 45. About 5% are due to translocation. The risk of Down syndrome in the offspring is 10%

when the translocation is carried by the mother and 2.5% when carried by the father. The recurrence risk is low if the parents are not carriers.

Chromosomal and Genetic Analysis

Chromosomal and genetic disorders can be suspected based on clinical features but diagnosis is confirmed by karyotype. The changes in the chromosomes are evident on light microscopy. They can be further subdivided as numerical problems (for example, trisomy 21, 13,) or structural problems (deletion or translocation). Karyotype is an analysis of chromosomes which differentiates the different types of chromosomes and also identifies their structure. It is therefore useful to identify abnormal number and structural abnormalities like deletions, inversions, insertions or translocations. Some recent modifications in karyotype include chromosome painting and fluorescent in situ hybridisation (FISH). Chromosome painting enables the identification of a particular chromosome directly, while FISH identifies specific sites along the chromosome. Specific DNA probes are used here with a fluorescent label. FISH can detect microdeletions, aneuploidies of 21, 13 and 18 and sex chromosomes. FISH can be used in uncultured amniocytes and therefore can be used to detect chromosome aneuploidies rapidly. Quantitative fluorescent polymerase chain reaction (QF-PCR) is a recent technology which helps detect sex and autosomal aneuploidies.

Indications for fetal karyotype

The indications for performing a fetal karyotype are:

- advanced maternal age
- previous child with aneuploidy
- structural fetal defects
- symmetrical IUGR
- positive triple test or biochemical screening.

Single gene disorders can only be diagnosed by DNA analysis and not by karyotype. They have a clear pattern of inheritance. For molecular analysis, DNA is extracted from amniocytes, chorionic villi or fetal blood cells. Most inborn errors of metabolism are autosomal recessive or X-linked. These can be diagnosed by DNA analysis, estimations of enzymes in the villi or amniotic fluid. Intermediate metabolite estimation can be used in some cases. Polymerase chain reaction (PCR) is useful for the amplification of tiny quantities of DNA and permits the identification of specific DNA sequences.

Recent Advances in Prenatal Diagnosis

Identification of fetal cells in the maternal circulation

Fetal cells gain access to maternal circulation through placental villi. If fetal cells from the maternal circulation can be identified and used, many invasive prenatal diagnostic tests can be avoided. Fetal cells are collected from maternal blood by week 18, though they can be collected from week 12 onwards. Nucleated fetal cells obtained from maternal circulation include lymphocytes, RBCs and trophoblasts. Fetal cells may persist from previous pregnancies and sometimes only a few cells may be present.

Preimplantation genetic diagnosis

This is possible in IVF programmes where only healthy embryos are transferred to the uterine cavity after ruling out certain genetic disorders. Biopsy of the embryos in early cleavage stages not only prevents the transfer of genetic disease but also improves implantation rates. Polar body analysis or blastomere biopsy is used to identify the genes responsible for disorders such as thalassemia, sickle cell disease and X-linked disease. Using FISH, cytogenetic analysis of even a single cell can be performed.

Population screening

This entails the testing of the whole population to detect those at risk of a genetic disease. However, this is not practical and cost-effective. Hence, there are other alternatives such as prenatal screening, carrier detection and neonatal screening. Population screening for heterozygous carriers aims at identifying carriers who are at risk of having an affected child if the other parent is also a carrier.

Neonatal screening is being done for phenylketonuria and hypothyroidism. Once a diagnosis is made, specific treatment such as a phenylalanine-restricted diet or the administration of the thyroid hormone will prevent severe mental retardation. This permits early treatment for infants, thereby decreasing morbidity.

Cascade screening is the screening of all the relatives of an affected individual. The carrier pick-up rate is high.

Genetic Counselling

This is a communication process whereby information and advice regarding the genetic condition, consequences of the disorder, the probability of developing and transmitting it and the ways in which it can be ameliorated are given. Genetic information is usually documented in a family tree or a pedigree chart which helps one understand the inheritance pattern. During these sessions, the counsellor presents facts, discusses options and helps the couple to make decisions. A nondirective counselling should be done after prenatal diagnosis. In couples with a family history of a genetic disorder, genetic counselling helps them discuss reproductive options. Parents should be informed regarding the limitations of the prenatal tests. No single test or even a combination can exclude all abnormalities.

Prenatal Diagnostic Technique (PNDT) Act, 1994

Gender bias and prejudice against female babies led to large-scale female feticide in some parts of India in the 1990s. Prenatal diagnostic techniques have been misused for sex determination and termination of pregnancies with female fetuses. Female infanticide, which has existed for generations in some Indian states, has been replaced by female feticide with the advent of ultrasound and other prenatal diagnostic methods. The declining sex ratio has forced the government to enact an Act. The Indian Parliament passed the Prenatal Diagnostic Techniques (Regulation and Prevention of Misuse) act on September 20, 1994; it was implemented in 1996. This act was modified in 2003 to overcome certain discrepancies. With the implementation of this act, the use of sex selection techniques before and after conception as well as misuse of prenatal diagnostic techniques for selective abortions has been banned.

Diagnosis for inheritable or other disorders done during the antenatal period helps to:

- confirm that the baby is normal.
- plan a pregnancy for carriers of genetic disease.
- terminate the pregnancy if the fetus is abnormal.
- be prepared mentally, for an abnormal baby.
- decide the route of delivery.
- decrease perinatal mortality and morbidity.
- refer on time to higher centres for neonatal surgery.
- implement fetal therapy, if feasible.

Antenatal screening for fetal anomalies is the standard care today. Termination of pregnancy is an option when lethal anomalies are diagnosed. If the anomaly is compatible with life, optimal treatment can be offered in the neonatal period. The patient can be referred to tertiary centres where facilities are available. Obstetric decision-making is influenced by the presence of anomalies. Cesarean section for IUGR or fetal distress can be avoided in the presence of certain chromosomal anomalies. Fetal therapy is becoming a reality today. Certain anomalies such as diaphragmatic hernia, and meningocele are being treated by fetal surgery. Prior knowledge about the anomaly helps the parents cope with the birth of an abnormal baby.

KEY POINTS

- The prenatal diagnostic tests available in the first and second trimesters are of two types: noninvasive and invasive.
- The noninvasive screening tests identify the group at risk from the general population. Invasive tests such as CVS, amniocentesis and fetal blood sampling are performed to confirm the diagnosis of genetic disorders.
- Neural tube defects are the most common structural anomalies reported in India. MSAFP is used for screening. USG is used for both screening and diagnosis.
- Some major structural defects are detectable by ultrasound as early as by 12 weeks. They include anencephaly, major limb defects and conjoined twins.
- Down syndrome screening involves natural tube (NT) thickness by ultrasound in the first trimester and biochemical screening in both the first and second trimesters.
- NT thickness and biochemical screening have a high detection rate of 90% for Down syndrome.
- Confirmation of Down syndrome after positive biochemical or ultrasound screening is by karyotype. This is obtained with CVS in the first trimester or amniocentesis/cordocentesis in the second trimester.
- Single gene disorders are identified by DNA analysis while chromosomal disorders are diagnosed by karyotype.
- The PNDT Act prohibits sex selection before or after conception.
- Genetic counselling is mandatory before and after prenatal diagnosis.
- Prenatal diagnosis reduces perinatal mortality and morbidity. It helps in obstetric decision-making and reassures couples at risk when the fetus is normal.

QUESTIONS

Select the single most appropriate answer:

1. First trimester screening for Down syndrome includes all of the following tests *except*
   a. chorionic villius biopsy   c. serum β-hCG
   b. nuchal translucency   d. PAPP-A
2. Raised maternal serum AFP indicates all of the following *except*
   a. down syndrome   c. neural tube defect
   b. gastroschisis   d. omphalocele
3. Which of the following is *not* an ultrasound marker for trisomy 18?
   a. choroid plexus cyst   c. fetal growth restriction
   b. diaphragmatic hernia   d. short femur
4. Which of the following imaging technologies is useful for the detection of fetal anomalies in the presence of oligoamnios?
   a. 2D ultrasound   c. CT scan
   b. 3D ultrasound   d. MRI
5. Limb defect is a complication of
   a. amniocentesis   c. cordocentesis
   b. chorionic villus biopsy   d. fetoscopy
6. Fetal fibroblasts are examined in
   a. amniocentesis   c. cordocentesis
   b. chorionic villi biopsy   d. cephalocentesis
7. The incidence of neural tube defects in India is
   a. 1–5.4 per 1,000   c. 12–17.4 per 1,000
   b. 6–11.4 per 1,000   d. 18–23.4 per 1,000
8. The risk of Down syndrome in the offspring when the mother is a translocation carrier is
   a. 10%   b. 15%   c. 20%   d. 25%
9. Karyotyping is used for the detection of
   a. sickle cell anemia   c. translocation carrier
   b. thalassemia   d. Tay–Sachs disease
10. The recurrence risk of a neural tube defect after one affected pregnancy is
    a. 3%–5%   b. 7%–10%   c. 12%–15%   d. 18%–20%
11. FISH is useful for the detection of all of the following *except*
    a. fetal sex
    b. hemophilia
    c. microdeletions
    d. Turner syndrome

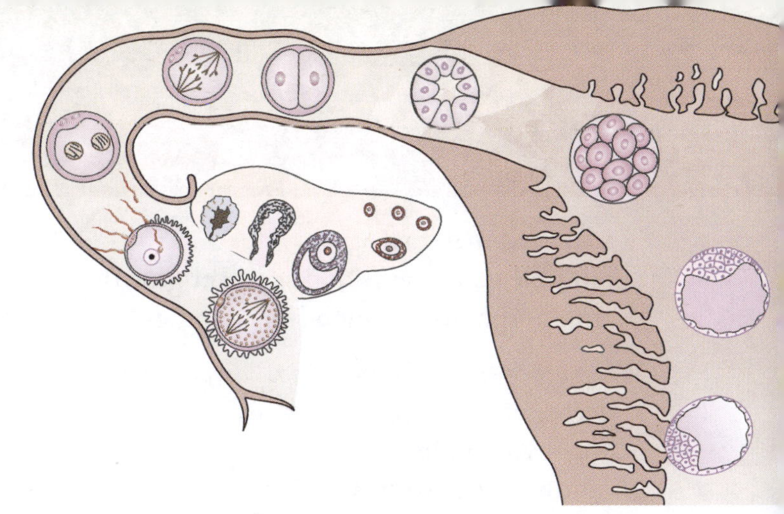

15

Antepartum Assessment of Fetal Wellbeing

S Habeebullah

LEARNING OBJECTIVES

At the end of this chapter, the reader should be able to:

- state the goal of fetal surveillance
- select women who need high-level surveillance
- enumerate the methods available for fetal surveillance
- state the period of gestation at which the tests should be initiated
- list the frequency of testing
- describe the procedure of the non-stress test (NST)
- list the components of a biophysical profile (BPP) and modified BPP
- interpret the results of the tests
- outline the management based on the test results

Introduction

Four decades ago, the mother was the only concern for obstetricians; the fetus was considered an accessory organ, and it was accepted that maternal wellbeing reflected fetal wellbeing. With a decrease in the maternal mortality rate, attention shifted to perinatal mortality. With advances in technology, it has become possible to understand fetal physiology and treat 'the fetus as a patient in its own right'. The clinical methods of assessment of fetal wellbeing have stood the test of time and continue to be of great value. Equipments such as ultrasound and cardiotocography machines provide an objective diagnosis and are also useful for their documentation value. However, it is pertinent to remember that the interpretation of the results of the tests is extremely important, and that most of them are useful in predicting '**fetal wellbeing**' rather than '**fetal distress**'.

Antepartum Fetal Monitoring

Over two-thirds of fetal deaths occur in the antepartum period: most of them occur in women who are at risk of uteroplacental insufficiency. This can be prevented by identifying the fetuses at risk and instituting maternal and fetal interventions. The goal of antepartum fetal surveillance is to avoid antepartum fetal death and perinatal morbidity by the early detection of fetal compromise.

The **indications** for antepartum fetal monitoring are:

High risk of uteroplacental insufficiency

prolonged pregnancy
hypertension complicating pregnancy
diabetes mellitus complicating pregnancy
previous stillbirth
IUGR

advanced maternal age
multiple gestation with discordant growth
antiphospholipid antibody syndrome

When other features suggest fetal compromise
decreased fetal movements
oligohydramnios
routine antepartum surveillance

Timing: In developed countries, antepartum fetal monitoring is initiated at 25–26 weeks of gestation; however, in developing countries like India, the monitoring starts at around 32 weeks. It may be initiated earlier in tertiary centres with intensive neonatal care facilities.

Methods: Clinical methods can assess fetal growth but cannot accurately predict fetal wellbeing.

Biochemical tests (serum HPL, urinary estriol) are timeconsuming and have poor sensitivity and hence are not useful for the assessment of fetal wellbeing in late pregnancy.

A number of biophysical tests have evolved during the last three decades. The basis for these tests is that an intact fetal central nervous system (CNS) is essential for any fetal biophysical activity. In the presence of hypoxia, the fetal CNS is depressed.

The biophysical tests include:

- Daily fetal movement count (DFMC)
- Contraction stress test (CST)
- Non-stress test (NST)
- Fetal biophysical profile (BPP)
- Doppler velocimetry.

Daily fetal movement count (DFMC)

The basis for this test is that 80% of the fetal movements are perceived by the mother. The periods of active movements last up to 40 minutes. Reduced fetal movement may be associated with fetal death in 24 hours. Fetal sleep state and administration of narcotic drugs to the mother may reduce the fetal movements.

Cardiff count to ten: The pregnant woman is asked to count the fetal movements starting from 9 am till she perceives ten movements. If it takes longer than 12 hours or no movements are perceived, she should report for further evaluation.

Sadovsky count: The pregnant woman is asked to count fetal movements for one hour after food three times in a day. That is multiplied by four to arrive at a 12-hour count. If the DFMC is less than 10 in 12 hours, it is taken as abnormal and should be followed by further evaluation.

The advantages of these tests are that they are simple, inexpensive and can be applied in routine antepartum surveillance in low-risk populations; however, the sensitivity of these tests is low.

Contraction stress test (CST)

It was first described by Ray and colleagues in 1972 and is also known as the oxytocin challenge test. It is a test of uteroplacental function and tests the ability of the fetus to withstand the stress of labour.

Principle: Physiologically, the reduction in blood flow to the intervillous space during uterine contractions does not compromise the fetal heart rate. In the presence of uteroplacental insufficiency, these contractions elicit late decelerations of the fetal heart rate. This correlates well with stillbirth, low Apgar score and IUGR.

Contraindications: History of preterm labour, PROM, placenta previa, cervical incompetence, multiple pregnancy and previous classical cesarean section contraindicate this test.

Procedure: After obtaining consent, external monitors to record fetal heart rate (FHR) and uterine contractions are connected, with the patient in the left lateral position. Dilute IV oxytocin is started at the rate of 0.5 mU/min and doubled every 20 minutes till 3 contractions in 10 minutes (each lasting for 40–60 seconds) are obtained. Alternatively, contractions can also be induced by rubbing the nipples through clothes for five minutes (**nipple stimulation test**).

Interpretation:

Negative	No late decelerations and normal FHR tracings
Positive	Presence of late decelerations with ≥50% of uterine contractions
Unsatisfactory	<3 contractions in 10 minutes

Hyperstimulation	5 or more contractions/10 min or each lasting more than 90 sec
Suspicious	Inconsistent late decelerations.

A positive test should be followed by other tests like BPP; negative test may be followed by weekly NST. Suspicious/unsatisfactory test has to be repeated within 24 hours.

Disadvantages:

- It has a high incidence of false positives: this may lead to unnecessary intervention.
- It is time-consuming (90 minutes) and cumbersome.
- It may result in preterm labour.

Non-stress test (NST)

Freeman and Lee (1975) introduced the NST to describe FHR accelerations in response to fetal movements as a sign of fetal health. Currently, NST is the most commonly used test for fetal wellbeing.

Principle: The sympathetic and parasympathetic components of the autonomic nervous system control fetal cardiac behaviour. A healthy fetus shows fluctuations and oscillations in the baseline FHR. Accelerations of FHR will occur with fetal movement, uterine contractions or in response to external stimuli. This appears to be a reflection of CNS alertness and activity. Fetal sleep, CNS depressants (narcotics), chronic smoking and hypoxia modify these responses.

Procedure: NST is performed on an outpatient basis using an external monitor. The fetal heart rate is recorded in the sitting or reclining position with lateral tilt. Fetal movements are marked on recording paper by the patient herself. The test may be continued for 20 minutes during which time at least two FHR accelerations of ≥15 bpm lasting for ≥15 seconds should be recorded. When there are no fetal movements, the test can be continued for up to 40 minutes keeping in mind the fetal sleep state. While evaluating the trace, baseline FHR, FHR variability, accelerations/decelerations and abnormal patterns if any, should be noted.

Interpretation:

Reactive : Normal baseline FHR (120–160 bpm), normal variability (5–20 bpm), at

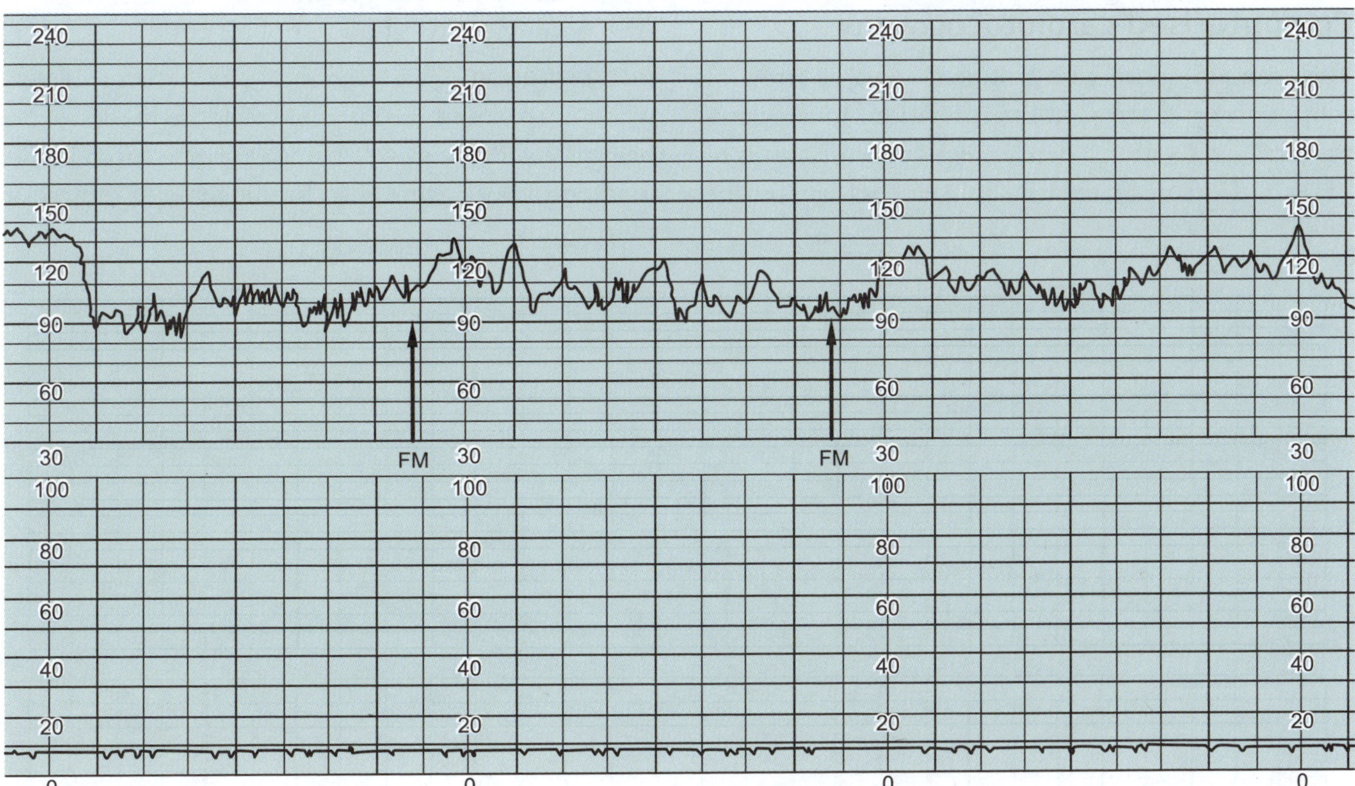

Fig. 15.1 Reactive NST.

least two accelerations and absence of spontaneous decelerations (**Fig. 15.1**)

Nonreactive : Baseline FHR <120 or >160 bpm, reduced baseline variability (<5 bpm), presence of decelerations and absence of accelerations even after 40 minutes (**Fig. 15.2**)

Unsatisfactory: No fetal movements even after 40 minutes of observation

If NST is reactive, it is usually **repeated weekly**. However, in high-risk conditions like PIH or diabetes, it may be repeated twice or thrice a week. **A nonreactive NST should be followed by CST or BPP.**

Disadvantages: NST carries a high false positive rate, especially if the test is performed on a preterm fetus.

Vibroacoustic stimulation test (VAST)

An unsatisfactory NST should be repeated using vibroacoustic stimulation which involves the use of electronic artificial larynx 82dB with a frequency of 80 Hz. Routine use of VAST reduces the testing time considerably.

Computerised cardiotocography

This test is short (10 minutes) and is free of subjectivity and errors in interpretation. It calculates the rate, accelerations, decelerations and variations of FHR and incorporates fetal movements felt by the mother.

Fetal biophysical profile scoring (BPPS)

This test was described by Manning et al (1980) using real-time ultrasound to monitor various fetal biophysical activities. In hypoxia and acidosis, the fetus loses the biophysical variables in the reverse order in which they are acquired in the course of fetal development: presence of late decelerations → absence of accelerations → reduced breathing movements → reduced body movements → absent fetal tone.

Components: They include NST, fetal movement (FM), fetal tone (FT), fetal breathing movement (FBM) and amniotic fluid volume (AF).

Test	Normal criteria
NST	≥2 accelerations ≥15 bpm for ≥15 seconds in 20–40 minutes
FBM	≥1 episode of rhythmic breathing lasting ≥ 30 seconds in 30 minutes
FM	≥3 discrete body or limb movements within 30 minutes
FT	≥1 episode of extension of extremity with return to flexion or opening and closing of hand within 30 minutes
AF	Single vertical pocket of ≥2 cm

Interpretation: Each variable gets a score of two when normal and zero if abnormal, the highest score being 10 and the lowest being 0. These variables are markers of both acute and chronic hypoxia (amniotic fluid volume).

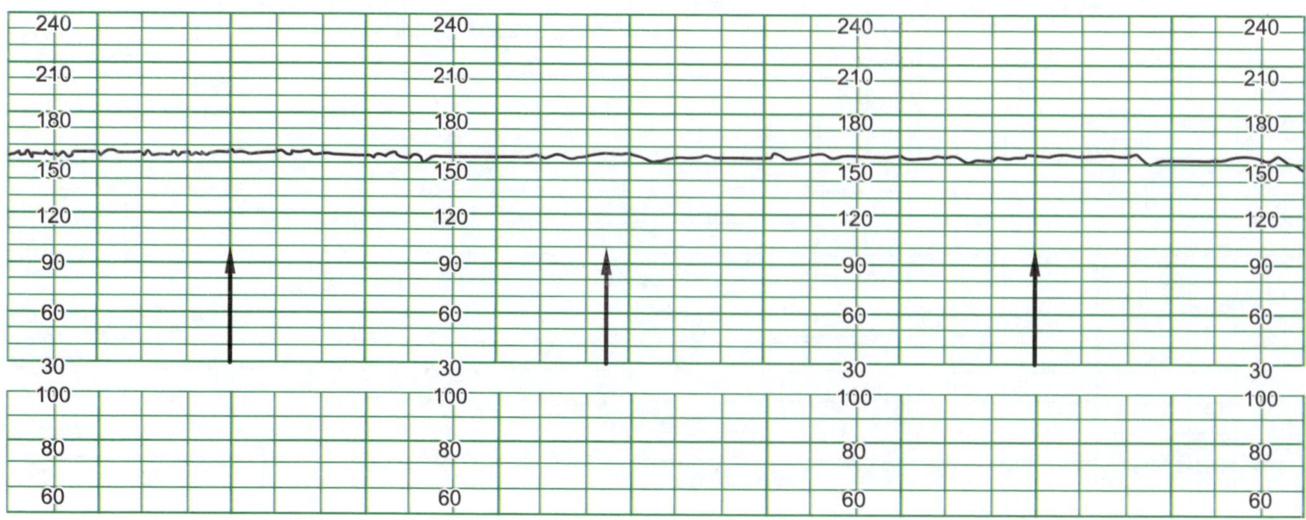

Fig. 15.2 Nonreactive NST.

Management based on BPP scores is shown in **Table 15.1**.

Advantages: The advantages are:

- Normal variables are highly predictive of good perinatal outcome.
- It can predict fetal jeopardy in terms of acute and chronic hypoxia.
- It can detect fetal anomalies and predict chorioamnionitis.

Disadvantages:

- The USG machine is required to perform the test.
- Time-consuming; the fetal sleep state can further prolong the test period.
- The test is not reliable in cases of polyhydramnios.

Modified biophysical profile

It consists of NST and amniotic fluid index (AFI); the former reflects acute, the latter chronic, hypoxia. An AFI below 5 cm is considered abnormal. Modified BPP reduces the duration of testing without affecting the benefits of BPP. It is observed that if the NST is reactive, the BPP will be ≥8 in 95% of cases. A reactive NST is generally associated with good perinatal outcome. If BPP is less than 5, there are no instances of reactive NST.

Doppler velocimetry

The principle of Doppler is that when sound waves strike a moving object (like RBCs in blood vessels) their frequency is changed proportional to the velocity and direction of the moving object. Various fetal blood vessels are used to measure Doppler flow velocity, the most common being the umbilical artery which reflects the resistance of blood flow within the placenta. The commonly used indices are: systolic (S)/diastolic (D) velocity ratio, pulsatality index (PI) and resistance index (RI). In normal pregnancy, as the pregnancy progresses, the S/D ratio and the PI decrease. Normal S/D ratio in the third trimester is 1.5–2.5. In pathological states with increased vascular resistance of fetoplacental unit like preeclampsia and IUGR, there is increase in S/D ratio and PI. In severe cases there may be absence (**Fig. 15.3**) or even reversal of end diastolic flow (**Fig. 15.4**) which warrants termination of pregnancy.

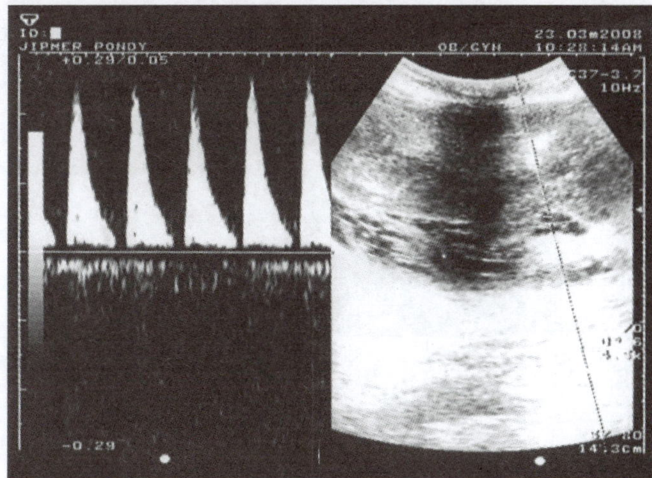

Fig. 15.3 Absent diastolic flow.

Table 15.1 BPP scoring and recommended management (Manning et al 1987)

BPP score	Interpretation	Recommended management
10	Normal, non-asphyxiated	Repeat weekly or twice weekly
8 with normalamniotic fluid	Normal, non-asphyxiated	Repeat testing depends on clinical situation
8 with oligohydramnios	Suspicious of chronic fetal hypoxia	If >37 weeks ⟶ deliver; otherwise repeat testing
6	Possible fetal hypoxia	If amniotic fluid volume is abnormal ⟶ deliver If amniotic fluid is normal ⟶ repeat test If repeat test ≤6 ⟶ deliver If repeat test >6 repeat testing as per protocol
4	Probable fetal hypoxia	Repeat testing on same day; if ≤6 ⟶ deliver
	Almost certain fetal hypoxia	Deliver

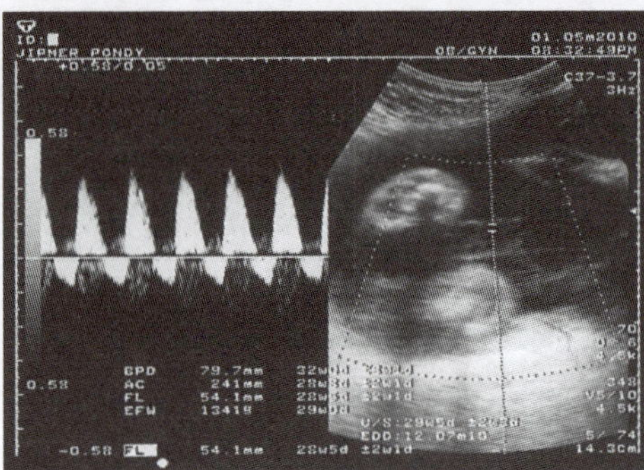

Fig. 15.4 Reversed end diastolic flow.

Prolonged fetal hypoxia due to uteroplacental insufficiency results in redistribution of blood flow to vital organs of the fetus, resulting in decreased resistance in the fetal brain (can be detected by imaging the middle cerebral artery) and increased resistance in the umbilical vein. These changes may occur three weeks before the FHR abnormalities manifest. So, Doppler velocimetry is not used as a screening test but as an adjunct to standard methods of fetal monitoring.

KEY POINTS

- Although subjective, DFMC is a simple, inexpensive method of fetal testing. If abnormal, it should be followed by other tests like NST.
- NST involves acceleration of FHR in response to fetal movement or stimulation. This is the most commonly used test in clinical practice.
- NST can be performed 2–3 times a week in high-risk conditions like IUGR and diabetes mellitus.
- VAST can be used for fetal stimulation in cases of unsatisfactory NST.
- NST is a test of fetal condition; CST is a test of placental insufficiency.
- BPP or modified BPP has higher positive predictive value than NST; they are the tests for both acute and chronic hypoxia.
- Doppler is mainly used in the evaluation of IUGR fetuses. Absent and reverse end diastolic flow velocity in the umbilical artery is associated with increased perinatal morbidity and mortality.

QUESTIONS

Select the single most appropriate answer:

1. During NST, if no fetal movements are noted, the test result is
   a. fetal distress
   b. nonreactive
   c. reactive
   d. unsatisfactory
2. In early labour, if the CTG shows persistent early decelerations, one should suspect
   a. cephalopelvic disproportion
   b. cord compression
   c. placental insufficiency
   d. fetal distress
3. In the CTG, a sinusoidal pattern of FHR indicates
   a. fetal distress
   b. cord compression
   c. fetal anemia
   d. placental insufficiency
4. Which of the following indicates oligohydramnios?
   a. amniotic fluid index <10 cm
   b. single vertical pocket <5 cm
   c. single vertical pocket <3 cm
   d. amniotic fluid index <5 cm
5. Modified biophysical profile refers to
   a. non-stress test + amniotic fluid index
   b. non-stress test + fetal breathing movement
   c. fetal breathing movement + fetal tone
   d. fetal tone + amniotic fluid index

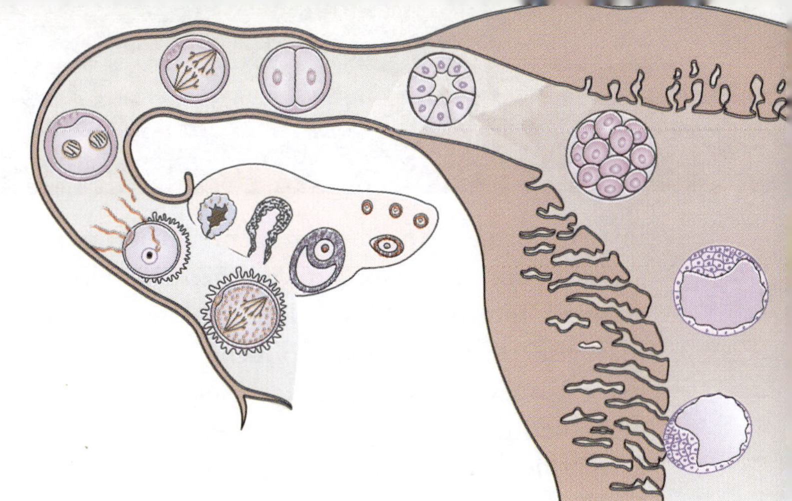

16

Abortion

Raksha Arora

LEARNING OBJECTIVES

At the end of this chapter, the reader should be able to:

- define abortion
- identify various causes of abortion
- understand the pathology of abortion
- enumerate different clinical types of abortions
- list the clinical features and investigations
- list the complications of abortion
- describe the management of abortion

Introduction

Human reproduction is relatively inefficient and abortion or miscarriage is the most common complication of pregnancy. The incidence is approximately 15% in pregnancies that are clinically recognised. Abortion is defined as the process of termination of pregnancy, either spontaneous or intentional, before the fetus develops sufficiently to survive (called the period of viability), that is, 20 weeks. This cut-off point varies according to state laws for reporting abortions, fetal and neonatal deaths. In India, the period of viability is considered to be 28 weeks; so, by definition, all pregnancies ending before 28 weeks are included under abortions.

Etiology

More than 80% of abortions occur in the first 12 weeks of pregnancy and approximately 50% result from chromosomal abnormalities. Abortions may be due to fetal, maternal and paternal factors.

Fetal factors

Abnormal zygote development: Early spontaneous abortions commonly demonstrate a developmental abnormality of the zygote, embryo, early fetus or sometimes the placenta.

Aneuploid abortion: About 50%–60% of embryos and early fetuses that are spontaneously aborted have chromosomal abnormalities. Autosomal trisomy is the most frequently identified anomaly associated with first trimester abortions. Trisomy 13, 16, 18, 21 and 22 has been found to be common. Monosomy X, triploidy, tetraploidy and chromosomal structural abnormalities are the other types of aneuploid abortions.

Euploid abortion: This usually occurs later in gestation and tends to increase with maternal age.

Maternal factors

Infections: Many severe maternal infections have been reported to cause spontaneous abortion, probably due to maternal pyrexia or bacteremia. Viral infections such as rubella and cytomegalovirus in early pregnancy produce congenital malformations and abortion. Influenza and the hepatitis virus and parasitic infections like malaria and toxoplasmosis may also cause abortion. Spirochetes cause second trimester abortions. Recently, bacterial vaginosis has been incriminated in second trimester abortions.

Endocrine abnormalities: Hypothyroidism and insulin-dependent diabetes with poor glycemic control increase the risk of abortion. Progesterone deficiency in terms of luteal phase defect has also been suggested as a cause of abortion.

Drugs and environmental factors: Teratogenic drugs, when used in the first trimester, may increase the risk of abortion. Tobacco, alcohol and caffeine, if consumed in large amounts, ionising radiation and environmental toxins like pesticides, arsenic, lead, formaldehyde, benzene and nitrous oxide are also abortifacients.

Stress: Abdominal trauma, extensive surgery and emotional stress can also increase the risk of abortion.

Immunological factors: Phospholipid antibodies such as lupus anticoagulant and anticardiolipin antibodies have been implicated in spontaneous abortion, particularly in the second trimester. Various alloimmune disorders have been shown to cause recurrent abortions.

Uterine malformations: Bicornuate or septate uterus, cervical incompetence and submucous fibroids may cause second trimester abortions.

Idiopathic: The exact cause may not be known in about 25% of cases.

Paternal factors

Little is known about paternal factors in the genesis of spontaneous abortion although abortion could be associated with chromosomal abnormalities in the sperm.

Pathology

There is hemorrhage into the decidua basalis, followed by necrosis of tissues adjacent to the bleeding. If it occurs early in the pregnancy, the ovum detaches and is expelled once the uterine contractions begin. When the gestation sac is opened, fluid is commonly found surrounding a small macerated fetus; sometimes no fetus is visible. This is generally referred to as 'blighted ovum'. In later abortions, either the retained fetus gets macerated or the fetus gets compressed and desiccated once the amniotic fluid is absorbed. This may lead to **fetus papyraceus.**

Types of Abortions

Abortions can be classified depending on the clinical stage, the reason for abortion and whether there is associated infection. It may also be classified based on local laws. The clinical types are shown in **Table 16.1**.

Threatened abortion

This is a common type of abortion diagnosed in as many as 25% of pregnant women in whom the process of abortion has just started and may not result in expulsion of the products of conception (**Fig. 16.1**).

Symptoms:

- amenorrhea
- vaginal bleeding
- lower abdominal pain or lower back pain
- may occur repeatedly over many days
- no history of passage of products of conception.

Signs:

- General condition depends on the amount of blood loss.
- Uterus corresponds to the period of amenorrhea and contractions may be perceived.
- Speculum examination reveals a congested cervix with or without bleeding.

Table 16.1 Types of abortion

Clinical types	Based on onset	Based on complication
• Threatened • Inevitable • Incomplete • Complete • Missed • Recurrent	• Spontaneous • Induced • Medical termination of pregnancy or legal abortion • Illegal abortion	• Febrile or septic • Non-septic

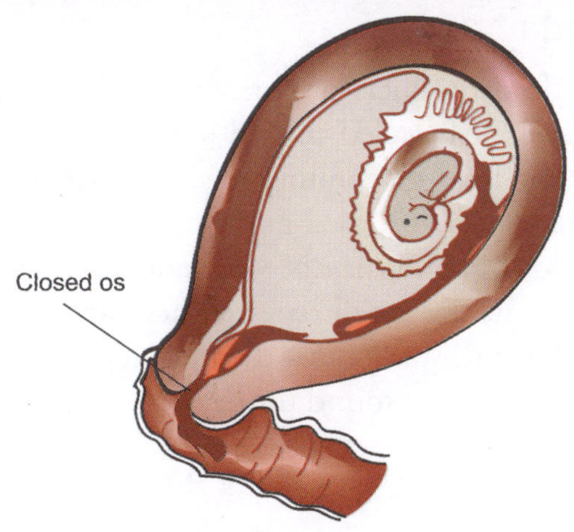

Fig. 16.1 Threatened abortion.

- On bimanual examination, the cervix is closed.

Investigations:
- to assess general condition
- ultrasound to ascertain if the embryo or fetus is alive and normal and to differentiate from other conditions.

Differential diagnosis:
- ectopic pregnancy to be ruled out in all women presenting with history of amenorrhea, pain and bleeding; in threatened abortion, bleeding starts before the onset of abdominal pain and is heavier.
- delayed period
- molar pregnancy and other types of abortions
- local lesions like cervical erosion, polyp or growth and severe vaginal infections.

Treatment: In a clinically diagnosed threatened abortion, the general condition of the mother and status of the embryo or fetus by ultrasound will determine the course of action. If blood loss is excessive or fetal cardiac activity is absent or the fetus shows major anomalies, pregnancy is terminated. The method of termination depends on the period of gestation.

If cardiac activity is present and the bleeding does not affect the condition of the mother, conservative treatment is adopted: bed rest, analgesics, sedatives and tranquilisers, that is, 30 mg of phenobarbitone or 5 mg of diazepam twice daily may be beneficial. A sympathetic attitude with continuing support and follow-up are very important. Strenuous physical activity and sexual intercourse should be avoided.

Inevitable abortion

When pregnancy cannot be continued due to separation of products from the uterine wall and the cervical os is open, it is termed inevitable abortion (**Fig. 16.2**).

Symptoms:
- excessive bleeding following a period of amenorrhea
- aggravation of pain in the lower abdomen which may be intermittent and severe in intensity.

Signs:
- General condition will depend on the amount of blood loss.
- Uterus corresponds to the period of pregnancy.
- Speculum examination shows fresh bleeding through a dilated os.
- When the duration of pregnancy is more than 12 weeks, a bag of membranes may be seen bulging through the os or drainage of liquor may be visible.

Treatment:
- This is an emergency and has to be managed very promptly to avoid excessive hemorrhage.
- An injection of morphine 10–15 mg is given intramuscularly as soon as the diagnosis is made.
- Intravenous access is secured and blood reserved.
- Suction evacuation is done if the pregnancy is less than 12 weeks.

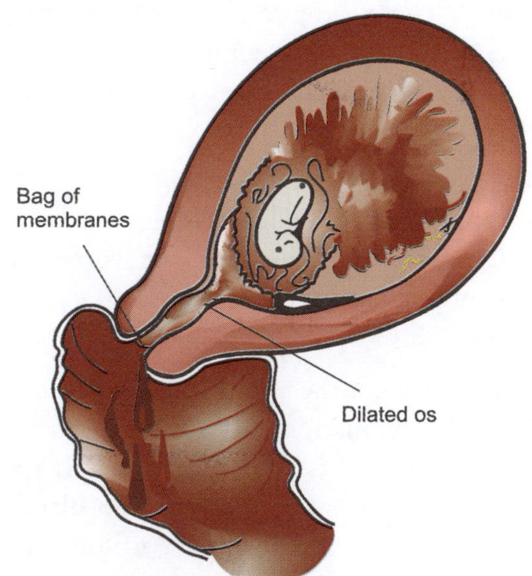

Fig. 16.2 Inevitable abortion.

- Oxytocin drip with 10–20 units in 500 ml of Ringer lactate is started if the pregnancy is more than 12 weeks. Intramuscular prostaglandin $F_2\alpha$ in doses of 250 μg 3–4 hourly is also useful to facilitate expulsion.
- Blood transfusion may be given if the patient is already anemic or is bleeding profusely.

Incomplete abortion

This condition is diagnosed when the products of conception are partly expelled.

Symptoms: In addition to those described above:

- history of expulsion of products of conception
- persistent vaginal bleeding and pain.

Signs:

- The general condition will depend on the blood loss.
- Speculum shows bleeding and products through the open os.
- Vaginal examination reveals that the cervix is open and uterus size is less than that for the corresponding period of pregnancy.

Treatment: It is similar to that for inevitable abortion since this condition is also an emergency.

Complete abortion

When the products of conception have been fully expelled, it is termed complete abortion.

Symptoms: There is a history of expulsion of products of conception accompanied by relief from pain in the abdomen and reduction in vaginal bleeding.

Signs:

- The general condition depends on the blood loss.
- Uterus is smaller than that for corresponding period of pregnancy.
- Os is closed.

Treatment: Once the products are completely expelled, the woman is advised to return for a follow-up visit, and is firm hematinics. If there is any doubt about the completeness, an ultrasound examination may be done. Antibiotics may be prescribed if there is a risk or presence of infection.

Missed abortion

When dead products of conception are retained in the uterus, it is called missed abortion. Beyond 12 weeks, the fetus gets mummified or macerated once the liquor gets absorbed and the placenta becomes pale, and thin and may become adherent. However, before 12 weeks, small repeated hemorrhages in the choriodecidual space cause disruption of the villi and the clotted blood around the dead ovum may remain as a fleshy or carneous mole.

Symptoms:

- amenorrhea followed by bleeding
- persistence of dark vaginal bleeding
- regression of pregnancy symptoms such as morning sickness and fetal movements.

Signs:

- Uterine size is less than that corresponding to the period of amenorrhea.
- Speculum examination shows thick dark bleeding through the closed os.
- On bimanual examination, the cervix does not feel soft as in a normal pregnancy, the uterus is smaller than it should be and feels firm.

Investigations:

- routine blood and urine examination as in threatened abortion
- USG to confirm missed abortion (empty gestation sac [blighted ovum] or fetus with no cardiac activity)
- plasma fibrinogen level to exclude coagulopathy.

Treatment: Management can be termination of pregnancy or expectant.

- Expectant treatment may be chosen with the hope of spontaneous expulsion of the products of conception. It may not be prolonged beyond 3–4 weeks to prevent coagulation defects or if the patient wishes for evacuation of the uterus.
- Before 12 weeks of pregnancy, medical treatment in the form of PGE_1 (vaginal misoprostol 200 μg, 4-hourly) can be given till the products are expelled. Alternatively, surgical treatment is by dilatation and evacuation.
- If it occurs after more than 12 weeks of pregnancy, abortion has to be induced with prostaglandin

E_2 or E_1 or laminaria tent followed by 250 µg of carboprost intramuscularly or oxytocin drip till the products are expelled.

Septic abortion

When the products of conception become infected followed by spread of infection to the endometrium, parametrium and peritoneum, it is called septic abortion. This is a common cause of maternal morbidity and mortality in India. It is commonly seen when an abortion is illegally induced (and is performed by untrained personnel); however, it may occur even after spontaneous abortion or medical termination of pregnancy.

Pathogenesis: The causative microorganisms are endogenous anerobes (Bacterioides, Streptococci, *Clostridium welchii* and *C tetani*) or aerobes (*E coli*, *Klebsiella*, *Staphylococcus* and *Pseudomonas*); these microorganisms are present in the vagina and become pathogenic whenever the patient's resistance is lowered or there is tissue trauma (for example, in induced abortion).

Clinicopathological grading: According to the extent of spread of infection, septic abortion may be classified as:

Grade I: The infection is localised to the products of conception or sometimes localised endomyometritis.

Grade II: The spread of infection goes beyond the uterus to the parametrium, fallopian tubes and ovaries or pelvic peritoneum.

Grade III: There is generalised peritonitis and/or septicemia, jaundice or acute renal failure.

Symptoms:
- history of abortion, spontaneous or induced
- fever
- pain abdomen
- offensive vaginal discharge
- symptoms of complications like shock and renal failure.

Signs:
- tachycardia, pyrexia, anemia and hypotension
- tenderness, guarding and rigidity in case of peritonitis
- speculum examination may reveal evidence of trauma or offensive purulent discharge
- uterus tender in grade I; thickening and tenderness in the fornices noted in grade II septic abortion.

Investigations:
- hematological tests like hemoglobin, hematocrit, total and differential counts and tests for coagulation status
- blood biochemistry for renal and liver function including serum electrolytes
- culture of blood, urine and cervical or high vaginal swab with antibiotic sensitivity
- ultrasound of abdomen and pelvis to exclude retained products or peritoneal fluid or pus.

Treatment: The aim of treatment is to control sepsis and to provide supportive therapy. The management will depend on the condition of the patient.

Grade I: A combination of ampicillin, gentamicin and metronidazole is given to cover Gram-positive, Gram-negative and anerobic organisms. The dose of ampicillin is 500 mg IV 6-hourly and that of gentamicin is 1.5 mg/kg IV 8-hourly. Metronidazole is given as 500 mg IV 8-hourly.
- Under cover of antibiotics, the source of infection (products of conception) should be removed by evacuation as early as possible.
- Blood transfusion, as indicated.

Grade II: In addition to antibiotics and evacuation of the uterus, colpotomy may be required if pus collects in the pouch of Douglas.

Grade III:
- Intensive clinical monitoring is done by noting the pulse, respiration, temperature, blood pressure and urine output.
- Supportive therapy is started to treat generalised peritonitis by gastric suction and intravenous fluids.
- Aggressive antibiotic therapy with higher antibiotics like cephalosphorins and amikacin is carried out.
- Laparotomy is indicated if perforation of the uterus, injury to viscera or peritonitis is suspected.

Recurrent abortion

Recurrent abortion or recurrent pregnancy loss is defined as a loss of three or more pregnancies. It is a distressing problem affecting about 1% of all women. Maternal age and previous number of abortions are two independent risk factors for further miscarriage.

Investigations:

- parental karyotyping: The couple should be referred to a geneticist if there is any abnormality
- cytogenetic analysis of products of conception after abortion
- pelvic ultrasound to rule out uterine malformations and submucous fibroids
- glucose tolerance test
- detection of antiphospholipid antibodies: Lupus anticoagulant (LA) and anticardiolipin antibodies (ACA)
- screening for bacterial vaginosis
- toxoplasma, rubella, cytomegalovirus and herpes
- routine TORCH screening is not recommended as these infections do not cause recurrent abortions.

Treatment: If the patient presents with a history of recurrent pregnancy loss, but is not pregnant, an attempt is made to find out and treat the cause, for example, metroplasty for bicornuate uterus, hysteroscopic removal of uterine septum or myomectomy for submucous fibroid.

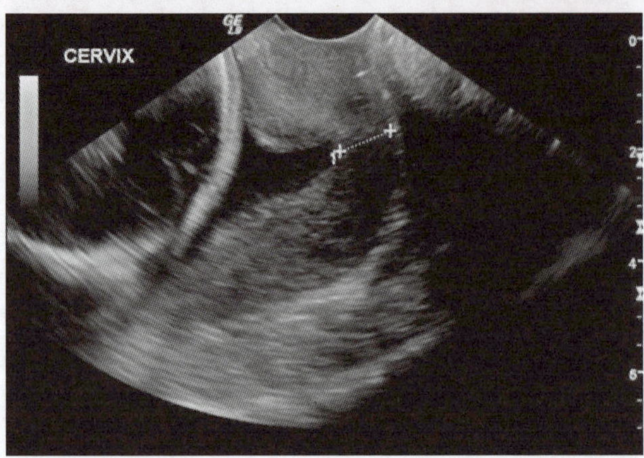

Fig. 16.3 Incompetent os.

If the patient has come in the first trimester, USG is done to confirm pregnancy and fetal cardiac activity. Investigations depend on the period of pregnancy when the patient had the previous loss. Patients with antiphospholipid antibodies are treated with heparin and low-dose aspirin.

In the second trimester of pregnancy, incompetent os (**Fig. 16.3**) may be suspected if the patient reports a history of painless abortion. Speculum examination may reveal the cervical os to be open and cervical length may be short. The treatment of incompetent os is cerclage operation in which a non-absorbable encircling suture is placed around the internal os. The suture is removed at 38 weeks of pregnancy or whenever the patient goes in to labour.

KEY POINTS

- Abortion is one of the most common complications of pregnancy, with an incidence of 15% among clinically recognised pregnancies.
- First trimester abortions are the most common and 50% result from chromosomal abnormalities. Maternal infections, drugs, uterine malformations and immunological factors are the other etiological factors.
- No cause may be found in about 25% of cases.
- Ectopic pregnancy must be ruled out.
- The different clinical types of abortions are threatened, inevitable incomplete, complete and missed.
- Septic abortion can result from spontaneous abortion; however, it commonly occurs following illegally induced abortion.
- Threatened abortion is managed conservatively, whereas termination is the intervention in inevitable and incomplete abortion.
- Recurrent abortion should be investigated before instituting treatment.

QUESTIONS

Select the single most appropriate answer:

1. Most spontaneous abortions occur before which week of pregnancy?
   a. 15 weeks
   b. 14 weeks
   c. 13 weeks
   d. 12 weeks
2. Approximately 50% of abortions are caused by
   a. maternal hypothyroidism
   b. chromosomal abnormalities
   c. maternal toxoplasmosis
   d. incompetent cervical os
3. An inevitable abortion can be clinically differentiated from a threatened abortion by
   a. closed cervical os
   b. increased bleeding
   c. absence of membranes
   d. open cervical os
4. What percentage of all clinically diagnosed pregnancies end in abortion?
   a. 5% b. 10% c. 15% d. 20%
5. The most common cause of early abortion is
   a. maternal diabetes mellitus
   b. abnormal zygote development
   c. corpus luteum insufficiency
   d. maternal thyroid disorder
6. All of the following are characteristic of threatened abortion *except*
   a. presence of vaginal bleeding
   b. pain in lower abdomen
   c. cervical os is open
   d. uterus corresponds to the period of gestation

In the following questions, there are two statements. Select the appropriate answer using the following key:

a. if both statements are true and causally related
b. if both statements are true but not causally related
c. if the first statement is true and the second is false
d. if the first statement is false and the second is true
e. if both statements are false

7. A woman with a missed abortion must undergo evacuation of the uterus *because*

   A woman with a missed abortion is likely to suffer from disseminated intravascular coagulation.
8. An incomplete abortion need not be evacuated *because*

   An incomplete abortion will always be completed spontaneously.

Select the appropriate answer using the following key:

a. if only responses 1, 2 and 3 are correct
b. if only 1 and 3 are correct
c. if only 2 and 4 are correct
d. if only 4 is correct
e. if all are correct

9. In a woman with recurrent pregnancy loss, which of the following laboratory investigations must be performed?
   1. glucose tolerance test
   2. immunological tests
   3. parental chromosomal studies
   4. screening for torch infections
10. The management of recurrent pregnancy loss in a woman who tests positive for antiphospholipid antibodies should be with
    1. cervical cerclage and low-dose aspirin
    2. progestogens and heparin
    3. progestogens and low-dose aspirin
    4. heparin and low-dose aspirin

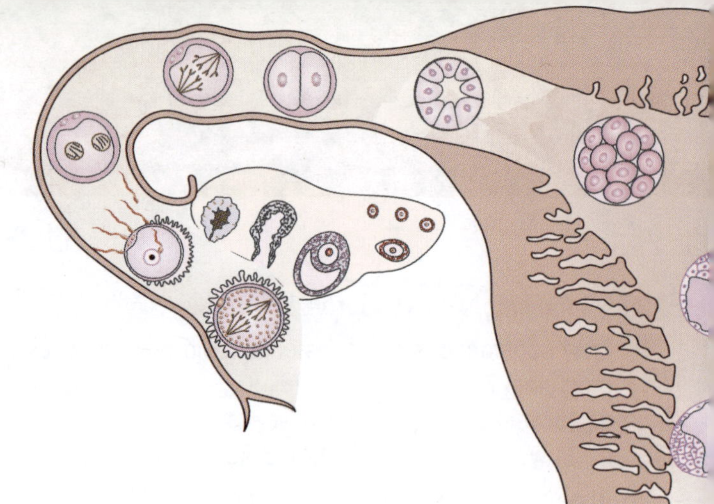

17

Medical Termination of Pregnancy

Kamala Ganesh

LEARNING OBJECTIVES

At the end of this chapter, the reader should be able to:

- define medical termination of pregnancy
- appreciate the reasons why the MTP Act was framed
- follow the guidelines for providing MTP
- list the indications for MTP
- enumerate the methods currently in use for terminating first and second trimester pregnancies
- describe the criteria for selecting women for MTP and understand the need for counselling
- describe briefly the procedures for the termination of pregnancy in the first trimester
- list the complications, their prevention and management
- provide follow-up services after MTP

Introduction

From time immemorial, abortion has been resorted to for unwanted pregnancies, often without legal and social sanction. Concerns were raised in India by Central Family Planning Board over the large number of illegal abortions performed in unsafe conditions, leading to significant mortality and morbidity among young women. In order to prevent the untoward consequences of unsafe abortion, the Medical Termination of Pregnancy Act (MTP Act) was passed by Parliament in 1971 and implemented in 1972. MTP Rules were notified in 1975 and were amended in 2003.

Medical termination of pregnancy (MTP) may be defined as the wilful termination of pregnancy before 20 weeks.

Guidelines for Providing MTP Services

The MTP Act and Rules have laid down specific conditions to ensure that voluntary abortion is made safe.

Indications for MTP

A pregnancy can be terminated when the doctor is convinced that:

- the continuation of pregnancy endangers the life of the woman or will cause grave injury to her physical and mental health.
- the baby is at risk of having serious physical or mental abnormalities.

- the pregnancy has resulted from rape.
- the pregnancy is due to failure of contraception.

Qualification and registration of the provider

A medical practitioner registered with the State Medical Council/Indian Medical Council with any one of the following qualifications is permitted to provide services for MTP if:

- He/she has completed six months of housemanship in obstetrics and gynecology. He/she has done a housemanship of one year at any hospital in the practice of obstetrics and gynecology.
- He/she possesses a postgraduate degree/diploma in obstetrics and gynecology.
- He/she has assisted a qualified practitioner in 25 MTP procedures in a training institution approved by the government.
- He/she has registered in the State Medical Council/ Indian Medical Council before the commencement of the MTP Act, with more than three years of experience in the practice of obstetrics and gynecology.

The place where pregnancy can be terminated

In order to provide MTP services, it is mandatory that a health centre or nursing home should have certain facilities. Therefore, MTP can be provided only at:

- a hospital established and maintained by the government
- a place or hospital approved for this purpose by the government.

Other guidelines

Other guidelines that need to be meticulously adhered to are as follows:

- MTP services are provided to the woman in strict confidence. The identity of the abortion-seeker is kept confidential.
- For pregnancy up to 12 weeks, the opinion of one qualified medical practitioner suffices. For pregnancy of 12–20 weeks, the opinion of two qualified medical practitioners is necessary.
- Written consent of the woman seeking MTP must be taken. The guardian's consent is necessary when the MTP seeker is less than 18 years of age or is mentally unsound.
- Prescription for medical abortion medications should bear the qualification and registration number of the doctor.

Counselling

Counselling is an integral part of safe abortion services. The woman undergoing MTP is under emotional and sociocultural stress. She may need help in making the decision. To avoid another unwanted pregnancy, she needs counselling on contraception too. The partner should be counselled whenever possible.

Pre-abortion counselling

Pre-abortion counselling is important for the following reasons:

- It helps her take a decision about MTP.
- The method used for termination of pregnancy, the chances of failure and any complications of the procedure and anesthesia are explained. Any doubts raised by the woman or her partner should be clarified, thus ensuring informed consent.
- It helps in adopting a contraceptive method after the procedure.

MTP should not be refused even if the woman refuses concurrent contraception.

Post-abortion counselling

Post-abortion counselling is done in order to:

- ensure that the woman understands post-abortion care, how complications are likely to manifest and the measures that need to be taken.
- reinforce the need to continue the chosen family planning method.
- counsel women who are undecided about accepting a contraceptive method.

The steps in counselling for MTP are the same as in counselling for other situations.

Assessment of the woman for MTP

A thorough assessment of the woman is useful in choosing the method of termination of pregnancy and also to avoid complications that may contribute to mortality and morbidity. It also helps to identify women who need to be referred to a health facility where complications can be managed. The assessment includes the following:

Confirmation of pregnancy: It is essential to confirm pregnancy because amenorrhea could be due to other causes as well.

Period of gestation: Assessment of the period of gestation is crucial as it determines the method of termination.

General health: The general health of the woman must be assessed in light of the information gathered from history, physical examination and results of laboratory investigations. An opinion from the physician/other specialist may be obtained if the woman has medical problems. A pre-anesthetic assessment is invaluable.

Associated gynecological disorders/infection: Any infection of the genital tract must be treated. Any presence of gynecological disorders like fibroid/ovarian tumour must be considered while making a decision to perform MTP.

Methods of MTP

The choice of method for terminating a pregnancy depends on the period of gestation. The methods or procedures of MTP are listed below. However, the focus will be on the methods used for the termination of pregnancy in the first trimester.

First trimester MTP

- Medical method
- Surgical method: Manual vacuum aspiration (MVA), Suction evacuation (SE)

Second trimester MTP

- Extra/intraamniotic instillation of drugs: Ethacridine lactate (marketed as Emcredil), prostaglandin ($PGF_2\alpha$)
- Introduction of devices through the cervix to induce abortion: Laminaria tent, catheters/bougies
- Surgical methods: Abdominal hysterotomy, abdominal hysterectomy (rarely)

Extraamniotic ethacridine lactate instillation is the most common method. Intraamniotic instillation of hypertonic saline or other solutions, which was preferred earlier, has been abandoned because of high rates of complications. Occasionally, hysterotomy may be required when other methods fail. Very rarely, abdominal hysterectomy with fetus in situ is performed if there is an associated condition warranting hysterectomy.

Medical Abortion

Mifepristone followed by misoprostol is a safe method for the termination of pregnancy till seven weeks, that is, 49 days. Only qualified medical practitioners approved under the MTP Act are permitted to prescribe mifepristone with misoprostol, and they should ensure that the woman has access to a health facility should she require emergency intervention. **Table 17.1** lists the advantages and disadvantages of medical abortion.

Mechanism of action: Mifepristone has an antiprogestational action: it acts on the decidua leading to necrosis and separation of the placenta. Misoprostol causes softening and dilatation of the cervix; it produces uterine contractions which expel the products of conception. **Table 17.2** lists the absolute and relative contraindications for the use of mifepristone and misoprostol for MTP.

Table 17.1 Advantages and disadvantages of medical abortion

Advantages	Disadvantages
Affords more privacy Abortion at an early stage Noninvasive Risk of anesthesia and surgery eliminated No effect on further fertility Providers do not require extensive training as for surgical procedures	At least three visits are required The bleeding lasts up to 15 days Side effect of the drugs Risk of fetal malformation if the method fails and the woman fails to return for follow-up

Table 17.2 Absolute and relative contraindications for using mifepristone and misoprostol for MTP

Absolute contraindications	Relative contraindications
Age above 35 years and smokes Has high blood pressure (160/100 mm Hg or more) Hemoglobin is below 8 g/dl Suffers from coagulopathy, angina, arrhythmias, hepatic and renal disorders, glaucoma, uncontrolled seizures Has no access to emergency services	Is pregnant with IUCD in situ (it should be removed) Has associated fibroid encroaching on endometrial cavity (the method is likely to fail/risk of heavy bleeding) Has a scar on the uterus Is on antitubercular drugs (risk of failure)

The provider must convince the client about the need for follow-up visits and that she will accept surgical intervention should the need arise.

Under some circumstances, it may be wiser to resort to the surgical method:

- The woman is unable to take the responsibility.
- She wants a 'quick abortion'.
- She has communication problems.
- She is not willing to under go medical abortion for fear of failure.
- The woman opts for tubal ligation along with MTP.

Dose schedule and route of administration: In India, the recommended protocol is mifepristone 200 mg on the first day (day 1), followed by misoprostol 400 µg on the third day (day 3). The dose of misoprostol is 800 µg if the period of gestation is more than 49 days and less than 63 days. For vaginal use, misoprostol tablets are moistened with a few drops of water.

Side effects: The following are frequently noted: vomiting, diarrhea, headache, feeling of warmth, chills and rigors, dizziness and fatigue

Clinical protocol: A clinical protocol for medical abortion is given below.

First visit (Day 1)

- After counselling and selection of the woman, informed consent is obtained.
- Mifepristone 200 mg is administered orally.
- In case the woman is Rh-negative, anti-D 50 µg is given.
- She has to maintain a record of the quantity and duration of bleeding.
- Back-up facility, address and phone number are given to the woman in case of any emergency.
- She must report to the clinic after 48 hours.
- Even if she expels the products (which may happen occasionally), the drug schedule with misoprostol should be completed.

Second visit (Day 3)

- Oral/vaginal misoprostol 400 µg is administered.
- With vaginal misoprostol, the woman should lie down on a bed for 30 minutes.
- She is observed for four hours in the health facility and her pulse and BP monitored. Side effects are recorded.
- Vaginal examination is performed to note if the cervical os has opened and the products are expelled partially. They are removed digitally.
- Analgesics are prescribed for pain relief, if required.
- She is advised to avoid coitus or to use condoms.
- She should not leave station.
- She should report to the health facility if there is excessive pain or bleeding.

Third visit (Day 15)

- History of symptoms is taken and a clinical examination is done to ensure that there are no complications.
- If history and examination do not conform to complete abortion, ultrasonography is recommended.
- If bleeding persists, curettage is done.
- She has to report to the doctor if her periods do not start in six weeks (she is informed that the first period may be delayed by a few days).
- Contraception advice is given and appropriate contraception is provided.

Adjuvant medications: Drugs may be required to treat side effects and to prevent infection.

Antibiotics: Routine prophylactic antibiotic therapy is not indicated. Women who need prophylactic antibiotic therapy are:

- those with vaginal infection
- nullipara
- those who have had home administration of abortion tablets

Analgesics: Pain occurs with the process of abortion and, therefore, analgesics like paracetamol or antispasmodics like dicyclomine may be prescribed. NSAIDs are avoided till the products have been expelled since they have an antiprostaglandin effect.

Antiemetics and antidiarrheals: Routine use of antiemetics and antidiarrheals is not required. Nausea and vomiting are generally mild and occur with varying frequency. An antiemetic is given:

- when the woman vomits within half an hour of taking the abortion tablets, followed by a second dose half an hour later.
- Antidiarrheals are generally not required as it is self-limiting.

Prevention and management of complications

Proper selection of woman, appropriate counselling and referral ensures the success of medical abortion. The complications are:

Failure: The term failure is used when surgical evacuation is performed for any reason including the clinician's decision, patient's choice or true drug failure. True drug failure is defined as the presence of fetal cardiac activity two weeks after RU-486 therapy. True failure is treated by surgical evacuation.

Missed ectopic pregnancy: Ectopic pregnancy is suspected when pain persists or the woman fails to pass the products.

Heavy bleeding: When bleeding is heavier than during menses, it is termed heavy bleeding. Some heavy bleeding with pain occurs during the process of abortion. If heavy bleeding persists, or the woman feels dizzy, surgical evacuation is done.

Abdominal cramps: Pain usually accompanies the abortion process and is relieved once the products are expelled. Pain persisting for several hours in spite of analgesic drugs warrants evaluation of other causes such as ectopic pregnancy, infection or incomplete abortion.

Fever or feeling of warmth: Prostaglandin analogue drugs cause fever or a feeling of warmth. It resolves spontaneously. Paracetamol given for pain relief also brings the dose takes care of fever. If the temperature exceeds 38 °C or persists for several hours despite antipyretics, infection is suspected.

Missed/incomplete abortion: Persistent gestational sac without cardiac activity two weeks after mifepristone and misoprostol administration is diagnosed as missed abortion or incomplete abortion. Usually, they expel the products spontaneously in about five weeks. Sometimes surgical evacuation is needed.

Risk of teratogenesis: If the woman does not abort following the administration of RU-486 with misoprostol and the pregnancy continues, the fetus may have teratogenic effects. Hence, if the drug fails and the pregnancy is viable, the abortus must be surgically evacuated. If the woman refuses surgical evacuation, the doctor must ensure that she makes a written statement concerning this.

Post-abortion contraception, counselling and follow-up

Follow-up is advised after the first period or if she does not have menses in 5–6 weeks. A contraceptive method is to be started as follows:

- Oral combined pills or depot medroxy progesterone acetate (DMPA) can be started on day 15 if abortion is complete.
- Copper intrauterine devices (IUD) are inserted after one normal period.
- Condoms should be used if the woman has had intercourse prior to day 15 (third visit). Abstinence is preferred.
- If the woman desires tubal ligation, she should be counselled for surgical abortion.
- The woman is counselled for the prevention of sexually transmitted infections including HIV/AIDS.

Surgical methods of first trimester MTP

The two surgical techniques used are manual vacuum aspiration and suction evacuation. Dilatation evacuation and dilatation and curettage are not advisable. The counselling and patient selection protocol is similar to that described above.

MVA technique: This is performed using a syringe which can hold vacuum (**Fig. 17.1**) and a flexible Karman's plastic cannula of an appropriate size (**Fig. 17.2**). The vacuum pressure produced in the syringe is 600–650 mm Hg. The vacuum level is almost the same produced by an electric suction machine for suction evacuation. The MVA technique should not replace existing methods of termination of pregnancy; it is an additional method.

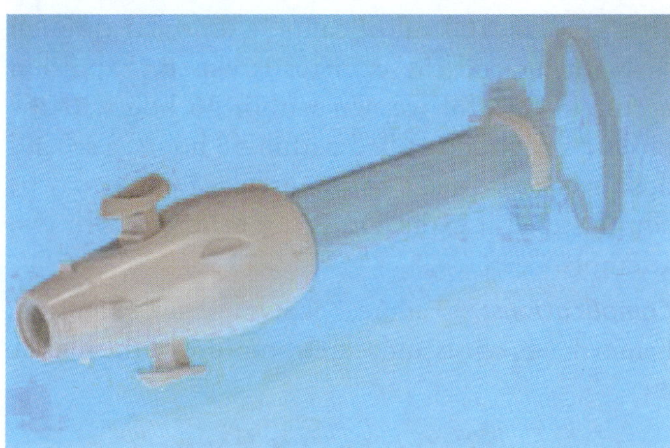

Fig. 17.1 MVA syringe.

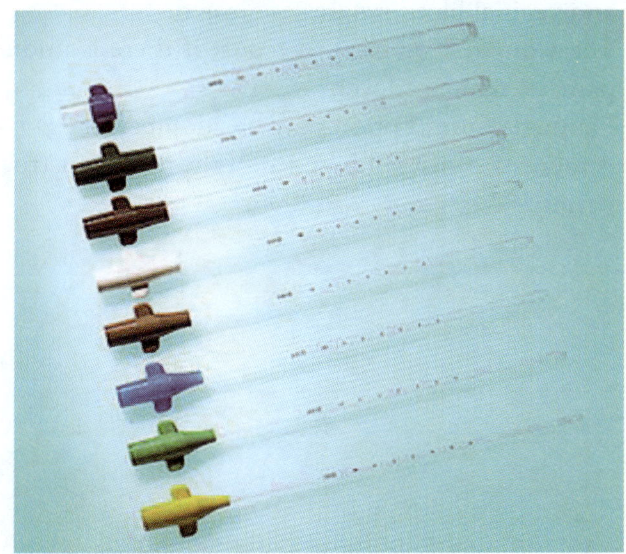

Fig. 17.2 Karman's cannula.

Advantages

- It is a simple, safe and effective method for the termination of pregnancy and evacuation of the uterus in inevitable and incomplete abortions.
- It does not depend on electricity.
- It can be performed at a PHC/any health facility where normal delivery or minor surgery can be conducted.
- It can be performed without anesthesia. In selected cases a paracervical block may be required.
- Pregnancy up to eight weeks can be terminated safely (though experienced persons can handle an abortion for a pregnancy up to 12 weeks).
- Effectiveness for complete abortion is reported to be more than 98%.
- Complication rate is low.

Disadvantages

- Syringe and cannula need to be replaced after about 30 procedures.
- As in any invasive procedure, serious complications such as hemorrhage, infection and perforation can occur.

Contraindications for use

MVA should not be used for the termination of pregnancy in the following conditions:

- uterine size more than eight weeks (even if reported duration of pregnancy is less than eight weeks)
- infection
- pregnancy with fibroid uterus
- pregnancy with uterine scar
- severe cervical stenosis
- caution is necessary in the following conditions: anemia with hemoglobin less than 8 g, bleeding disorders, hypertension (>160/100 mm Hg), heart disease, renal disease, diabetes mellitus, young adolescent, nulliparous woman.

Procedure

1. The woman is asked to empty her bladder before lying on the table in the lithotomy position.
2. All aseptic and antiseptic precautions are taken.
3. Vacuum is created within the syringe and maintained.
4. Examination per vaginum is done to reassess the size of the uterus.

5. The anterior lip of the cervix is held with vulsellum forceps.
6. Paracervical block is given if necessary.
7. The cannula is inserted into the uterine cavity.
8. The prepared syringe is attached to the cannula.
9. The vacuum is released into the uterine cavity.
10. The syringe and the cannula are rotated and moved back and forth to evacuate the uterus.
11. When a gritty sensation is felt and no more tissue is seen in the cannula, it is withdrawn and the syringe is detached.
12. The contents of the syringe are emptied into a strainer.
13. IUCD is inserted if the client has agreed to it.

Suction and evacuation (SE) procedure: In suction evacuation, vacuum is created by a suction machine and in MVA by a syringe. For the effective suction of the products, the suction machine used for the termination of pregnancy should rapidly develop a negative pressure of 600–700 mm Hg and should also have free air displacement of 25–30 ml/minute. When suction pressure is less than 600 mm Hg, incomplete evacuation may occur. A flexible lightweight plastic tubing, which does not collapse with high vacuum, is used to connect the suction machine to the suction cannula.

Second Trimester MTP (at 13–20 Weeks)

It is important to understand that MTP in the second trimester is associated with more complications than that in the first trimester. Patients should be selected on the basis of strict criteria and termination should be undertaken only if unavoidable. Currently, the extraamniotic instillation methods are widely practised. These act by prostaglandin effect either from the drug instilled or that released from the decidua–membrane separation. Results from methods using 200 μg of vaginal misoprostol every three to four hours with a maximum of six doses or till expulsion are promising.

Extraamniotic instillation: The period of gestation is carefully assessed. The woman lies in lithotomy position; after local asepsis, the cervix is held with a vulsellum. A 20 or 22 Foley catheter is inserted through the cervix beyond the internal os. The balloon is inflated with 30 ml saline. Ten percent ethacridine lactate in a dose of 10 ml per week of pregnancy up to a maximum of 150 ml, or 250 μg of $PGF_2\alpha$ in 100 ml of saline is injected through the catheter and the catheter is closed. Expulsion occurs in 90% of women within 36 hours. If the products are not expelled within 48 hours, a second dose may be instilled. Intramuscular $PGF_2\alpha$ may be administered if expulsion is not achieved with two attempts.

Complications: Failure, incomplete expulsion, hemorrhage, sepsis and, rarely, rupture of the uterus.

Post-abortion Care

- Immediately after the procedure, the vital signs and vaginal bleeding are monitored.
- The woman is advised to report if there is undue pain, bleeding or fever.
- Planned contraception may be adopted.
- A follow-up visit is advised after the next menstrual period.

KEY POINTS

- The Medical Termination of Pregnancy Act was introduced in 1972 to prevent morbidity and mortality resulting from unsafe abortion. The guidelines clearly indicate the personnel who can provide MTP, the health facility where it can be provided and lay emphasis on confidentiality.
- MTP is the voluntary termination of pregnancy provided under the MTP Act and Rules before 20 weeks, gestation.
- Counselling and assessment of the woman for MTP help in selecting the appropriate method.
- Clinical assessment is adequate to confirm pregnancy and to assess the period of gestation. Urine pregnancy test and ultrasound examination may be needed in certain cases.
- Duration of pregnancy of more than eight weeks is associated with more complications. Hence, it must be done in a place with emergency facilities.
- In case of gestation up to seven weeks, the medical method is preferred, although the surgical method may also be offered as an option.
- Selection of method for terminating a pregnancy is made after considering the methods available for the duration of pregnancy, indications and contraindications, advantages and disadvantages and the side effects.
- Medical abortion is done by administering oral RU-486 (mifepristone) 200 mg followed by vaginal/oral misoprostol 400 μg 48 hours later.
- Surgical methods available for the first trimester pregnancy are suction evacuation and manual vacuum aspiration.
- Methods of second trimester abortion are extraamniotic instillation of ethacridine lactate. Prostaglandins are also useful.
- Pre- and post-abortion counselling are important components of abortion services.

QUESTIONS

Select the single most appropriate answer:

1. In which year was the Medical Termination of Pregnancy Act enacted?
   a. 1971 b. 1972 c. 1973 d. 1974
2. According to the Medical Termination of Pregnancy Act and Rules, a pregnancy can be terminated for all of the following indications *except*
   a. continuation of pregnancy is detrimental to the mother's health.
   b. the baby is at risk of malformations.
   c. the woman did not use any contraception.
   d. pregnancy resulted from rape.
3. Medical termination of pregnancy can be performed by which one of the following according to the Medical Termination of Pregnancy Act and Rules
   a. doctor with MBBS degree
   b. general surgeon
   c. doctor who has done 25 procedures under supervision
   d. ANM with training in MTP procedures
4. All of the following are absolute contraindications to medical abortion *except*
   a. an IUCD in place
   b. presence of hypertension
   c. presence of coagulation disorders
   d. absence of access to emergency medical services
5. It is recommended that for best results, a medical method of abortion should not be used beyond
   a. 5 weeks c. 9 weeks
   b. 7 weeks d. 11 weeks
6. In a primary health centre, the best method of MTP at eight weeks of gestation is
   a. dilatation and curettage
   b. manual vacuum aspiration
   c. medical abortion
   d. suction evacuation

In the following questions, there are two statements. Select the appropriate answer using the following key:

a. if both statements are true and causally related
b. if both statements are true but not causally related
c. if the first statement is true and the second is false
d. if the first statement is false and the second is true
e. if both statements are false

7. In India, the problem of unskilled abortion is non-existent *because*
   In India, abortion has been liberalised.
8. Medical method of abortion should never be recommended *because*
   Surgical method of MTP is a 'quick method' of abortion.
9. For medical abortion, mifepristone and misoprostol must be given under medical supervision *because*
   The selection of the client for medical abortion must be done according to strict criteria.

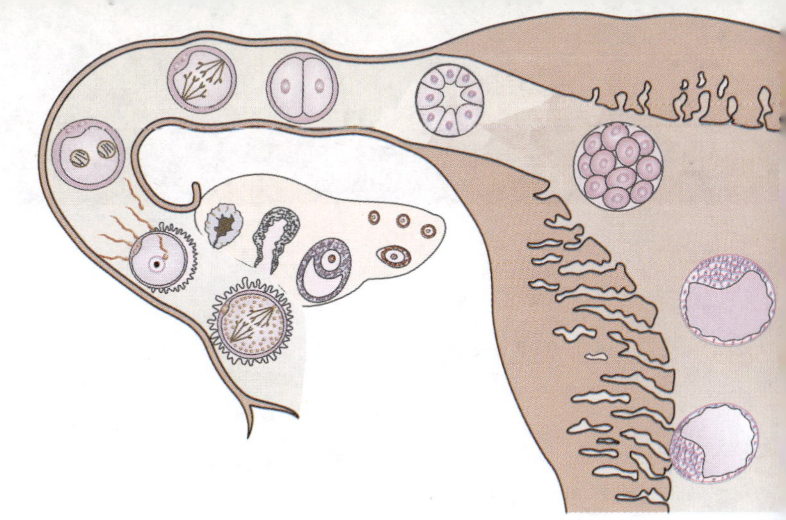

18

Ectopic Pregnancy

Asha Oumachigui

LEARNING OBJECTIVES

At the end of this chapter, the reader should be able to:

- define ectopic pregnancy
- describe the pathogenesis of ectopic pregnancy
- list the factors that predispose to EP
- describe the modes of termination of EP
- identify the clinical features and the differential diagnosis
- list the investigations for confirmation, describe the treatment and outline the management of unruptured EP

Introduction

The fertilised ovum is normally implanted in the uterine cavity, resulting in an intrauterine pregnancy. If it gets implanted at any other location, the pregnancy is said to be **ectopic**. The fertilised ovum may fail to reach the uterine cavity and be implanted in the fallopian tube; very rarely, it may be implanted in the ovary, the cervix or any other site.

Ectopic pregnancy (EP) can be an acute life-threatening condition. The incidence of EP is 1 in 250 to 1 in 150 conceptions; it is on the rise due to the increased prevalence of pelvic inflammatory disease, and is now easily diagnosed because of better diagnostic techniques. In recent years, mortality due to EP has declined markedly because of early diagnosis and intervention, and the ready availability of blood transfusion facilities.

Tubal Ectopic Pregnancy

The fallopian tube is the most common site of ectopic pregnancy.

Pathogenesis

Changes in the uterus: The fertilised ovum can become implanted when the zona pellucida is partially or completely shed. This normally happens in the uterine cavity. However, when there is a delay in the fertilised ovum reaching the uterine cavity, it is implanted in the fallopian tube during its passage. Implantation can occur in any part of the tube and the frequency is: ampulla 70%, isthmus 12%, fimbrial part 11% and interstitial part 2%. Very rarely, the ovum gets implanted in the ovary (3%), in the abdominal cavity (1%) and cervix (<1%) (**Fig. 18.1**).

Unlike in the uterus, the decidual reaction in the tube is minimal. Therefore, when the ovum gets implanted, the trophoblast burrows through the tubal epithelium and the ovum lies in the muscular wall. The peripheral active trophoblast invades and erodes the muscular layer; subsequently, it erodes into maternal blood vessels, leading to hemorrhage within the trophoblast or between it and the adjacent tissues. The tubal wall ruptures, resulting in hemorrhage.

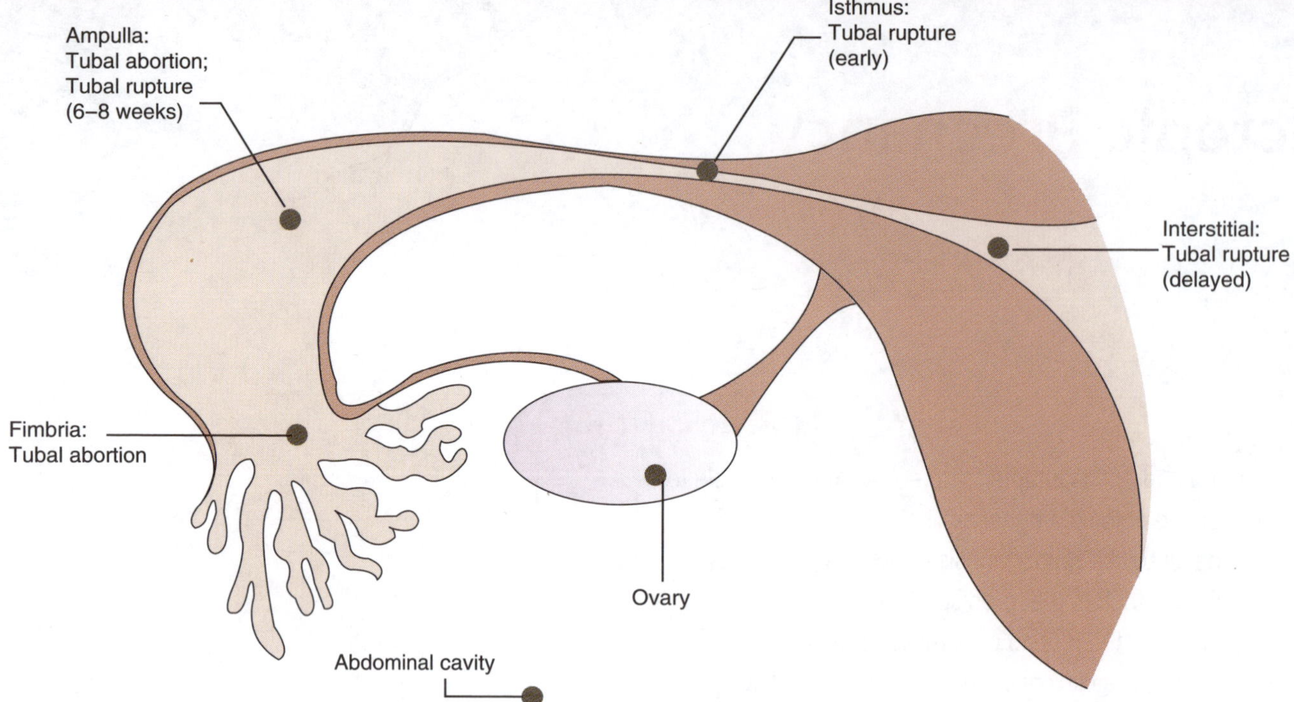

Fig. 18.1 Sites of ectopic pregnancy.

Therefore, a tubal pregnancy rarely progresses beyond eight weeks.

Changes in the uterus: Consequent to an increase in the level of hormones, the uterus becomes soft and may be enlarged, as in early intrauterine pregnancy. The extent of decidual reaction is variable; the presence of decidual reaction and absence of trophoblast suggest an EP. The endometrium shows the Arias–Stella reaction, characterised by large epithelial cells with hyperchromatic, irregular and lobulated nuclei.

Etiology

The exact etiology of EP remains unknown. Several factors prevent or delay the passage of the fertilised ovum into the uterine cavity. They can be classified as mechanical and functional.

Mechanical factors: These consist of structural defects like narrowing, kinking and other anatomical abnormalities:

Surgery on the fallopian tubes: It is the most important risk factor. Women who have had tubectomy, especially by laparoscopy, tuboplasty for tubal block and surgery for previous EP are at high risk.

Pelvic inflammatory disease: It can result in endosalpingitis and loss of cilia consequent to gonorrheal infection. Exosalpingitis leads to kinking of tubes and formation of pockets; tuberculosis causes this condition. Chlamydial infection, appendicitis and endometriosis also make a woman prone to EP.

Anatomical abnormalities: Congenitally long tubes, the presence of diverticula and double ostia are known to predispose a woman to EP.

Functional factors: The factors known to delay the passage of the fertilised ovum are:

Hormonal contraceptives: Women on progestogen-only pills or fitted with IUCDs impregnated with progestogen (Progestasert) seem to be predisposed to EP.

Assisted reproductive techniques: A higher incidence of EP has been noted in women who undergo assisted reproduction, particularly the zygote intrafallopian transfer (ZIFT) technique.

Delayed ovulation: It is possible that an ovum released just before menstruation is fertilised and its passage down the tube is delayed by the backflow of menstrual blood.

Other factors: Although the exact mechanism is not understood, smoking, douching and age below 18 years appear to be associated with an increased incidence of EP.

Modes of termination

It is clear from the previous discussion that an EP ends in the early part of pregnancy. The modes of termination are largely determined by the site of implantation in the fallopian tube.

Tubal abortion: This is the most common mode of termination and occurs in about 65% of cases. The implantation is usually in the ampullary or fimbrial parts of the tube. The invading trophoblast erodes capillaries, leading to small hemorrhages that separate the placenta from the tubal wall, resulting in death of the zygote. The zygote is then absorbed completely or aborted completely or incompletely into the peritoneal cavity. In some instances, it forms a tubal mole as blood collects around the zygote.

The blood that trickles through the tube collects in the pouch of Douglas giving rise to a **pelvic hematocele** (Fig. 18.2).

Tubal rupture: This mode of termination is seen in about 20% of cases. As the products of conception grow, the tube distends progressively and the trophoblast invades and weakens the muscularis and further penetration leads to rupture. Tubal rupture is most often seen when the zygote is implanted in the isthmic part of the tube.

Secondary abdominal pregnancy: Very rarely, the expelled zygote continues to grow after getting re-implanted in the abdominal cavity. In some cases, the fetus dies early and is converted into a lithopedian, but in a few exceptional cases it can reach term.

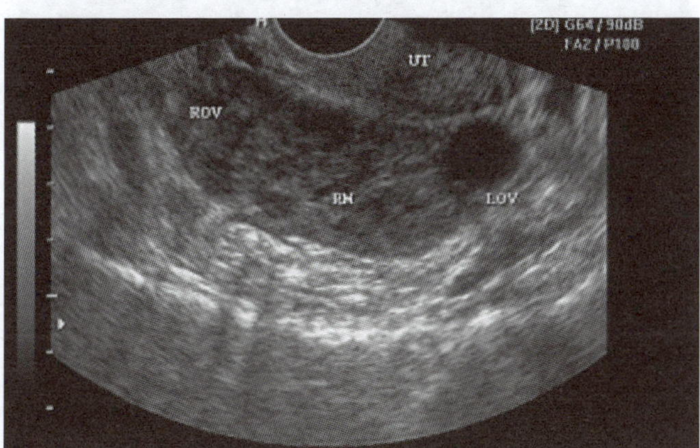

Fig. 18.2 Pelvic hematocele.

Clinical features

The clinical manifestations of EP are extremely diverse and depend on the site of EP in the tube and the mode of termination. The possibility of EP must always be considered in a woman of reproductive age. History is of great importance and should be taken meticulously.

Symptoms: The cardinal symptoms of EP are amenorrhea, abdominal pain and vaginal bleeding.

- **Abdominal pain** is the most constant feature of EP and is present in 95% of cases. The location and character of the pain depend on the mode of termination. A woman with tubal abortion is likely to complain of pain localised to the lower abdomen.
- **Amenorrhea** is of short duration; it may be absent in 20% of cases.
- **Vaginal bleeding** usually follows pain. It is scanty, brownish and continuous following a short period of amenorrhea. Sometimes, it starts as normal menstruation, but the bleeding is minimal.
- There may be a history of syncopal attacks.

Signs: The general condition of the patient will depend on the presence and extent of intraabdominal bleeding and will be disproportionate to external bleeding. Pallor, tachycardia and hypotension indicate severe intraabdominal bleeding.

Abdominal examination may reveal free fluid and tenderness. Bluish discolouration around the umbilicus, called the **Cullen sign**, is not often appreciable in dark-skinned women.

Pelvic examination may reveal an adnexal mass, which may be pulsatile and tender. Movement of the cervix is extremely painful. In pelvic hematocele, the pouch of Douglas feels boggy.

Types of clinical presentation

Subacute presentation: Around 60% of cases of EP belong to this category. The patient presents with a history of mild lower abdominal pain or discomfort. Occasionally, there may be an episode of sharp pain and fainting due to an intraperitoneal bleed, followed by constant pain which may or may not be severe. The patient is usually hemodynamically stable. On examination, there is tenderness in the lower abdomen and vaginal examination reveals tenderness in the fornices. Further, an attack of severe pain recurs and the patient collapses or the pain subsides depending on whether the tube has ruptured or tubal abortion is complete.

A pelvic mass in the posterior or lateral fornix is present in 15%–20% of patients. It feels soft if it is due to a pelvic hematocele; a firm mass (felt more through the lateral fornix) is caused by infiltration of blood in the tube.

Acute presentation: This presentation is seen in about 20% of patients. The woman presents with sudden collapse following severe pain; there is marked pallor, tachycardia and hypotension. On examination of the abdomen, there is severe tenderness; movements of the cervix are very painful, described as 'yelling tenderness'.

Culdocentesis is a simple technique used to aspirate fluid from the pouch of Douglas. EP is confirmed if the fluid aspirated is blood that does not clot, or fluid with fragments of blood clots. **A negative culdocentesis does not rule out an EP.**

Differential diagnosis

It is important to differentiate EP from other conditions so that treatment can be instituted at the earliest.

First trimester abortions: The three symptoms of amenorrhea, pain and vaginal bleeding are present. But the intensity of pain is much less and the vaginal bleeding is much more than in EP. On examination, the uterus corresponds to the period of gestation in case of threatened and inevitable abortion and less than the period of gestation in incomplete abortion. The movements of the cervix are not tender. The cervical os is open in inevitable and incomplete abortions. The general condition is proportionate to the perceived blood loss.

Other causes: There are several causes of acute abdomen, but acute salpingitis and acute appendicitis are the most important. Fever is a feature in these conditions, but not in case of EP. However, conditions like corpus luteum cyst rupture, twisted ovarian cyst and surgical causes of acute abdomen should also be kept in mind.

Diagnosis

In acute cases with internal bleeding, the diagnosis of EP is not difficult. However, in those with subacute presentation, the diagnosis can be quite intriguing. Laboratory tests are useful when interpreted in light of clinical findings. An immunological pregnancy test may be positive in 75% of cases which are not very specific. Estimation of serum of β-hCG is more accurate; if the serum level is ≤1500 mIU/ml and the uterus is empty, no definitive diagnosis can be made.

If transvaginal sonography reveals an empty uterus and serum level of β-hCG is ≥1500 mIU/ml, the diagnosis of EP is made. The diagnosis is more certain if sonography shows a sac and/or a fetus in the adnexal region (**Fig. 18.3**).

Unruptured ectopic pregnancy: EP must be suspected in women who have risk factors. An early diagnosis of EP, before it is disturbed, is possible by estimation of serum level of β-hCG and transvaginal sonography. Although β-hCG can be detected from day 22 of the cycle, a gestational sac cannot reliably be identified until five weeks after the last menstrual period. During this critical period, serial estimation of serum level of β-hCG is extremely useful. In an intrauterine pregnancy, the mean doubling time for serum levels of β-hCG is 48 hours. In case of an EP, the increase is less than 66% in 48 hours.

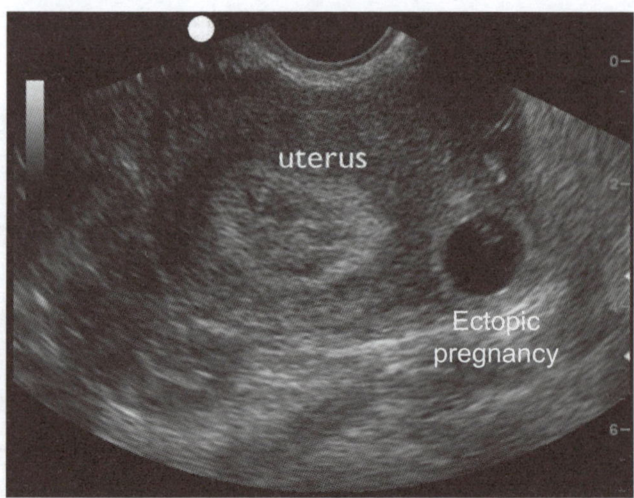

Fig. 18.3 USG of EP showing sac.

Laparoscopy is very useful in making a definitive diagnosis of EP. It can also be used to surgically treat the condition in a hemodynamically stable patient.

Treatment

General measures: Whenever EP is suspected, the woman must be admitted/referred to a well-equipped health facility. If she is in shock, it is mandatory to institute immediate resuscitative therapy, including intravenous fluids or blood, and administer morphine or pethidine to reduce pain.

Surgical management

Laparotomy: Once a diagnosis of ectopic pregnancy is made, a laparotomy should be performed by a subumbilical midline incision. After opening the abdomen, the uterus is lifted out, the affected tube is identified and the other tube and ovary are inspected. A partial salpingectomy is done. If the woman desires to maintain her fertility, efforts should be made to conserve the tube by resorting to:

- excision of the ruptured segment (segmental resection),
- fimbrial expression in case of tubal abortion or
- salpingostomy, where an incision is made on the tube and the products removed.

Laparoscopy: This is used in diagnosis and surgical management of EP unless the patient is hemodynamically unstable.

Besides performing surgical procedures like salpingectomy and salpingostomy, methotrexate can be injected directly into EP.

Medical management: With the availability of sophisticated diagnostic aids, EP is being diagnosed at an early stage before it is disturbed. As described above, unruptured EP can be treated with conservative surgical procedures such as laparoscopy or laparotomy. Medical management is being resorted to more frequently. However, meticulous selection of patients and follow-up are required. The drug of choice is methotrexate.

A patient for methotrexate therapy should be selected very carefully. The following criteria must be fulfilled:

- The patient should be hemodynamically stable.
- The size of the gestational sac should be ≤ 3.5 cm and cardiac activity should be absent.
- The serum β-hCG concentration should be preferably ≤1000 mIU/ml. When concentrations are higher, failure rates of medical management increase.
- The patient's hemogram, renal and hepatic function should be within normal limits.

Before administering methotrexate, the following guidelines must be adhered to strictly:

- The patient must be informed that medical therapy may fail, and she may require re-treatment with methotrexate or surgery.
- She must be instructed to report to the hospital immediately if she has any symptoms like abdominal pain or giddiness.
- She must abstain from sexual intercourse.
- She should not take any multivitamins or folic acid.

Methotrexate is an anticancer drug, being a folic acid antagonist. It is administered in a single dose of 50 mg/m^2 intramuscularly. The patient is monitored by estimation of serum β-hCG on days 4 and 7; if the difference is 15% or more, estimation is repeated weekly till it reaches ≤ 15 mIU/ml. If the difference is less than 15%, another dose of methotrexate is given. The patient should be monitored for methotrexate toxicity.

Other Types of Ectopic Pregnancy

Secondary abdominal pregnancy

This occurs subsequent to implantation of the zygote expelled from a tubal abortion or ruptured tubal pregnancy. The pregnancy may advance to varying periods. The woman may provide a history of a sudden severe episode of pain earlier in pregnancy which later on subsided. On examination, the fetal parts are felt superficially and the presenting part is not felt through the os. Ultrasound examination shows the fetus to be outside the uterus. A laparotomy is planned, keeping enough blood available. The placenta may be implanted on other organs or the pelvic vessels. After delivery of the baby, if difficulty is anticipated in removing the placenta, it is best to leave it after tying the cord and monitor its involution using ultrasound. Fetal survival is very poor.

Ovarian pregnancy

Implantation on the ovary is very rare. It is important that Spiegelberg's criteria be fulfilled to diagnose an ovarian pregnancy:

- The tube on the affected site must be healthy.
- The fetal sac must be in the position of the ovary.
- The ovary must be connected to the uterus by the ovarian ligament.
- Definite ovarian tissue must be found in the fetal sac wall.

Clinically ovarian pregnancy may present just like a tubal pregnancy. Treatment is surgical in the form of ovariectomy, wedge resection or excision of the sac.

Cervical pregnancy

Pregnancy at this site is uncommon, but its incidence seems to be on the rise. The cervix is eroded by the trophoblast and the pregnancy grows in the fibrous tissue of the cervix, leading to a barrel-shaped enlargement of the cervix. Hysterectomy used to be the treatment of choice because of massive hemorrhage. Currently, medical management with methotrexate and arterial embolisation are being used to manage cervical pregnancy.

KEY POINTS

- Ectopic pregnancy is the condition when the zygote fails to reach the uterine cavity and gets implanted in the fallopian tube.
- Previous EP, surgery on the tubes and pelvic inflammatory disease are risk factors associated with EP.
- There is no submucosa in the tube and the decidualisation is minimal so that the trophoblast invades the muscularis and blood vessel, and the pregnancy ends.
- Ampulla is the most common site for ectopic pregnancy and the most common mode of termination is tubal abortion.
- Tubal rupture is common when the zygote is implanted in the isthmus.
- Clinically 60% or more present as a subacute condition and 20% present as acute.
- The possibility of EP must be kept in mind whenever a woman of the reproductive age presents with abdominal pain.
- The diagnosis can be difficult in subacute presentation. Estimation of serum β-hCG and vaginal ultrasound are invaluable tools.
- Hemodynamically unstable cases must be subjected to laparotomy; others can be managed laparoscopically.
- When cases are diagnosed with an intact EP, they can be treated medically after careful selection.
- Early diagnosis, early intervention and availability of blood transfusion have reduced mortality due to EP significantly.

QUESTIONS

Select the single most appropriate answer:

1. In which part of the fallopian tube does ectopic pregnancy occur most frequently?
   a. interstitial part　c. ampullary part
   b. isthmus　d. fimbrial part
2. Tubal rupture is common when the ectopic pregnancy is situated in the
   a. isthmus　c. interstitial part
   b. ampullary part　d. fimbrial part
3. Which of the following contraceptives is most associated with an increased risk of ectopic pregnancy?
   a. combined oral pills　c. copper-T
   b. progestasert　d. vaginal diaphragm
4. The symptom of amenorrhea could be absent in approximately what percentage of women with ectopic gestation?
   a. 5%　b. 10%　c. 15%　d. 20%

5. For an early diagnosis of ectopic pregnancy on TVS, the uterine cavity should be empty and the serum β-hCG level should be
   a. more than 1,500 mIU/ml
   b. less than 1,500 mIU/ml
   c. more than 1,000 mIU/ml
   d. less than 1,000 mIU/ml
6. Which of the following statements is false regarding the medical the manangement of tubal pregnancy?
   a. should be hemodynamically stable
   b. serum β-hCG level should be less than 1000 mIU/ml
   c. the sac should measure 4.5 cm
   d. the woman should be willing to return for follow-up

In the following questions, there are two statements. Select the appropriate answer using the following key:

a. if both statements are true and causally related
b. if both statements are true but not causally related
c. if the first statement is true and the second is false
d. if the first statement is false and the second is true
e. if both statements are false

7. On culdocentesis, aspiration of blood is essential to confirm ectopic pregnancy *because*

   In disturbed ectopic pregnancy, blood collects in the pouch of Douglas.
8. The incidence of ectopic pregnancy is high in women with pelvic inflammatory disease *because.*

   Fallopian tubes are damaged in pelvic inflammatory disease.
9. The incidence of ectopic pregnancy is on the rise *because.*

   The incidence of pelvic inflammatory disease is on the rise.
10. In ectopic pregnancy, the fertilised ovum is implanted in the fallopian tube *because*

    The zona pellucida is partially or completely shed when the fertilised ovum reaches the uterine cavity.

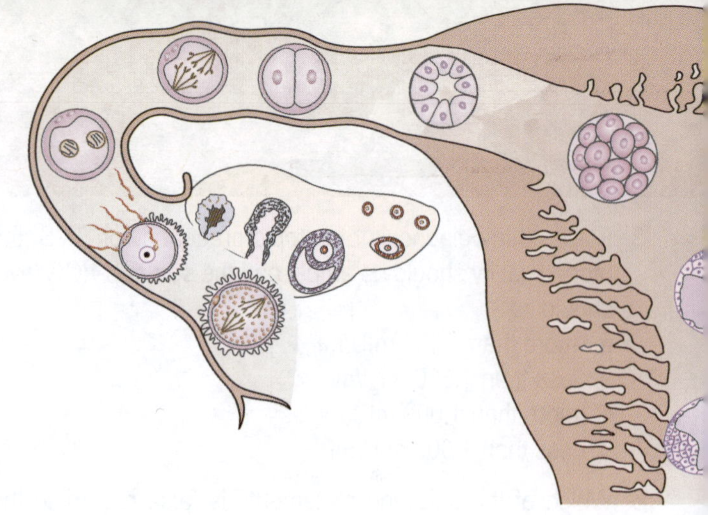

19

Gestational Trophoblastic Disease

Raj Narayan

LEARNING OBJECTIVES

At the end of this chapter, the reader should be able to:

- list the risk factors associated with hydatidiform mole (H. mole)
- describe the histopathological and cytogenetic features of the various types of GTD
- enumerate the symptoms and signs of H. mole
- list the methods available to diagnose this condition
- describe the management options for H. mole
- describe the protocol for follow-up after evacuation of H. mole
- categorise postmolar GTD into risk categories
- outline the management of GTT

Introduction

Gestational trophoblastic disease (GTD) includes a unique group of neoplastic conditions occurring in the mother but arising from fetal tissue, namely, the trophoblastic epithelium of the placenta. It represents a spectrum of diseases that includes complete and partial hydatidiform mole, invasive mole, choriocarcinoma, and placental site trophoblastic tumour (PSTT), whereas gestational trophoblastic tumour (GTT) includes invasive mole, choriocarcinoma and PSTT. Therefore, it is important to remember that GTD and GTT are not synonymous. The term gestational trophoblastic neoplasia (GTN) is sometimes used in place of GTT.

These tumours are unique in two aspects: human chorionic gonadotrophin (hCG) is synthesised by the trophoblastic cells and the β subunit of hCG is, therefore, a very sensitive marker for the disease. Gestational trophoblastic tumour is the most curable gynecologic malignancy and the majority of the patients with this disease can be cured with chemotherapy alone. Moreover, it does not need histopathological confirmation.

Epidemiology

The incidence of H. mole varies between different geographic areas. It ranges from 1 in 60 pregnancies in Indonesia to 1 in 5,000 in Paraguay, with Europe and USA in the low-to-intermediate range. In India, it occurs in about 1 in 500 to 1,000 pregnancies.

Risk factors

Following are the risk factors for H. mole:

Parental age: Risk is higher in women under the age of 20 years and over the age of 40 years.

Previous H. mole: The risk of another H. mole in a subsequent pregnancy is 1% and may increase to about 25% in women who have had more than one molar pregnancy.

Oral contraceptive use: There is approximately a twofold increase in the incidence of H. mole with oral contraceptive use for more than four years. However, the risk of developing GTD was unchanged in a randomised trial when oral contraceptive was used after evacuation of H. mole.

Environment and lifestyle factors: Some studies have shown an increased risk of developing GTD in smokers and in women who had high alcohol intake while others did not find a similar association. The association of GTD with malnutrition, folic acid deficiency, diet deficient in animal protein and animal fat are unproven.

The risk factors for GTT/choriocarcinoma are:

Size of uterus: Women with H. mole and normal-size or large-for-dates uteri have a 25% chance of developing invasive disease while those with small-for-dates uteri have an 11% chance of developing invasive disease.

Size of ovaries: Women with H. mole and enlarged ovaries have an approximately 50% risk of developing invasive disease.

Histopathology and Cytogenetics

Trophoblasts are epithelial cells derived from the outermost layer of the blastocyst. There are three types: cytotrophoblast, syncytiotrophoblast and intermediate trophoblast. Cytotrophoblast is on the surface of the chorionic villi and differentiates into syncytiotrophoblast on the villous surface and intermediate trophoblast in the placental bed. The syncytiotrophoblast is a polynuclear structure without any proliferative activity. Intermediate trophoblast infiltrates the decidua, the myometrium and the maternal arteries to create an effective maternal–fetal circulation.

Hydatidiform mole: The chorionic villi in the case of H. mole are found to have hydropic swelling and there is evidence of trophoblastic proliferation. There are two types of H. mole: complete and partial. The differences between complete and partial H. mole are listed in **Table 19.1**.

Complete molar pregnancy occurs:

- when an anuclear ovum is fertilised by a haploid sperm which then duplicates, its chromosomes resulting in 46XX karyotype, or
- when an empty ovum is fertilised by two haploid spermatozoa, resulting in 46XX or 46XY karyotype.

Partial molar pregnancy occurs when an ovum with a haploid set of chromosomes is fertilised by two spermatozoa, resulting in 69XXX, 69XXY or 69XYY karyotype. There are two sets of chorionic villi seen in partial H. mole: normal villi and hydropic villi with focal hyperplasia.

Invasive mole: It occurs when enlarged hydropic villi penetrate deep into the myometrium. It may closely mimic choriocarcinoma with vaginal or lung metastatic lesions. Karyotype is usually diploid but may occasionally be aneuploid too.

Choriocarcinoma: It consists of masses of cells invading adjacent tissues, blood vessels and lymphatic spaces. There is complete **absence of villi** with proliferation of syncytiotrophoblasts and cytotrophoblasts with abnormal mitotic figures.

Table 19.1 Features of complete and partial mole and choriocarcinoma

Characteristic	Complete mole	Partial mole	Choriocarcinoma
Chorionic villi	Diffuse edema	Focal edema	Absent villi
Trophoblastic hyperplasia	Diffuse	Focal	Diffuse, with necrosis, hemorrhage
Embryo	None	Abnormal fetus	None
Karyotype	Paternal origin 46 XX (90%) 46 XY (10%)	Maternal/paternal origin (triploid), 69XXY, 69XXX, 69XYY	Aneuploidy
Malignant potential	20%	4%	100%

Significant hemorrhage and necrosis are also seen. The karyotype is aneuploid.

Placental site trophoblastic tumour (PSTT): This is a condition where trophoblastic infiltration is confined to the endometrium and myometrium of the placental implantation site. The tumour is composed of sheets of intermediate trophoblasts. Necrosis is not significant.

Clinical Features and Treatment

Hydatidiform mole

Hydatidiform mole is suspected when the following clinical features are seen.

Presenting features: A woman with H. mole presents with the following features:

- Amenorrhea followed by vaginal bleeding is the most common presentation in complete molar pregnancy.
- Passage of grape-like tissue from the vagina may be noticed by the patient.
- Symptoms of preeclampsia may be noticed.
- Severe nausea and vomiting may also be the presenting complaints in women with complete H. mole.
- Symptoms of hyperthyroidism are rarely a presenting feature.
- Partial molar pregnancy often presents as missed abortion or incomplete abortion.

Clinical examination: On examination, the following findings are associated with a diagnosis of molar pregnancy:

- Pallor is frequently noted in women who present with vaginal bleeding.
- Hypertension, tachycardia and edema may be seen if preeclampsia or hyperthyroidism are present.
- The abdomen may reveal a palpable uterus larger than estimated for gestational age with no palpable fetal parts and a 'doughy' feel. Enlarged ovaries with theca-lutein cysts may be palpable in some cases.
- Speculum examination may reveal vaginal bleeding, open cervical os and, occasionally, molar tissue in the vagina.
- Bimanual pelvic examination will confirm an enlarged uterus which is disproportionate to the expected gestational age, and ovaries may also be palpably enlarged.

Investigations: The following tests are helpful in the management of H. mole:

- Urine pregnancy test is positive. Presence of significant protein in urine suggests preeclampsia.
- Baseline quantitative serum β-hCG using a sensitive assay shows markedly elevated levels. In partial H. mole, there is less marked elevation. This test is important for the evaluation of risk as well as for follow-up.
- Complete blood count and a coagulation profile are required as these patients are at a high risk of massive blood loss.
- Ultrasound examination of the pelvis reveals a characteristic 'snow storm' appearance within the uterus (**Fig. 19.1**). However, in early pregnancy, the heterogeneous opacity may be mistaken as a missed abortion. Although fetal structures are absent in complete H. mole, they may be seen in partial H. mole. The ovaries may be enlarged and cystic.
- Histopathologic examination of products of conception that are spontaneously expelled will also confirm the diagnosis.
- The ABO and Rh blood groups and cross-matching of packed red blood cells for possible transfusion are necessary as hemorrhage is a common complication.

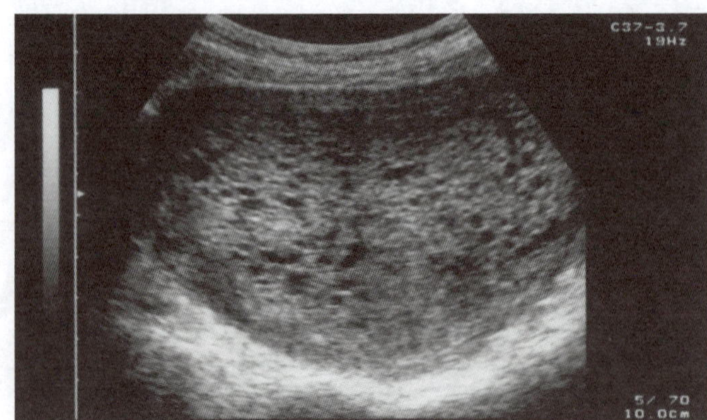

Fig. 19.1 Ultrasound image of uterus with H. mole showing 'snow storm' appearance.

- In patients with features suggestive of high-risk molar pregnancy (**Table 19.2**), preeclampsia, hyperthyroidism or severe nausea and vomiting will need other tests such as serum levels of electrolytes, urea, creatinine and uric acid, liver function tests and thyroid function tests.
- Chest radiography is included in the initial evaluation of molar pregnancy to detect metastatic lesions.

Treatment: The patient should be treated expeditiously. Dilatation of the cervix followed by suction evacuation with an atraumatic cannula is the procedure of choice even when the uterus is of more than 20 weeks, gestation. Evacuation of a large uterus may result in uterine atony and hemorrhage. Oxytocin infusion commences before starting the evacuation. Intraoperative blood transfusion may be needed and cross-matched packed red blood cells should be readily available before starting the procedure. Other complications of uterine evacuation include uterine perforation and trophoblastic embolisation resulting in acute respiratory distress syndrome. Hemorrhage may be multifactorial and may result from uterine atony, retained trophoblastic tissue, uterine perforation and, rarely, disseminated intravascular coagulation.

Total hysterectomy may be offered to women who are 40 years or older and who do not want to retain future fertility options. However, theca-lutein ovarian cysts should be left in situ as they regress completely when the hCG levels return to normal. Anti-Rh (D) immune globulin is administered to Rh (D) negative women as trophoblastic tissue contains the Rh (D) antigen.

Follow-up: Serum β-hCG is a sensitive marker and all women who have been diagnosed with hydatidiform mole (complete or partial) must be followed by serial measurements of serum levels of the β subunit of hCG by a sensitive assay. This is required even in women treated with hysterectomy. Initially, this should be performed at 1–2 week intervals until there are two normal values. This occurs in about 80% of women with complete H. mole. The serial measurements must continue every month for a total of six months. Serial pelvic examinations are also recommended every two weeks until the β-hCG levels are normal, followed by examinations every three months for a year. Evidence of vaginal metastasis or subinvolution of the uterus indicates persistent or progressive disease (also known as GTT) and needs additional prompt intervention.

Effective contraception must be used for six months. Combined low-dose contraceptive pills or barrier methods should be used.

Chest radiography need not be repeated unless the β-hCG levels plateau or begin to rise. Women who have metastases or in whom β-hCG levels plateau or rise after initial treatment should be treated with chemotherapy. Sometimes, D&C done for persistent bleeding may reveal histopathological diagnosis of choriocarcinoma. The treatment for persistent GTD and choriocarcinoma is the same.

Table 19.2 Features of high-risk gestational trophoblastic disease

- Uterine size >20 weeks' gestation, or more than the period of amenorrhea
- Theca–lutein cysts (≥6 cm)
- Marked trophoblastic proliferation
- Tumour anaplasia
- Hyperthyroidism
- β-hCG levels $>10^5$ mIU/ml

Invasive mole

This condition (also known as **chorioadenoma destruens**) is diagnosed when a rising or persistent serum β-hCG level is noticed after evacuation of complete or partial H. mole. Persistence is defined as detectable levels (>5 mIU/ml) more than six months after evacuation of H. mole. Ultrasound or CT scan may help to diagnose invasion. These lesions mimic choriocarcinoma with lymphovascular invasion and vaginal or lung metastases. However, unlike choriocarcinoma, invasive mole can regress spontaneously. A complete evaluation for the detection of metastatic disease is also necessary. Chemotherapy with a single agent such as methotrexate or actinomycin D is initiated and continued for one or two cycles after serum β-hCG is negative. Serum levels of β-hCG should be followed for at least

12 months after chemotherapy. Effective contraception is necessary to confirm persistent remission from disease. Occasionally, emergency hysterectomy may be needed for a bleeding invasive mole.

Choriocarcinoma

Choricarcinoma is a histological diagnosis. It is a malignant tumour which can arise from any type of trophoblastic tissue. The most common site of origin is the uterus. Hydatidiform mole precedes malignant disease in 50% of women. Approximately 25% of the patients have an antecedent normal pregnancy and another 25% have a preceding abortion or ectopic pregnancy. Choriocarcinoma is easily suspected if it follows soon after H. mole or a pregnancy. However, the preceding pregnancy may have occurred years earlier. The presenting symptom may be persistent vaginal bleeding or symptoms of metastasis like vaginal nodule (vaginal metastasis), hemoptysis, shortness of breath, chest pain (lung metastasis), jaundice, abdominal pain (liver metastases) and altered sensorium, headache, seizures or stroke (brain metastasis). Abnormal uterine bleeding in a premenopausal woman should always be investigated with a sensitive serum β-hCG assay. Indications for chemotherapy are listed in **Table 19.3**.

A complete work-up for metastasis is essential in patients with suspected invasive disease. The recommended evaluation is shown in **Table 19.4**.

The last three tests are required **only if the first six tests indicate possible metastatic disease.** Once the work-up is done, the cases need to be classified into risk categories.

Classification of GTD: The commonly used classifications are National Institute of Health (NIH) classification and modified FIGO scoring (2000). All these systems help identify patients at risk of poor response to single-agent chemotherapy. About 90% of the patients at low risk attain remission.

Table 19.3 Indications for chemotherapy

Rising hCG after evacuation of H. mole
Plateauing hCG over three weeks
Serum hCG >20,000 mIU/ml, four weeks after evacuation of H. mole
Elevated hCG even six months after evacuation
Histology suggesting choriocarcinoma
Metastases in the lungs or vagina with increased β-hCG
Metastases in the liver or brain

Table 19.4 Recommended evaluation of gestational trophoblastic disease

Complete history and physical examination
Serum quantitative β-hCG assay
Complete blood count
Liver function tests
Renal function tests
Chest radiography
Computed tomography of the brain
Pelvic ultrasound
Computed tomography of the liver

NIH classification of GTT

- Non-metastatic
- Metastatic
  1. Good prognosis, low risk
  2. Poor prognosis, high risk (presence of any risk factor)
     a. duration >4 months
     b. pretreatment serum β-hCG 40,000 mIU/ml
     c. brain or liver metastases
     d. GTT after term gestation
     e. previous failed therapy

Non-metastatic and metastatic good prognosis tumours can be treated with single-agent chemotherapy. Metastatic poor prognosis patients need multiagent chemotherapy. The FIGO scoring system is shown in **Table 19.5**.

Treatment of choriocarcinoma/GTT: The primary treatment modality is chemotherapy. Surgery along with chemotherapy is reserved for women who are at high risk, women who have completed their childbearing and those who have persistent disease even after chemotherapy. Radiation therapy may also be used in conjunction with chemotherapy, particularly for arresting bleeding from the vaginal nodule, brain and liver metastasis.

Chemotherapy: It is the mainstay of treatment and the regimen chosen will be according to the risk status indicated above.

Table 19.5 FIGO risk scoring (2000)

Prognostic factors	Score			
	0	1	2	4
Age (years)	≤39	>39		
Antecedent pregnancy	H. mole	Abortion	Term	
Months from last pregnancy	<4	> 4–6	7–12	>12
Pretreatment–hCG (mIU/ml)	$<10^3$	10^3–10^4	10^4–10^5	$>10^5$
Largest tumour size (cm)	3–4 cm	5 cm		
Site of metastasis	Lungs, vagina	Spleen, kidneys	GI tract	Brain, liver
Number of metastases		1–4	4–8	>8
Prior failed chemotherapy			Single agent	≥2 drugs
Total Score	≤6 low risk; ≥7 high risk			

Single-agent chemotherapy: Methotrexate was the first drug to be used for this purpose and is very effective. It should not be used in women with liver dysfunction as it is metabolised in the liver. It is an antimetabolite, and folinic acid is the antidote. It is administered intramuscularly or intravenously either as a daily, alternate day or weekly dose. High-dose alternate day therapy can be alternated with folinic acid as a rescue for normal epithelial cells. Side effects are bone marrow suppression, megaloblastic anemia, diarrhea, stomatitis and vomiting.

Actinomycin D is an antibiotic given as a daily intravenous dose. Side effects include bone marrow suppression, stomatitis and diarrhea.

5-Fluorouracil (5-FU) is also an antimetabolite and has been used successfully as a single agent in choriocarcinoma. It is given by slow intravenous infusion. Side effects include bone marrow suppression, stomatitis, diarrhea and alopecia.

Multiple-agent chemotherapy: This is the treatment of choice in poor prognosis metastatic disease and a multimodality treatment is often necessary. Initially, a triple therapy may be used consisting of methotrexate, actinomycin D and chlorambucil or cyclophosphamide (MAC). Many other complicated multidrug regimens, for example, etoposide, methotrexate, actinomycin D, cyclophosphamide and oncovin/vincristine (EMA-CO) are used in patients with advanced disease. Intracranial metastasis may be treated with intrathecal methotrexate and whole brain irradiation. Surgery may be required in some cases.

Surgery: Hysterectomy is reserved for the elderly, those with high-risk GTT and in cases of uterine perforation. However, the ovaries need not be removed. In these patients, the number of chemotherapy cycles may be reduced.

Prognosis: The overall cure rate for patients with non-metastatic disease is nearly 100%. The cure rates for good prognosis metastatic disease are also high, up to 84%. In patients with poor prognosis metastatic GTT, the mortality rate is about 20%. It is important that all women with GTT be monitored with serial measurements of serum levels of β-hCG for 12–24 months after completion of chemotherapy. Patients should be on effective contraception for a minimum of one year following treatment.

Placental site trophoblastic tumours (PSTT)

These are rare tumours which arise from the intermediate trophoblast. They present months to years after a term pregnancy or an abortion. The presenting symptom is typically abnormal uterine bleeding. Findings include uterine enlargement which may be diffuse or nodular or a large endometrial polyp with myometrial invasion may be found. Serum β-hCG levels are elevated but not markedly. Serum human placental lactogen (hPL) is elevated. Biopsy shows intermediate trophoblast and stains for human placental lactogen. It is locally invasive and may invade the adnexae. Metastasis has been reported, though rarely. These are relatively insensitive to chemotherapy. Treatment is hysterectomy.

KEY POINTS

- Gestational trophoblastic disease comprises a spectrum of diseases including hydatidiform mole, invasive mole, choriocarcinoma and placental site trophoblastic tumour
- Complete and partial hydatidiform mole behave differently and need early diagnosis, treatment and appropriate follow-up.
- β-hCG is a sensitive marker and the amount of β-hCG is directly proportional to tumour mass.
- Choriocarcinoma is the most curable gynecologic malignancy.
- The gestational trophoblastic tumours are extremely sensitive to chemotherapy.
- Individualisation of treatment based on risk score results in high cure rates, even in advanced disease.

QUESTIONS

Select the single most appropriate answer:

1. Human chorionic gonadotrophin (hCG) levels are increased in all of the following *except*
   a. complete mole b. partial mole
   c. endodermal sinus tumour
   d. embryonal carcinoma
2. Which is the best method to diagnose a vesicular mole?
   a. uterine size more than period of amenorrhea
   b. presence of ovarian cyst
   c. hCG estimation
   d. ultrasound examination
3. In vesicular mole, all the following are risk factors for the development of choriocarcinoma *except*
   a. initial serum hCG > 100,000 mIU/ml
   b. bilateral theca-lutein cysts > 6 cm
   c. uterine size more than 20 weeks
   d. features of preeclampsia
4. The treatment of choice for choriocarcinoma in a 35-year-old woman is
   a. hysterectomy
   b. radiotherapy
   c. chemotherapy
   d. dilatation and evacuation
5. Which of the following is the most common site of metastatsis of choriocarcinoma
   a. vagina b. lung c. liver d. brain
6. Human chorionic gonadotrophin is primarily secreted by
   a. syncytiotrophoblast c. cytotrophoblast
   b. decidual cells d. fetal kidneys

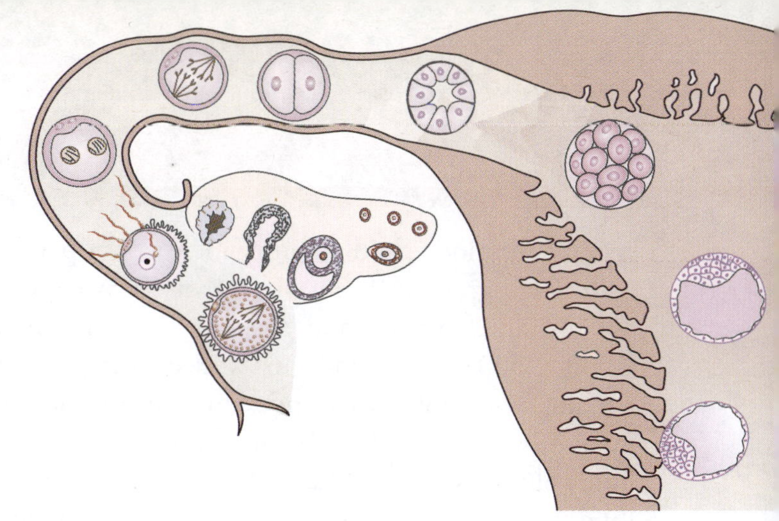

20

Amniotic Fluid and its Abnormalities

Lavanya Rai

LEARNING OBJECTIVES

At the end of this chapter, the reader should be able to:

- describe the normal physiology, constituents and functions of amniotic fluid
- enumerate the criteria for the ultrasound assessment of amniotic fluid and its abnormalities
- appreciate the significance of amniotic fluid in the evaluation of fetal health in pregnancy and labour
- list the complications associated with amniotic fluid abnormalities
- outline the management of polyhydramnios
- outline the management of oligohydramnios

Introduction

Amniotic fluid surrounds the fetus in the amniotic cavity and is essential for its growth and development. This low-resistance environment allows fetal movements and prevents compression of the umbilical cord. Quantitative assessment of amniotic fluid by ultrasound has become an important test for fetal surveillance. Abnormalities in amniotic fluid are associated with perinatal morbidity and mortality. Both excessive as well as deficient amniotic fluid may be markers for underlying fetal or maternal pathologic conditions.

Physiology of Amniotic Fluid

Production

Both the fetus and the mother contribute to the production of amniotic fluid. There is a continuous movement of the constituents of the amniotic fluid between the fetus, the mother and the amniotic cavity. Thus, a balance is maintained between these three compartments for adequacy of amniotic fluid.

Early pregnancy:

- Amniotic fluid is secreted from the cells of the amnion.
- Fetal plasma transudation through the non-keratinised fetal skin and umbilical cord is seen.

Late pregnancy:

- Transudation occurs from the maternal serum across the fetal membranes.
- Fetal urine forms the main source of amniotic fluid from the second trimester onwards.
- Fetal lung and oral-nasal secretions also contribute considerably.

Dynamics

Fluid is reabsorbed through the fetal membranes. The fetus swallows about 400 ml of fluid per day and it is partly reabsorbed from the fetal gut. This promotes the development of the gastrointestinal system. Amniotic fluid quantity increases in parallel with fetal growth, from 30 ml at 10 weeks to 400 ml at 20 weeks, and then to a maximum of 1,000–1,500 ml around 36 weeks; thereafter, it remains steady for a while and reduces to around 800 ml at 40 weeks and then decreases further. Amniotic fluid volume is thus maintained by a balance between fluid production (urine, lung secretions) and fluid resorption through swallowing, and flow across fetal membranes. Maternal hydration can affect the quantity of amniotic fluid. Thus, amniotic fluid is not in a static but a dynamic state.

Composition

The composition is similar to that of extracellular fluid; it is hypotonic with respect to maternal plasma. Concentrations of most of the substances are less than that of serum. As gestational age advances, amniotic fluid composition as well as volume changes. Many hormones and enzymes are present which help in the diagnosis of fetal inborn errors of metabolism.

Functions

The amniotic fluid protects and contributes to fetal development in the following ways:

- It protects the fetus. Its cushioning effect prevents trauma or the pressure of uterine contractions on the cord and fetus and serves to maintain an even temperature.
- It is necessary for lung development from 20 weeks onwards. Fetal breathing movements allow the movement of amniotic fluid in and out of the lungs. Oligohydramnios is often associated with pulmonary hypoplasia.
- Amniotic fluid allows fetal functions such as body movements, breathing movements and swallowing which are required for the growth of the musculoskeletal and gastrointestinal systems.
- It has antibacterial activity which inhibits the growth of certain potentially pathogenic bacteria. It flushes the birth canal during labour, preventing ascending infection.
- Amniotic fluid provides about 25% of fetal protein requirements in late pregnancy.

Ultrasound Assessment of Amniotic Fluid

Amniotic fluid is seen as an echo-free space between the uterus and the fetus on ultrasound. Definitions of increased or decreased amniotic fluid are based on sonographic criteria. A number of methods of amniotic fluid assessment have been described. The important ones are discussed below.

Subjective impression: Qualitative assessment is made by visualising echo-free spaces and fetal crowding. This is reliable if performed by a skilled person.

Maximum vertical pocket (MVP): The largest cord-free vertical pocket is measured in centimetres. An MVP of less than 2 cm or greater than 8 cm represents oligohydramnios and polyhydramnios, respectively. This method is preferred in multiple pregnancies.

Amniotic fluid index (AFI): Amniotic fluid measured as AFI is a semiquantitative assessment of the amniotic fluid volume. The gravid uterus is divided into four quadrants arbitrarily using the umbilicus as the centre point. The deepest vertical pocket in each quadrant is measured in centimetres. The sum of the four quadrants is referred to as the AFI. In a normal pregnancy, the values are 8–24 cm. It is not useful in multiple gestations. AFI is widely used for monitoring high-risk pregnancies.

Abnormalities of amniotic fluid complicate about 7% of pregnancies. If the AFI is **less than 5 cm**, it is **oligohydramnios**, while an **more than 24 cm** indicates **polyhydramnios.** AFI is more reliable in the diagnosis of polyhydramnios than oligohydramnios.

Amniotic Fluid for Evaluation of Fetal Health

During pregnancy

Prenatal diagnosis: Amniocentesis is done for karyotyping, DNA studies and the diagnosis of several inborn errors of metabolism.

Lung maturity: Levels of phospholipids are estimated. In recent years, this test is rarely used because corticosteroid prophylaxis is routine whenever preterm labour is anticipated.

Severity of Rh isoimmunisation: This is detected by spectrophotometry of the amniotic fluid to detect bilirubin levels which indicate severity of hemolysis in Rh isoimmunisation.

Fetal wellbeing test: AFI is used widely for monitoring high-risk pregnancies. As a component of the biophysical profile, it is used to conclude that reduced amniotic fluid volume reflects long-term placental insufficiency.

During labour

Meconium-stained fluid: It is an indicator of fetal distress in some, while in others it may indicate maturity of the gut. Heavy or thick meconium-stained liquor is associated with lower Apgar scores at birth and is associated with the risk of meconium aspiration.

Amniotic fluid embolism: It is a rare, life-threatening complication where the sudden entry of a large amount of amniotic fluid into the maternal circulation results in the development of respiratory distress, shock, disseminated intravascular coagulation and maternal death. Amniotic fluid and fetal cells trigger an anaphylactic reaction, causing cardiorespiratory collapse.

Polyhydramnios

Polyhydramnios is a pathological accumulation of excessive amniotic fluid due to an imbalance between its production and removal. The incidence in clinical practice is about 1% of singleton pregnancies. However, with ultrasound diagnosis, the incidence rises to 8%. When hydramnios is clinically evident, the quantity of amniotic fluid exceeds 2 litres. Based on the rapidity of accumulation of fluid, hydramnios can be classified into two types. Slow accumulation or **chronic hydramnios** is ten times more common than the acute variety, where there is rapid accumulation of fluid over a short period of time.

- **Acute hydramnios** forms 2%–5% of all cases of hydramnios. This is seen in monozygotic twin pregnancies in the second trimester. Maternal symptoms like pain, discomfort and dyspnea are more severe compared to that in chronic hydramnios. It is a common manifestation of twin-to-twin transfusion syndrome and is generally seen prior to 26 weeks of gestation. The prognosis is poor because pregnancy ends in abortion or preterm delivery.
- **Chronic hydramnios** accounts for 95% of all hydramnios cases and is usually seen in the third trimester. Women tolerate this well as the fluid accumulation is gradual, symptoms are less intense and the prognosis is good.

Causes

The etiology of polyhydramnios is diverse and involves many maternal and fetal conditions, as depicted in **Table 20.1**. If none of these causes is identified, then a diagnosis of idiopathic polyhydramnios is made and this is seen in 40%–50% of cases. In a severe degree of polyhydramnios, the cause is identified in almost 90% of cases, while in mild to moderate degree, the cause is evident in only 15% of cases. Fetal anomalies are seen in 20%, the majority being in the central nervous and gastrointestinal systems. Polyhydramnios is seen at times with fetal growth restriction in chromosomal abnormalities. Maternal lithium therapy has been associated with hydramnios secondary to fetal diabetes insipidus. Neuromuscular disorders cause polyhydramnios due to impaired fetal swallowing. In twin-to-twin transfusion syndrome, polyhydramnios in the recipient sac is associated with oligohydramnios in the donor sac.

Clinical features

Symptoms: The woman is asymptomatic in the case of mild to moderate hydramnios. She may suffer from abdominal discomfort, pain and dyspnea. Many patients are unable to lie down. She may report with preterm labour or preterm rupture of membranes.

Signs

- pedal edema due to compression of major veins
- abdominal skin shiny and stretched

Table 20.1 Causes of polyhydramnios

Fetal (20%)
Fetal anomalies
Gastrointestinal tract obstruction
Esophageal atresia
Duodenal atresia
External compression
Diaphragmatic hernia
Failure to swallow
Anencephaly, neck tumours, musculoskeletal dysfunction
Exposure of meninges: meningocele, anencephaly
Fetal anemia
Hydrops fetalis immune/non-immune
Large-for-date baby
Twins with/without twin-to-twin transfusion syndrome
Maternal (20%)
Diabetes
Rh isoimmunisation
Syphilis
Lithium therapy
Placental
Chorioangioma of the placenta
Large placenta

- overdistended uterus appears tense and may be tender in acute hydramnios
- abnormal increase in fundal height
- fetal parts not clearly visualised
- fluid thrill is present
- fetal heart sounds may not be audible

There is difficulty in diagnosing malpresentation, high floating head and unstable lie, which are often present. Vaginal examination may a reveal shortened cervix with a partially open os through which a tense bag of membranes may be felt.

Investigations

Ultrasound: It is an indispensable tool in the management of polyhydramnios for the following reasons:

- confirmation of diagnosis: AFI exceeds 24 cm
- indicates severity of hydramnios
- detects causes such as fetal anomalies, placental chorioangioma and twins

A detailed survey is essential to rule out anomalies. Some anomalies such as esophageal atresia and musculoskeletal disorders may be easily missed. Fetal movements are checked to rule out neuromuscular disorders. In multiple pregnancies, besides anomalies, chorionicity and evidence of twin-to-twin transfusion syndrome are looked for.

- Differentiates hydramnios from ascites or a large ovarian cyst
- Essential for amnioreduction as well as for fetal monitoring during medical therapy

Other investigations: Blood group, Rh type and indirect Coombs test in Rh-negative women are done to rule out isoimmunisation. Glucose tolerance test and VDRL are performed to rule out some of the maternal causes like diabetes and syphilis.

Complications

Polyhydramnios is associated with a number of complications for the mother as well as her fetus (**Table 20.2**). Unengaged head and malpresentations are responsible for the increased incidence of operative deliveries. Overdistended uterus results in the increased incidence of uterine atony, which leads to postpartum hemorrhage. Hydramnios

Table 20.2 Complications of polyhydramnios

Pregnancy
Discomfort, dyspnea
Unstable lie
PROM
Malpresentation
Preterm labour
Mirror syndrome
Labour
Unengaged head
Cord prolapse
Abruptio placentae
Dysfunctional labour
Postpartum hemorrhage
↑ Operative delivery
Fetal
Prematurity
↑ Perinatal mortality

associated with fetal hydrops may cause **mirror syndrome**, wherein the mother develops proteinuria and edema.

Management

The objectives of management are to:

- determine the cause and correct it if possible
- prevent preterm labour and intrapartum complications
- relieve the mother of discomfort by reducing the liquor by medical or surgical therapy.

A comprehensive fetal evaluation and a work-up to rule out maternal factors are essential in the management of polyhydramnios. Conservative or expectant line of management is adopted for a mild degree of hydramnios where patients are generally asymptomatic.

When a specific cause is not identified, no treatment is indicated unless maternal problems arise. Treatment of causes like diabetes and Rh isoimmunisation will correct the problem. A detailed assessment of fetal anatomy is mandatory to rule out structural anomalies in every case of hydramnios. If a lethal anomaly is detected, labour is induced.

Medical management

Indomethacin and sulindac are nonsteroidal antiinflammatory drugs (NSAIDs) used for treating hydramnios in symptomatic patients. These prostaglandin synthetase inhibitors not only decrease amniotic fluid but also prevent preterm labour. They act by decreasing fetal urine output and enhance fluid absorption across the fetal lungs and membranes.

Indomethacin is used in the dose of 25 mg, 6-hourly. However, the side effects limit its use beyond 32–34 weeks of gestation. It induces closure of the ductus arteriosus, causes cerebral vasoconstriction and impaired renal function, and also increases the risk of necrotising enterocolitis. Sulindac has a selective effect of reducing amniotic fluid with a favourable side effect profile compared to indomethacin. It takes about four days for these drugs to be effective. Hence, if immediate relief is required, in symptomatic cases, amnioreduction is preferred and thereafter medical therapy may be instituted.

Surgical management

Amnioreduction or slow decompression by therapeutic amniocentesis is the option for acute hydramnios or whenever the patient is uncomfortable and the medical method fails. Ultrasound-guided slow release of liquor using an 18-gauge needle with an infusion set is preferable. Fluid is removed till the mother has symptomatic relief and fetal parts are readily palpable. Risks of this procedure include preterm labour, preterm rupture of membranes and abruptio placentae.

Obstetrical management depends on the period of gestation and the cause of polyhydramnios.

No detectable cause and preterm fetus

- bed rest to prevent preterm labour
- steroid prophylaxis if less than 34 weeks of gestation

Term fetus

- delivery after controlled rupture of membranes to prevent cord prolapse
- prophylactic oxytocics given in labour to prevent atonic postpartum hemorrhage

After delivery, the baby is examined thoroughly. A catheter is passed into the stomach to rule out esophageal atresia. The severity of polyhydramnios should be taken into account when counselling patients about fetal prognosis. The more severe the degree of polyhydramnios, the higher the perinatal mortality rate. Prognosis is generally good in the idiopathic group occurring near term. Perinatal mortality is high because of prematurity, malformations and other complications of hydramnios.

Oligohydramnios

Oligohydramnios is the decreased quantity of amniotic fluid for the gestational age and can develop at anytime in pregnancy though it is more common in the last trimester. It is generally associated with poor perinatal outcome when severe and occurs in the second trimester. Oligohydramnios is diagnosed when AFI is less than than 5 cm and the volume of amniotic fluid may be less than 200 ml.

Causes

- Maternal conditions like hypertensive disorders, dehydration and the intake of drugs like NSAIDs where placental circulation is compromised cause oligohydramnios.
- In the presence of oligohydramnios, there is a fourfold increased risk of fetal growth restriction. When fetal malformations cause oligohydramnios, it occurs early in pregnancy. A compromised fetus will preferentially shunt blood away from the trunk and periphery to the major organs like brain, heart and adrenals. This reduces renal perfusion, resulting in oliguria which manifests as oligohydramnios in IUGR. The smaller fetal vascular volume in an IUGR fetus also contributes.
- The incidence of fetal anomalies is 51% in midtrimester oligohydramnios and 22% in the third trimester. Fetal deformities occur as a result of prolonged oligohydramnios. Thus, fetal anomalies can be the cause or the result of oligohydramnios.
- Premature rupture of membranes results in reduced liquor.

Oligohydramnios is a common finding in postterm pregnancy and is a marker of declining placental function. Here, the reduction in amniotic fluid is progressive and rapid. When no apparent anomaly or growth restriction is evident, premature rupture of membranes should be ruled out. **Table 20.3** summarises the causes of oligohydramnios.

Table 20.3 Causes of oligohydramnios

Fetal causes

Fetal growth restriction
Postmaturity
Premature rupture of membranes (PROM)
Fetal anomalies
  Renal agenesis/dysplasia
  Lower urinary tract obstruction
  Sirenomelia
Chromosomal anomaly: Trisomy 13, 18

Maternal causes
Preeclampsia Dehydration Drug ingestion: Angiotensin converting enzyme (ACE) inhibitors like captopril NSAIDs: Indomethacin Placental causes: Circumvallate placenta

Effects and complications

The effects and complications of oligohydramnios depend on the gestational age: the earlier the manifestation, the worse the fetal prognosis. When it occurs very early due to leaking of amniotic fluid, amniotic bands develop. Entanglement of fetal parts in amniotic bands results in constrictions and amputations. The spectrum of deformation anomalies include craniospinal, abdominal wall and limb reduction defects. Prolonged oligohydramnios can lead to deformation sequence in 10%–15% of cases. Pulmonary hypoplasia is an important complication of second trimester oligohydramnios. Perinatal mortality is high even in third trimester oligohydramnios due to prematurity or complications of fetal growth restriction (**Table 20.4**).

Oligohydramnios is a warning sign that the placental reserve is low. Hence, there is an increased risk of fetal distress either due to placental insufficiency or to cord compression. Reduced fluid with meconium staining in labour is likely to cause meconium aspiration syndrome in the neonate. Prognosis depends on the cause, period of gestation and severity of oligohydramnios. Prolonged, early onset oligohydramnios with fetal anomalies has the worst prognosis. Survival has improved with antepartum surveillance and timely delivery for late onset oligohydramnios, with IUGR and post-dated pregnancies.

Table 20.4 Effects and complications of oligohydramnios

First and second trimester	Third trimester and labour
Amniotic band syndrome • Amputation of limbs/digits • Abdominal wall defects Pulmonary hypoplasia Fetal anomalies: Talipes, wry neck, joint contracture, Potter sequence Abortion	Preterm labour Cord compression Fetal growth restriction Fetal death Malpresentation: Breech Operative delivery increased Placenta: Amnion nodosum High perinatal mortality Meconium aspiration syndrome

Clinical diagnosis

The woman is often asymptomatic; in rare cases, she may complain of decreased fetal movement. Detailed history should be taken and clinical examination performed with a view to establishing the cause.

Signs

- inadequate weight gain
- reduced fluid on palpation
- fundal height generally less than normal for the period of gestation
- fetal parts may not be easily palpable as the fetus is gripped by the uterus

Management

The objectives of management are to:

- find the cause
- perform a fetal surveillance
- ensure timely delivery.

Investigations: Ultrasound confirms the diagnosis of oligohydramnios when the amniotic fluid index is less than 5 cm; it is also used to detect/rule out anomalies associated with oligohydramnios. Fetal growth parameters along with biophysical profile are measured serially in IUGR with oligohydramnios in the third trimester. Due to lack of fluid and poor acoustic window, the ultrasound view is often suboptimal. Fetal flexion and compression further impair visualisation of fetal anatomy. Amnioinfusion may be attempted to improve the acoustic window, for better diagnosis.

Treatment: There is no specific treatment though many methods such as bed rest to improve uteroplacental circulation, maternal hydration and uterine relaxants have been tried empirically with no proven benefit. Maternal intravascular fluid status is linked to that of the fetus. Thus, hydrating the mother may have some transient effect on amniotic fluid volume and may be beneficial.

Oligohydramnios at term or near term requires aggressive fetal monitoring, and delivery is considered if fetal maturity is present. The likelihood of cesarean section in labour is high because of fetal distress. At times, elective cesarean section is preferred in severe oligohydramnios and IUGR. If anomalies are present, pregnancy can be terminated depending on the type of anomaly, prognosis and gestational age. In IUGR with oligohydramnios, close monitoring with antepartum fetal surveillance is required from the beginning of the third trimester. Steroid prophylaxis, and rest with hydration may allow the pregnancy to continue for a few more days or weeks to improve the neonatal outcome.

Normal saline or Ringer lactate is infused into the uterine cavity to prevent cord compression during labour. This is done to optimise the neonatal outcome and to decrease the chance of meconium aspiration syndrome and cord compression. The dilutional effect of infused fluid is believed to prevent meconium aspiration syndrome.

KEY POINTS

- The amniotic fluid plays an important role in protecting the fetus.
- Increased liquor is polyhydramnios and decreased liquor oligohydramnios.
- Abnormalities in amniotic fluid are seen in 7% of pregnancies.
- Ultrasound is invaluable in the management of abnormalities of amniotic fluid.
- Midtrimester polyhydramnios or oligohydramnios have poor prognosis.
- In oligo/polyhydramnios, fetal malformations should be ruled out.
- Amnioreduction and medical management with indomethacin/sulindac are used in the treatment of polyhydramnios.
- Fetal growth restriction and renal anomalies are to be ruled out by ultrasound in the presence of oligohydramnios.
- Fetal surveillance and timely delivery improve outcome in oligohydramnios without anomalies.

QUESTIONS

Select the single most appropriate answer:

1. The amniotic fluid has all of the following characteristics *except*
   a. composition similar to extracellular fluid
   b. hypotonic compared to maternal plasma
   c. has antibacterial activity
   d. provides 75% of the fetus protein requirements
2. Amniotic fluid embolism is *not* characterised by
   a. anemia
   b. disseminated intravascular coagulation
   c. respiratory distress
   d. hypovolemic shock
3. Acute hydramnios is a feature of
   a. dichorionic twins
   b. gastroschisis
   c. multicystic kidneys
   d. twin-to-twin transfusion
4. The drug which causes hydramnios is
   a. alpha methyldopa c. indomethacin
   b. digoxin d. lithium
5. Fetal aneuploidy should be suspected when polyhydramnios is associated with
   a. anencephaly c. macrosomia
   b. growth restriction d. skeletal dysplasia
6. Which of the following anomalies is not associated with polyhydramnios?
   a. congenital diaphragmatic hernia
   b. esophageal atresia
   c. non-immune hydrops
   d. Potter sequence
7. Oligoamnios can cause all of the following complications *except*
   a. cord compression
   b. deformation sequence
   c. postpartum hemorrhage
   d. pulmonary hypoplasia
8. The quantity of amniotic fluid at 20 weeks is approximately
   a. 200 ml b. 400 ml c. 600 ml d. 800 ml
9. Functions of amniotic fluid include all of the following *except*
   a. cushioning effect to the fetus
   b. improves urine output
   c. maintains even temperature for the fetus
   d. promotes development of fetus
10. Oligoamnios is a feature of
    a. diaphragmatic hernia
    b. omphalocele
    c. spina bifida
    d. sirenomelia
11. Amniotic fluid studies help in the diagnosis of all of the following *except*
    a. fetal gestational age
    b. karyotype
    c. lung maturity
    d. Rh isoimmunisation

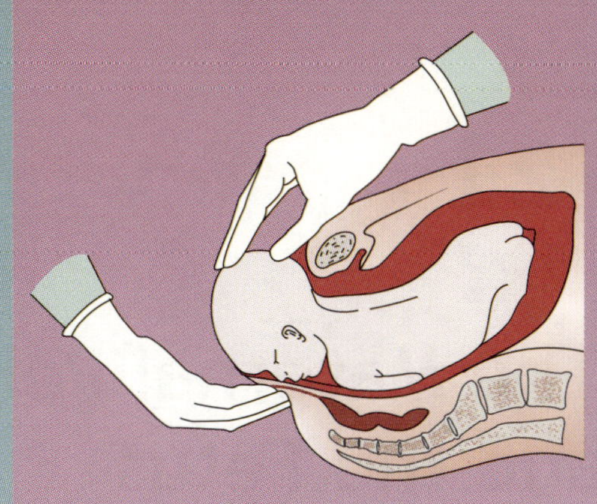

Part III Labour

21

The Maternal Pelvis and the Fetus

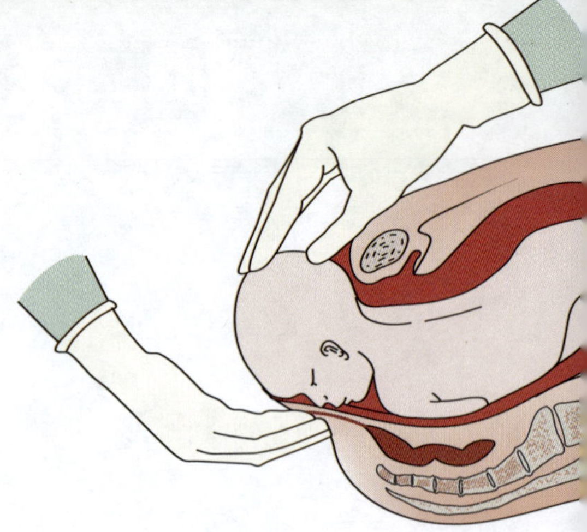

Asmita Rathore

LEARNING OBJECTIVES

At the end of this chapter, the reader should be able to:

- appreciate the importance of the maternal pelvis and fetal skull in obstetrics
- describe the anatomy of the bony pelvis and its dimensions
- list the different types of pelvis
- enumerate the steps of pelvic assessment
- describe the essential musculature of the pelvis and its role in labour
- describe the anatomy of the fetal skull and its bony landmarks
- list the important measurements of the fetal skull

Introduction

Knowledge of the anatomy of the maternal pelvis and fetus is essential to the understanding of obstetrics. In women, the pelvis is specially adapted to childbearing. The size and shape of the female pelvis and of the fetal skull are of great importance in obstetrics as the mechanism of labour is essentially a process of accommodation of the fetus to the bony passage through which it must pass. In this chapter, we will discuss the maternal pelvis and fetus from the obstetric point of view.

The Maternal Pelvis

The female pelvis is shaped like a basin: it contains and protects the internal organs of reproduction and the fetus passes through it during parturition. It is composed of bones and soft tissue.

Bony pelvis

The bony pelvis consists of bones and ligaments stripped of the muscular coverings (**Fig. 21.1**).

The pelvis is formed by four bones: two hip bones or innominate bones at the sides with the sacrum and coccyx behind. The hip bones are composite bones formed by the union of the ilium, ischium and pubis on each side and give origin to the levator ani muscle. The important points on the ilium are the anterior superior iliac spine and the iliac crest. The ischium is a part of the sacrosciatic notch and has a prominent ischial spine, which is an important landmark in the pelvis. The ischial tuberosity is the lower part of the ischium. The pubic crest and tubercle are part of the pubic bone; they are used as points of reference for fetal position. The sacrum is a triangular bone with the base above, and consists of five fused vertebrae. The sacral promontory,

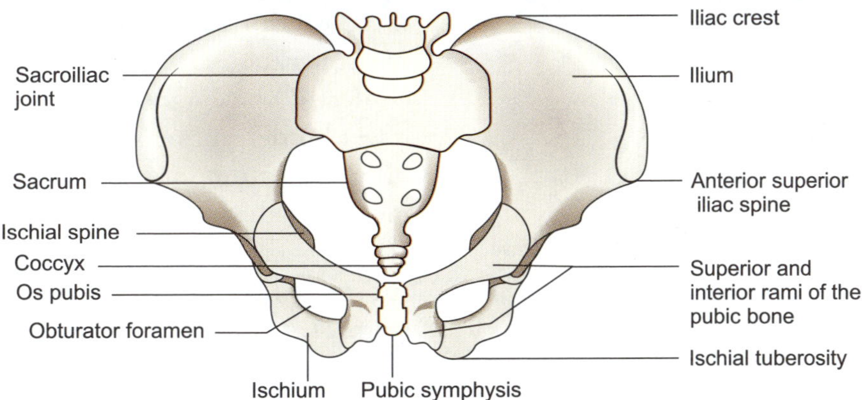

Fig. 21.1 Bony pelvis.

which is the anterior superior edge of the sacral bone, protrudes slightly into the cavity of the pelvis. The anterior surface of the sacrum is concave and forms the posterior wall of the pelvic cavity. The **coccyx** articulates with the lower end of the sacrum and provides attachment to the coccygeus muscles, levator ani and sphincter ani externus muscles. Joints articulate with the four pelvic bones and the union is completed by strong ligaments.

Joints

There are four joints: two sacroiliac joints, the pubic symphysis and the sacrococcygeal joint.

Sacroiliac joints: On either side, the iliac and sacral bones are applied to each other by their large articular surfaces, with a plate of hyaline cartilage covering both surfaces. It is a synovial joint united by fibrocartilaginous adhesions in its upper part and by a small cavity containing synovial fluid at the lower end. It is strengthened by ligaments in front and behind.

Pubic symphysis: This fibrocartilaginous joint has no capsule and no synovial membrane. It connects the ends of the two pubic bones and has superior and inferior pubic ligaments. Normally, there is very little movement at this joint. The separation of bones during pregnancy can cause difficulty and pain on walking.

Sacrococcygeal joint: This is a synovial joint between the sacrum and the coccyx and allows movement of the coccyx backwards during labour.

Ligaments

The ligaments that take part in the formation of the pelvis are the sacrotuberous and sacrospinous ligaments, obturator membrane, inguinal ligaments and ligaments covering the various joints. The sacrotuberous ligament is attached at one end to the side the of sacrum and the posterior iliac spines, and to the ischial tuberosity on the other. The sacrospinous ligament is a triangular ligament with its base attached to the sacrum and coccyx and its apex to the ischial spine. They form the posterolateral wall of the pelvic cavity. During pregnancy, the ligaments of the pelvis are softened to allow a slight degree of stretching and increase the range of movement. This softening may be due to increased vascularity or the effect of hormones like progesterone and relaxin.

The Pelvis and its Dimensions: Obstetric Importance

From the obstetric point of view, the pelvis is divided into the false pelvis and the true pelvis, separated by the arcuate line formed by the upper margin of the symphysis pubis, iliopectineal lines and the promontory of the sacrum. It is the true pelvis that is of obstetric significance.

True pelvis

This is the bony canal, roughly cylindrical, bent forwards, through which the fetus has to pass. It is divided into an inlet, midcavity and outlet (**Fig. 21.2**).

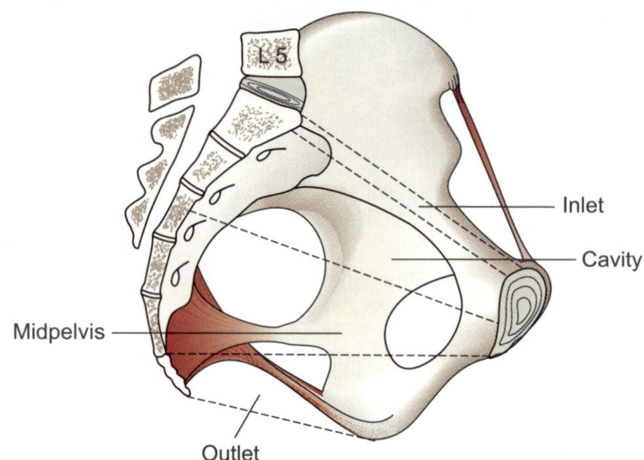

Fig. 21.2 Lateral view of the pelvis showing the brim, cavity and outlet.

The inlet or brim of the pelvis is bound by the sacral promontory posteriorly, the ala of the sacrum, and on either side the iliopectineal lines, iliopectineal eminences and upper border of the pubic bones. It is oval and has a posterior projection due to the sacral promontory. The plane of the inlet has an inclination of about 60 degrees with the horizontal.

Diameters of the inlet

The various diameters of the pelvic inlet are as follows (**Fig. 21.3**):

Anteroposterior diameters: The anatomical conjugate or true conjugate is measured from the middle of the sacral promontory to the top of the symphysis pubis and measures about 11 cm. The **obstetric conjugate** is measured from the middle of the sacral promontory to the nearest point on the posterior surface of the symphysis pubis and measures about 10.5 cm. This cannot be measured clinically. The **diagonal conjugate** extends from the lower border of the pubic symphysis to the middle of sacral promontory and this is the diameter measured during clinical pelvimetry; it measures 12–12.5 cm; to obtain the obstetric conjugate, subtract 1.5 cm from the diagonal conjugate (**Fig. 21.4**).

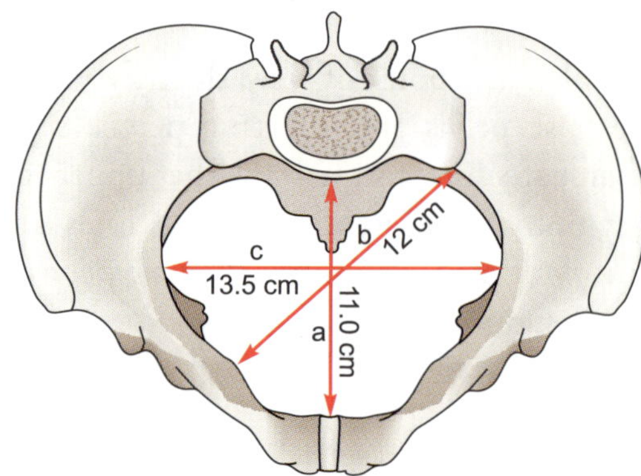

Fig. 21.3 Diameters of the pelvic inlet
a: Anteroposterior b: Oblique c: Transverse

Oblique diameters: On both the right and left sides, oblique diameters are measured from the corresponding sacroiliac joint to the iliopectineal eminence of the opposite side (about 12 cm).

Transverse diameter: It is the greatest distance between the two arcuate lines; measures about 13 cm.

The important diameters of the bony pelvis can be summarised as follows:

	Anteroposterior	Oblique	Transverse
Brim	11	12	13
Cavity	12	12	12
Outlet	13	–	11

Midcavity

It extends from the inlet to the outlet. Its anterior wall is formed by the posterior surface of the symphysis

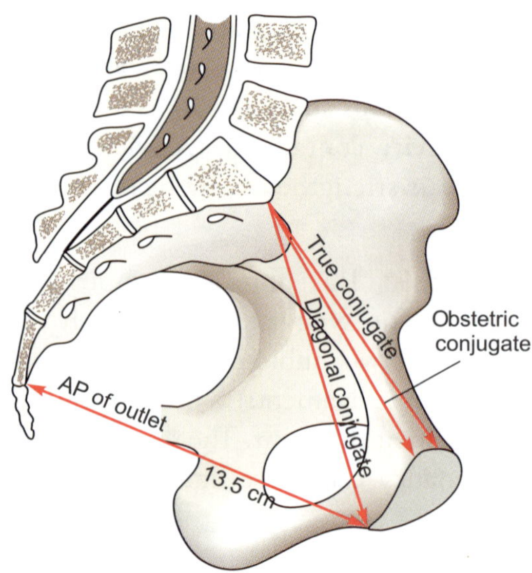

Fig. 21.4 Sagittal section of the pelvis with conjugate diameters.

pubis, the side walls by ischial spines and part of the ilium and the sacrotuberous and sacrospinous ligaments posteriorly. The posterior wall of the cavity is formed by the anterior surface of the sacrum and coccyx and is curved from above downwards and from side to side.

The ischial spines are the important bony landmarks of the midcavity. The distance between the two ischial spines forms the transverse diameter of the midcavity of the pelvis (**Fig. 21.5**). The ischial spines also form the point of reference for assessing the status of the presenting part with reference to the pelvis.

Pelvic outlet

The outlet of the pelvis is bound posteriorly by the coccyx and the sacrotuberous and sacrospinous ligaments and anteriorly by the lower edge of the symphysis pubis and the rami of pubes. At the sides, it is bound by ischial tuberosities.

Diameters of the outlet: The anatomic anteroposterior diameter of the outlet extends from the inferior margin of the symphysis pubis to the tip of the coccyx and measures about 13.5 cm. The transverse diameter extends between the medial surfaces of the ischial tuberosities and measures about 11 cm (**Fig. 21.6**).

Planes and diameters

The plane of **greatest pelvic dimensions**, which is the roomiest part of the pelvis, passes from the centre of the posterior surface of the symphysis pubis to the

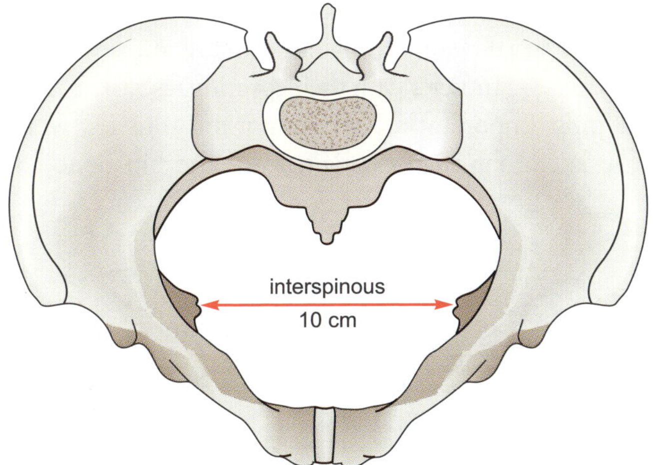

Fig. 21.5 Transverse diameter of the midcavity.

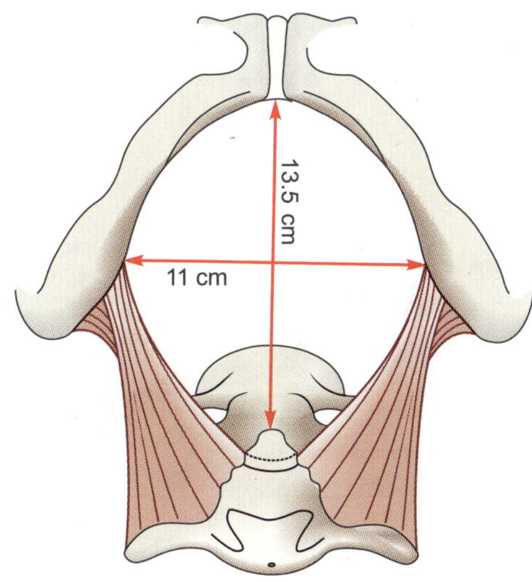

Fig. 21.6 Diameters of the pelvic outlet

junction of the second and third sacral vertebrae. At the level of the plane of greatest pelvic dimensions, the shape of the cavity is roughly circular and all anteroposterior, oblique and transverse diameters measure about 12 cm.

The plane of least pelvic dimensions passes through the lower margin of the symphysis, tips of the ischial spines to the tip of the fifth sacral piece (**Fig. 21.7**). The interischial spinous diameter or transverse diameter of the plane of least pelvic dimensions is measured between the medial surfaces of the ischial spines, and measures about 10 cm.

Axis of the pelvis

This is the theoretical path traversed by the centre of the fetal head during birth. At any of the levels, it is represented roughly by a perpendicular passing through the centre of that plane and as a whole is a curved line formed by the combination of such axes. Due to the curve of the sacrum, the upper portion of the cavity is directed downwards and backwards, middle part downwards and the lower part downwards and forward (**Fig. 21.8**). This is known as the curve of Carus.

Pelvic shapes

Caldwell and Moloy classified the female pelvis by shape as gynecoid, android, anthropoid and

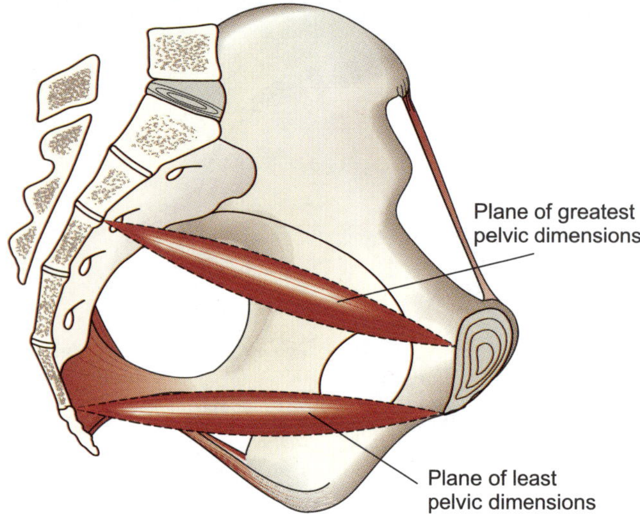

Fig. 21.7 Planes of pelvis.

platypelloid (**Fig. 21.9**). Of these, the gynecoid type is the most common, seen in about 50%; the android type is seen in about 20%, anthropoid in 25% and platypelloid in 5% of women. However, in most women, the pelvis does not exclusively conform to one type. The characteristic of the posterior segment determines the type and the anterior segment determines the tendency. For example, a pelvis could be, of the android type with a tendency for the gynecoid type. The mechanism of labour may vary in different types, with gynecoid being the most favourable for normal labour. The ideal pelvis is the gynecoid type where the inlet is oval in shape with no undue projection of the sacral promontory. The anteroposterior diameter is 11–11.5 cm, and is inclined about 60 degrees to the horizontal. The cavity itself is shallow; in fact, it is described as **a narrow segment of a long cone,** the side walls are minimally convergent and the ischial spines are not prominent. The sacrum has a smooth curve, the subpubic arch is rounded and the intertuberous

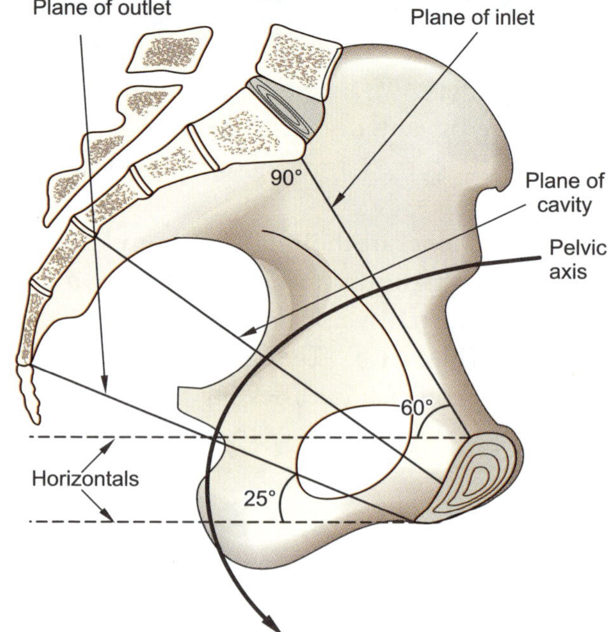

Fig. 21.8 Axis of pelvis.

diameter is 11 cm. The main characteristics of these types and their effect on labour are summarised in **Table 21.1**.

Soft Tissues of the Pelvis

The pelvis is a dynamic structure during life. The soft tissues of the pelvis encroach to a considerable extent upon the space in the true pelvis and play an important role in the mechanism of labour.

Pelvic floor

It is a muscular diaphragm, also known as pelvic diaphragm, that separates the pelvic cavity above from the perineal space below. It mainly contains the levator ani and coccygei muscles with their covering fascia. Of these, the most important are the levator ani muscles, which have lateral fan-shaped origin from the hip bone and

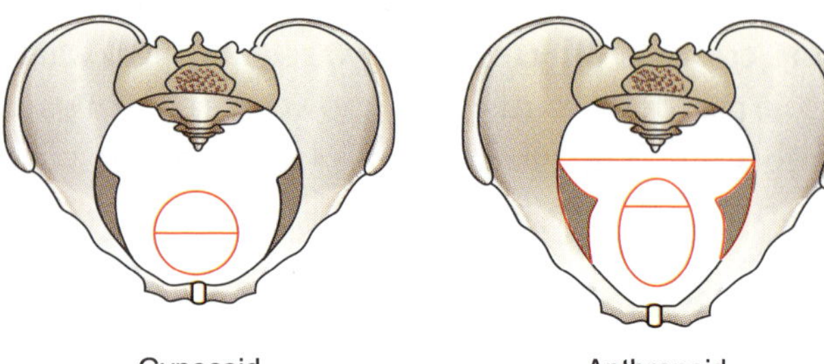

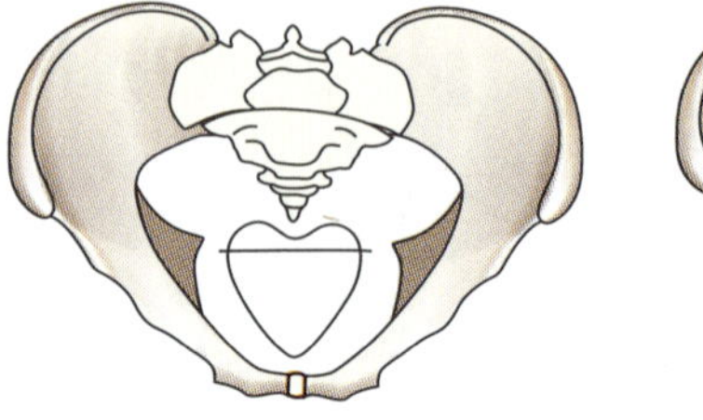

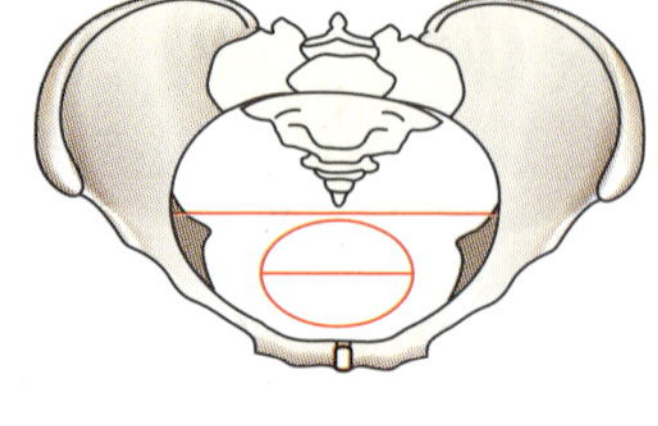

Fig. 21.9 Types of pelvis.

Table 21.1 Caldwell-Moloy classification of the pelvis

	Gynecoid	Android	Anthropoid	Platypelloid
Inlet				
Shape	Round or transversely oval	Heart-shaped or wedge-shaped	Anteroposterior oval	Transverse oval
Cavity				
Sacrum	Wide, short, deep curve	Flat, long, narrow, inclined forward	Narrow, long inclined backward	Wide, deep curve, angulated
Side walls	Straight, parallel	Convergent/funneled	Straight	Parallel/divergent
Ischial spines	Not prominent	Prominent	Variable	Variable
Sacrosciatic notch	Wide, short	Narrow, long	Wide	Short
Capacity	Adequate	Reduced in all diameters	Adequate long	Reduced short
Outlet				
AP diameter	Long	Short	Long	Short
Pubic arch	Wide, round	Narrow, deep	Normal or narrow	Very wide
Effect on labour				
Engagement of head	In transverse or oblique diameter	In transverse or post diameter	In AP diameter, or occipitoposterior position common	In transverse diameter, with asynclitism
Problems during labour	None	Deep transverse arrest common	Easy delivery, Face-to-pubis delivery common	Delay at inlet, then easy birth

central insertion where it joins with the corresponding muscle of the opposite side. Each levator ani comprises pubococcygeus, iliococcygeus and ischiococcygeus muscles. They pass from the pubes back to their insertion, embracing the rectum and vagina and acting as a sling to hold them in position, and form a fibrotendinous raphe between the anus and the coccyx (**Fig. 21.10**).

The pelvic floor supports the pelvic viscera and helps in building effective intraabdominal pressure. The displacement of the anterior and posterior segments of the pelvic floor during labour plays an important role in the mechanism of labour, helping in internal rotation of the presenting part.

Perineum

The perineum is the diamond-shaped area between the medial aspects of the thighs. It is bound laterally by bones and joints of the pelvic outlet, the pubic symphysis anteriorly, ischiopubic rami and ischial tuberosities anterolaterally, sacrotuberous ligament posterolaterally and the coccyx posteriorly.

Anterior triangle: A line joining through the ischial tuberosities divides the perineum into two triangles: the anterior triangle known as the urogenital triangle and the posterior triangle termed the anal triangle.

The boundaries of the anterior triangle are pubic rami superiorly, the ischial tuberosities laterally and the superficial transverse perineal muscle posteriorly.

Urogenital triangle: In addition to the opening of the urethra and vagina, the urogenital triangle contains the urogenital diaphragm, crura of clitoris and bulbs of vestibule, Bartholin glands and their ducts, perineal body, superficial perineal muscles, superficial fascia of perineum with its membranous and fatty layer and blood vessels, nerves and lymphatics. The urogenital diaphragm, which is also known as the triangular ligament, is made up of the deep transverse perineal muscles with its internal and external fascial covering and constrictor urethra. The superficial muscles of the perineum include the superficial transverse perineal muscles, ischiocavernosus muscles and bulbocavernosus muscles and have an attachment to the perineal body. These muscles, along with vaginal mucosa and skin, are incised during episiotomy. The anal

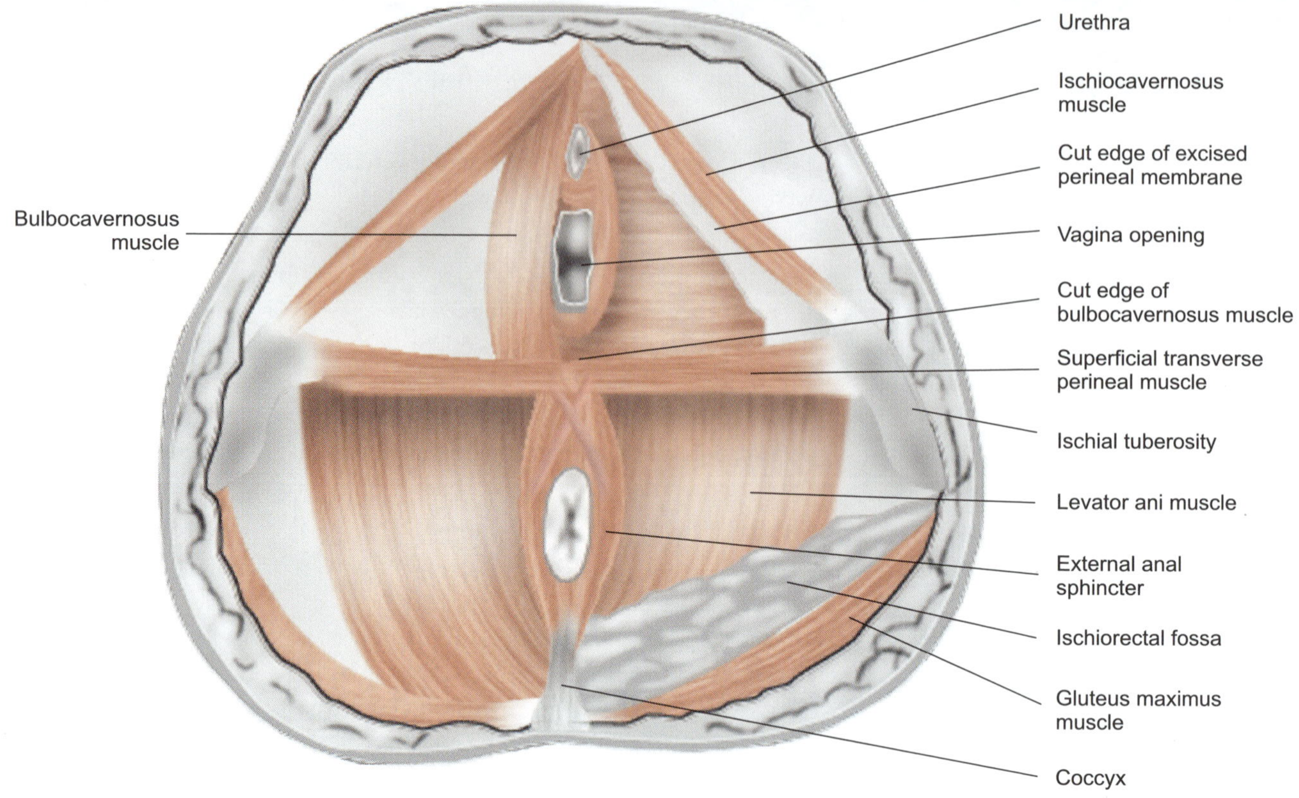

Fig. 21.10 Pelvic floor.

triangle contains the lower end of the anal canal and its sphincters, anococcygeal body, ischiorectal fossa, blood vessels, lymphatics and nerves.

Perineal body: This is the central tendon of the perineum and lies between the anus and the vagina. It is formed by the median raphe of the levator ani, the superficial and deep transverse perineal muscles, the bulbocavernosus muscles and the external sphincter ani muscles. The perineal body provides support for the perineum. During childbirth, the anterior fibres of the levator ani, perineal body, muscles and skin become enormously stretched, and are liable to be torn. Such injury, especially if it involves the levators, favours subsequent prolapse of the uterus and vaginal walls. In the case of complete perineal tear, the perineal body along with the rectal sphincter are torn and if not appropriately repaired can lead to anal incontinence.

Blood supply to the perineum is mainly by the internal pudendal artery and its branches. The innervation is primarily through the pudendal nerve originating from S2, 3, 4 and its branches.

THE FETUS

By weeks 38–40, the fetus is fully mature. It measures about 50 cm in length and weighs 3,000 g. The circumference of the head and the shoulder are almost the same. The fetus influences the course of labour by its size, presentation and position. The fetal head is the most voluminous, least compressible part, and is the leading part during labour in the majority of cases. It is therefore important to study the fetal skull and its relevant dimensions.

The Fetal Skull

The fetal skull is more ovoid in shape than that of the adult and the face is a relatively smaller part of the whole head. The skull is divided into the vault and base of the skull by an imaginary line drawn from the orbital ridges to just behind the foramen magnum. The base of the skull is mainly bony, not compressible and protects the vital centres in the medulla and pons. The vault of the skull is more compressible and can withstand a good deal of pressure and undergoes adjustments during labour.

Bones and sutures

The bones that form the vault of the fetal skull are two frontal bones, two parietal bones, two temporal bones laterally and one occipital bone at the back. The bones of the vault are laid down in membrane and are not completely ossified at birth. The edges of the bones are membranous and separated from each other by definite spaces known as sutures (**Fig. 21.11**). They permit moulding during labour and their identification on vaginal examination during labour helps in determining the position and progress during labour. The important sutures are: the **sagittal suture** separating the two parietal bones, the **lambdoid suture** between the occipital and parietal bones, the **coronal suture** between the frontal and parietal bones, and the **temporal suture** between the temporal and parietal bones.

Fontanelles

These are the areas of membranes at the junction of sutures. There are two fontanelles, which are identified by their shape and the presence of radiating sutures and serve as important landmarks during labour.

- The anterior fontanelle or bregma is a lozenge-shaped area at the junction of the coronal suture with the sagittal and frontal sutures and measures about 3 cm × 2 cm.
- The posterior fontanelle is a small triangular area at the junction of the posterior end of the sagittal suture and lambdoid suture.

Important landmarks on the fetal skull

For convenience of description, obstetricians define certain regions of the fetal skull in terms of the following landmarks (**Fig. 21.11**).

Vertex: It is the region bound in front by the anterior fontanelle, behind by the posterior fontanelle and on either side by the parietal eminences. It is the presenting part in case of normal labour.

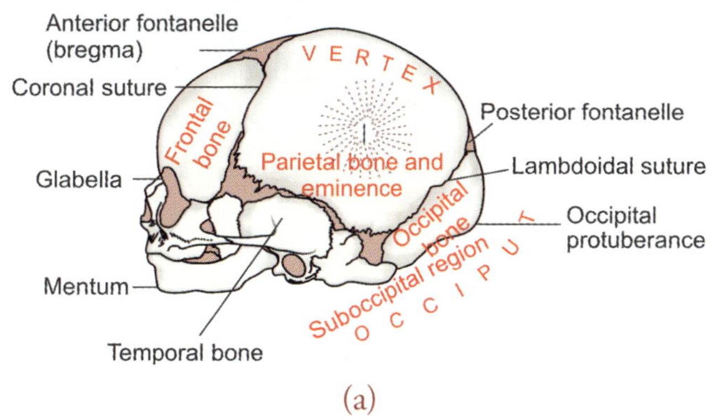

(a)

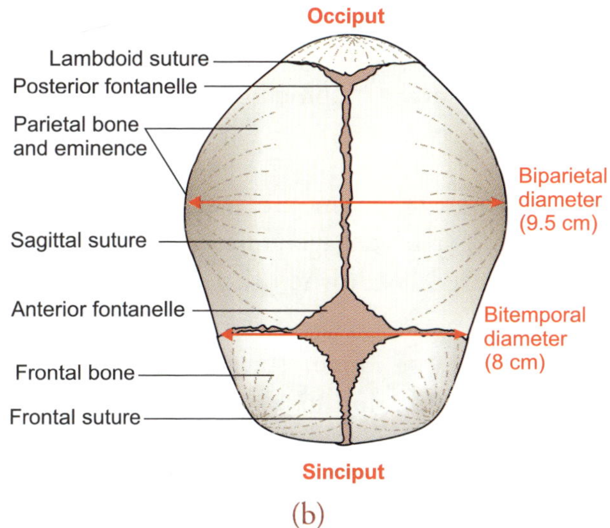

(b)

Fig. 21.11 Bones and sutures of fetal skull
a: Lateral view b: Superior view.

Occiput: The occiput comprises the area behind the posterior fontanelle and lambdoid suture.

Sinciput: It is the region in front of the anterior fontanelle and coronal suture and extends up to the orbital ridges.

Face: It is the area below the orbital ridges.

Glabella: It is the elevated area between the orbital ridges and can be easily felt in brow and face presentations.

Diameters of the fetal skull

Just as in the maternal pelvis, the imaginary planes and their diameters are defined in the fetal skull in order to facilitate its description (**Fig. 21.12**).

Suboccipito-bregmatic diameter: It extends from the centre of the bregma to the midpoint between the occipital protuberance and the posterior margin

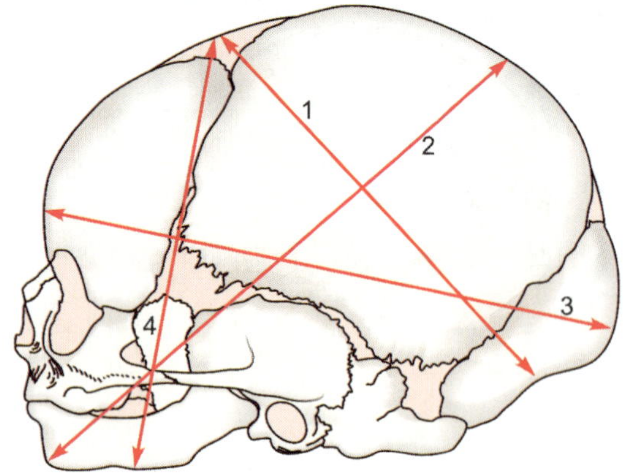

Fig. 21.12 Diameters of the fetal skull
1: Suboccipito-bregmatic 2: Mento-vertical
3: Occipito-frontal 4: Submento-bregmatic.

of the foramen magnum and measures 9.5 cm. It is the diameter of engagement in normal labour with well-flexed head, when the presenting part is the vertex.

Suboccipitofrontal diameter: It extends from the suboccipital point to the root of the nose. It measures 10.5 cm.

Occipitofrontal diameter: It passes through the occipital protuberance and the glabella or the root of the nose and measures 11.25 cm. It is the diameter of engagement in labour with vertex when the head is deflexed.

Mento-vertical diameter: It passes through the posterior fontanelle and the midpoint of mentum or the chin and measures 13.5 cm. It is the diameter of engagement in brow presentation when the head is extended halfway. This is the largest diameter of the skull and cannot negotiate the maternal pelvis, making vaginal delivery impossible.

Submento-bregmatic diameter: It extends from the angle of the neck to the midpoint of the bregma and measures 9.5 cm, the same as the suboccipito-bregmatic diameter. It is the diameter of engagement in face presentation when the head is completely extended.

Biparietal diameter: It extends between the two parietal eminences and measures 9.5 cm. It is the largest transverse diameter of the skull. The fetal head is said to be engaged when the biparietal diameter crosses the pelvic brim (**Fig. 21.11b**).

Bitemporal diameter: It passes vertically through the lower end of the coronal sutures and is not of much significance in obstetrics (**Fig. 21.11b**).

Moulding

The skull is subjected to considerable pressure as it passes through the pelvis. As described earlier, the bones of the fetal skull are mobile and under pressure in the pelvis; the shape of the head is modified to mould into the pelvis. During moulding, the parietal bones slip under each other, and the occipital and frontal bones slip under the parietal bones (**Fig. 21.13**).

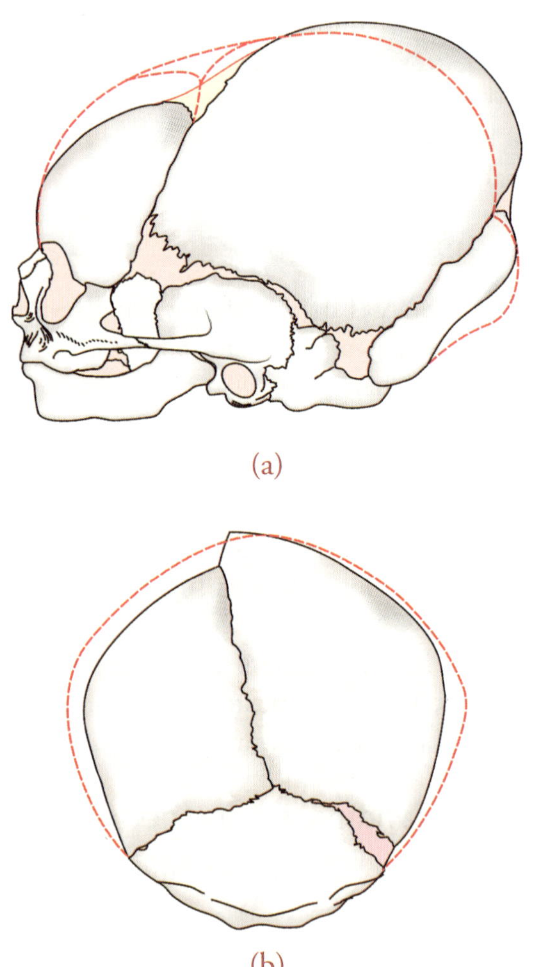

Fig. 21.13 Moulding of fetal head a: Lateral view b: Superior view.

KEY POINTS

- The anatomy of the female pelvis and fetal skull is important in obstetrics as, during labour, the fetus has to accommodate to the maternal pelvis.
- The pelvis is formed by the two hip bones with the sacrum and coccyx behind, which are united by four joints. Important ligaments taking part in the formation of the pelvis are the sacrotuberous ligament, sacrospinous ligament and the ligaments covering various joints.
- The bony pelvis is divided into the inlet or brim, midpelvis or cavity and outlet.
- Pelvic shapes are classified into gynecoid, android, anthropoid, platypelloid and mixed types. The mechanism of labour may vary in different types of pelves; the gynecoid type is the most favourable for normal labour.
- Pelvic size can be assessed with reasonable accuracy clinically and the relative size of fetal head to the pelvis is more important than the absolute size of either.
- Soft parts of the pelvis play an important role in the mechanism of labour.
- The pelvic floor, which mainly contains the levator ani muscles, supports the pelvic viscera and helps in internal rotation of presenting part during labour.
- The perineum lies below the pelvic floor and is liable to be torn during labour due to stretching.
- The bones forming the fetal skull are the two frontal, parietal and temporal bones and one occipital bone. Important sutures in the fetal skull are sagittal, lambdoid and coronal sutures.
- Important landmarks of the fetal skull are occiput, sinciput, vertex, brow, glabella and face.
- The important diameters of the fetal skull are suboccipito-bregmatic diameter (9.5 cm), mento-vertical diameter (13.5 cm) and submento-bregmatic diameter (9.5 cm) which are diameters of engagement in vertex, brow and face presentations, respectively.
- The biparietal diameter, when it crosses the pelvic brim, is used to indicate engagement and measures 9.5 cm.

QUESTIONS

Select the single most appropriate answer:

1. The sacrococcygeal joint is
   a. synovial joint
   b. fibrous joint
   c. cartilagenous joint
   d. fibrocartilagenous joint
2. The angle of inclination of the pelvic brim is
   a. 15°
   b. 30°
   c. 45°
   d. 60°
3. The diameter of engagement in brow presentation is
   a. occipito-frontal
   b. mentobregmatic
   c. mento-vertical
   d. submento-bregmatic
4. Face-to-pubis delivery is common in which type of pelvis?
   a. android
   b. anthropoid
   c. gynecoid
   d. platypelloid
5. The denominator in face presentation is the
   a. nose
   b. mentum
   c. glabella
   d. orbital ridge

Mark true (T) or false (F) against each statement:

6. The anatomical conjugate of the pelvic inlet indicates the space available to the fetus.
7. The interischial spinous diameter is the smallest diameter of the pelvis.
8. X-ray pelvimetry is more accurate than clinical pelvimetry in predicting vaginal delivery.
9. The axis of the pelvis is a straight line.
10. The left occipitoposterior position is the commonest position in normal labour.

22

Physiology of Labour

Raj Narayan

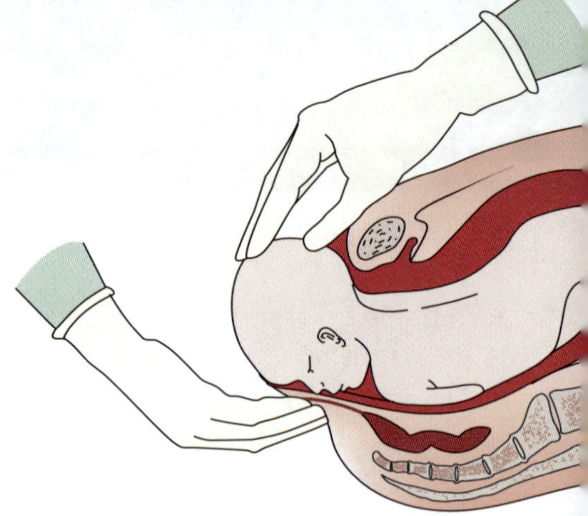

LEARNING OBJECTIVES

At the end of this chapter, the reader should be able to:

- define labour
- describe the changes in the uterus and the cervix
- define the clinical stages of labour
- list the duration of each stage
- describe the molecular basis of myometrial contraction
- describe the biochemical processes involved in the activation of the myometrium
- describe the regulation of uterine activity during pregnancy and labour
- list the various methods of measuring uterine activity

Introduction

Labour is the climax of the reproductive process. It is a physical and an emotional stress for the mother and a 'hazardous journey' for the fetus. Labour is defined as the physiological process by which the fetus and placenta are expelled from the uterus. The process consists of a complex sequence of events which results in a change in the pattern of myometrial activity, change in consistency and structure of the cervix and a gradual descent of the fetus through the birth canal and delivery to the outside world.

Changes in the uterus and cervix prior to labour

The pregnant uterus is in a state of quiescence till 36 to 38 weeks. During pregnancy, the cervix becomes soft, but remains closed with a mucus plug. This not only protects the pregnancy from infection, but more importantly, it maintains its physical integrity as the uterus enlarges through pregnancy.

Before the actual onset of labour, the unresponsiveness of the uterus is suspended and the cervix undergoes some remodelling by which it responds to myometrial contractions and dilates to allow the passage of the fetus.

During pregnancy, the uterus narrows continuously to accommodate the products of conception and its blood flow is increased. The uterine musculature remains refractory to any stimuli till 36 to 38 weeks of gestation. However, a few, infrequent contractions of low intensity are noted near the end of pregnancy; they are not effective enough to produce cervical dilatation.

The cervix, during this period, softens due to increased vascularity, stromal and glandular hyperplasia and change in the composition of the extracellular matrix.

The myometrium undergoes changes by which its quiescence is suspended and it is ready to respond to stimuli and contract. Changes in the expression of key proteins like contraction-associated proteins (CAPs), which include oxytocin and PGF receptors, play an important role in the onset and continuation of labour. There is a marked increase in the number of oxytocin receptors. This, along with an increase in gap junction proteins, removes the refractoriness of the myometrium and effective uterine contractions set in. It is important to remember that the myometrium contracts and retracts, which means that the fibres shorten when they contract, but do not return to the original length after relaxation. It is this property of the myometrium which is responsible for fetal propulsion through the birth canal. The lower uterine segment develops from the isthmus of the cervix, which is the part of the uterine wall between the anatomical and histological internal os (**Fig. 22.1**). As pregnancy advances, the lower uterine segment stretches and thins out.

The cervix softens further, becomes shorter and thinner, leading to **effacement**; it is also dilatable. Such a cervix is designated as a **ripe cervix**. In other words, it is a cervix that is ready to go into labour. In a primigravida, effacement precedes cervical dilatation whereas in a multigravida, effacement and dilatation occur simultaneously during labour (**Fig. 22.2**).

The changes noted so far in the uterus and the cervix are followed by the onset of active labour marked by a progressive increase in the frequency and intensity of uterine contractions. This is associated with cervical dilatation and expulsion of the fetus.

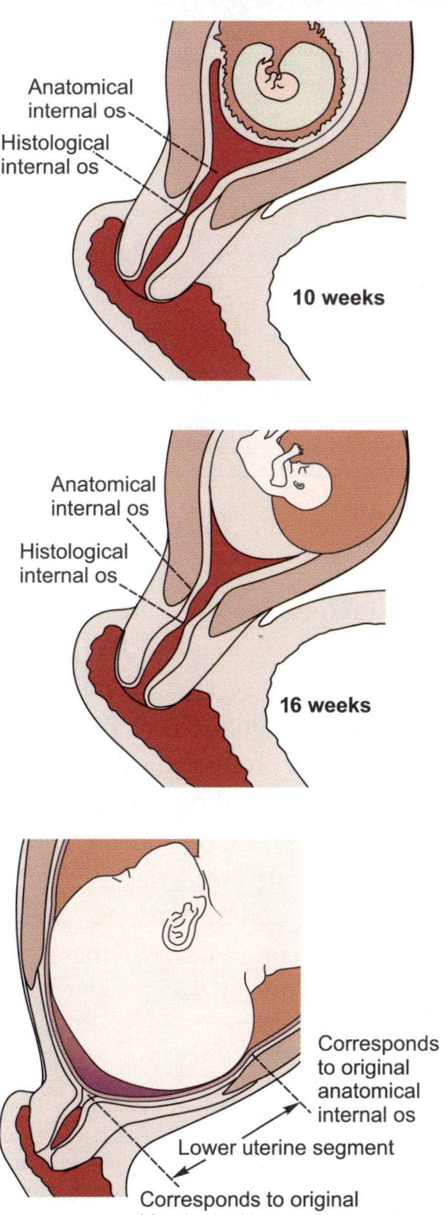

Fig. 22.1 Formation of lower uterine segment.

Clinical course of labour

From a clinical perspective, labour is divided into three stages. **The first stage** starts with the onset of effective uterine contractions, qualified as three contractions in 10 minutes and each lasting for 45 to 50 seconds with complete relaxation in between. The cervix gets thinner and shorter and is said to be **effaced.** This stage ends with the full dilatation of the cervix, which corresponds to 10 cm. The **second stage** begins with the full dilatation of the cervix and ends with the expulsion of the fetus. The **third stage** begins with the expulsion of the fetus and ends with the expulsion of the placenta.

The first stage of labour: Uterine contractions increasing in intensity and duration mark the onset of the first stage. The woman complains of colicky pain which starts in the lumbar region and moves anteriorly to the umbilicus and then radiates downwards towards the medial aspect of the thighs.

Effacement of the cervix is enhanced as labour progresses, leading to the conversion of the narrow cylindrical cervix to a funnel with a small opening at the external os. Further, the effaced cervix gets incorporated into the lower segment. The cervix and the lower segment are passive and yield to the contractions of the upper segment by thinning and

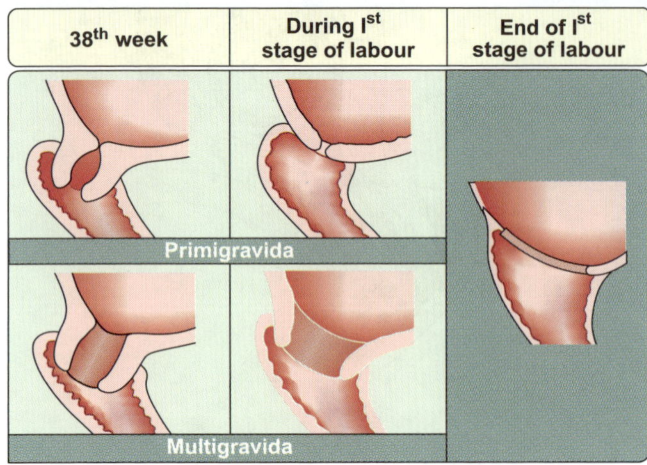

Fig. 22.2 Cervical effacement and dilatation.

dilating. As uterine activity continues, the cervix dilates progressively to reach full dilatation.

Factors that promote cervical dilatation are pressure on the cervix by the amniotic bag of membranes and the presenting part. This pressure on the cervix enhances uterine contractions, leading to further dilatation (Ferguson's reflex). Early rupture of membranes is associated with difficulty in cervical dilatation.

From **Fig. 22.3** it is clear that cervical dilatation is divided into the latent and active phases. The active phase is subdivided into three phases:

- phase of acceleration
- phase of maximum slope
- phase of deceleration.

The duration of the latent phase is variable and is affected by factors like sedation. Once the cervix is fully dilated, further progress in labour will be determined by the descent of the fetus.

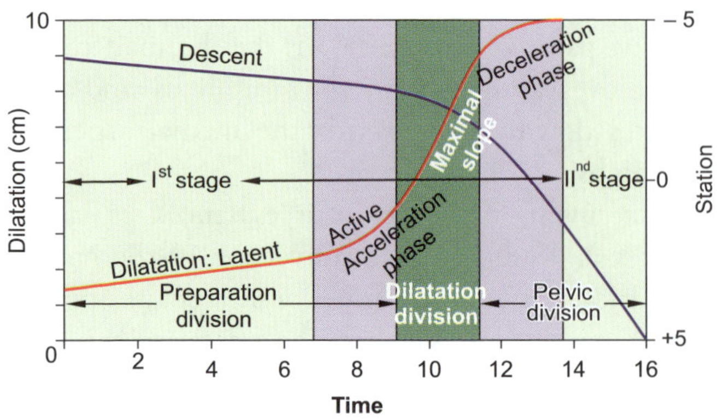

Fig. 22.3 Phases of labour.

The second stage of labour: The uterine contractions become intense, leading to the descent of the fetal head into the pelvic cavity. If not engaged earlier, the fetal head gets engaged during this stage. Further descent and expulsion are aided by voluntary efforts of the mother. The stretching of the levator ani and the thinning of the central part of the perineum aid in the delivery of the fetus.

The third stage of labour: This is the stage of expulsion of the placenta and membranes. After the delivery of the fetus, there is a sudden decrease in the size of the uterus. The uterus is palpable as a hard mass just at the umbilicus. Placental separation occurs consequent to reduction in the area of placental attachment on the uterine surface, while the placental surface, remains unchanged (**Fig. 22.4**). Further contraction of the uterus and formation of retroplacental hematoma also contribute to placental separation. The retroplacental hematoma pushes down the central part of the placenta. As the placenta is expelled, it drags down the membranes with it (**Fig. 22.5**).

The process of labour is initiated by a complex mechanism. The myometrial activity is controlled by several molecular and biochemical factors.

Molecular basis of myometrial contractions

Labour is the onset of painful uterine contractions coming at a regular interval of about three minutes associated with progressive cervical effacement and dilatation along with fetal descent. Uterine contractions occur when myocytes shorten as a result of actin sliding over myosin. This in turn results from the phosphorylation of the myosin light chain by myosin light chain kinase (MLCK). MLCK is activated by the calcium–calmodulin complex which is created when there is a sudden increase in intracellular calcium. The factors that influence the calcium content of myocytes are shown in **Fig. 22.6**.

The factors which increase intracellular calcium are:

- oxytocin, which works by increasing, the release of stored intracellular calcium as well as the influx of extracellular calcium into the cell

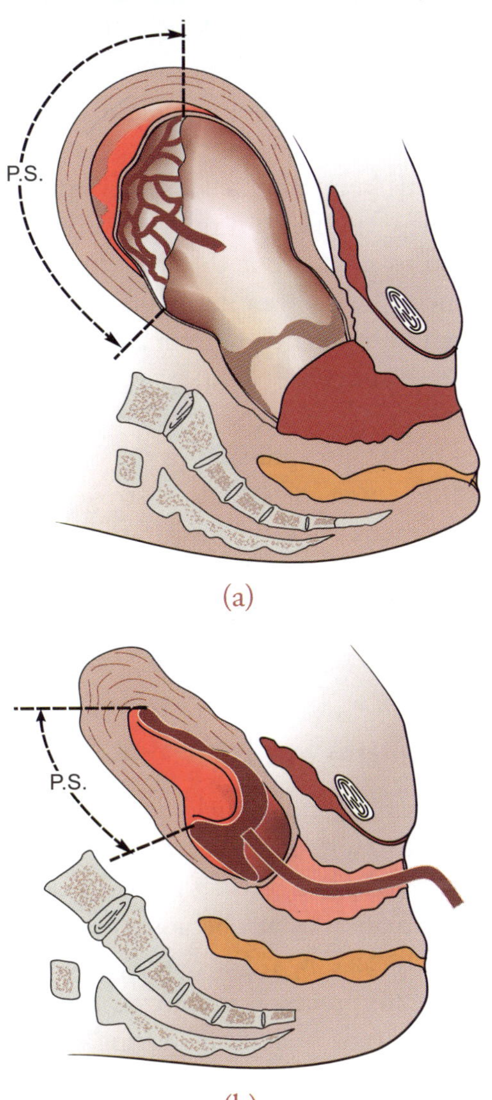

Fig. 22.4 Reduction in placental site
PS: Placental surface a: Before delivery of the baby
b: After the delivery of the baby.

- Prostaglandins (E_2 and $F_2\alpha$), which activate L-type calcium channels into the cell and decrease cyclic AMP(cAMP) and cyclic GMP(cGMP) levels.

The processes which decrease intracellular calcium are:

- increasing levels of cyclic AMP: beta receptor agonists, prostacyclin, relaxin, nitric oxide
- calcium channel blockers such as nifedipine
- magnesium probably works by blocking calcium channels but the exact mechanism is unclear.
- endothelin decreases the receptor-mediated influx of Ca^{2+} into the cell.

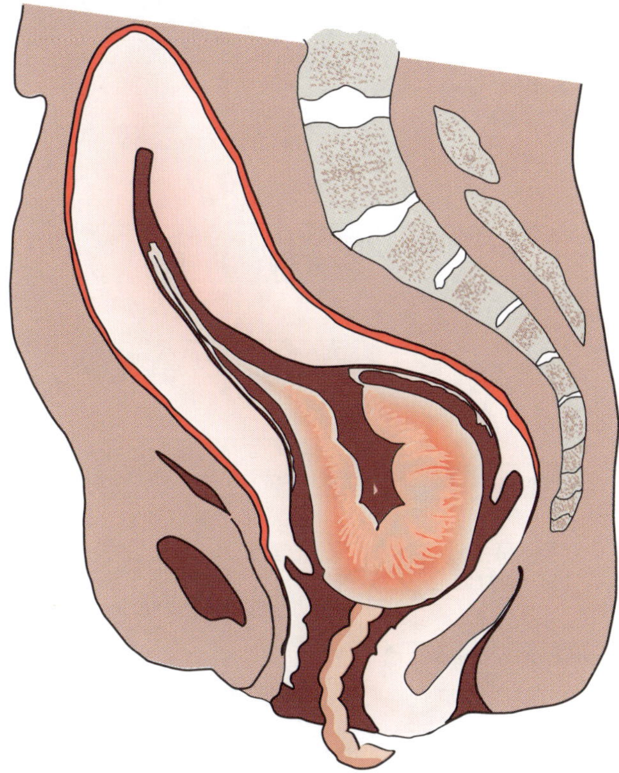

Fig. 22.5 Expulsion of the placenta.

Activation of myometrial contractions

During pregnancy, the myometrium is in a state of quiescence till term when the uterine contractions set in. This myometrial activation is the process by which the myometrium switches from its inactive state in pregnancy to an excitable state responsive to agonists. It has been proposed that activation results from the expression of a cassette of proteins termed CAPs. These CAPs include ion channels, receptors for agonists and gap junctions.

It appears that the CAPs may be regulated by genetic control, endocrine factors and mechanical changes. Activation of the fetal hypothalamo-pituitary-adrenal axis results in an increase in fetal cortisol, placental estrogen and increased prostaglandin production, leading to uterine activity in pregnant sheep. The fetal genome determines the time for the stimulation of the fetal hypothalamo-pituitary-adrenal axis. Additionally, the mechanical changes resulting from uterine stretch result in myometrial activation and initiation of labour (**Fig. 22.7**).

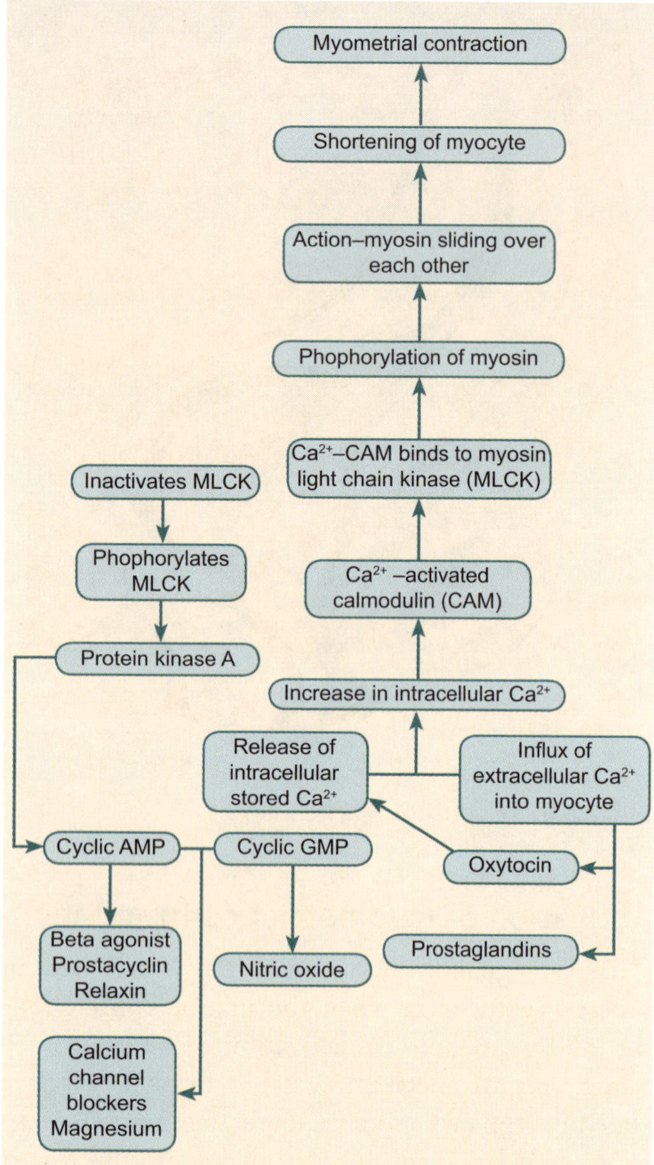

Fig. 22.6 Biochemical pathways regulating myometrial contractions.

Onset of labour

The onset of labour occurs when activation of the myometrium results in increased response of the uterus to stimulants. Research confirms that there is activation of the fetal hypothalamo-pituitary-adrenal axis which in turn stimulates placental production of the corticotrophin releasing hormone (CRH). Placental CRH stimulates fetal cortisol production; fetal cortisol increases myometrial prostaglandin synthesis. There is a resulting increase in the estrogen—progesterone ratio. This shift results in the expression of CAP, and increased production and decreased breakdown of prostaglandins in the myometrium.

The levels of prostaglandin in plasma and amniotic fluid have been found to increase in labour. The prostaglandins are rapidly metabolised by prostaglandin dehydrogenase (PGDH) in the chorion and very few prostaglandins cross from the fetal to the maternal compartment. It has been noted that PGDH activity is decreased in spontaneous, term and preterm labour and also in the presence of infection.

Oxytocin plays a significant role as shown by increased oxytocin expression in the chorio-decidual layer at the onset of labour. Estrogens produced during myometrial activation also stimulate oxytocin production from the pituitary and increase oxytocin receptors in the myometrium. Progesterone increases PGDH activity which results in lower levels of prostaglandins.

Changes in the cervix

The cervix is firm and unyielding during pregnancy and changes to a soft, dilatable structure just before the onset of labour. Such a cervix is known as a ripe cervix. This transformation occurs because the collagen fibres in the cervix break down. The exact mechanism for the initiation of this process is unknown. The biophysical changes that occur include increasing breakdown of collagen fibres, rearrangement of collagen bundles,

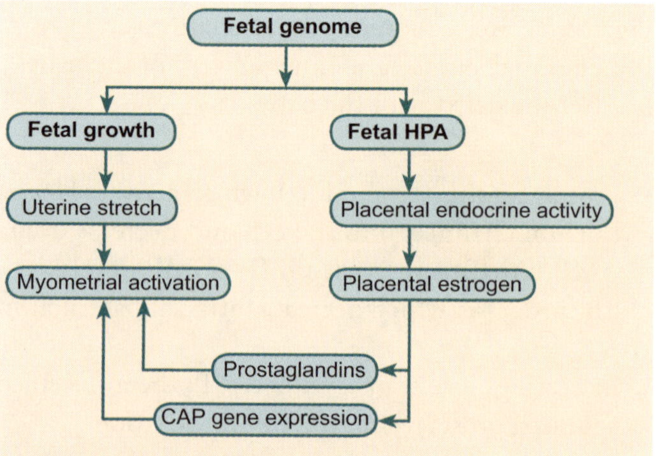

Fig. 22.7 Myometrial activation
HPA: Hypothalamo-pituitary-adrenal axis
PG: Prostaglandins
CAP: Contraction-associated protein

an increase in the amount of hyaluronic acid in the cervical stroma and a decrease in dermatan sulphate. Local release of prostaglandins and, probably, lowering of progesterone levels may be the events that initiate the change in the cervix.

Labour at term

Myometrial contractility prior to onset of labour is characterised by irregular, low frequency, low intensity, long duration contractions. These change to regular, high intensity, high frequency, short duration contractions. There is accompanying cervical dilatation and effacement and eventually expulsion of the fetus from the uterus. At the onset of labour at term, there is cessation of the inhibitory effects of pregnancy like progesterone, prostacyclin, relaxin, nitric oxide, parathyroid hormone-related peptide, corticotrophin releasing hormone, and many other agents. There is activation of the myometrium, as described above, followed by stimulation of myometrial activity by uterotonic agents such as oxytocin, prostaglandin E_2 and $PGF_2\alpha$. Following delivery of the fetus and the placenta, uterine involution occurs primarily through the oxytocin effect.

Measurement of uterine activity

Uterine contractions can be monitored in several ways. Clinical evaluation of the intensity, frequency and duration of contraction by palpation is a reliable method of determining the adequacy of uterine contractions. In 1957, Caldeyro-Barcia and colleagues measured uterine activity by amniotic fluid pressure catheters introduced through the abdominal wall and reported that the frequency and intensity of contractions varied considerably but that the product of the two measurements remained constant. Intensity is measured by the rise in pressure above the baseline. The Montevideo unit is the product of average intensity in millimetres of mercury and the number of contractions in 10 minutes. Intrauterine pressure catheters are used to measure intraamniotic pressure and these are introduced into the uterine cavity through the cervix after rupture of membranes. When levels of Montevideo units are 200 or above, uterine contractions are considered adequate. El-Sahwi and colleagues modified it to create the Alexandria unit which included the duration of contraction in the calculation.

External pressure transducers are a noninvasive method of evaluating the frequency and duration of uterine contractions. Although external monitors do not provide data on intraamniotic pressure, when combined with the clinical assessment of intensity of contractions, they provide adequate data for the continuous monitoring of uterine activity.

KEY POINTS

- Labour is a physiological process by which the fetus and the placenta are expelled from the uterus.
- Till 36 to 38 weeks of pregnancy, the uterus is maintained in a quiescent state by several endocrine factors.
- Uterine contractions occur when myocytes are shortened as a result of myosin sliding over actin. This involves a complex biochemical mechanism.
- Labour is initiated when the activated myometrium is influenced by stimulatory factors and by the removal of inhibitory factors.
- The fetal hypothalamo-pituitary-adrenal-placental axis plays a significant role in the initiation of labour.
- The cervix undergoes changes in its architecture prior to onset of labour.
- Uterine activity may be measured clinically, by external pressure transducers applied to the abdominal wall or through internal monitoring of the intrauterine pressure.

QUESTIONS

Select the single most appropriate answer:

1. The factors responsible for the suspension of uterine refractoriness at 36 to 38 weeks are all of the following *except*
   a. oxytocin
   b. prostaglandin F
   c. progesterone
   d. gap junction proteins
2. The most important change in the cervix before the onset of labour is due to
   a. softness
   b. increased vascularity
   c. glandular hyperplasia
   d. change in the composition of extracellular matrix
3. A 'ripe cervix' is characterised by which of the following changes in the cervix?
   a. softening
   b. dilatability
   c. shortening
   d. all of the above
4. Which of the following statements about the onset of uterine contractions is correct?
   a. oxytocin increases the release of stored intracellular calcium
   b. oxytocin decreases the influx of extracellular calcium into the cell
   c. prostaglandins do not activate the L type calcium channels
   d. prostaglandins increase cyclic AMP levels
5. All of the following are factors that decrease intracellular calcium in the myocyte *except*
   a. salbutamol
   b. prostaglandin F_2
   c nifedipine
   d. magnesium sulphate
6. Myometrial activation results when genes for contraction-associated proteins (CAP) are expressed in myocytes. Myometrial activation occurs due to all of the following *except*
   a. fetal hypothalamo-pituitary-adrenal-placental axis
   b. placental estrogen
   c. uterine stretch
   d. progesterone
7. Uterine activity can be monitored by all of the following *except*
   a. intrauterine pressure catheter
   b. external tocodynamometer
   c. clinical palpation
   d. fetal scalp electrode
8. All of the following may be used to induce labour *except*
   a. oxytocin
   b. indomethacin
   c. prostaglandin E2
   d. prostaglandin F_2

Select the appropriate answer using the following key:

a. if only responses 1, 2 and 3 are correct
b. if only 1 and 3 are correct
c. if only 2 and 4 are correct
d. if only 4 is correct
e. if all are correct

9. The enzyme prostaglandin dehydrogenase decreases in
   1. the presence of infection
   2. post-term pregnancy
   3. preterm labour
   4. oligohydramnios
10. At the onset of labour, there is cessation of which of the following factors?
    1. progesterone
    2. relaxin
    3. prostacyclin
    4. hPL

23

Mechanism of Normal Labour

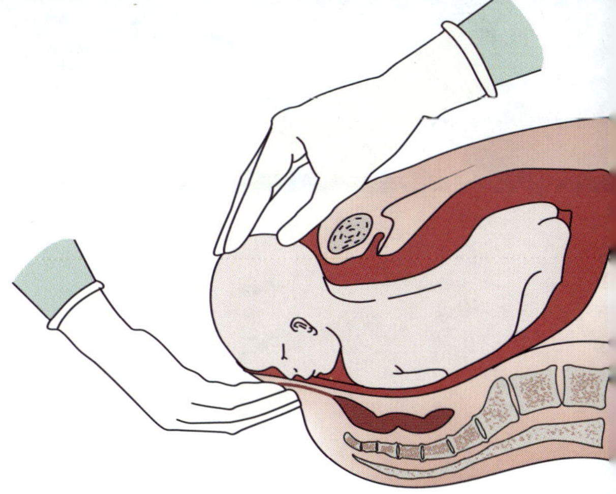

Manorama Purwar

LEARNING OBJECTIVES

At the end of this chapter, the reader should be able to:

- define fetal lie, presentation, position and attitude
- enumerate the steps in obstetric palpation
- enumerate important clinical findings to be noted during vaginal examination
- define engagement of the fetal head
- enumerate the symptoms and signs of labour
- define the three stages of labour
- define the mechanism of labour
- enumerate the cardinal fetal movements during labour
- define caput and moulding

Introduction

Labour is the process by which the products of conception are expelled spontaneously (via naturalis) from the uterine cavity after the period of viability. It begins with the onset of uterine contractions and ends with the expulsion of the placenta. The fetal head is the most voluminous and least compressible part of the fetus. The shape and diameters of the pelvis vary from the inlet to the outlet. In order to descend, the fetal head therefore adapts to the pelvic cavity by several movements. This process is known as the mechanism of labour. A sound knowledge of the mechanism of labour helps in proper conduct of labour.

Fetal lie

Fetal lie is defined as the relation of the long axis of the fetus to the long axis of the maternal spine (**Fig. 23.1**).

Longitudinal lie: The lie is said to be longitudinal when the long axis of the fetus is parallel to the maternal spine. It occurs in 99% of cases.

Transverse lie: The lie is said to be transverse when the long axis of the fetus is perpendicular to the maternal spine.

Oblique lie: The lie is said to be oblique when the fetal and maternal axes cross at 45°.

Fetal presentation

The part of the fetus that occupies the lower pole of the uterus is known as presentation. The presentation may be **cephalic** (96.5%), **podalic** (3%) or **shoulder** (0.5%). Rarely, when more than one part of the fetus is presenting, it is known as **compound presentation**.

Presenting part

It is the most dependent part of the fetus lying nearest to the cervix and felt first during vaginal examination.

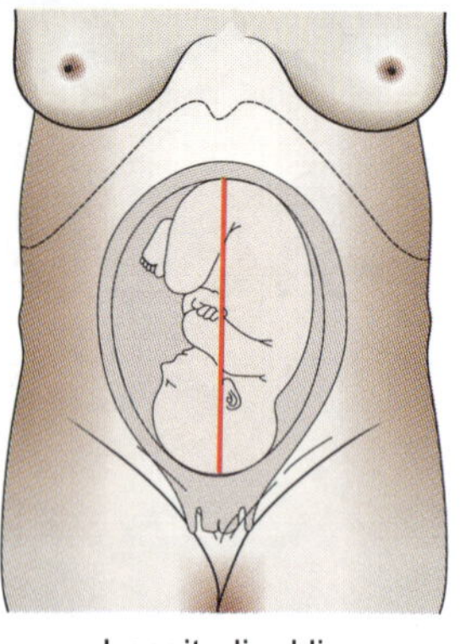

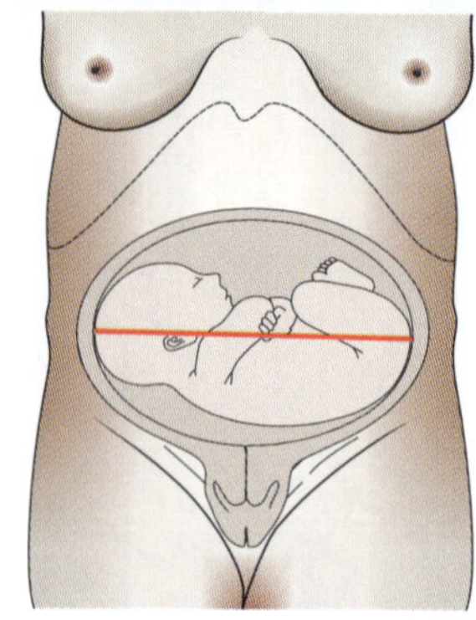

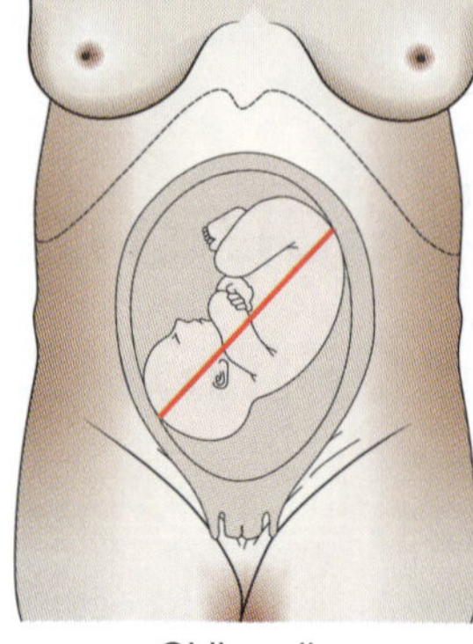

Fig. 23.1 Fetal lie.

Attitude

Attitude is the relation of the various parts of the fetus to each other. In general, the fetus is in an attitude of universal flexion. The back is arched, the head bent down towards the chest, the limbs folded in front with all the joints flexed (**Fig. 23.2**). The fetus forms an ovoid mass to accommodate itself to the shape of the uterine cavity and occupies the least possible space.

In case of longitudinal lie, the presentation may be cephalic (head) or podalic (breech). Cephalic presentations are classified according to the degree of flexion of the head (**Fig. 23.3**).

- **Vertex** is the presenting part when the head is flexed sharply, the chin is in contact with the thorax; the vertex is the area bound by the coronal suture, lambdoid suture and two parallel lines passing through the parietal eminences.
- **Face** is the presenting part when the fetal neck is sharply extended, and the occiput comes in contact with the back.
- **Brow** is the presenting part when the fetal head assumes a position between the extremes of flexion and extension.

A breech presentation may be a flexed (complete breech), extended (frank breech), footling or knee, according to the degree of flexion of the lower limbs. In the transverse lie, the presentation is usually the shoulder.

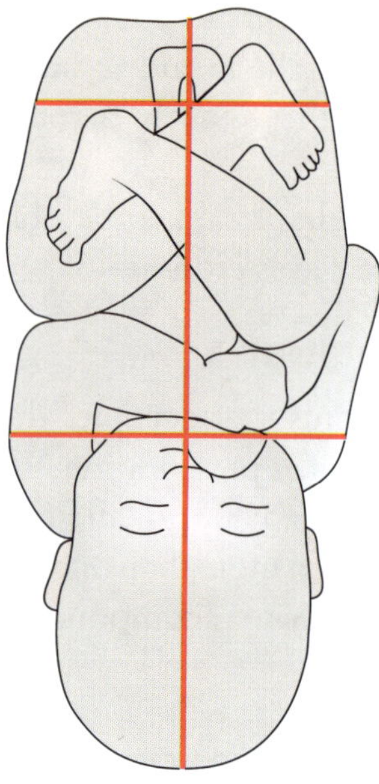

Fig. 23.2 Attitude of universal flexion.

Denominator

The denominator is a fixed point on the presenting part of the fetus used for describing the position. Each presentation has its own denominator (**Table 23.1**).

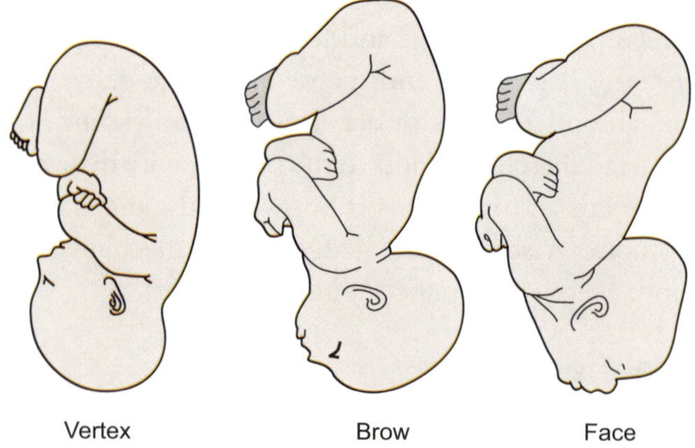

Fig. 23.3 Types of cephalic presentation.

Table 23.1 Denominator for different types of presentation

Presentation	Denominator
Vertex	Occiput
Breech	Sacrum
Face	Mentum (chin)
Brow	Frontal eminence
Shoulder	Acromion (scapula)

Position

The pelvic girdle has a circumference of 360°. For descriptive purpose, the pelvis is divided into equal segments of 45° each; iliopectineal eminences, sacroiliac joints and the sacral promontory are used as reference points to describe the fetal position.

The position is anterior when the denominator is opposite the iliopectineal eminence, transverse if it lies between the sacroiliac joint and the iliopectineal eminence, posterior if it is opposite the sacroiliac joint and direct posterior if it is opposite the sacral promontory. **Figure 23.4** shows the various positions in vertex presentation.

All terms of direction refer to the mother in the standing position. Upper means towards, maternal head while lower indicates towards the feet. Anterior, posterior, right and left position are in relation to the maternal pelvis.

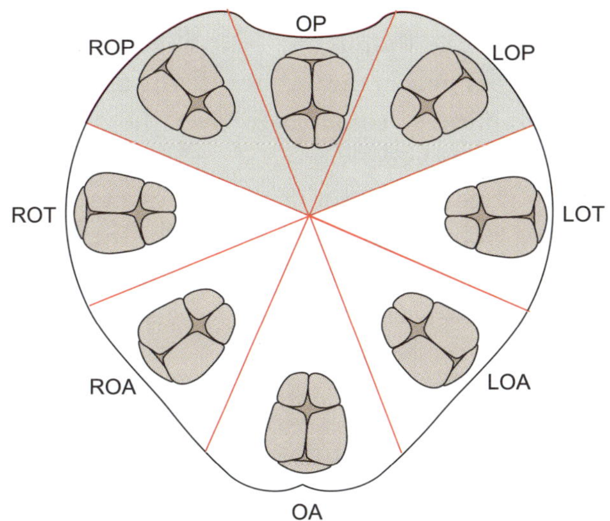

Fig. 23. 4 Various positions in vertex presentation.

Engagement

The fetal head is considered to be engaged when the biparietal diameter has crossed the brim. Engagement mostly takes place during labour, but in some primigravidas, it could occur in the last few days of pregnancy.

The most frequently encountered position of vertex is left occipito-anterior (LOA), when the occiput is in the left anterior quadrant, opposite the left iliopectineal eminence. This is the most favourable postion for vaginal delivery.

Diagnosis of Presentation and Position

Clinical examination is sufficient in most instances to diagnose fetal presentation and position and its wellbeing. The examination consists of abdominal palpation, vaginal examination, combined examination and auscultation. Ultrasonography is a useful tool when clinical examination findings are inconclusive.

Abdominal Examination

The woman lies with the head slightly raised and knees drawn up to relax the abdominal muscles. The abdomen is fully exposed and the examiner stands on the right side facing the woman.

Inspection

- The uterine ovoid at term just reaches up to the xiphisternum in the longitudinal lie.
- If the uterus appears unusually broad in its lower part, the lie may be transverse.
- In the occipito-posterior position, there may be subumbilical flattening of the abdomen.
- The presence of any scar is noted.

Palpation

After reassuring the patient, palpation should be carried out with utmost gentleness. Manipulations should be suspended during uterine contractions.

While palpating, one hand is used to palpate while the other hand is used to steady the uterus or to press the fetus against the first hand. Palpation is best effected by using the flat of the plam and/or fingers.

Height of the uterus: Using the ulnar border of the left hand, the fundal height of the uterus is palpated by passing the hand gently from below upwards till a lack of resistance is detected, while the right hand corrects the dextrorotation of the uterus, if present.

The uterus is just palpable above the symphysis pubis at 12 weeks and reaches the umbilicus at 24 weeks of gestation. The distance between the symphysis pubis and the umbilicus is divided into three parts, marking 16, 20 and 24 weeks of gestation. The uterus is at the xiphisternum at 36 weeks of gestation. The distance between the umbilicus and the xiphisternum is divided into three parts, marking 28, 32 and 36 weeks of gestation (**Fig. 10.1**).

Symphysio-fundal height (SFH): The fundal height is marked, the pregnant woman then extends her lower limbs to avoid errors due to tilting of the pelvis. The distance between the symphysis pubis and the fundal height is measured in centimetres. Ideally, SFH is measured throughout pregnancy and the values are plotted on a gravidogram to monitor fetal growth. If the measurements are below the 50th percentile, IUGR is suspected and the woman should be referred for further evaluation. A single measurement in centimetres corresponds to the gestational age in weeks between 18 and 30 weeks.

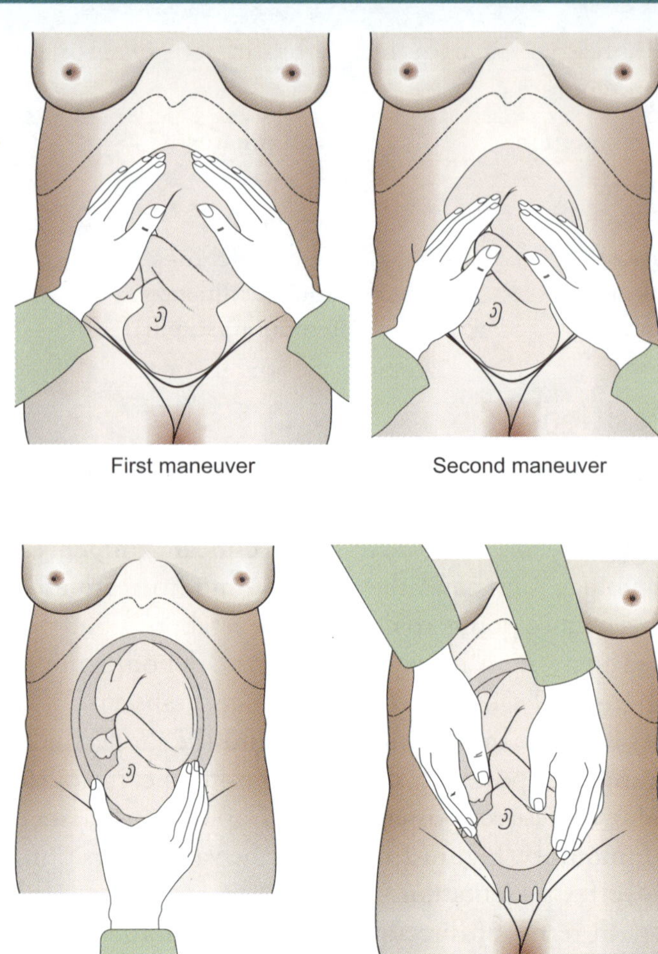

Fig. 23.5 Steps in obstetric palpation (Leopold's maneuvers).

Obstetrical grips or maneuvers

The different types of grips are discussed below (**Fig. 23.5**).

Fundal grip or first maneuver: The fundus of the uterus is palpated with both hands. This maneuver identifies the fetal pole: whether breech or head that occupies the fundus. Breech is felt as a broad, firm, irregular and non-ballotable mass, compared to the head which is well defined, hard, globular and ballotable.

Lateral/umbilical grip or second maneuver: Both hands are placed on either side of the abdomen and gentle deep pressure is exerted. On one side, a firm resistant structure is felt (this is the back); on the other side, numerous small, irregular, mobile parts are felt, indicating the fetal limbs.

First pelvic grip (Pawlik's grip) or third maneuver: The thumb and four fingers are placed over the lower pole of the uterus with the ulnar border of the examiner's hand placed over the symphysis pubis. The fetal pole is grasped and its side to side mobility is assessed. In a cephalic presentation, the head feels globular, hard and ballotable. The grip also helps in finding out whether the head is engaged; when the head is engaged, either the sinciput alone or no part of the head is palpable.

Second pelvic grip or fourth maneuver: The examiner faces the mother's feet. Both the hands are placed on the either side of lower abdomen parallel to the inguinal ligament, the cephalic pole is palpated and the occiput and the sinciput are felt. The occiput is broad and is felt on the same side as the back of the fetus, as compared to sinciput, which is smaller, sharper and is on the opposite side of the fetal back. When the head is fully flexed, the occiput is at a lower level than the sinciput. If the head is deflexed, the occiput and the sinciput are at the same level; the occiput is felt at a higher level when the head is extended.

Auscultation of fetal heart sound

This should be done at the junction of the lateral third and medial two-thirds of a line joining the umbilicus to the anterior superior iliac spine (spino-umbilical line), in a vertex anterior position, at the side of the back of the fetus, as this is where the fetal heart sound is heard best.

Abdominal examination may confirm the lie, presentation and position, as well as whether labour has begun and how far it has advanced.

Vaginal Examination

The woman should empty the bladder and lie in the lithotomy or dorsal position. Observing septic precautions, two fingers of a gloved hand are introduced into the vagina.

If the os is sufficiently dilated, admitting one or more fingers, the nature of the presenting part is determined by identifying the sutures and fontanelles. The diameter of the pelvis in which the sagittal suture lies is ascertained and both fontanelles are located.

Points to be noted during vaginal examination

- **Palpation of the cervix:** Position, consistency, dilatation and effacement
- **Presentation:** Cephalic/breech or shoulder presentation, station of the presenting part
- **Bag of membranes:** Intact or ruptured
- **Position:** Identification of the sagittal suture and its course
- Location of the anterior and posterior fontanelle
- Pelvic assessment
- Cephalopelvic relationship

Ultrasonography may be used to complement abdominal examination in identifying the fetal position especially in obese women or when there is an excess amount of amniotic fluid.

Labour

Labour begins with the onset of uterine contractions. Contractions are said to be effective when there are three contractions in 10 minutes and each contraction lasts for 40–50 seconds. Labour progresses, culminating in the delivery of the fetus followed by delivery of the placenta. The first stage begins with the onset of uterine contractions and ends with full dilatation of the cervix. The second stage begins with full dilatation of the cervix and ends with the delivery of the fetus. The third stage begins with the delivery of the fetus and ends with the delivery/expulsion of the placenta. One hour after the third stage is the fourth stage when the risk of hemorrhage is high and one needs to be vigilant.

In a primigravida, the average duration of labour is 14–16 hours. The duration of the second stage is one hour and that of the third stage is 15–20 minutes.

With effective uterine contraction and retraction during labour, the fetus is pushed into the pelvis and the fetal head accommodates itself to the shape of the birth canal, which varies at different levels. The series of movements by which the head adjusts itself to the shape of the pelvis during its journey through the birth canal is known as the **mechanism of labour**.

Mechanism of labour

As discussed earlier, the left occipito-anterior (LOA) is the most favourable fetal position, because the lie is longitudinal with the fetus in an attitude of complete flexion. The denominator is the occiput, with the sagittal suture in the right oblique diameter of the pelvis (**Fig. 23.6**).

The cardinal movements of labour are listed below (**Fig. 23.7**):

- descent
- engagement
- flexion
- internal rotation
- extension
- restitution
- external rotation
- expulsion of trunk.

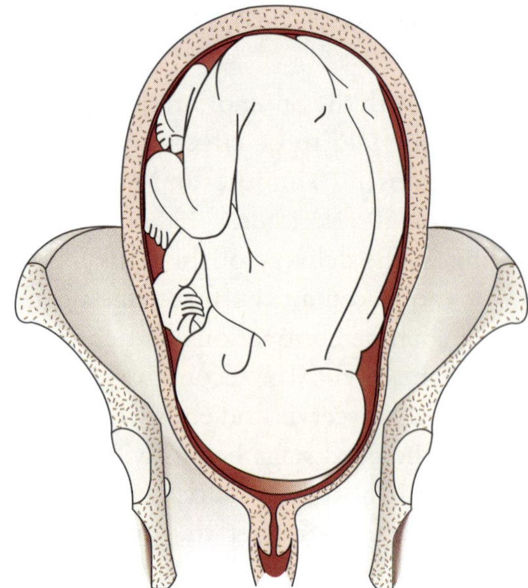

Fig. 23.6 Left occipito-anterior (LOA).

Descent: This is a universal movement throughout labour. It is therefore associated with every other movement. Considerable descent occurs during the first stage of labour. As the head descends, there is further flexion.

The factors facilitating descent are:

- effective uterine contraction and retraction
- amniotic fluid pressure before rupture of membranes
- extension and straightening of fetal ovoid after rupture of membranes
- bearing down efforts by the mother.

Engagement: When the biparietal diameter, the greatest transverse diameter of the fetal head, passes through the pelvic inlet, it is known as **engagement**. The fetal head engages in the last few weeks of pregnancy in primigravida, and usually after the commencement of labour in multigravida. In some primigravidas and many multigravidas, the head is freely movable above the pelvic inlet at the onset of labour and is known as **floating head**.

Engagement of the head indicates that the pelvic inlet is adequate and the presenting part is at the level of the ischial spine on vaginal examination.

Asynclitism: The fetal head enters the pelvis with the sagittal suture in the transverse diameter of the inlet, being equidistant from the sacral promontory and the symphysis pubis: this is called synclitic engagement.

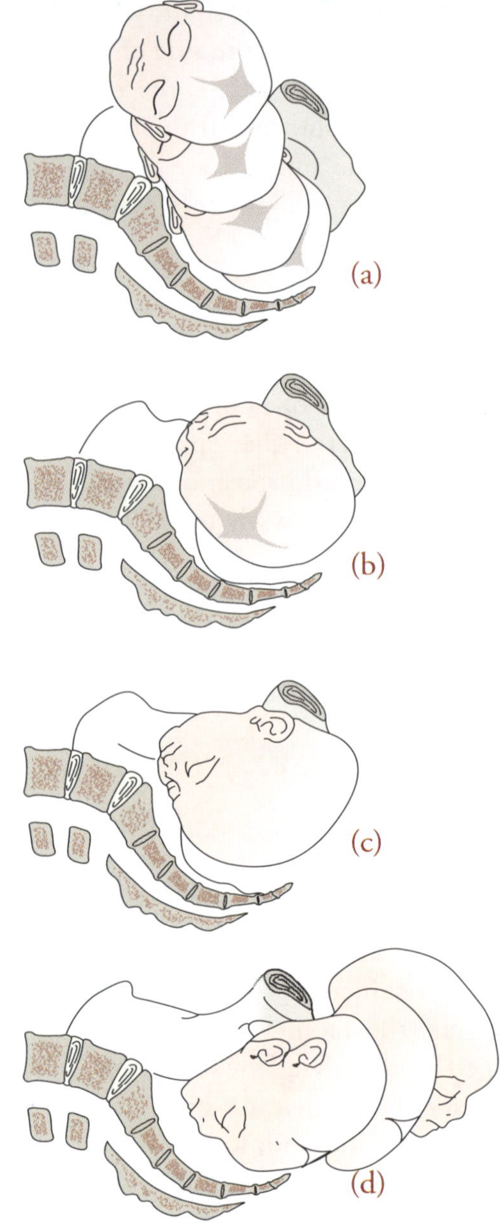

Fig. 23.7 Left occipito-transverse (or lateral) position of the vertex a: Descent with further flexion b: Internal rotation beginning c: Internal rotation almost completed, head in the lower strait d: Birth of head by extension.

If the sagittal suture is closer to the pubic symphysis, the posterior parietal bone presents to the examining finger and is called posterior asynclitism (Litzman's obliquity). If the sagittal suture is closer to the sacral promontory, the anterior parietal bone presents; this is called anterior asynclitism (Naegle's obliquity). Moderate degrees of asynclitism are common when

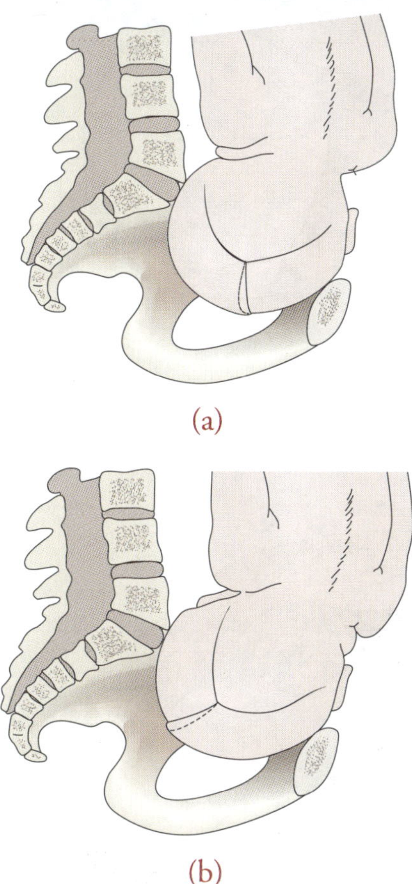

Fig. 23.8 Asynclitism a: Posterior b: Anterior.

the fetal head negotiates through the maternal bony pelvis (**Fig. 23.8**).

Flexion: Whenever the descending head meets any resistance from the birth canal, from the cervix, walls of the pelvis or pelvic floor, there is an increase in preexisting flexion.

The effects of flexion are:

- Presenting diameter is changed from occipito-frontal (11 cm) to smaller and rounder suboccipito-bregmatic (9.5 cm). Thus, a smaller area of fetal head is thrown across the pelvis.
- The occiput becomes the leading part of the fetus.

Flexion is explained by the two-arm lever theory. The spinal column is articulated to the head nearer the occiput than the sinciput. If the fulcrum is represented by the spine, the occiput forms the short arm and the sinciput the long arm. According to the law of mechanics, when resistance is encountered, the short arm (occiput) descends and the long arm (sinciput) ascends, resulting in flexion of the head.

Internal rotation: This is a movement of great importance without which there will be no further descent. Once the cervix is fully dilated, the head descends rapidly to the level of the ischial spines, where it meets the grooved gutter of the pelvic floor and begins to rotate. Further, flexion of the head occurs and anterior rotation of the occiput takes place through 45° in the occipito-anterior, 90° in the occipito-transverse and 135° in the occipito-posterior position. Thus, the occiput lies under the pubic arch, with the sagittal suture in the antero-posterior diameter of the pelvis; the shoulders continue to remain in the oblique diameter, leading to a twist in the fetal neck (**Fig. 23.9**). The effect of internal rotation is that the long diameter, of the head is brought into the largest diameter of the pelvic outlet (anteroposterior).

The causes of internal rotation are:

- Absence of a bony wall makes the pubic arch the direction of least resistance.
- Elastic recoil of the pelvic floor (Hart's rule): The two halves of the levator ani muscle form a gutter. The fibres of the levator ani muscle are directed downwards, forward and medially. During each contraction, the occiput stretches the levator ani; after the contraction passes off, the elastic recoil of the levator ani forces the occiput forward and towards the midline. This process is repeated till the occiput is rotated anteriorly.

Extension: After internal rotation, with further uterine contractions and by the voluntary contraction of the diaphragm and the abdominal wall muscles, the head is forced down towards the vulva, and the vertex appears stretching the vulval orifice. With further contractions, extension of the head occurs and the forehead, base of the nose, mouth and chin sweep over the perineum to release the head (**Fig. 23.10**).

Restitution: Once the head is free outside the vulva, it is untwisted and resumes its normal relation with the shoulders (**Fig. 23.11**).

External rotation: This is the outward manifestation of the internal rotation of the shoulder. The effect is that the bisacromial diameter of the trunk is brought into the largest anteroposterior diameter of the outlet (**Fig. 23.12**).

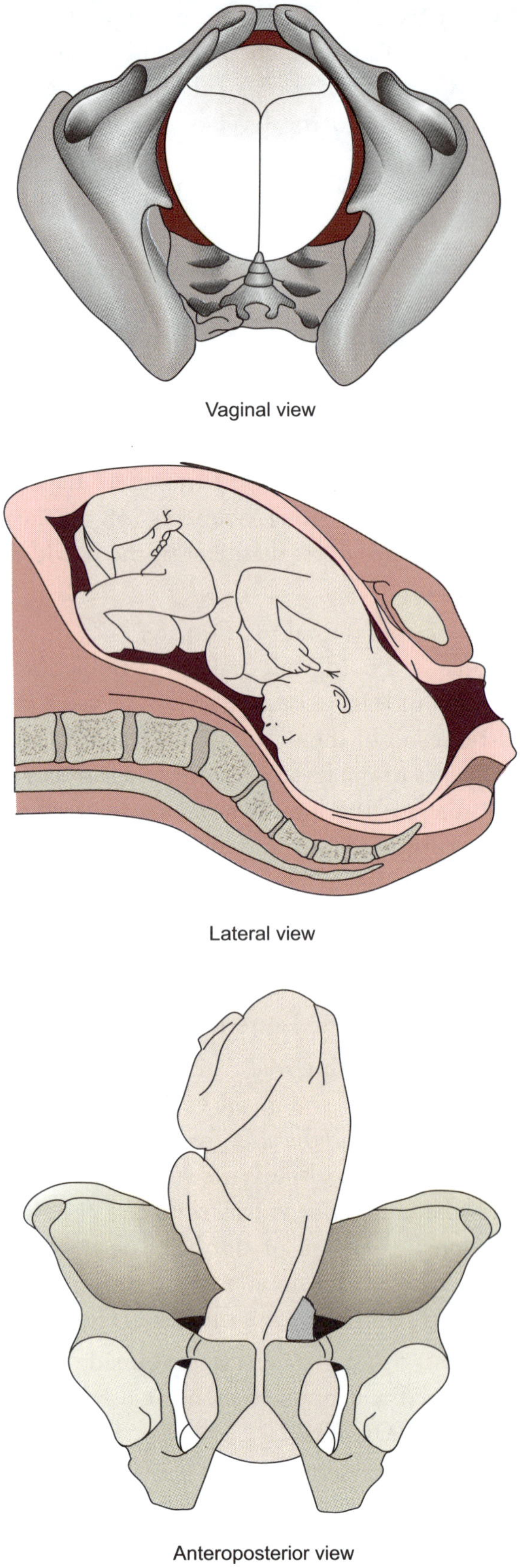

Vaginal view

Lateral view

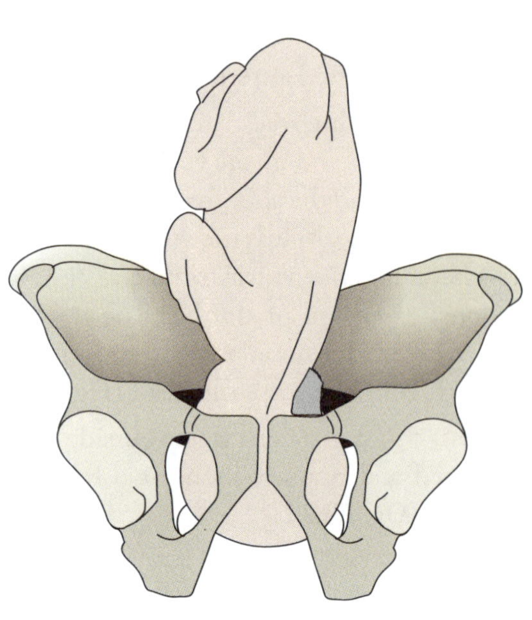

Fig. 23.9 Internal rotation.

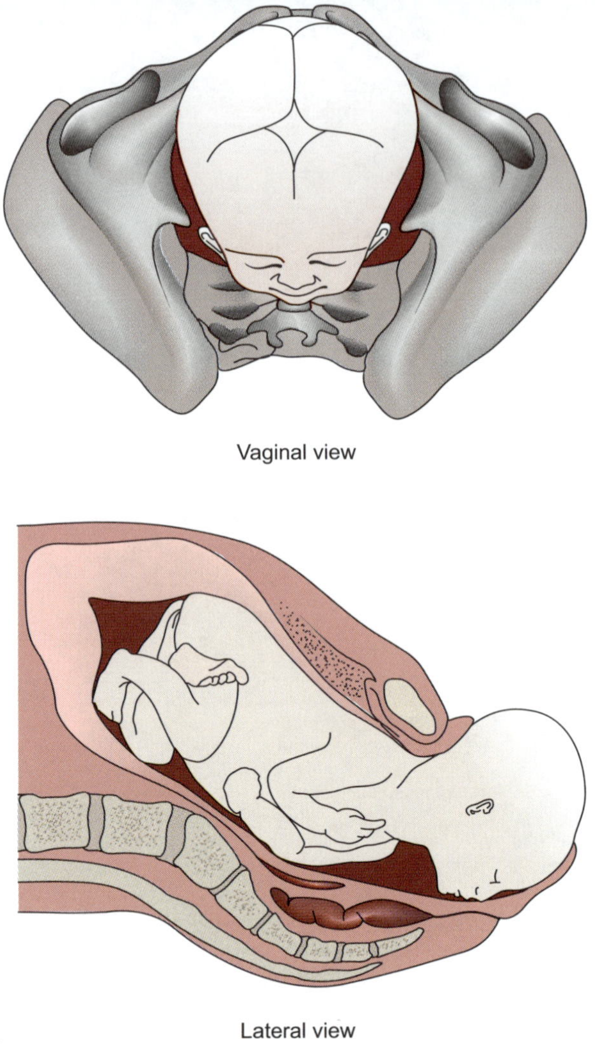

Vaginal view

Lateral view

Fig. 23.10 Extension of the head.

Expulsion/delivery of the shoulders and remainder of the fetus: Immediately after external rotation, the descent continues, with the anterior shoulder hitching under the symphysis pubis. The posterior shoulder then sweeps over the perineum by the movement of lateral flexion and is delivered first. This is followed by the delivery of the anterior shoulder and the rest of the body.

The fetal head is subjected to considerable pressure during its passage through the pelvis. Because of the mobility of the skull bones, the parietal bones slip under each other, and the occipital and frontal bones slip under the parietal bones. Thus, the shape of the fetal head is modified so that it can mould itself to the pelvis. This phenomenon is known as physiological moulding.

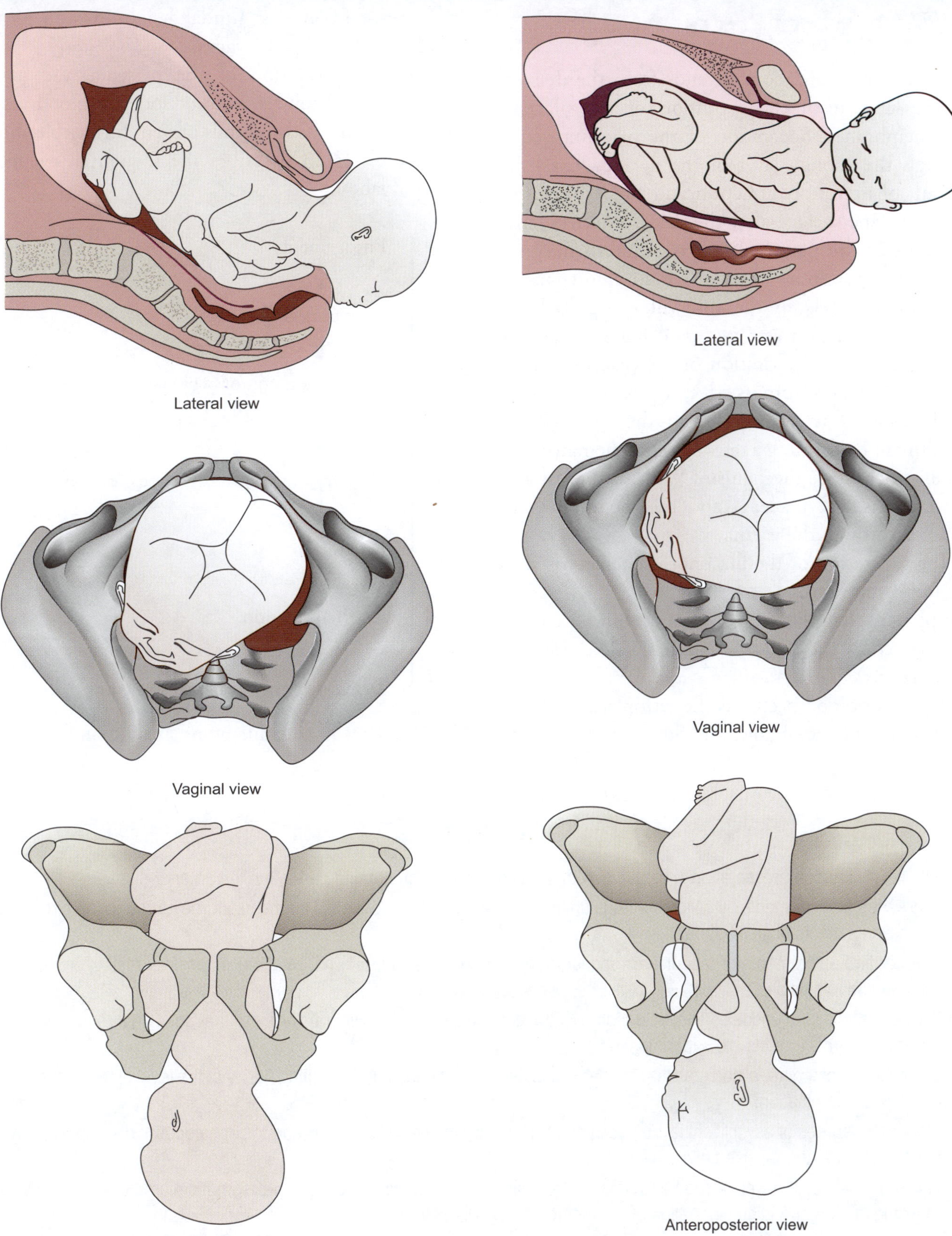

Fig. 23.11 Restitution.

Fig. 23.12 External rotation.

Mechanism of Placental Delivery

The third stage of labour extends from the delivery of the fetus until the expulsion of the placenta and membranes. Separation of the placenta occurs through the spongy layer of the decidua basalis as a result of uterine contraction and sudden decrease in the uterine surface after the delivery of the fetus. The area of the placental bed is reduced markedly while the placental surface remains unchanged. The blood vessels in the intervillous space break down giving rise to retroplacental hemorrhage and leading to further separation of the placenta. If the placenta separates from its edge, it is called Duncan's mechanism. If it separates from the centre of its attachment by forming a retroplacental hematoma, it is called Schultze's mechanism. With further uterine contractions, the placenta and the membranes are expelled through the vagina.

The separation of the placenta is characterised by the following signs:

- Apparent lengthening of the umbilical cord is observed as the separated placenta descends into the cervix.
- A gush of blood occurs as the retroplacental blood separates the membranes and flows into the vagina.
- Increase in uterine fundal height is seen as the placenta reaches the vagina.

After the expulsion of the placenta, the uterus contracts powerfully so as to occlude the blood vessels in the placental bed and thus prevent further bleeding.

Figure 23.13 describes the sequential events of normal labour.

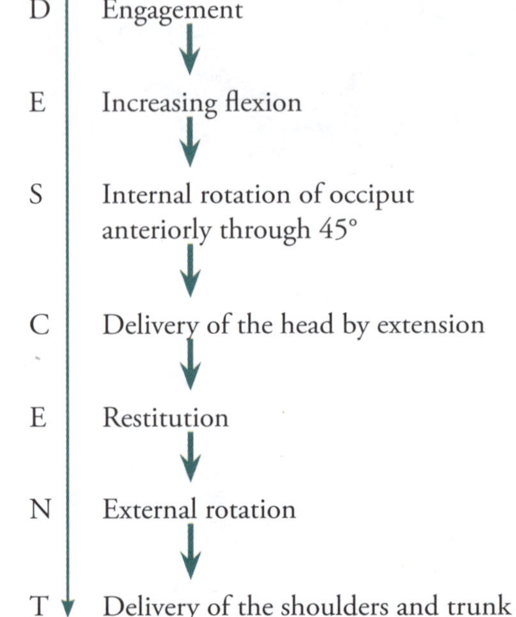

Fig. 23.13 Events during normal labour.

KEY POINTS

- The most common presentation is cephalic, with the vertex as the presenting part in the left anterior position.
- The series of movements by which the fetus adjusts itself to the shape of pelvis during its journey through the birth canal is known as mechanism of labour.
- The cardinal movements of labour are: engagement, descent, flexion, internal rotation, extension, restitution, external rotation and expulsion
- Provided there is no undue soft tissue or bony obstruction, descent is a continuous process that goes on throughout labour and all other movements are superimposed on it.
- Engagement of the head indicates that the pelvic inlet is adequate and the presenting part is at the level of the ischial spine on vaginal examination.
- Moderate degrees of asynclitism is the rule in normal labour, but, if severe, it may lead to cephalopelvic disproportion even in an otherwise normal-size pelvis.
- During moulding, in a well-flexed head of the LOA position, the engaging suboccipito-bregmatic diameter is compressed, resulting in corresponding elongation of the mento-vertical diameter.
- Location of caput gives an indication about the position of head in the pelvis and the degree of flexion achieved. In the left position, the caput is on the right parietal bone.

QUESTIONS

Select the single most appropriate answer:

1. All of the following are denominators for various cephalic presentations *except*
   a. occiput c. frontal eminence
   b. mentum d. acromion
2. Incidence of longitudinal lie at term pregnancy is
   a. 85% b. 90% c. 95% d. 99%
3. In the left occipitoanterior position, the engaging diameter is
   a. suboccipito-bregmatic
   b. biparietal
   c. submento-bregmatic
   d. mento-vertical
4. During moulding, in the left occipitoanterior position, which corresponding diameter of the head is elongated?
   a. suboccipito-bregmatic c. biparietal
   b. mento-vertical d. submento-bregmatic
5. In the left occipitoanterior position, internal rotation of the occiput occurs through
   a. 90° b. 45° c. 180° d. 135°
6. After birth, within how many hours does the caput succedaneum disappear spontaneously?
   a. 16 hours c. 24 hours
   b. 12 hours d. 48 hours
7. The visible passive movement of the head due to untwisting of the neck sustained during internal rotation is known as
   a. external rotation c. restitution
   b. extension d. flexion
8. In the left occipitoanterior position, as the head delivers by extension, the last part of the head to be seen is
   a. bregma c. chin
   b. vertex d. nose
9. Which of the following movements occurs throughout labour in the mechanism of labour?
   a. restitution c. internal rotation
   b. external rotation d. descent
10. Hart's rule explains which of the following movements of labour?
    a. descent c. internal rotation
    b. external rotation d. restitution

24

Conduct of Normal Labour

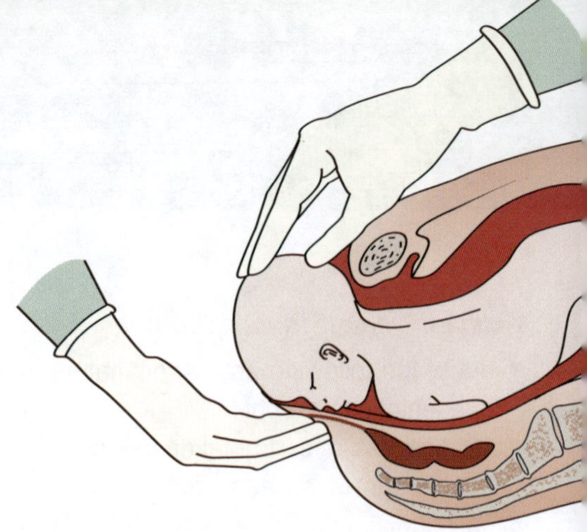

VP Paily

LEARNING OBJECTIVES

At the end of this chapter, the reader should be able to:

- diagnose labour
- perform an initial assessment of a woman in labour
- provide hydration, pain relief and support to a woman in labour
- monitor the progress of labour using a partogram
- understand the steps of delivery of the baby and placenta
- make and repair episiotomy
- enumerate the measures to prevent postpartum hemorrhage

Introduction

Every pregnant woman awaits the onset of labour with anxiety. The fear of unbearable labour pains is usually foremost in her mind. Her concern about the welfare of her baby will only add to her anxiety and affect the smooth progression of labour.

The caregivers in the labour room should help allay these fears and instil confidence in her. As such, the way the woman is received on arrival at the labour ward will make all the difference. It is essential to welcome her with a smile and maintain a friendly, helpful attitude throughout.

Initial assessment

If the woman's case records are available, they are studied and any special points like drug allergies, diabetes mellitus and previous surgeries are noted.

A brief history is taken and the duration of pregnancy reconfirmed. Importance should be given to factors like the time of onset of pain, and whether any leakage of liquor or bleeding has occurred.

After recording the vital signs, an abdominal palpation is undertaken for obstetric details. Fetal heart sounds should be auscultated. The presentation and the presenting part are noted.

If facilities are available, a short strip of cardiotocographic (CTG) recording, known as 'admission test' is done. This helps to record the status of the fetus on admission and can have medico-legal significance. In high-risk cases, more frequent CTGs may be performed.

Initial assessment is not complete until a vaginal examination is performed. However, unless there is an urgent need to assess the state of labour, the vaginal examination can be delayed until the patient is prepared for labour.

Preparation for labour

The pubic hair is clipped, if needed. The practice of giving enema is no longer universally followed. The advantage of giving enema is that the rectum and anal canal will be empty. But, if the woman is late in labour, this can lead to liquefied stool coming out at the most inopportune time, when the woman is straining, thus soiling the field. Even so, enema is usually given except in cases of antepartum hemorrhage or when the woman arrives in the labour room in advanced labour.

The woman is asked to change into a clean, loose and comfortable dress.

Vaginal examination

Before deciding on the vaginal examination, the possibility of placenta praevia is excluded. Similarly, if the patient has a history of ruptured membranes in a preterm pregnancy and conservative management is planned, digital examination may not be appropriate.

Aseptic precautions are followed while conducting the vaginal examination. A sterile kit containing items required for vaginal examination like gloves, cotton balls, forceps and pads can be kept.

- Speculum examination is performed to rule out any discharge, leaking of liquor or local abnormality.
- After cleansing with an aseptic solution like povidone iodine, the fingers of the left hand are used to separate the labia; thereafter, the middle finger of the right hand is introduced into the vagina gently. Once the patient is relaxed, the index finger is also introduced gently, and the vagina and cervix palpated systematically. The following points are noted:

- unusual findings in the vagina
- cervix: position, consistency, length and dilatation
- presence or absence of membranes
- presenting part: identity, station in relation to ischial spines, position, features like moulding and caput
- other features: placental tissue, cord or escaping meconium or liquor (this should be noted).

Pelvic assessment

Many experts believe that there is no evidence to support routine pelvic assessment prior to onset of labour. The best parameter of pelvic size is descent of the head in labour. However, in some cases like breech presentation or previous pelvic fractures, it may be useful. In regions where contracted pelvis is a common problem, routine assessment of the pelvis at 38 weeks or later may be justified. The following points are noted:

- ease of reaching the sacral promontory
- prominence of the ischial spines and the bispinous diameter
- pelvic side walls and sacrosciatic notches
- type of sacrum
  - whether it is smoothly curved
  - whether its tip or coccyx is jutting forward
  - relation of the presenting part to the spine, whether at or below the spine

The distance between the ischial tuberosities is assessed by seeing how many knuckles can be inserted between them. If the head has reached the spine level, disproportion is almost ruled out. However, if it is above the spine, an attempt can be made to push it from above and check if it can be brought to the level of the spines (**Müller–Hillis maneuver**).

The details of the findings are entered in the chart along with the doctor's signature.

Admission to the labour room

Diagnosing true labour can sometimes be difficult. The ideal arrangement is to admit to the labour room only those who are in labour, particularly in institutions with a paucity of beds. A prolonged stay in the labour room is not advisable for any woman. On an average, the stay in the labour room prior to delivery is about 4 or 5 hours.

An effaced, dilated cervix, along with regular contractions, indicates true labour and justifies a woman's stay in the labour room. If in doubt, after the initial assessment, the woman may be sent to the waiting room or her own room.

Monitoring and Care in the First Stage of Labour

It is important to ensure that the patient is comfortable and relaxed during the first stage of labour. If the membranes are intact, she may be allowed to walk around or sit. She may be encouraged to lie on her side to avoid supine hypotension syndrome.

During the first stage of labour, she may drink liquids. An intravenous line can be deferred until the second stage of labour. However, if there is vomiting or a reluctance to take fluid orally, or if anesthesia is likely to be given, the IV line may be started earlier. The fluid used should preferably be normal saline or Ringer lactate rather than 5% dextrose.

Analgesia during labour

Appropriate analgesia is provided for during labour, depending on the facilities available and the institutional practice. Epidural analgesia is a useful method, but requires expertise for administration and monitoring. Narcotic drugs are commonly used IM for labour analgesia, for example, pethidine 2 mg/kg body weight, morphine 0.3 mg/kg body weight or tramadol 100 mg.

Companion in labour

It is very reassuring for the pregnant woman to have a companion in the labour room, especially in the case of a primipara. In Western countries, it is usually the partner/spouse who stays with the woman. In India, the woman's mother or another close female relative who has experienced labour before may stay since it does not invade the privacy of other women in the labour room.

During the first stage, the woman can use the toilet without help. Close to the second stage, caution needs to be exercised since the pressure of the head on the perineum may create a sensation similar to that of passing stools. At that stage, a bed pan may be a better choice.

Monitoring maternal and fetal wellbeing

Periodically, the maternal pulse, BP and fetal heart sounds are recorded. In the early first stage, this is done every hour; as labour progresses and contractions are more frequent, this is recorded every 15 minutes. In the second stage, fetal heart is checked every 15 minutes.

The fetal heart is auscultated immediately after a contraction. This will help pick up any significant late deceleration. If available, a cardiotocograph is used in labour. In high-risk cases, like intrauterine growth restriction, it is used continuously.

The presence of early decelerations (**Fig. 24.1**) indicates head compression which is physiological during the second stage of labour. However, in early labour, if early decelerations are noted, one has to rule out CPD. Late decelerations are usually due to placental insufficiency (**Fig. 24.2**). Persistent late decelerations warrant immediate delivery. Since fallacies are common, if facilities are available, scalp pH should be done to rule out fetal acidosis. Variable decelerations (**Fig. 24.3**) are due to umbilical cord compression. They may disappear on change in maternal position. If they are persistent and severe (drop of FHR by 60 bpm or to 60 bpm lasting for 60 seconds), immediate delivery should be contemplated.

Assessing progress of labour

The simplest way of monitoring progress is watching the frequency and duration of contractions, which will increase as the second stage approaches. It is also possible to assess the descent of the vertex by abdominal examination, noting how much of head is palpable above the symphysis.

Vaginal examination is a more accurate way of assessing progress. However, very frequent vaginal examination will be an unpleasant experience for the woman and add to the risk of infection. A compromise is to conduct a vaginal examination once every 3–4 hours. During vaginal examination, progressive shortening of the cervix and later, dilatation, indicate progress. Descent of the presenting part is another parameter to monitor.

Usually, the second stage is suspected when the patient starts to bear down with contractions. This should be confirmed by a vaginal examination unless the head is already pressing on the perineum. In the occipito-posterior position, the woman may begin to bear down prematurely. Similarly, some multigravida also may bear down before full dilatation. This will be harmful as the cervix may get edematous or the ligaments and vaginal walls may get stretched and the pelvic floor may be damaged. In addition, premature pushing is harmful to the fetus

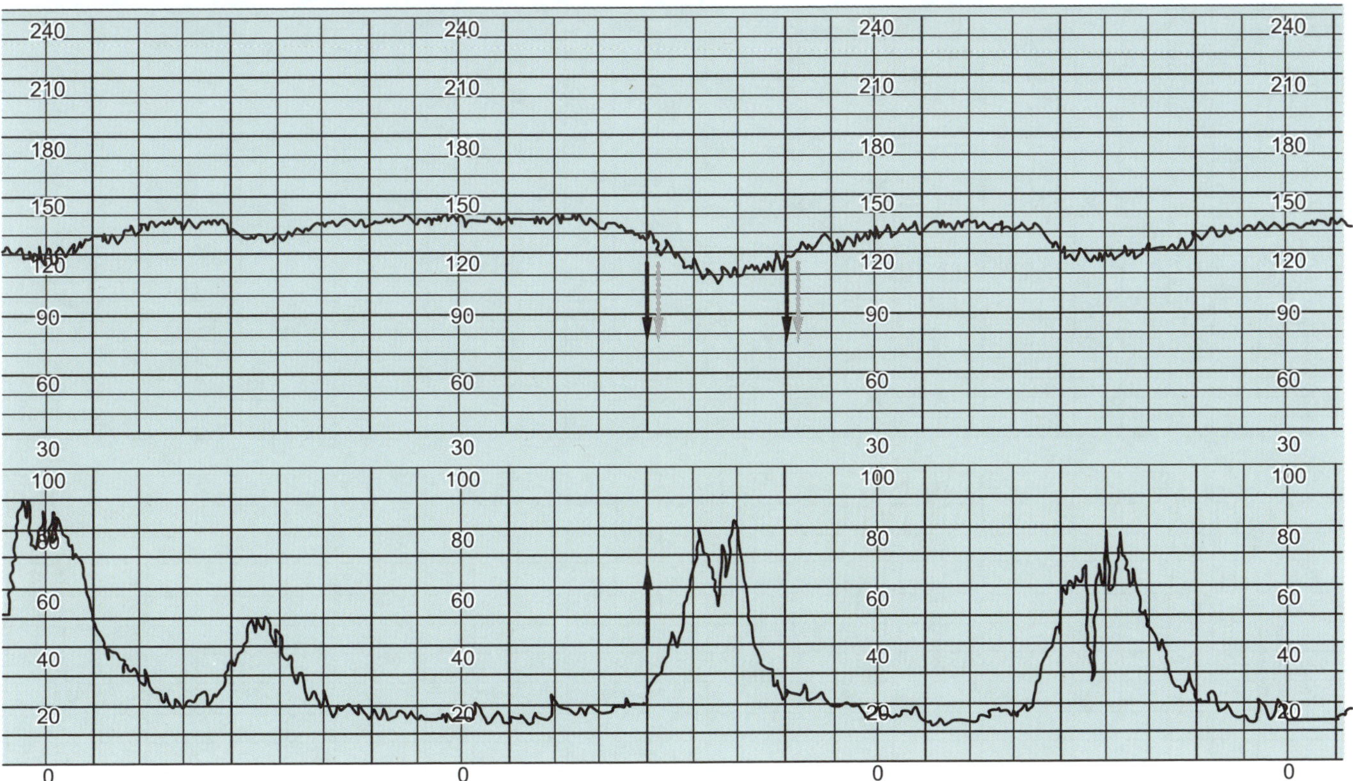

Fig. 24.1 Early decelerations.

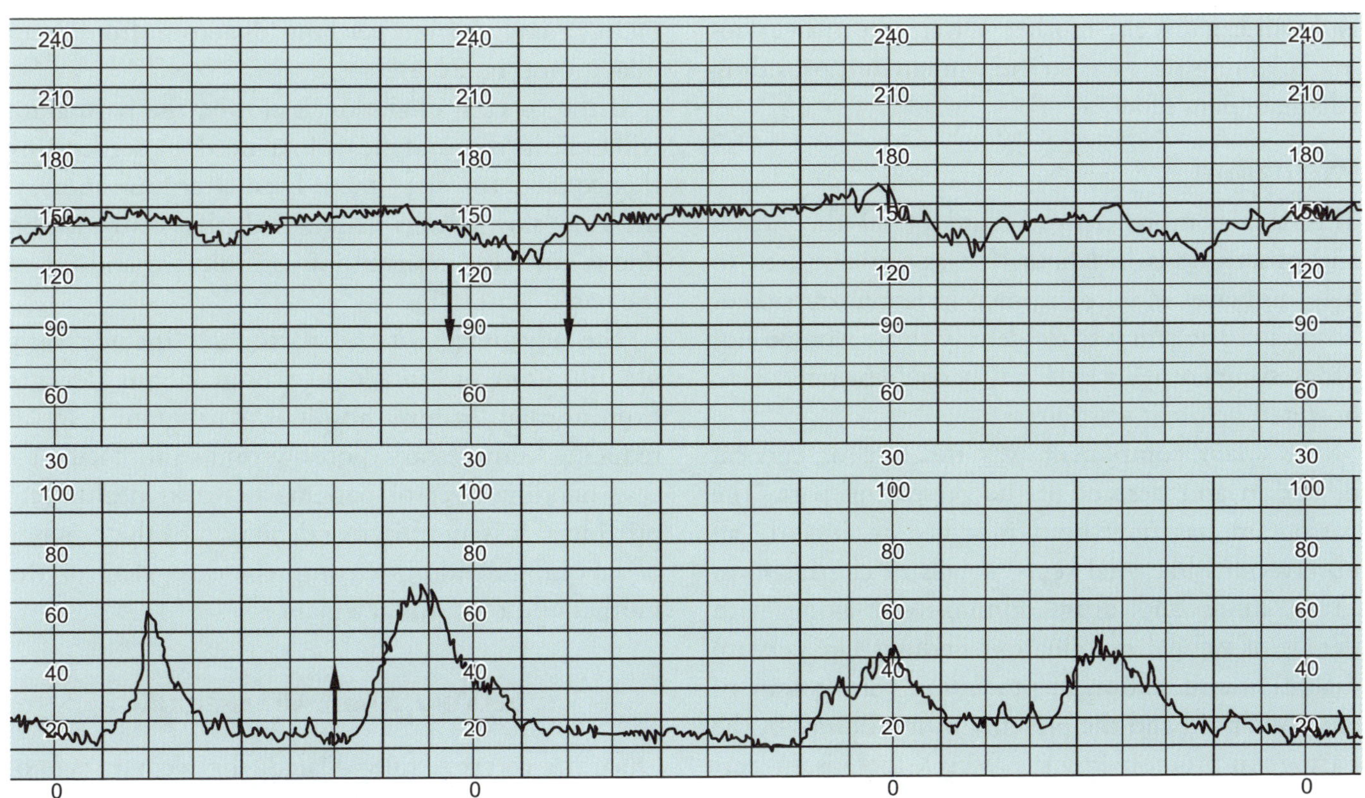

Fig. 24.2 Late decelerations.

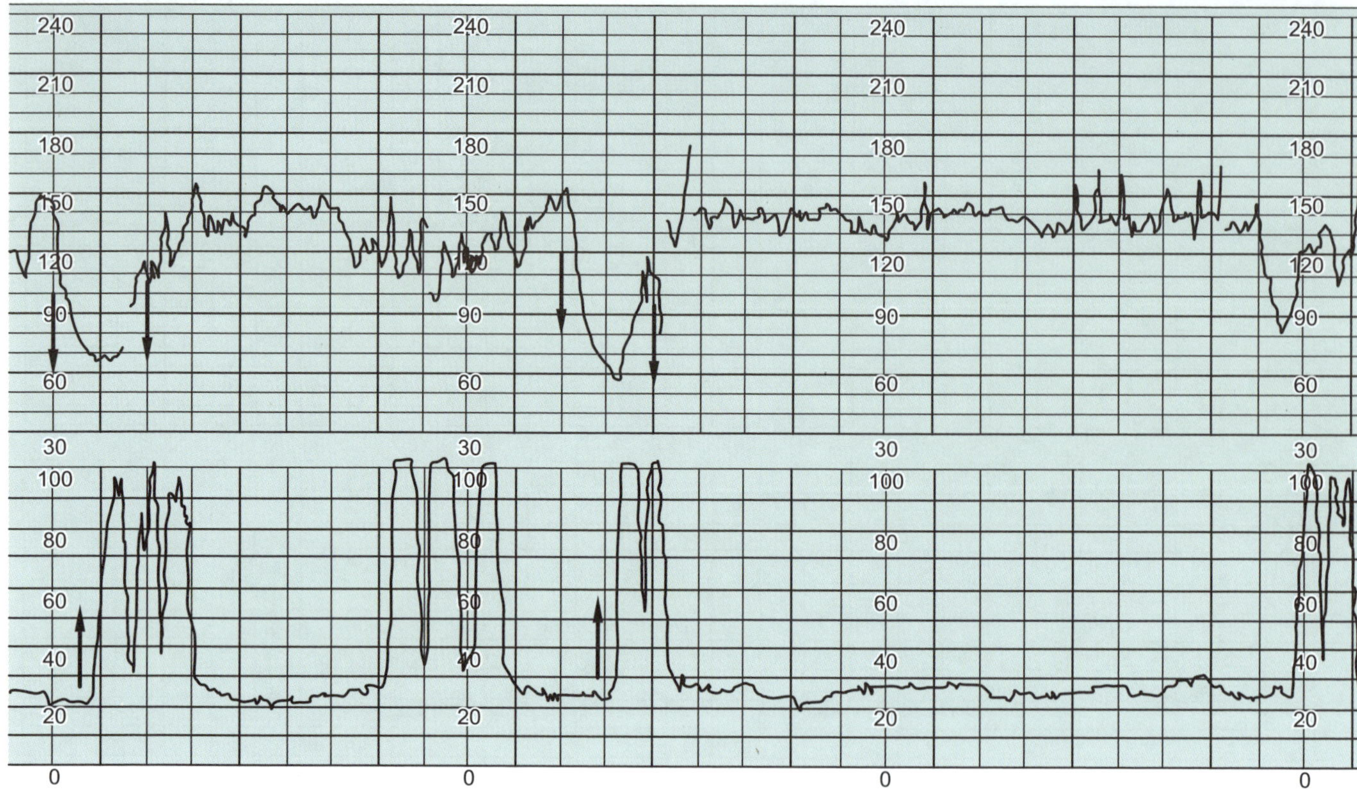

Fig. 24.3 Variable decelerations.

and will exhaust the mother. Often, the answer lies in explaining the facts to the woman and prosiding adequate pain relief.

Partogram

This is a comprehensive record of all the events and observations in labour. It was initially used to help midwives monitor women in labour outside of hospitals. The aim was to identify those women not progressing normally so that they could be referred to hospitals before it was too late.

The main component was the rate of cervical dilatation and descent of the presenting part. The partogram has now been modified to include all observations like vital signs, details of contractions, FHR, fluids and drugs administered along with details of vaginal examination findings like cervical dilatation and station of presenting part, colour of amniotic fluid and the presence of moulding. In the partogram promoted by the WHO, there is an alert line, and an action line drawn four hours later. The alert line in the cervical dilatation graph is marked taking a rate of 1 cm per hour dilatation from 3 cm dilatation (**Fig. 24.4**).

If the cervical dilatation is slower, the partogram will indicate that and the woman needs closer scrutiny (hence the term 'alert line'). Even after four hours, if the same slow pace is maintained (that is, the action line is crossed), intervention is indicated and hence the name 'action line'.

The advantages of the partogram include early identification of women in whom labour deviates from normal. In busy hospitals, partogram helps in reducing unnecessary notes-writing and facilitates easy handing over of patients between health care providers. It is an objective depiction of the progress of labour, providing a comprehensive view of the mother and the fetus at a glance.

Second Stage of Labour

Once the cervix is fully dilated, the second stage of labour is reached. Usually, along with dilatation of the cervix, descent of the presenting part and internal

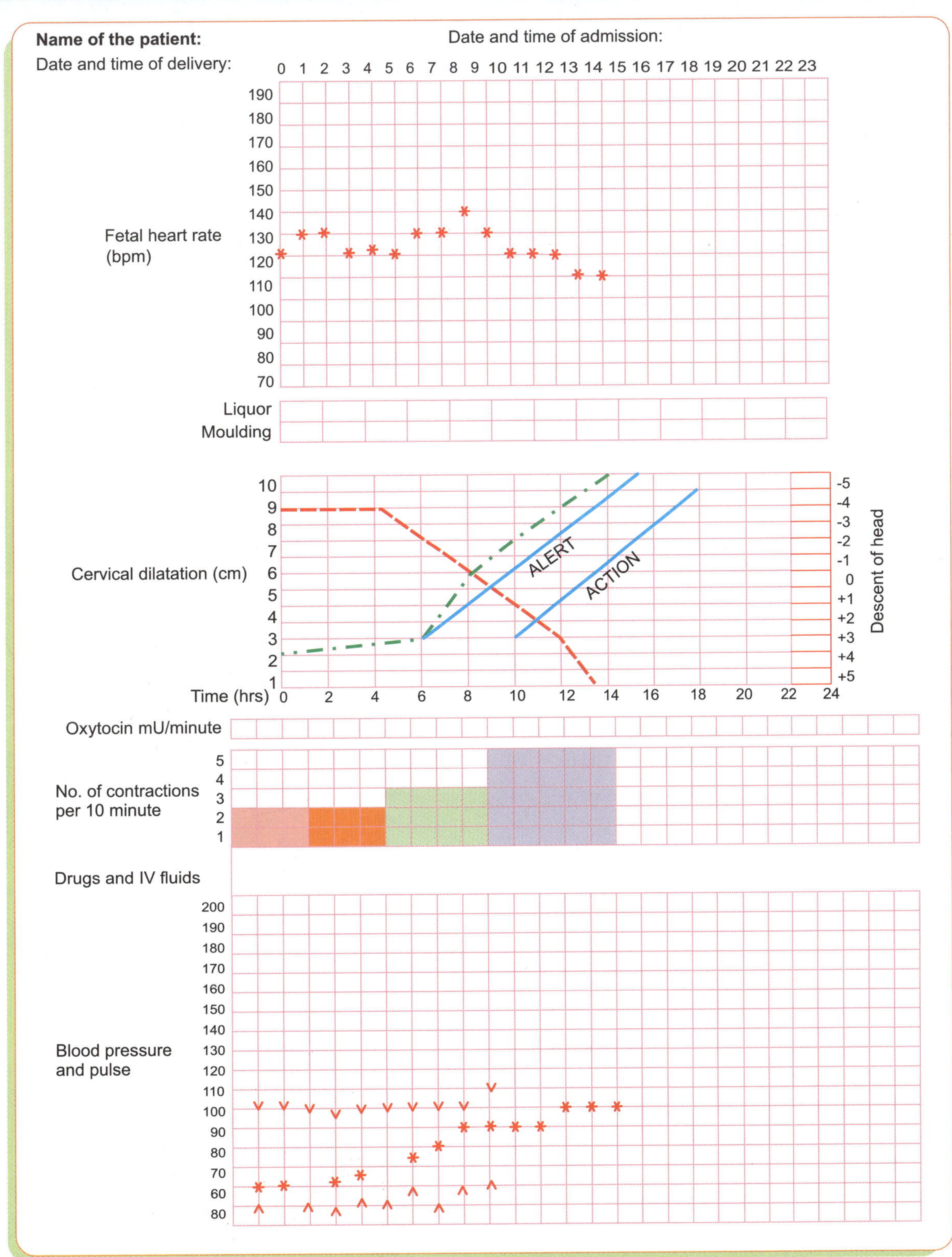

Fig. 24.4 Partogram in normal labour.

rotation would have occurred. The woman gets the urge to push with each contraction. Arrangements for conducting the delivery should be made at this point.

In many labour rooms, the woman is now shifted to a table specially used for conduct of labour. Such a shift can be avoided if the bed she had been using can be converted to a delivery table.

Adequate lighting is essential; a light coming from behind the obstetrician and adjustable at different angles is useful.

Delivery pack

A sterilised all-inclusive kit should be readily available for conducting the delivery. The common practice of assembling linen, bowls, cotton and instruments from different containers is not desirable. It can lead to the loss of valuable time. The pack should already have all the necessary linen, trays and instruments.

Maternal position

The position adopted by the woman in labour varies in different cultures and countries. The most widely practised is the dorsal position, with the woman drawing up the lower limbs and holding them with her hands. Between contractions, the feet may be rested on the tabletop or on special supports. The other maternal positions practised include sitting or squatting, standing or lying on the side.

Delivery of the head

Once the perineum has been cleaned with antiseptics and the patient draped with sterile clothes, she is encouraged to bear down with contractions. When the head has come low enough, the vertical slit of the introitus has become circular, and the head does not recede between contractions, it is called **crowning** (**Fig. 24.5**). From this point onwards, the descent and delivery of the head should be in a controlled manner. The palm of the right hand is used to support the perineum and the thumb and index finger of the left hand used at the occiput of the head to prevent sudden extension of the head (**Fig. 24.6**).

The head is allowed to escape slowly with the perineum gradually stretching and yielding (**Fig. 24.7**). If the soft tissue is resisting the escape

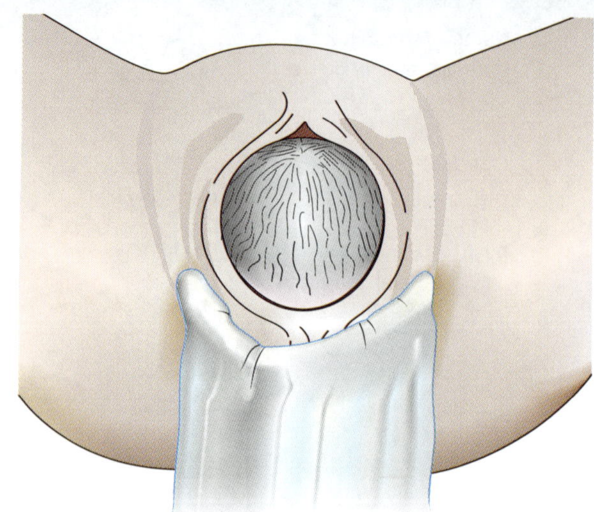

Fig. 24.5 Crowning.

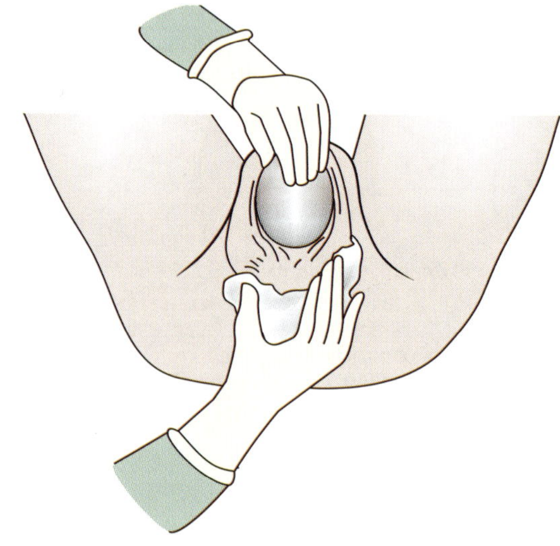

Fig. 24.6 Prevention of sudden extension of the head.

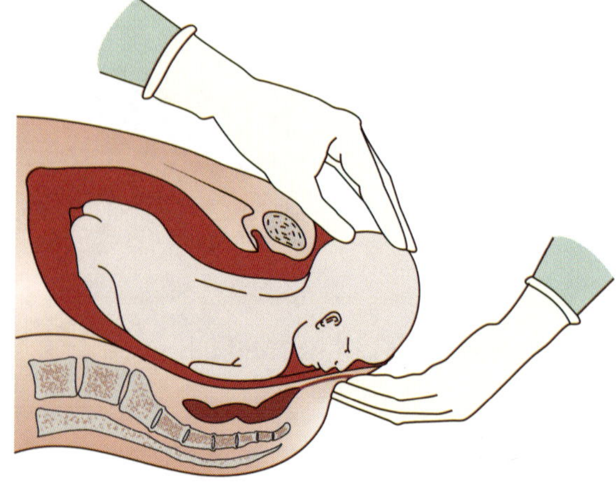

Fig. 24.7 Controlled delivery of the head.

of the head and appears to be at risk of tearing, an episiotomy is made.

Once the head is delivered, the neonate's eyes are cleaned with sterile gauze. A suction catheter tip may be used to clean the mucus, first from the mouth and then the nostrils.

While the eyes, mouth and nostrils are being cleared, the head would have undergone restitution and external rotation.

Delivery of the shoulders

The next step is conducting the delivery of the shoulder. The fingers of either hand are kept on the sides of the neck anteriorly and posteriorly, and gentle traction given, first gently downwards until the anterior shoulder hitches under the symphysis (**Fig. 24.8**). Traction is then directed gently anteriorly so that the posterior shoulder is delivered. This too must be done slowly and gently, otherwise perineal tears can occur during the delivery of the shoulders. Prophylactic intravenous methyl ergometrine in a dose of 0.2 mg helps in quick separation of the placenta and reduces blood loss during the third stage as well as the possibility of postpartum hemorrhage.

Delivery of the trunk

The delivery of the trunk usually follows without problems. The baby is then either allowed to lie on its side between the legs of the mother or held with its head tilted down slightly. It is advisable to wait a few seconds before clamping the cord so that about 50–70 ml of blood will flow to the fetus from the placenta. If the fetus is kept at a higher level on the maternal abdomen, much blood may pool at the placental site from the baby.

The cord may be clamped first close to the vulva after making sure there are no loose loops inside the vagina. The second clamp may be applied about 2–3 cm from the umbilicus. The segment between can now be cut. It is a good habit to cover the scissors with the operator's hand so that it will prevent blood spurting.

Episiotomy

Episiotomy is a deliberate incision of the perineum during labour to widen the introitus (**Fig. 24.9**). This may be used when the obstetrician feels that the perineum will tear or when additional space is required, as in cases of forceps delivery, breech delivery or shoulder dystocia. Episiotomy should always be performed after infiltrating the perineum with local anesthetic, unless a pudendal block has been given for operative delivery.

Traditionally, three types of episiotomy are considered: median, mediolateral and lateral. Lateral episiotomy is not advisable as it involves cutting too many tissues without a proportionate increase in the space available. The median episiotomy gives maximum increase in space but carries the risk of

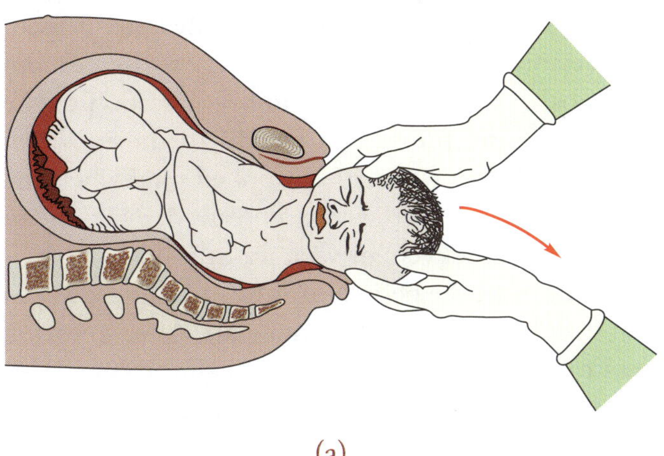

(a)

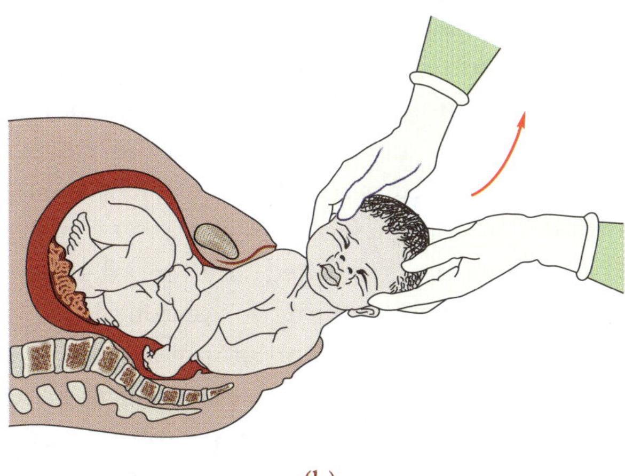

(b)

Fig. 24.8 a: Delivery of the shoulder b: Delivery of the trunk.

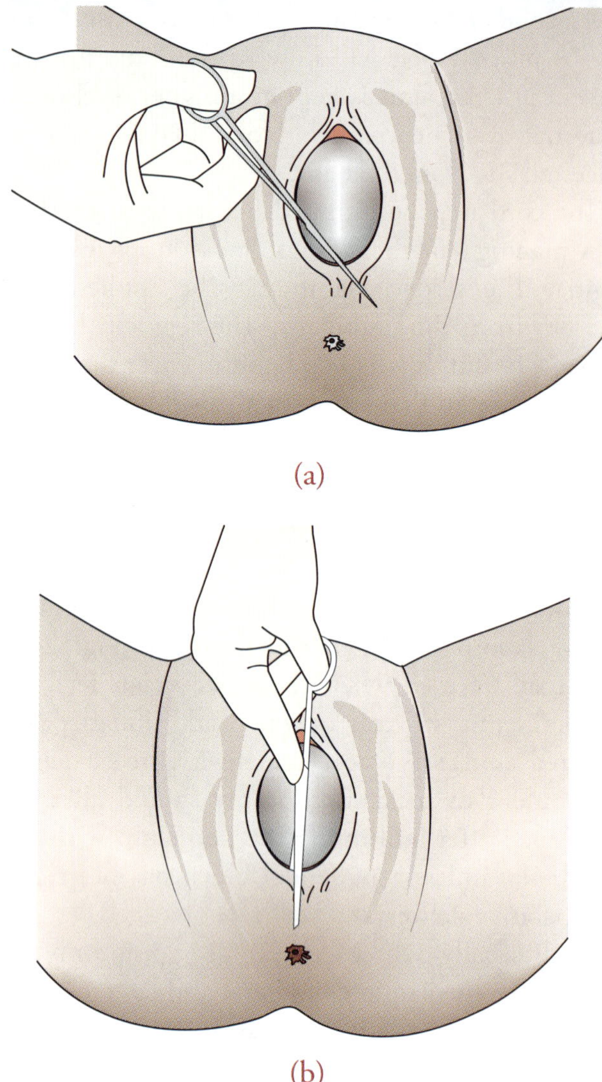

(a)

(b)

Fig. 24.9 Episiotomy a: Mediolateral b: Midline.

extending to involve the anal sphincter and mucosa. A compromise is the mediolateral episiotomy, which is made about 15–20 degrees from the midline, towards the right or the left. Even after mediolateral episiotomy, meticulous care should be taken to support the perineum as any extension is likely to involve the anal sphincter.

The episiotomy is repaired after the delivery of the placenta or while waiting for placental delivery. Any spurting vessel at the episiotomy wound should be tied separately. Venous bleeding will stop with tissue compression upon suturing. Suture material should be absorbable; a synthetic suture is preferred (polyglycolic acid) since it may get absorbed in a week. Catgut may also be used.

A continuous stitch is taken for the mucosa, taking care that the apex is not missed. The bites should be thick and, as it progresses towards the introitus, the bites should be adjusted so that the edge of the hymenal rim on one side is approximated with the edge on the other side. This will help in bringing back proper alignment of the two sides. The knots at the end of the mucosal running stitch may be buried deep. Two or three stitches may be used to appose the muscles. The skin may be closed with interrupted stitches with the same material. Alternatively, the sutures can be subcuticular so that there will be less discomfort. It is imperative that if there is any extension of the episiotomy, that too should be repaired while suturing. In such cases, a rectal examination must be performed to ensure that the anal sphincter and mucosa are intact.

Fundal pressure and ironing out the perineum

Any discussion on the conduct of labour would be incomplete without comments on these two very common practices. Both can be distressing and unsafe unless done carefully and properly.

'Fundal pressure' is the pressure applied to the fundus of the uterus to aid in the expulsion efforts of maternal pushing. It is important to remember that pressure should be applied to synchronise with the peak of uterine contraction. With the operator standing by the woman's side, the palms of the hands (rather than the tips of the thumb and fingers) should be used to apply pressure. If the latter is used, the pressure will be localised to a very small area and echymosis and even uterine injury may occur. The purpose of the pressure is to add to the maternal expulsive effort: it should be applied only when the head has started to crown, as a means of avoiding an outlet forceps delivery or vacuum help-out.

'Ironing out the perineum' is to stretch it slowly so that it slides over the presenting part. After smearing the introitus with a lubricating jelly or oil, the index and middle fingers are used to stretch the perineum by moving the fingers from one side to the other, stretching it posteriorly. In some centres, ironing out the perineum has even been advised as a preparation for labour in the last few days of pregnancy. However, it is more common to use it late in labour when the head has come to the pelvic floor. Prolonged ironing out leads to edema and even tearing of the perineum and, unless done gently, can be very distressing.

Delivery of the Placenta: Third Stage of Labour

The placenta is separated within a few minutes so the obstetrician should watch for signs of separation of the placenta. These are:

- lengthening of the cord outside the vulva
- fresh bleeding
- contracting uterus that appears prominently in the suprapubic region.

Once these signs appear, the obstetrician can push up and hold the contracted body of the uterus with the left hand and pull on the cord clamp with the right hand. (Traction on the cord with countertraction on the body of the uterus.) This method of delivery of placenta is called the Brandt–Andrews technique (**Fig. 24.10**). Once the body of the separated placenta has come out of the introitus, the abdominal hand can be released and both hands used to hold the placenta and rotate it so that the membranes inside will be rolled and come out entirely. Sometimes, a sponge-holding forceps may be required to hold the remnants of the membrane.

The placenta should be held in the palms of two hands and inspected before disposal. Any missing cotyledon can thus be noted. Inspection of the fetal surface of the placenta should be undertaken to see if any vessel abruptly stops at the edge of the placental disc: it could be an indication of a missing succenturiate lobe of placenta. If cord blood is required for investigation, it should be collected from the placental end before the placenta is delivered.

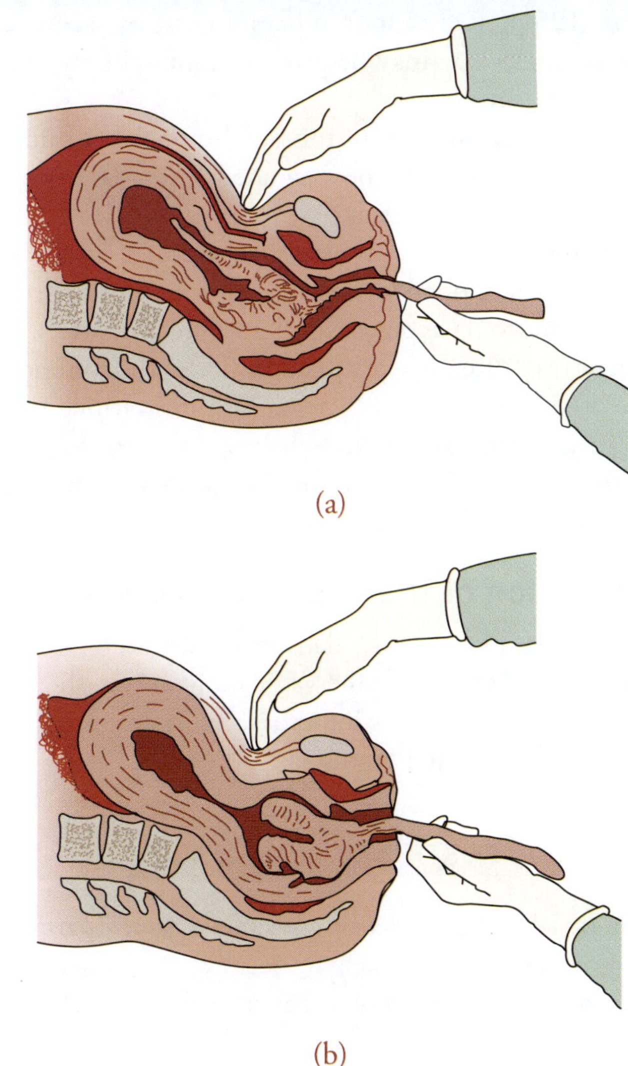

Fig. 24.10 Brandt–Andrew's method of placental delivery

Prevention of postpartum hemorrhage

It is now routine to recommend an oxytocic agent in the third stage of labour. If the oxytocin drip was on flow to stimulate uterine contraction, it may be continued at a higher dose (20 units per litre). In women at high risk of PPH like prolonged labour or prolonged use of oxytocin, an oxytocin drip may be used over 4 hours (40 units in 500 ml of normal saline at 125 ml/hour).

Other oxytocic agents that may be used are:

Methyl ergometrine: Given 0.2 mg slow IV or IM. The standard recommendation is to give it intravenously at the delivery of the anterior shoulder. It is crucial to time this well as the trunk of the fetus still inside the uterus will prevent hourglass spasm. Very often, the timing is not estimated accurately. If the fetus is already delivered, it is preferable to give it intramuscularly or intravenously at the time of delivery of the placenta.

Carboprost tromethamine: This prostaglandin analogue is a powerful uterotonic and can be administered intramuscularly. As a prophylactic dose, 125 µg (0.125 mg) suffices. In case of excessive bleeding, 250 µg may be given intramuscularly and repeated, if necessary.

In patients with a history of bronchial asthma, carboprost should be avoided as dangerous bronchospasm can result.

Misoprostol: This is available as a tablet and was originally developed for treating peptic ulcer. The drug was found to have powerful uterotonic properties. It can be used after delivery to make the uterus contract; the dose is 600–800 µg by rectal administration. This is particularly useful in non-hospital settings like domiciliary midwifery as no injection is required. Chills may occur in 25%–40% of cases.

Inspection of the vagina and cervix

After the placenta is delivered and before the episiotomy is sutured, the vagina and cervix should be inspected, especially if there is significant bleeding despite a contracted uterus.

Fourth Stage of Labour

The first hour after delivery is crucial as postpartum hemorrhage is most likely to occur at this time. The woman has to be closely supervised to check for bleeding. Vital signs should be recorded and the uterus should be checked for any relaxation.

Breastfeeding

The advantages of early breastfeeding are now well accepted. If the baby is active and crying, it can be put to breast immediately after delivery. The main advantage is that sucking will release more oxytocin, leading to uterine contraction and reduced blood loss. It will also be a boost to bonding between the mother and the baby.

After the delivery is complete, the woman is usually given a warm drink. Once she is cleaned and dressed, she can eat a snack. However, the woman should be kept in the labour room under observation for about three hours and sent to the ward only after she has passed urine. If she complains of inability to pass urine or severe pain at the episiotomy site, the possibility of a vulval or vaginal hematoma should be considered.

Labour is a stressful situation. The birth of the baby and the compassionate behaviour of the attending staff make it a pleasant and fulfilling experience for the woman. The joy of the family percolates to everybody around and is the best reward for the stress and strain of the caregivers.

KEY POINTS

- When a woman is admitted to the labour room, every effort should be made to make her comfortable.
- An initial assessment is made to confirm labour and to exclude abnormalities.
- The condition of the mother and the fetus, and progress of labour are carefully monitored using a partogram.
- Hydration, nutrition and analgesia are taken care of.
- The delivery of the fetus and placenta are conducted with required assistance.
- Prophylactic oxytocin is administered to reduce blood loss and prevent postpartum hemorrhage.
- An epsiotomy is made if required.

QUESTIONS

Select the single most appropriate answer:

1. The most reliable indicator of true labour is
   a. uterine contractions
   b. softness of cervix
   c. pain in the lumbar area
   d. effaced and dilated cervix
2. The preferred IV fluid for a patient in labour is
   a. 5% dextrose
   b. 10% dextrose
   c. ringer lactate
   d. dextran
3. The active phase of labour, as per WHO recommendations, is when
   a. cervix is 4–9 cm
   b. cervix is 3–10 cm
   c. regular painful contractions start
   d. full dilatation of cervix has occurred
4. In a partogram, all of the following are true *except*
   a. interval between alert line and action line is 3 hours
   b. interval between alert line and action line is 4 hours
   c. in the active phase of labour, the cervical dilatation is at the rate of 2 cm/hour
   d. once the head has reached the perineum, it is said to be at zero station
   e. if the graph of cervical dilatation is towards the left of the alert line, oxytocin drip should be started immediately
5. Crowning refers to the
   a. caput succedaneum on the scalp
   b. marks on the scalp after ventouse is applied
   c. appearance of the head at the introitus, seen between contractions
   d. distortion of head; extreme degree of moulding
6. Regarding delivery in occipitoanterior position all of the following statements are true *except*
   a. the head finally comes out by a process of flexion
   b. after the head comes outside the introitus, it undergoes restitution and then external rotation
   c. as soon as the head is delivered, the nose and then the mouth of the fetus should be cleaned
   d. normally, the posterior shoulder delivers before the anterior shoulder

Mark true (T) or false (F) against each statement:

7. The commonly performed episiotomy in India is median episiotomy.
8. A mediolateral episiotomy is made in a direction 15 to 20 degrees away from the midline.
9. If an episiotomy is made, perineal support is not needed during delivery of the head.
10. The risk with a median episiotomy is that it may lead to a third degree perineal tear.
11. Suture material used for episiotomy suturing should be delayed absorbable.
12. The most reliable sign of placental separation is the globular contracted uterus suprapubically.
13. Traction on cord while pushing down the contracted fundus of the uterus is the best method.
14. The placenta should be inspected after the episiotomy is sutured.
15. If cord blood is required for investigations, it should be collected before the cord is cut.
16. The missing succenturiate lobe of the placenta can be diagnosed by proper inspection of the placenta.
17. In patients with hypertension, routine administration of methergin should be avoided.
18. Carboprost tromethamine is given intravenously at the delivery of the anterior shoulder.
19. Misoprostol is inserted in the vagina as prophylaxis against PPH.
20. Oxytocin can be administered intravenously or intramuscularly.
21. The cervix and upper vagina must be inspected if bleeding persists in spite of a contracted uterus.

25

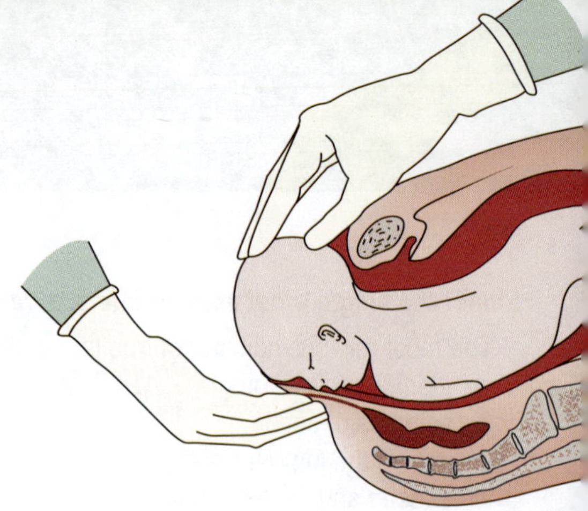

Obstetric Analgesia and Anesthesia

M Ravishankar

LEARNING OBJECTIVES

At the end of this chapter, the reader should be able to:

- explain the mechanism and effects of pain during labour
- appreciate the need to offer pain relief during labour
- list the non-pharmacological methods of pain relief
- enumerate the different pharmacological methods
- list the advantages and disadvantages of each method
- list the types of anesthesia for instrumental delivery
- explain the special concerns in anesthesia for cesarean section
- describe the types of anesthesia for obstetric surgery including cesarean section

Introduction

Labour pain or the pain of childbirth is believed to be one of the worst pains suffered by women. It is true that pain is a protective biological mechanism, abolition of which can expose an individual to unrecognised injury. This protective mechanism produces biological changes that, when excessive, can produce harmful effects by themselves. Pain during labour, when it exceeds a certain intensity and duration, produces harmful effects both on the mother and the fetus and some form of analgesia should be offered to all parturients.

Pain During Labour

Mechanisms and pathways of labour pains

For a long time, the pain during the first stage of labour was believed to be either due to compression of nerve endings between muscle fibres or due to ischemic myometrium (**uterine angina**). Now it has been established that the pain of the first stage is predominantly a result of dilatation of the cervix and lower uterine segment. The nociceptive afferents travel via the sympathetic nerves to be associated with the T10, T11, T12 and L1 spinal nerves.

With the commencement of the second stage, the contribution of the lower uterine segment and cervix to nociception decreases, while there is a progressive increase in the contribution from the pelvic parietal peritoneum, perineum, bladder, urethra and rectum. Hence, the neural pathways mainly involve the pudendal nerves (S_{2-4}) with a smaller contribution from the genitofemoral nerve and posterior cutaneous nerve of the thigh. From this, it can be deduced that the pain of the first stage overlies the skin of the lower abdomen and the lumbar vertebrae and that of the second stage is felt in the perineum, anus and thighs.

Factors influencing pain

Visualising the pain only in terms of intensity is akin to seeing the world in shades of grey. There are numerous other factors, which modify the pain sequence of a parturient. Pain increases as labour progresses. The severity of pain could be correlated with the woman's weight and height; there are also significant individual differences in the perception of pain. An uninformed, teenage primigravida experiences more pain. A large mother or a large baby can predispose to increased pain during labour. Parturients with abnormal presentation experience more pain. Likewise, fear, apprehension, anxiety, unfamiliar circumstances and the absence of a partner/supportive attendant can also enhance pain perception.

Effects of pain

It has been widely believed that labour is a natural process and that the accompanying pain must be benign. Labour pain produces deleterious effects both on the mother and the fetus. The effects are mediated at three levels: **cortical, suprasegmental** and **segmental**. Cortical effects are mediated by impulses arriving in the somatosensory cortex through the neospinothalamic tract. The suprasegmental effects are mediated by the connections of the paleospinothalamic tract with the reticular formation. Local neuronal connections at the spinal dermatome are responsible for the segmental effects.

Cortical effects include anxiety, fear, emotional arousal and behavioural changes like verbalisation and motor activity. Anxiety itself can produce incoordinate uterine action and depression. Suprasegmental effects include hyperventilation and an endocrine response, increasing the ACTH, cortisol and aldosterone levels. The segmental effects are mainly due to increased sympathetic tone leading to decreased GI motility, delayed gastric emptying, ileus, nausea and vomiting.

Analgesia for Vaginal Delivery

The ideal technique of pain relief during labour should fulfil the following criteria. It should be:

- safe
- effective
- easy to administer
- have no effect on the progress of labour
- successful
- have minimal side effects on the mother or fetus.

The methods that are in use to provide pain relief during labour are given in **Table 25.1**.

Non-pharmacological Methods

Psychoprophylaxis

Lamaze first reported success using psychoprophylaxis for obstetric analgesia in 1958. This method is based on the concept of reorganisation of cerebral cortical activity, thereby suppressing the pain of labour. It was believed that any natural process or event would be associated with no pain, and pain perception during labour was due to conditioning of the mother. Hence, pain relief, it was thought, could be achieved by creating positive conditioned reflexes in the mother and educating her about the process of natural childbirth.

Preparation of the woman usually begins six weeks before delivery. The woman is taught to take a

Table 25.1 Methods of pain relief for vaginal delivery

Non-pharmacological	
• Psychoprophylaxis • Hypnosis • Transcutaneous electrical nerve stimulation (TENS) • Acupuncture • Audioanalgesia • Electroanalgesia	
Pharmacological	
Systemic	**Regional/local**
• Narcotic analgesics • Sedatives • Ketamine • Inhalational agents	• Lumbar epidural block • Caudal epidural block • Subarachnoid block • Combined spinal epidural (CSE) block • Lumbar sympathetic block • Paracervical block • Pudendal block

deep breath when the contraction begins (cleansing breath), to concentrate on the release of muscle tension and to listen to reassuring words from the physician. This method, which was believed to be effective in relieving pain, was shown to modify pain perception but produced incomplete analgesia.

Hypnosis: Hypnotic procedures have been used to ameliorate labour pain since the nineteenth century. It is time-consuming and women with high hypnotisability report less pain.

Transcutaneous Electrical Nerve Stimulation (TENS): The intensity of labour pain has been successfully reduced by TENS. Electrical current is delivered by the stimulator, which provides a biphasic asymmetrical square waveform current. This method of pain relief is thought to work by 'gate control theory', whereby activation of fast conducting A fibres by TENS closes the gate for the transmission of the slow conducting visceral C fibres. Lumbosacral pain is controlled well with TENS but not the suprapubic pain. This may be due to the stretching of the perineal structures: the resulting painful sensations themselves are transmitted by A fibres. No adverse effects on the fetus or the mother have been reported; TENS can be used as a complement to conventional methods.

Acupuncture: This traditional form of Chinese medicine involves the insertion of needles at selected points to get desired results. Four main points are used. During the first stage, needles should be passed through all the points. Electrical stimulation of dense and disperse types should be used. With this, the pain relief is achieved in around 90% of cases to a satisfactory level. Electro-acupuncture did not adversely affect the uterine contractions and had no harmful effects on the mother or the neonate. The technique is time-consuming, limits the patient's movements and interferes with electronic monitoring.

Pharmacological Methods

Systemic analgesics

Systemically administered opioids, sedatives, tranquillisers and ketamine have been used for relief of labour pain with varied results. Among these, opioids are the most widely used drugs. Systemic medications have the advantage of ease of administration and patient acceptability. However, the drug, dose, time and route of administration must be chosen carefully to avoid adverse maternal and neonatal effects.

Opioids: These are substances that work by binding to opioid receptors in the CNS and the GI tract (**Table 25.2**). The receptors in these two systems mediate the beneficial and side effects of opioids. The analgesic effects of opioids are due to a decrease in the perception of pain, decreased reaction to pain and increased tolerance to pain. Side effects include sedation, respiratory depression and constipation.

Intramuscular pethidine continues to be the standard opioid analgesic used in labour. However, this produces incomplete pain relief in more than 50% of parturients.

Morphine is a powerful opiate but frequently causes nausea and vomiting and is a potent depressor of neonatal respiration. When an equianalgesic dose was used, it caused more respiratory depression than pethidine. Delayed onset of analgesia and the greater sensitivity of the newborn's respiratory centre make it unsuitable for labour analgesia.

Fentanyl has been used for labour analgesia IM or IV in doses of 50–100 μg per hour. This regimen was shown to be preferable to intravenous pethidine as it produced equivalent analgesia, though not complete, and there was no prolonged sedation or vomiting in the mother; requirement for neonatal naloxone was less.

The potent narcotic agonists when used for labour analgesia tend to slow labour and may adversely affect the mother and the child. Hence, the dosage range is limited. Pentazocine is a synthetic opiate with a partial agonist–antagonist profile. It is not a potent analgesic but nausea and vomiting is claimed to be

Table 25.2 Types of opioids, dose and effect

Opioid	Dose	Peak effect	Duration
Pethidine	50–150 mg	15 min	3 hours
Morphine	5–10 mg	1–2 hours	4–6 hours
Fentanyl	50–100 μg	3–5 min	30–60 min
Pentazocine	30–60 mg	15 min	2–4 hours

less and neonatal respiratory depression is less severe even with repeated intramuscular doses.

Complications of opioid analgesics: Nausea, vomiting and drowsiness are the most distressing complications following the use of opioids in labour. They cause decreased beat-to-beat fetal heart variability. Neonatal respiratory depression and low Apgar scores occur 2–3 hours after administration, as the neonatal plasma concentrations reach a peak at this time. Delayed neurobehavioral scores can be found 2–3 days after delivery probably due to the metabolite norpethidine.

Naloxone, a pure opioid antagonist can be administered to treat the respiratory depression in the mother or the neonate following opioid administration. But it should not be administered to the mother shortly before delivery because it may cause neonatal ventilatory depression. Although this may be effective, it reverses maternal analgesia at a time when it is most needed and in some instances has caused maternal pulmonary edema and even cardiac arrest.

Ketamine: Ketamine may be administered intravenously either as intermittent boluses or as a continuous infusion. Used as a continuous titrated infusion after a 0.2 mg/kg bolus intravenously, it has been shown to produce adequate analgesia during the first stage of labour. Safe and effective analgesia can be achieved with an infusion rate of 0.5–1 μg/kg/min.

The use of ketamine for labour analgesia was found to be associated with amnesia and a 10%–20% rise in systolic and diastolic blood pressure. Higher doses and administration for longer duration may result in maternal complications like apnea, laryngospasm, increased uterine tone, hypertension and fetal respiratory depression requiring positive pressure ventilation. Other complications include dryness of mouth, visual disturbances, hallucinations, dreams, restlessness, dizziness and nystagmus. The use of this drug for obstetric analgesia is not popular due to the unpredictability of complications.

Tramadol: Tramadol hydrochloride is a centrally acting drug with low affinity for opioid receptors and acts through activation of the descending monoaminergic non-opioid pathway. Tramadol 100 mg is shown to be as effective as 75 mg of pethidine in labour analgesia and has a superior safety profile. It produces a low incidence of respiratory and cardiac depression in the neonate. Rectal administraton of 100 mg tramadol suppositories has nearly the same analgesic effect as parenteral administration.

Nonsteroidal anti-inflammatory drugs (NSAIDs): These are not generally used for labour analgesia as the oral preparations have unpredictable absorption and cause vomiting. Due to antiplatelet action, this group of drugs can increase bleeding during delivery.

Benzodiazepines: Benzodiazepines are used as sedatives or adjuncts to narcotics in labour analgesia. They reduce maternal anxiety and narcotic requirements without prolonging labour or increasing the risk of neonatal respiratory depression. Diazepam crosses the placenta and maternal and fetal blood levels are approximately equal within minutes of an intravenous dose. The principal adverse effects of large doses of diazepam are hypotonia, lethargy, decreased feeding and hypothermia in the newborn (**floppy baby syndrome**); hence it is not widely used in labour analgesia.

Midazolam: The attractive pharmacokinetic profile of midazolam (shorter duration of action and rapid elimination) makes it a favoured alternative for diazepam. When used as intravenous bolus in 5-mg doses, it causes antegrade amnesia in the mother and respiratory depression in the neonate. It is used safely in a dose of 2–4 mg intravenously as an adjunct to epidural analgesia without complications.

Inhalational agents

Inhalation analgesia is widely preferred; even though it does not relieve pain completely, it makes pain tolerable. The agents commonly used are 50% nitrous oxide in oxygen (entonox), 0.35% methoxyflurane or 0.5% trilene. Enflurane 0.25%–1% in oxygen, isoflurane 0.2% with entonox and desflurane 1.0%–4.5% in oxygen are also being used. Proper timing of starting inhalation is essential for success. The inhalation agents are usually administered intermittently. Inhalation is begun at the start of each contraction and is discontinued at the end of the contraction. The start should not be delayed till the woman perceives the pain. The desired level of analgesia can be rapidly achieved or terminated.

In order to circumvent the difficulties associated with synchronising the maximal effects of intermittent analgesia with the peak of contraction, the continuous inhalation method was proposed. This is usually given during the second stage under the supervision of an anesthesiologist. The woman inhales the agent even during the interval between contractions and the anesthesiologist should make sure that the woman is awake, cooperative, and is able to bear down with each uterine contraction.

The use of inhalational agents increases the risk of environment pollution and needs a scavenging system. Inadvertent overdose can lead to loss of consciousness, vomiting and aspiration of gastric contents. Uterine activity is usually not affected by the analgesic concentrations. However, anesthetic concentrations are known to depress myometrial contractility. When used properly, inhalational agents produce good analgesia in one-third and partial relief in another one-third of parturients.

Regional analgesia

This method is the most commonly used technique for labour analgesia worldwide. The various methods are listed in **Table 25.1**.

Continuous lumbar epidural analgesia: It can be administered once the labour is well established (**Fig. 25.1**). It is mandatory to get an adequate intravenous access and infuse approximately 1,000 ml of a crystalloid before block is established, in order to decrease the incidence of hypotension following sympathetic block. A catheter is inserted and the tip (3 cm) is left in the lumbar epidural space. A test dose of 3 ml of 1.5% lidocaine with 5 µg/ml of adrenaline is used to exclude intravascular or subarachnoid placement of the catheter. After confirming the position of the catheter, the total dose of the drug is administered in fractional amounts of 4–5 ml. Left lateral tilt or lateral positioning of the parturient to prevent supine hypotension is mandatory. Arterial blood pressure and the heart rate should be monitored every 1–2 minutes for the first

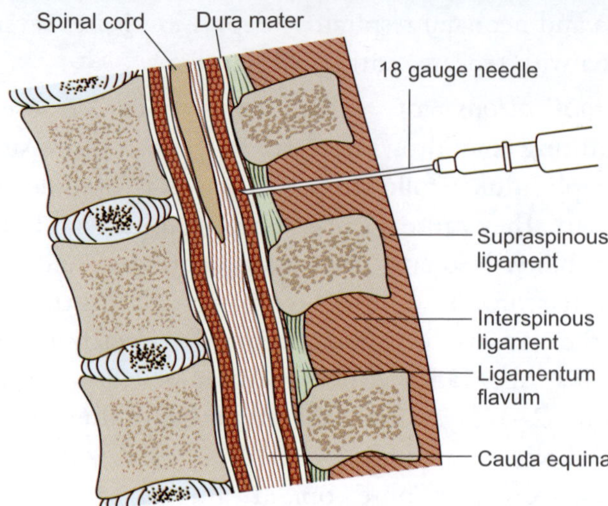

Fig. 25.1 Technique for epidural analgesia.

10 minutes and then every 5–15 minutes. During the second stage of labour, an additional drug is injected in the sitting position.

Epidural opioids in combination with local anesthetics help to decrease the concentration of the local anesthetic used, thus minimising the complications associated with higher concentration of local anesthetics, and act in synergism with them as the sites of action of these two groups of drugs are different.

Advantages of epidural block: These are listed below:

- Complete relief of pain is possible. Even partial relief of pain decreases hyperventilation, peripheral vascular resistance and improves uteroplacental circulation.
- Pain-induced reflexes are obliterated and lumbar epidural block stops the nociceptive input and decreases the release of catecholamines, beta-endorphins, ACTH and cortisol.
- Epidural analgesia ablates the detrimental increase in cardiac output and blood pressure produced by pain. This is particularly useful in women with heart disease and preeclampsia.
- Any form of analgesia decreases oxygen consumption, but epidural analgesia is superior to parenteral opioids in decreasing maternal work, oxygen consumption and metabolic acidosis.
- Epidural analgesia nearly eliminates the psychological and emotional reaction to pain.

- Effective pain relief can change incoordinate uterine contraction into an effective one and improve placental circulation.

Disadvantages:

- Technical expertise is necessary for its administration.
- Urge to bear down is decreased.
- Complications like maternal hypotension, total spinal and local anesthetic toxicity are possible.
- There is an increased probability of failed rotation of fetal head.
- Incidence of instrumental delivery is increased.
- Bladder atony leads to voiding difficulties.
- The method is not fail-proof.

Walking epidural analgesia: Extradural analgesia for labour pain causes motor block. Several techniques have been used to reduce or even abolish the motor blockade to facilitate spontaneous deliveries. Reducing motor block and encouraging walking is associated with a decreased rate of instrumental and operative deliveries. Walking in labour may:

- improve the rate of cervical dilatation
- encourage correct positioning of the fetal head and increase spontaneous delivery rate due to pelvic movements
- being upright may decrease any tendency to aorto-caval compression.

Continuous infusion epidural: Continuous infusion of low concentrations of local anesthetics provides a continuous and stable anesthetic level and the extent of motor blockade is reduced because of lower concentrations used. There are also fewer hypotensive episodes due to fewer fluctuations in sympathetic blockade compared to that seen with intermittent boluses. Potential complications are intravascular and subarachnoid migration of the epidural catheter.

Patient-controlled epidural analgesia (PCEA): During epidural analgesia for labour, any delay in administering the top-up injections will result in a higher pain level. This epidural 'catch-up' phenomenon can be overcome by PCEA. The patient is given control over the doses delivered while the dose and the interval are preset.

Subarachnoid block: The more rapid and reliable analgesia achieved by the intrathecal administration of drugs makes this route attractive. Opioids are preferable to local anesthetics as they have the advantage of providing safe analgesia without any motor block, hypotension or effect on uterine contractility. The minimal doses used do not produce serious fetal and neonatal effects. Intrathecal opioids produce effective analgesia during the first stage of labour but are inadequate during the second stage. Common side effects include pruritus, nausea, vomiting, urinary retention and respiratory depression.

Combined spinal epidural block: Pure spinal opioid analgesia often does not offer optimal analgesia; epidural analgesia usually has a slow onset. Combined spinal epidural (CSE) technique combines the advantages of rapid onset and reliability of spinal block, and the reinforcement of the anesthetic level; continuous administration of epidural block for longer duration has therefore come into practice.

Local blocks

Paracervical block: It is used for analgesia during the first stage of labour. This technique involves the injection of the local anesthetic into the lateral fornix of the vagina to provide analgesia by blocking all the visceral sensory fibres from the uterus, cervix and upper vagina. It is an easy method and needs minimum preparation: pain relief is achieved very rapidly. Around 8 ml of local anesthetic is injected into each fornix (**Fig. 25.2**). This produces adequate analgesia for the first stage in 80% of cases. Fetal bradycardia and death have been reported.

Pudendal block: It is an effective method of perineal analgesia for the second stage of labour. This block is administered just before delivery. Both sides have to be blocked by a transperineal or transvaginal route. The transvaginal approach is technically simpler, less painful and, has a higher success rate; there is less risk of damage to the fetus or to the rectum. The ischial spine is palpated, the needle (20 G) is placed below the spine, the sacrospinous ligament is pierced and the drug deposited (**Fig. 25.3**). Ten ml of 1%

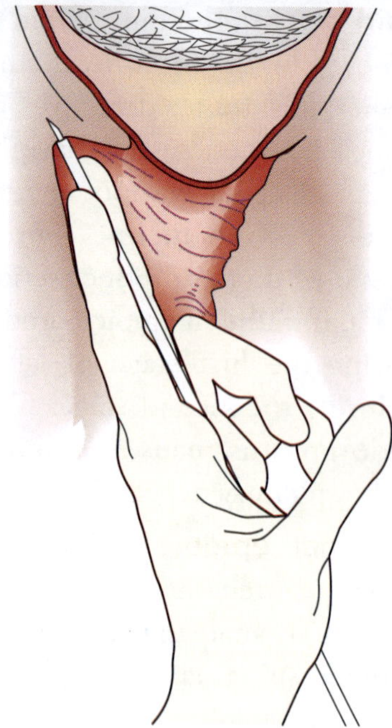

Fig. 25.2 Paracervical block.

lignocaine, 0.5% bupivacaine, 1% mepivacaine or 2% chloroprocaine is used to block each side. It provides analgesia in the lower portion of the vagina and perineum and permits forceps delivery and episiotomy.

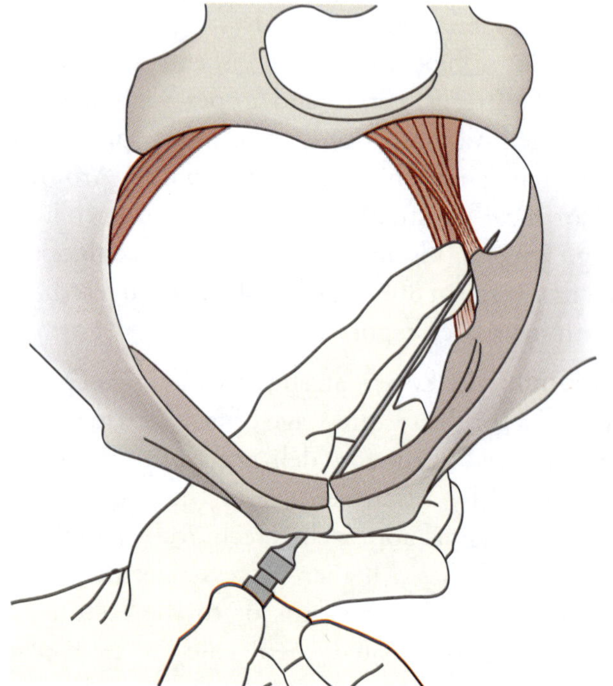

Fig. 25.3 Pudendal block.

Anesthesia for Operative Delivery

Concerns during pregnancy

Changes in smooth muscle tone occur early in pregnancy as a result of an increase in progesterone levels. There is significant reduction in lower esophageal sphincter tone. Combined with increase in abdominal mass, this predisposes the pregnant woman to increased risk of regurgitation and pulmonary aspiration of gastric contents. **Mendelson syndrome** is a condition where chemical pneumonitis is caused by pulmonary aspiration of acid gastric contents during induction of anesthesia.

Aorto-caval occlusion syndrome is another concern. The bulk of the gravid uterus presses on the aorta and inferior vena cava when the woman lies supine. This can lead to reduction in venous return to the heart and cardiac output. Added to this, the compression of the aorta decreases uteroplacental blood flow. All women should be nursed in the lateral position during labour. During anesthesia, precautions must be taken to prevent aorto-caval occlusion by keeping a wedge under the right side so the uterus is displaced to the left side.

Premedication

The operative delivery could be an elective or an emergency procedure to be performed under general or regional anesthesia. Concerns of acid aspiration and aorto-caval occlusion are genuine and precautions must be taken to prevent them. It is the usual practice to premedicate the woman with a H_2 blocker like ranitidine 150 mg orally to reduce the acidity of gastric secretions. Metclopramide 10 mg can be used to prevent vomiting. Narcotic premedication is avoided as it can depress the baby. Benzodiazepines in small doses may be used to allay anxiety.

Regional anesthesia

Regional anesthesia is the technique of choice for elective cesarean section. The techniques available are:

- spinal anesthesia
- epidural anesthesia
- combined spinal epidural anesthesia (CSE).

Spinal anesthesia is the most popular choice for elective cesarean section with increasing popularity of the combined spinal epidural (CSE) technique. The technique of performing the blocks is the same as that for labour analgesia but the drugs and the concentration used differ.

Spinal anesthesia: Most spinal anesthetics are performed with the patient on the operating table as this reduces the need to move. The following points are mandatory:

- routine preanesthetic equipment check
- monitoring of arterial pressure, ECG and pulse oximetry
- intravenous infusion of crystalloid, 500 ml loading in 10 minutes followed by 500 ml/hour
- vasopressor-like ephedrine should be readily available
- aseptic technique.

Spinal anesthesia may be performed with the patient in either the sitting or the lateral position. The choice of needle is important to minimise the incidence of post-dural puncture headache; a small (25 or 26 G) Quincke tip needle may be used.

Hyperbaric bupivacaine 0.5% is the drug of choice and 1.8–2.0 ml is usually sufficient. An opioid may be added to the local anesthetic as this may improve the quality of the anesthesia and provide postoperative analgesia. The block should be tested for loss of sensation to pinprick. The level of the block should be T4 bilaterally. Hypotension is treated with rapid infusion of Ringer lactate solution, ephedrine in boluses of 3 mg or as an infusion. The patient should be carefully observed at all times. Oxytocin 5–10 units is normally administered intravenously after the delivery of the baby to assist myometrial contraction. Blood loss should be monitored and blood replaced if it exceeds 15% of estimated blood volume. Routine postoperative care should take place in a well-equipped recovery area.

Epidural anesthesia: It was the regional anesthetic of choice until pencil-point spinal needles were introduced. The disadvantages of epidural anesthesia are that the onset of the block is prolonged and the spread of the block may be patchy, often giving poor anesthesia. The cardiovascular stability with an epidural is excellent and is the method of choice in women with heart disease or preeclampsia. The following combination of drugs can be used for an epidural anesthetic:

- bupivacaine 0.5% 12–16 ml with 1 in 2,00,000 epinephrine
- lidocaine 2% 12–16 ml with 1 in 2,00,000 epinephrine
- fentanyl 50 μg may be administered in addition to the local anesthetic and has been shown to improve the quality of the anesthesia

It is essential to test the block thoroughly from the thoracic level down to the sacral roots.

Combined spinal epidural (CSE) anesthesia: In the CSE technique, the spinal is usually conducted using the same dose of drugs as listed above, and the epidural, although placed as an 'insurance', is often used only for postoperative pain relief. The CSE may also be used as a sequential block, with a smaller intrathecal dose of local anesthetic, followed by an epidural top-up to achieve full anesthesia. This method provides greater cardiovascular stability, while an excellent sacral block is achieved with the spinal anesthetic.

Post-dural puncture headache (PDPH): One of the distressing complications of regional anesthesia is the development of PDPH. The clinical presentation is of an occipital headache which may radiate anteriorly, aggravated by the sitting position. This may possibly be associated with nausea, photophobia and, rarely, diplopia resulting from stretching of the 6th cranial nerve as it passes through the dura.

Management of PDPH consists of:

- bed rest, as the sitting position aggravates headache
- intravenous and oral fluids to prevent dehydration
- analgesics, for example, paracetamol, 500 mg 4-hourly
- antidiuretic hormone.

a sample of the patient's own venous blood collected under aseptic conditions and injected into the same or an adjacent epidural space to seal the CSF leak (epidural blood patch); it is 90% effective.

General anesthesia (GA)

Though regional anesthesia is the first choice, GA is required in the following situations:

- in an extreme emergency, for example, severe fetal distress or maternal haemorrhage
- there is a contraindication to regional anesthesia
- the woman refuses to have a regional anesthetic.

The main risk is aspiration of acidic gastric contents (as little as 25 ml with pH less than 2.5 may lead to a 50% mortality rate) and hypoxemia resulting from airway difficulties.

Preparation:

- The equipment including the suction apparatus is checked; the table tilts head-down.
- A quick preanesthetic check on the patient is done with particular attention to the airway and gastric contents.
- An assistant who can give cricoid pressure is ready.
- The patient is positioned, paying particular attention to aorto-caval compression and tracheal intubation.
- Intravenous access with a large bore cannula is obtained.
- Full routine monitoring is ensured.
- Preoxygenation for three minutes is carried out.
- Rapid sequence induction is followed.

Technique: It is standard practice to use thiopental to induce anesthesia in a dose of at least 4 mg/kg rapidly followed by succinylcholine 1–1.5 mg/kg. Cricoid pressure should be applied as the patient begins to lose consciousness and continued until the tracheal tube is in place. Anesthesia should be continued using 50% nitrous oxide and a volatile agent in oxygen and positive pressure ventilation. Halothane or isoflurane may be used. If the fetus is compromised, there is evidence that use of 100% oxygen with a volatile agent may be beneficial to the fetus because it increases oxygen transfer across the placenta. After the delivery of the baby, an opioid such as morphine, may be given with oxytocin, as well as an antibiotic to prevent wound infection. Additional non-depolarising muscle relaxant (for example, vecuronium 0.1 mg/kg) may be administered after the effect of the succinyleholine has worn off. Residual neuromuscular block should be antagonised before tracheal extubation, with the patient in the lateral position and with a slight head-down tilt. Routine postoperative care in a fully equipped recovery area is essential. At this time, postoperative pain relief should be effective and the baby should be handed over to the mother whenever possible.

KEY POINTS

- Labour pains are one of the most severe forms of pain.
- The pain has an adverse effect on the mother and the fetus.
- Pain relief makes the mother comfortable and labour pleasant.
- The ideal agent for labour analgesia should be easy to administer, effective, with no adverse effects on the mother, fetus or labour.
- Non-pharmacological methods have a role in select cases.
- Systemic opioids are most commonly used for labour analgesia.
- Epidural is a near-ideal labour analgesic, but is technically difficult to administer and needs expertise.
- Local blocks are useful for vaginal operative deliveries.
- Obstetric anesthesia has a risk of aspiration, which has high mortality; adequate preparation to neutralise gastric acidity reduces the risk.
- Regional anesthesia, particularly combined spinal epidural, is the preferred technique for obstetric anesthesia.
- When general anesthesia is needed, quick sequence induction is followed.

QUESTIONS

Select the single most appropriate answer:

1. Pain during the first stage of labour is attributed to
   a. myometrial ischemia
   b. dilatation of the cervix
   c. compression of nerve fibres
   d. accumulation of lactic acid
2. The nociceptive fibres responsible for labour pains travel through
   a. autonomic nerves
   b. sympathetic fibres of T4–T6
   c. parasympathetic fibres of S2–S4
   d. sympathetic fibres of T10–L1
3. Pain during the second stage of labour mainly involves
   a. pudendal nerves c. T10–L1 nerves
   b. T4–T6 nerves d. obturator nerve
4. Labour pains may be perceived to be more severe in all of the following *except*
   a. malpresentations
   b. young pregnant woman
   c. a bigbuilt mother with a large baby
   d. a multigravida
5. Which one of the effects of labour pains is cortically mediated?
   a. nausea and vomiting c. verbalisation
   b. hyperventilation d. bowel distension
6. The methods of labour analgesia likely to have least adverse effects on the mother and the fetus are
   a. opioid analgesics
   b. transcutaneous nerve stimulation (TENS)
   c. paracervical block
   d. spinal analgesia
7. The drug most commonly used for labour analgesia is
   a. ketamine c. midazolam
   b. propofol d. pethidine or morphine
8. The drug that causes maximum respiratory depression in the neonate is
   a. morphine c. pentazocine
   b. pethidine d. fentanyl
9. The inhalational agent that has the disadvantage of causing significant uterine relaxation is
   a. nitrous oxide c. halothane
   b. trilene d. methoxyflurane
10. The best method for relief of pain during labour is
    a. spinal analgesia
    b. epidural analgesia
    c. combined epiduralspinal analgesia
    d. caudal analgesia
11. For an uncomplicated instrumental or assisted breech delivery, the most suitable analgesia is
    a. paracervical block c. inhalational analgesia
    b. spinal analgesia d. pudendal block
12. A disadvantage of epidural analgesia is that
    a. there may be postnatal retention of urine
    b. pain relief is often unsatisfactory
    c. it is not useful in women with heart disease
    d. it worsens emotional reaction to pain
13. The presence of which of the following is most dangerous when general anesthesia is planned for an emergency cesarean section?
    a. abnormal uterine action
    b. neonatal depression
    c. full stomach
    d. aorto-caval compression
14. The disadvantage of epidural anesthesia for cesarean section for fetal distress is
    a. hypotension is inevitable
    b. there is delayed onset of action
    c. it may cause uterine atony
    d. neonatal depression
15. Post-spinal headache may be treated with all of the following *except*
    a. analgesia c. blood patch
    b. hydration d. corticosteroids

26

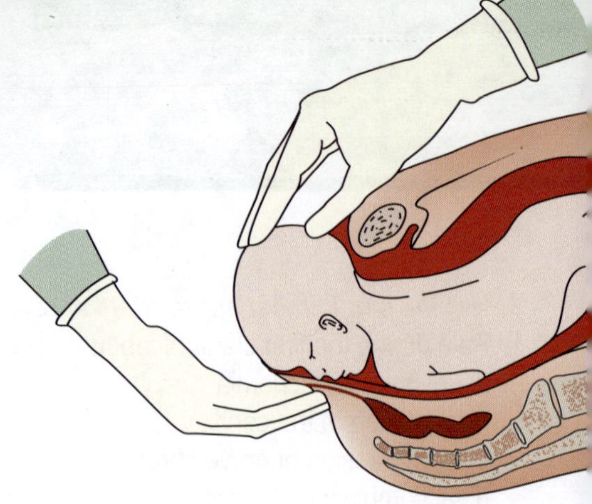

Prolonged Labour

Asha Oumachigui

LEARNING OBJECTIVES

At the end of this chapter, the reader should be able to:

- define prolonged labour and obstructed labour
- enumerate the causes of prolonged labour
- list the adverse effects on the mother and her child
- anticipate the possibility of prolonged labour from history and physical examination
- interpret a normal partogram and appreciate deviation
- outline the management of prolonged labour
- enumerate the sequelae of obstructed labour
- describe the steps in the prevention of obstructed labour

Introduction

The term 'prolonged labour' includes a wide spectrum of conditions ranging from an apparently harmless prolonged latent phase of labour to the more dangerous condition of obstructed labour. It accounts for significant maternal and perinatal morbidity and mortality in developing countries.

The partogram, a graphic documentation of the progress of labour in relation to time, is a useful tool for the prevention and early detection of prolonged labour. A multicentric WHO study documented that the use of a partogram reduced the incidence of prolonged labour.

Definition

The normal duration of labour in a nulliparous woman is 14–16 hours; in a multiparous woman, it is 7–8 hours. Labour is said to be prolonged if it lasts beyond this duration.

Labour is said to be **obstructed** when the descent of the presenting part is arrested and delivery is impossible without professional assistance. The condition is dangerous, leading to rupture of the uterus, a catastrophe that reflects gross negligence in obstetric care.

Etiology

The following factors can lead to prolonged labour:

- Insufficient uterine contractions are responsible for most cases of prolonged labour.
- Malpositions like occipito-posterior; cephalopelvic disproportion (CPD) could be due to contracted pelvis, or average pelvis and big baby.
- Malpresentations like transverse lie, brow presentation.

Insufficient Uterine Contractions

It is the main cause of 70% of cases of prolonged labour; mainly the latent and early active phases of the first stage are affected. Rarely, the second stage of labour may also be prolonged due to insufficient contractions.

Prolonged latent phase

The latent phase varies widely from 12 to 20 hours in nulliparas, and 6 hours to 8 hours in multiparas. The frequency of uterine contractions during the latent phase is two in 10 minutes and the duration is 20 seconds or less. In this phase, a woman, with a cervical dilatation of 1–2 cm may fail to reach the active phase at the end of 8 hours for a nullipara and 4 hours in a multipara. However, at this stage it is important to ensure that the woman is actually in labour; the following criteria are indicators:

- progressive increase in the frequency and duration of uterine contractions
- complete effacement of the cervix
- presence of 'show'
- formation of 'bag of membranes'.

Management: Essentially conservative. In case the woman is not in labour, she must be transferred to the ward. It is likely that she will develop uterine contractions after a period of rest.

If the woman is in labour, one must reassure her, ensure hydration and nutrition; she may be allowed to ambulate. It is **essential** at this stage to rule out malpresentations and cephalopelvic disproportion.

Oxytocin must be used judiciously, after ensuring that the cervix is completely effaced and/or has dilated at least 3 cm. Membranes may be ruptured artificially (ARM) at this stage.

Prolonged active phase

The active phase begins with a 3 cm cervical dilatation. If the rate of dilatation is less than 1 cm/hour, it is termed prolonged active phase. Alert line in the partogram is drawn from 3 cm at the rate of 1 cm/hour (**Fig. 26.1**).

Management: Essentially conservative. The woman must be reassured and pain relief must be provided. She should be hydrated and given food. Oxytocin augmentation must be instituted with proper titration and adequate monitoring (see Chapter 30). If membranes are intact, ARM may also help to augment labour. An action line is drawn four hours after the alert line in the partogram. If labour is progressing slowly, one may wait for four hours or till the action line is reached if the fetal condition is good. Cesarean section is indicated if there is no progress in cervical dilatation, descent of presenting part or there are signs of fetal distress.

Prolonged second stage

This should be anticipated in women who have experienced prolonged latent and active phases of labour, those with an occipito-posterior position and those who have been administered epidural anesthesia for pain relief. Therefore, if the second stage lasts beyond one hour, it is essential to perform a review keeping in mind the conditions mentioned earlier; most importantly, cephalopelvic disproportion must be ruled out. Delayed descent or arrest of descent usually indicates CPD.

Management: If insufficient uterine contractions are the only reason, it is useful to enhance the contractions with oxytocin. Ventouse or forceps may be applied, provided the conditions for their use are fulfilled. If there is suspicion of CPD, cesarean section should be resorted to.

Obstructed Labour

Of the three elements—power, passage and passenger—involved in the mechanism of labour, the faults in the first have been discussed. Faults in the last two are mechanical in nature and could be due to a disproportion between the maternal pelvis and the fetal head or abnormal presentation of the fetus. In such cases, labour does not progress due to mechanical factors and is said to be **obstructed**. While most cases of obstructed labour are prolonged, not all cases of prolonged labour are obstructed.

Causes

The commonest causes of obstructed labour are cephalopelvic disproportion, specific pelvic deformities and generally contracted pelvis. These conditions are closely associated with ill health and malnutrition in childhood and adolescence. When minor disproportion is combined with an occipito-

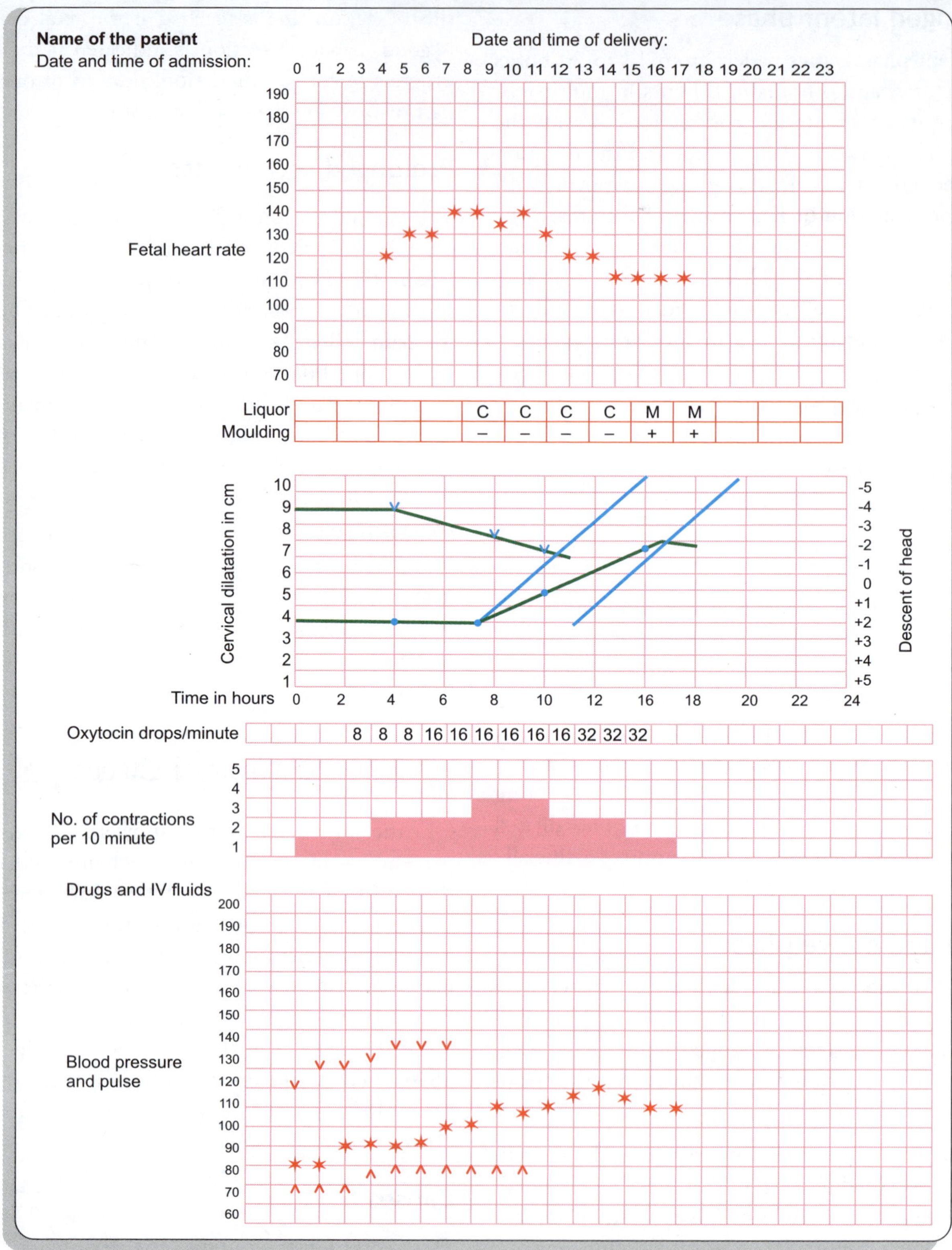

Fig. 26.1 Partogram in prolonged labour.

posterior position, major difficulties are likely because of the deflexed head.

The other important cause of obstructed labour is neglected shoulder presentation. Breech presentation can lead to obstructed labour if the baby is large or the pelvic inlet is small. Other fetal malpresentations that lead to obstruction are brow, mento-posterior and compound presentations. Congenital anomalies in the fetus like hydrocephalus may cause obstructed labour. Rarely, there may be soft tissue abnormalities in the genital tract, or tumours like fibroids or ovarian tumours impacted in the pelvis causing obstruction.

Pathology

The uterus responds to the obstruction by increasingly stronger contractions, which is subsequently followed by tonic contraction. The retraction meanwhile continues, and the lower segment thins out, elongates and becomes thinner as the lower end is wedged between the fetus and the symphysis pubis (**Fig. 26.2** and **Fig. 26.3**). In multiparous women, the retraction continues and the lower segment continues to stretch till it ruptures. In primigravidas, labour usually comes to a standstill when the uterus experiences a firm spasm.

Metabolic changes: A woman in obstructed labour is often dehydrated, due to inadequate intake and fluid loss. Metabolic acidosis develops from the accumulation of lactic acid produced by the contracting uterus and the skeletal muscles. Other detrimental changes are hypoglycemia, hyponatremia and hypokalemia.

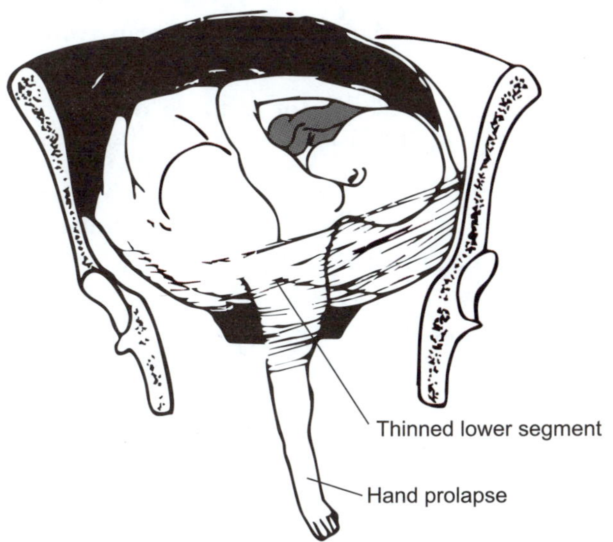

Fig. 26.2 Neglected shoulder presentation.

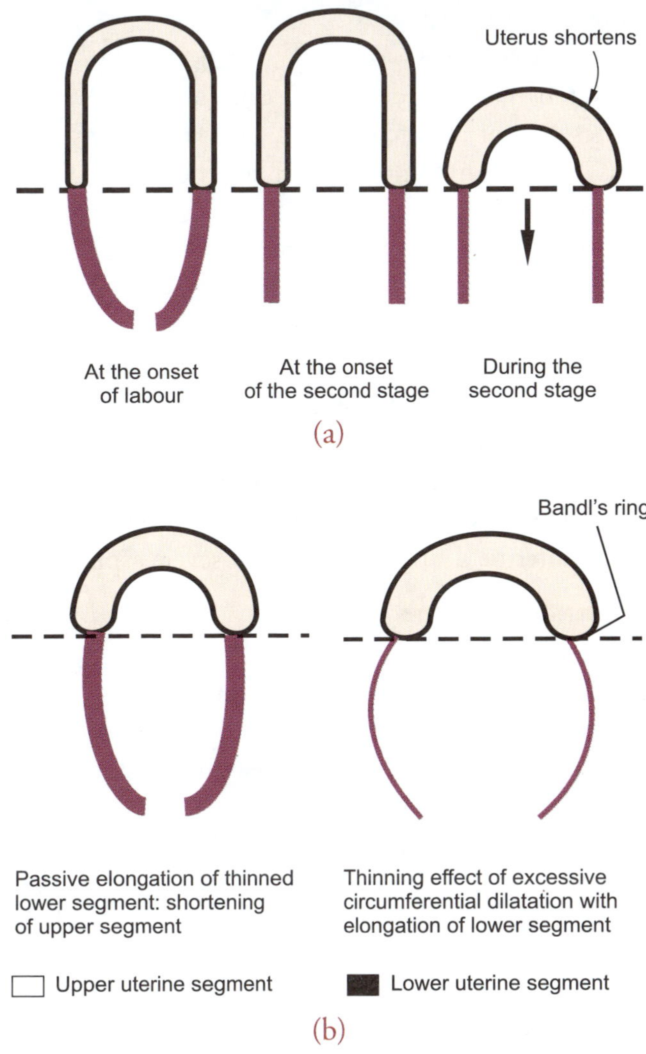

Fig. 26.3 Changes in the upper and lower uterine segments in a: Normal and b: Obstructed labour

Infection of the birth canal is consequent to early rupture of membranes, frequent vaginal examinations and possible 'manipulation' by untrained birth attendants; it is common in developing countries.

Diagnosis of obstructed labour

The woman is anxious, febrile and dehydrated; there could be hypotension, especially if the uterus has already ruptured.

Other features are:

- elongated uterus
- stretched and tender lower segment
- presence of retraction ring or Bandl's ring seen as an oblique indentation at the level of the umbilicus
- distended bladder (the woman is unable to empty the bladder as it is compressed between the fetal head and the symphysis pubis)
- edema/injury of the lower vagina and vulva
- the presenting part 'jammed' in the pelvis
- marked moulding of the fetal head
- presence of a large caput succedaneum
- cervix not well applied to the presenting part
- intrauterine death of the fetus or severe asphyxia.

Maternal sequelae

- mortality at about 5%
- hemorrhage due to atony or rupture of the uterus
- infection
- injury to the genital tract: vaginal and perineal lacerations
- vesicovaginal fistulae occur due to pressure necrosis caused by compression of the vagina and the bladder, and between the fetal head and the symphysis pubis.

Fetal sequelae

- perinatal mortality in 80%–100%
- intrauterine death due to severe asphyxia
- intracranial injury can occur due to severe moulding of the head.

Management

The following steps for general and specific management are necessary.

General care:

- The woman is kept nil orally as surgical intervention under anesthesia will probably be required.
- There is a need to administer sedatives as the woman is anxious and in pain.
- Dehydration must be corrected with intravenous Ringer lactate or normal saline.
- Blood transfusion is warranted if there is evidence of blood loss.
- Hyponatremia and hypokalemia are corrected.
- Appropriate antibiotics are administered.
- Prolonged catheterisation is needed to prevent urinary fistulae.

Specific care: Specific intervention depends on whether features of the impending rupture of the uterus are present, and whether the fetus is alive or dead.

- In the presence of signs of threatened rupture, vaginal intervention is likely to result in rupture of the uterus.
- If the fetus is dead and there is no suspicion of impending rupture, one may attempt to deliver the fetus vaginally to avoid a scar on the uterus. Ensure full dilatation of the cervix before planning to deliver the woman per vaginum.

The options are:

- Vacuum extraction or forceps delivery, after a liberal episiotomy if the fetus is presenting by the vertex and the head is at the level of the ischial spines.
- Destructive operations are performed with the intention of reducing the fetal bulk and delivering vaginally. The most frequently performed procedure is craniotomy for hydrocephalus or a dead fetus with cephalic presentation. Decapitation may be resorted to in case of shoulder presentation.

A cesarean section is planned when there is a suspicion of threatened rupture of the uterus, as denoted by a thinned out and tender lower segment or the presence of Bandl's ring. Cesarean section is also indicated when the fetus is alive. During the procedure, the possibility of injuring other organs, especially the bladder, is considerably high as it is distended and edematous and there is a need for extreme care. After delivering the fetus and closing the uterus, one must check the posterior aspect of the uterus for the presence of any injury, possibly caused by an attempted vaginal delivery.

Rupture of Uterus

Rupture of an unscarred uterus is the worst catastrophe for a pregnant mother and reflects gross negligence in obstetric care.

Clinical features

Besides the usual features described for obstructed labour, the following are also seen.

- The woman in labour will say that the labour pains have stopped.
- She is pale and there are symptoms of tachycardia.
- There is hypotension due to blood loss.
- The contour of the uterus is lost and the fetal parts are felt superficially.
- The fetus is usually dead.
- On vaginal examination, the presenting part is seen to have receded.
- Vaginal bleeding.

Management

After instituting resuscitatory measures, a laparotomy must be performed at the earliest. The objective of the intervention is to achieve hemostasis **quickly**. The surgical procedures are:

- Subtotal hysterectomy is acceptable since the main aim is to secure hemostasis in a short time.
- If the rent is well defined and hemostasis can be achieved quickly by suturing it, repair is advocated.
- Repair of other organs like the bladder if they are involved in the process of rupture of the uterus or injured during surgery.
- Particular attention must be paid to the prevention of urinary fistulae during postoperative care; prolonged catheterisation is usually needed to rest the urinary bladder.

Prevention

'An ounce of prevention is better than a pound of cure' is best applied to obstructed labour, which is largely preventable. One needs to be vigilant during pregnancy and labour. Most cases of obstructed labour can be prevented by **intelligent anticipation**.

The factors that predispose to obstructed labour.

- adolescents
- short women (height <145 cm)
- women with a history of prolonged labour/difficult delivery in the past.
- women with abnormalities of the lower limbs and spine
- abnormal presentation or position of the fetus
- mobile head at term in a primigravida
- large baby/large head.

Anticipation during labour: Using a partogram to monitor labour can prevent the condition. It also records other information: frequency and intensity of uterine contractions, maternal pulse, temperature and blood pressure, fetal heart sounds, colour of liquor, moulding and fluids and drugs administered to the mother.

Even if conditions that predispose to obstructed labour are not identified during the antenatal period, competent monitoring during labour should anticipate trouble well before the stage of obstruction. The criteria for caution are:

- Secondary onset of inefficient uterine contractions in a primigravida, calls for a careful re-evaluation.
- Cervical stasis for four hours despite good uterine contractions; on a partogram, a protracted active phase is a pointer to possible obstructed labour.
- Failure of descent of the presenting part.

By paying due attention to the points mentioned above it is possible to prevent obstructed labour by appropriate intervention.

Facilities for referral: Many of the cases of obstructed labour take place at home or in peripheral health centres and reach referral hospitals in the late stages or with rupture of the uterus. Therefore, it is necessary to:

- train skilled birth attendants in anticipating obstructed labour during pregnancy and labour by detecting deviation from the normal
- provide facilities for transport
- develop links with institutions in the vicinity with the resources to perform cesarean section.

KEY POINTS

- Labour is said to be prolonged if it lasts for more than 14–16 hours in a primigravida and 7–8 hours in a multigravida.
- Labour is prolonged due to a fault in the uterine contractions, and mechanical factors like abnormalities in the fetus and the maternal pelvis.
- Attention must be paid to fluid and electrolyte balance and pain relief.
- Monitor labour with a partogram; it helps in the early detection of prolonged labour.
- When progress of labour is arrested due to mechanical factors, the labour is said to obstructed, and it can end in rupture of the uterus.
- In obstructed labour, both maternal and perinatal morbidity and mortality are unacceptably high.
- Obstructed labour can be anticipated during pregnancy and labour.
- The use of the partogram has significantly reduced the incidence of prolonged labour.
- Training skilled birth attendants in how to use a partogram and developing links for appropriate referral is the keystone in the prevention of obstructed labour and its complications.

QUESTIONS

Select the single most appropriate answer:

1. In a primigravida, labour is said to be prolonged if the duration is more than
   a. 18–20 hours c. 10–12 hours
   b. 14–16 hours d. 6–8 hours
2. The most common cause of prolonged labour is
   a. cephalopelvic disproportion
   b. occipito-posterior
   c. transverse lie
   d. inefficient uterine contractions
3. When a woman presents with a history of being in labour for a long period, which one of the following must be done first?
   a. monitor uterine contractions
   b. give sedation
   c. rule out malpresentation
   d. start oxytocin
4. What is the permissible duration of the second stage of labour in a primigravida?
   a. half an hour c. one and a half hours
   b. one hour d. two hours
5. In case of prolonged active phase of labour, the rate of cervical dilatation is
   a. less than 1 cm/hour c. less than 2 cm/hour
   b. 1 cm/hour d. 2 cm/hour
6. The presence of which of the following in a woman who is in labour is most characteristic of obstructed labour?
   a. hypotonic uterine contractions
   b. hypertonic uterine contractions
   c. retraction ring
   d. cervix not well applied to the presenting part
7. Obstructed labour can be complicated by
   a. metabolic acidosis c. hypokalemia
   b. hyponatremia d. all of the above

In the following questions, there are two statements. Select the appropriate answer using the following key:

a. if both statements are true and causally related
b. if both statements are true but not causally related
c. if the first statement is true and the second is false
d. if the first statement is false and the second is true
e. if both statements are false

8. Vesicovaginal fistula is a complication of obstructed labour *because*
   In obstructed labour, the vagina and the urinary bladder undergo necrosis due to compression of the vagina and bladder between the fetal head and the symphysis pubis.
9. In India, obstructed labour accounts for significant maternal morbidity *because*
   In India, the rate of cesarean section has increased.
10. Spontaneous rupture of the uterus following obstructed labour is considered the worst catastrophe in obstetrics *because*
    It reflects the total neglect of both antenatal and intranatal care.

27

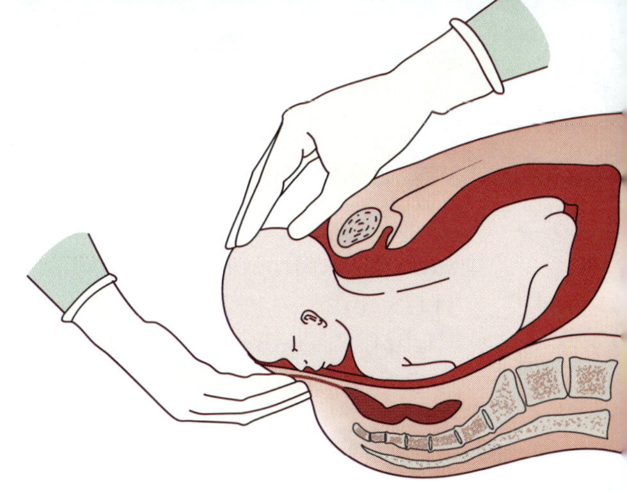

Occipito-posterior Position and Face and Brow Presentations

Asha Oumachigui

LEARNING OBJECTIVES

At the end of this chapter, the reader should be able to:

- define the occipito-posterior (OP) position
- enumerate the factors that influence the occurrence of OP
- describe the clinical features of OP
- describe the mechanism of labour in OP
- list the factors that favour an anterior rotation
- describe the management of labour
- enumerate the maternal and fetal complications
- define face and brow presentations
- enumerate the factors that favour these presentations
- describe the clinical features of face and brow presentations
- describe the mechanism of labour in face presentation

Introduction

The occipito-posterior position of the vertex is a fairly common occurrence in the last few days of pregnancy and at the onset of labour. It may complicate about 10% of labours. The incidence is remarkably reduced late in labour, as the vertex rotates anteriorly in most cases. It is very important to anticipate the cases in which the vertex may fail to rotate anteriorly and lead to complications.

Face and brow are abnormal presentations and are more prone to difficulties during labour. The mechanism of birth is complicated and the real problem is the timing of intervention while awaiting a normal delivery. In the case of brow presentation, vaginal delivery is impossible if both the baby and the maternal pelvis are of average size.

Occipito-posterior Position

Definition

In an occipito-posterior (OP) position, the presenting part of the fetus is the vertex, as in the occipito-anterior position, but the occiput is in the posterior segment of the pelvis. It could be opposite the **sacroiliac joint or the sacrum (Fig. 27.1)**. The OP differs from the OA as follows:

- The fetal attitude of universal flexion is disturbed.
- The head is deflexed.

- The engaging diameters are larger: suboccipito-frontal (10.5 cm) and occipito-frontal (11.5 cm).
- Right OP is more common because of the presence of the maternal rectosigmoid on the left.

Factors favouring OP

In the anthropoid and android types of pelvis, the anterior segment cannot accommodate the occiput; this favours the occurrence of OP.

Diagnosis

1. On inspection there is 'flattening' of the abdomen in the subumbilical region.
2. On palpation:
   - The back is far from the midline, in the flanks.
   - The anterior shoulder is also far from the midline and well above the symphysis pubis.
   - The fetal limbs are felt on both sides of the midline.
   - The part of the head that is most easily felt is the sinciput.
   - The occiput and the sinciput are found to be at the same level on Pawlik's grip.

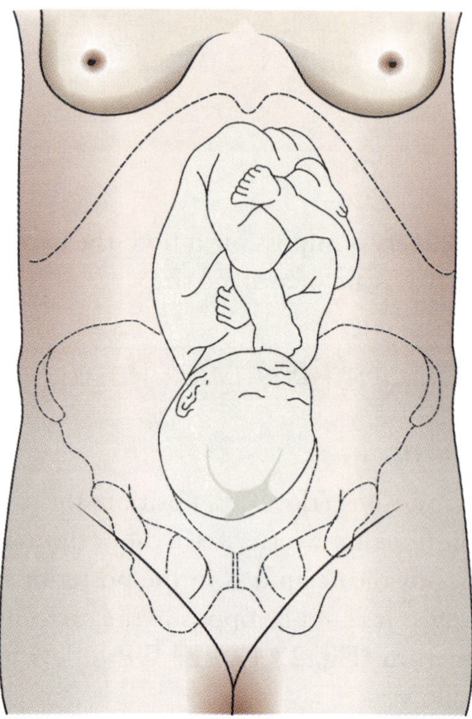

Fig. 27.1 Occipito-posterior position.

3. On auscultation, the fetal heart sounds are best heard far out in the flank. During labour, when the cervix is dilated, the sagittal suture is in the oblique diameter of the pelvis and the posterior fontanelle is near the sacroiliac joint.

Mechanism of labour

The process of labour is influenced unfavourably by the posterior position, which in turn leads to deflexion and an altered angle between the axis of the fetus and the maternal pelvis.

The steps in the mechanism of labour are:

1. Descent
2. Flexion
3. Internal rotation: 135° compared to 45° in the occipito-anterior position
4. Extension
5. Restitution
6. External rotation

In about 90% of the cases, the occiput rotates through 90° and delivers as occipitoanterior (**Fig. 27.2**). In some cases, the occiput rotates by 90° to the transverse position; in a few, it rotates in the opposite direction by 45° and the occiput comes to lie directly against the sacrum. Factors that favour or hinder anterior rotation are listed in **Table 27.1**.

Management of labour

It is worth remembering that labour is likely to be prolonged in case of OP, and that if managed properly, about 70% of women will deliver normally. Management calls for a thorough evaluation of the woman in the last week of pregnancy and during labour so as to make an appropriate decision for obstetric intervention.

Last week of pregnancy: One must check for 'dystocia-dystrophia' syndrome (short and stout) in women who are likely to have an android type of pelvis. Tall women often have an anthropoid type of pelvis. In women with short stature, the pelvis, even if the gynecoid type, will have a reduced capacity. At this stage, the weight of the baby must also be estimated.

During labour: The parameters listed during pregnancy must be assessed, if not already done

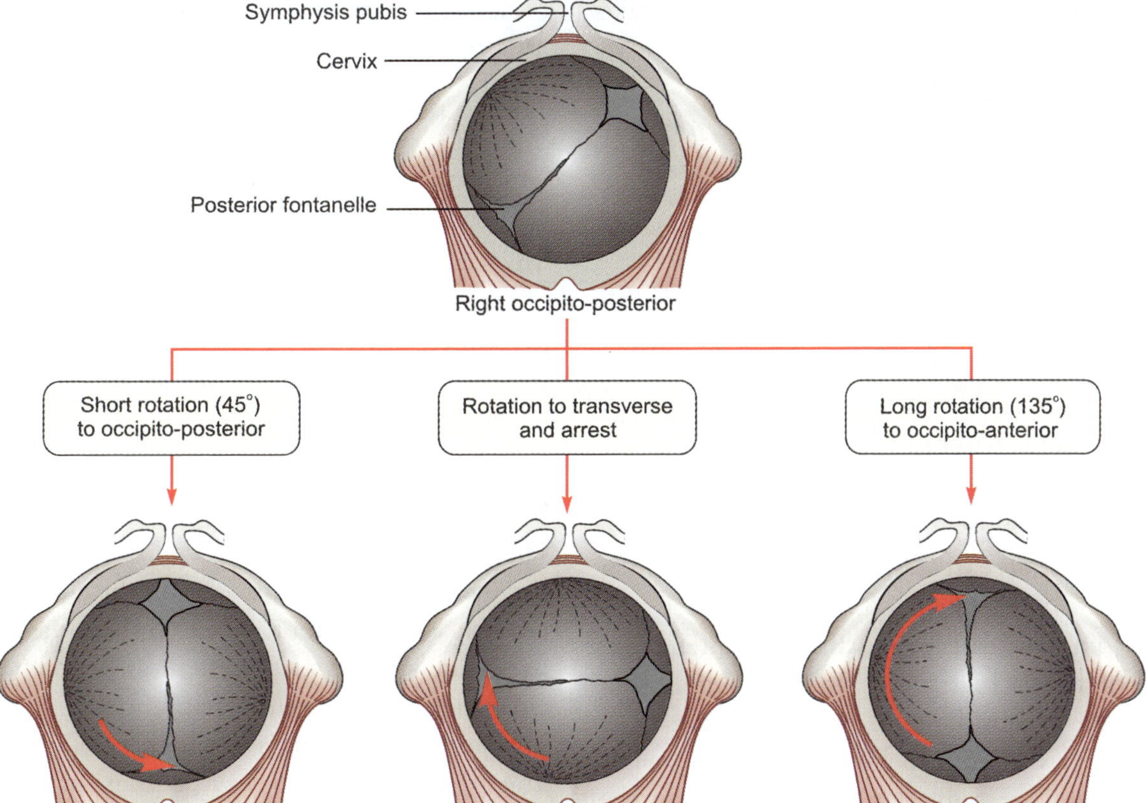

Fig. 27.2 Possible methods of rotation of the head.

Table 27.1 Favourable and unfavourable factors for anterior rotation

Favourable
Early entry of the fetal head in the pelvis
Minimal or no deflexion of head
Anterior shoulder not too deep in the flanks
Gynecoid pelvis of good capacity
Good uterine contractions
Baby of average size
Rupture of membranes at or near full dilatation of the cervix
Pelvic muscles with good tone
Unfavourable
Delay in entry of fetal head in the pelvis
Significant deflexion
Anterior shoulder far away from the midline
Anthropoid or android type of pelvis
Poor uterine contractions
Large baby
Rupture of membranes early in labour
Poor tone of pelvic muscles

so. It is important to perform a thorough obstetric examination to diagnose OP, assess the size of the baby and look for CPD which is assessed better during labour. The type and capacity of the pelvis should be ascertained.

Monitoring of labour: Once a vaginal delivery is planned, particular attention must be paid to hydration, nutrition and pain relief as the duration of labour is expected to be longer. The progress of labour is monitored using a partogram and obstetric intervention is instituted appropriately.

Failure to rotate to OA: If there is failure to rotate anteriorly, there are three possible outcomes:

Posterior rotation to the occipito-sacral position: The occiput makes a short posterior rotation of 45° to the lie opposite the sacrum. This happens when the woman has an anthropoid type of pelvis in which the antero-posterior diameter is the longest. Vaginal delivery may be planned. The mechanism of labour differs from OA in that the baby delivers by flexion as face-to-pubis (unlike OA where the head is delivered by extension) with the root of the nose or sinciput hitched under the symphysis pubis. The biparietal diameter of the baby negotiates the perineum (unlike the bitemporal in OA) predisposing to perineal injuries.

Persistent OP: The occiput does not undergo any rotation and continues to be at the sacroiliac joint. The woman must be reassessed for cephalopelvic disproportion; if present, the baby is delivered by cesarean section. If there is no cephalopelvic disproportion and the head is below the level of the ischial spines, ventouse and/or forceps are used for rotation of the head, followed by extraction.

Deep transverse arrest: This is said to occur when the occiput rotates partly and lies between the sacroiliac joint and the ileopectineal eminence, at the level of the ischial spines after full dilatation of the cervix for one hour or more. In such cases it is absolutely essential to look for cephalopelvic disproportion; if present, cesarean section must be resorted to. If there is no disproportion, application of ventouse may be used for rotation of the head followed by extraction.

Complications in the mother and her baby

- The mother is likely to suffer from perineal injuries if the baby is delivered as face-to-pubis or due to instrumental delivery.
- The baby is prone to suffer from asphyxia as the labour may be prolonged.
- Greater chance of birth injury to the baby

Face Presentation

Face presentation is rare (1 in 500 deliveries).

Definition

The head is fully extended as a result of which, the face is felt on vaginal examination; the denominator is the mentum (chin) of the fetus.

The positions are designated as left mento-anterior (LMA), right mento-anterior (RMA), left mento-posterior (LMP) and right mento-posterior (RMP). The engaging diameter is submento-bregmatic and measures 9.5 cm, which is the same as in a fully flexed head (suboccipito-bregmatic).

Factors favouring face presentation

The classical factor often quoted, but rarely seen now, is anencephaly in the fetus. Others are the presence of tumours in the neck or multiple loops of cord round the neck that promote extension of the fetal head.

Diagnosis

On obstetric palpation, there is a distinct groove between the fetal spine and the head; the cephalic eminence, the occiput, is felt on the same side as the back, unlike in vertex presentation where the cephalic eminence, the sinciput, is felt on the opposite side of the back. The occiput is also higher than the sinciput. The spine assumes an S curve, because of the extension of the head (**Fig. 27.3**).

During labour, when the cervix is dilated, the orbital ridges, malar eminences, nose, mouth and chin

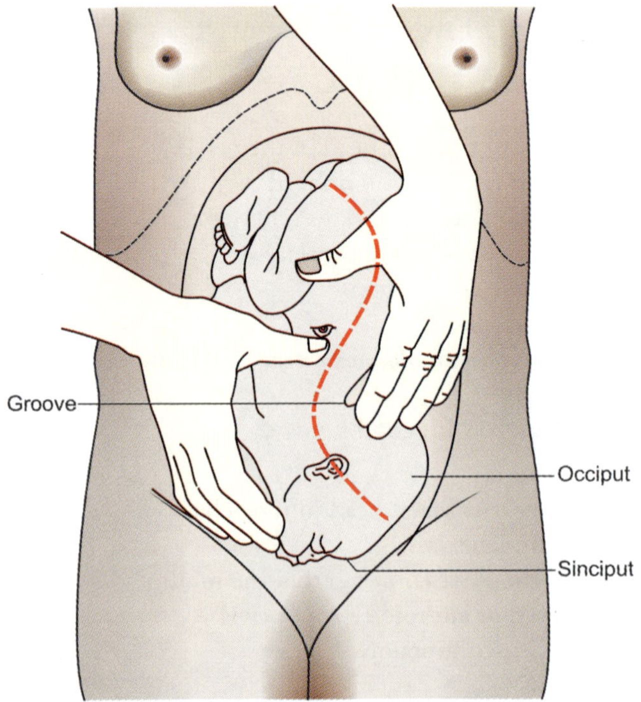

Fig. 27.3 Abdominal palpation in face presentation.

are felt. The face may occasionally be mistaken for a breech, but the difference is that the mouth forms a triangle with the malar eminences, while in breech the anus is in the same line as the ischial tuberosities.

Mechanism of labour

The steps in the mechanism of labour are:

1. descent
2. extension
3. internal rotation
4. flexion
5. restitution

In case of LMP or RMP position, a long internal rotation is the rule, as in OP. However, if the face does not rotate or it makes a short internal rotation to the sacral position, vaginal delivery is impossible, as the chin cannot negotiate through the sacral hollow, leading to an impacted mento-posterior position and obstructed labour.

Management of labour

Whenever a face presentation is diagnosed, efforts must be made to rule out any congenital anomalies, if not checked for earlier. Face, unlike vertex, does not press on the cervix evenly and therefore prolonged labour must be anticipated. This is particularly important if the position is posterior, when birth by flexion is impossible (**Fig. 27.4**). Labour must be monitored using a partogram and attention must be paid to the woman's hydration, nutrition and pain relief. Liberal episiotomy may be needed to avoid perineal injury.

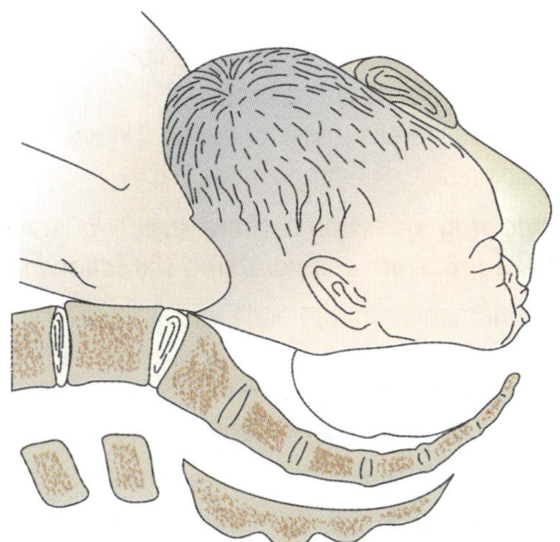

Fig. 27.4 Impacted mento-posterior position. Birth of the head is impossible.

Unlike in vertex, vacuum cannot be used in face presentation. However, forceps can be applied in carefully selected cases. Cesarean section is indicated whenever the chin rotates to the sacral position or there is persistent LMP/RMP.

Complications in the mother and her baby

Mother: Morbidity is increased as there is a need for operative intervention in 20% of cases.

Child: It is more prone to facial edema and hypoxia due to decreased venous return from the head and neck.

There is a greater risk of injury to the fetus, particularly to the face.

Brow Presentation

It occurs in 1 in 1,000 to 1 in 2,000 deliveries. Brow presentation is the most unfavourable of all cephalic presentations as the mento-vertical diameter measuring 13.5 cm is the presenting diameter, whereas the **largest diameter** in an **average pelvis** is 13 cm.

Definition

Brow occurs when there is partial extension of the head, where the anterior fontanelle is the presenting part; the root of the nose and orbital ridges also present. The mouth or chin is not felt in the vaginal examination.

Factors favouring brow presentation

These are essentially the same as that favouring face presentation. Brow can occur when the extension of the head is partial.

Mechanism of labour

Early in labour, in 30%–40% of cases, the brow may convert to face or vertex and deliver vaginally if there is no cephalopelvic disproportion. There is no mechanism of labour in brow presentation and cesarean section is required in more than 70% of cases when the maternal pelvis and baby are of average size.

If no action is taken, brow presentation will result in obstructed labour and rupture the uterus.

KEY POINTS

- The occipito-posterior position is a common malposition.
- Labour may be prolonged because of a long internal rotation.
- Non-rotation, malrotation and incomplete rotation lead to increased obstetric intervention.
- Face and brow presentations are uncommon.
- The mento-posterior position and brow presentation often require cesarean section.
- There is an increased risk of maternal and fetal injury.

QUESTIONS

Select the single most appropriate answer:

1. Which one of the following statements about the occipito-posterior position is true?
   a. sinciput is at a higher level than the occiput
   b. occiput is at a higher level than the sinciput
   c. occiput and sinciput are at the same level
   d. occiput is easily felt
2. For a normal delivery to occur in a case of ROP, the occiput rotates through
   a. 45° b. 90° c. 135° d. 180°
3. If deep transverse arrest is noted during delivery in an OP, one must think of
   a. anthropoid type of pelvis
   b. cephalopelvic disproportion
   c. inefficient uterine contractions
   d. gynecoid pelvis
4. Which of the following statements is not true about face presentation?
   a. it is usually associated with multiple loops of cord around the neck
   b. it may rotate posteriorly to become persistent mento-posterior
   c. cesarean section must be performed for all cases
   d. the engaging diameter of the fetal head is submento-bregmatic

Select the appropriate answer using the following key:

a. if only responses 1, 2 and 3 are correct
b. if only 1 and 3 are correct
c. if only 2 and 4 are correct
d. If only 4 is correct
e. If all are correct

5. OP is most frequently seen in which type of pelvis?
   1. android
   2. gynecoid
   3. anthropoid
   4. platypelloid
6. What are the factors that favour anterior rotation in OP?
   1. head mildly deflexed
   2. anterior shoulder close to midline
   3. good pelvic capacity
   4. rupture of membranes early in labour
7. Which statements are true about the occipito-sacral position?
   1. delivery of the head occurs by flexion
   2. vaginal delivery is not possible
   3. there is an increased risk of perineal injury
   4. birth injuries are common in the baby

In the following questions, there are two statements. Select the appropriate answer using the following key:

a. if both statements are true and causally related
b. if both statements are true but not causally related
c. if the first statement is true and the second is false
d. if the first statement is false and the second is true
e. if both statements are false

8. In brow presentation, cesarean section is the recommended mode of delivery *because*

   In about 30% of cases, brow presentation may convert to face or vertex presentation.

9. In face presentation in the mento-sacral position, vaginal delivery is impossible *because*

   The chin cannot negotiate through the sacral hollow.

10. In brow presentation, cesarean section is the mode of delivery *because*

    The largest pelvic diameter is 13 cm.

28

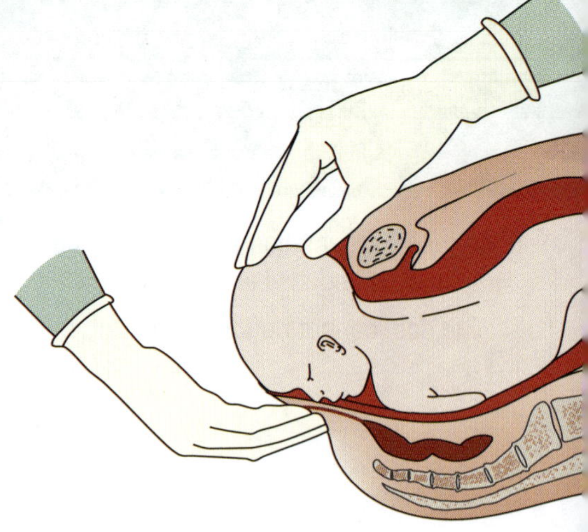

Breech and Shoulder Presentations

V Mathini

LEARNING OBJECTIVES

At the end of this chapter, the reader should be able to:

- describe the breech and shoulder presentations
- enumerate the obstetrical findings characteristic of these presentations
- describe the mechanism of labour in breech presentation
- explain the principle governing the procedures of external cephalic version (ECV) and internal podalic version (IPV)
- discuss the management of breech
- discuss the management of transverse lie
- describe the maternal and fetal complications

Introduction

Towards term pregnancy, the buttocks of the fetus being bulky compared to the head move towards the fundus of the uterus where more space is available, and the fetal head comes to occupy the lower segment. Therefore, the incidence of breech presentation decreases as pregnancy advances and at term the incidence of breech presentation is just 3%–4%. Vaginal delivery must be planned very carefully as the head, which is the most voluminous and vital part of the fetus, enters the pelvis last and there is hardly any time for the head to adapt to the pelvis.

Definition

Breech presentation: The lie of the fetus is longitudinal, and the podalic pole of the fetus or the buttocks occupies the lower pole of the uterus.

Shoulder presentation: The lie of the fetus is perpendicular to the long axis of the uterus. It is also referred to as transverse lie.

Etiology

The most important factors predisposing to breech and transverse lie are those that hamper stabilisation of the head in the lower pole of the uterus. Therefore, the following factors are considered in the occurrence of the above presentations:

Preterm labour: When labour sets in before term, the incidence of breech or transverse lie is higher. Before term, the fetus is mobile and the presentation changes because the volume of amniotic fluid is much more than the volume of the fetus. Multiparity contributes by undue relaxation of the abdominal wall.

Uterine factors: Malformations like bicornuate/arcuate uterus and placenta previa are significant. Tumours of the uterus, like fibroids, may also predispose to breech or shoulder presentations.

Contracted pelvis: This predisposes to breech or shoulder presentations as the head cannot be accommodated in the pelvis.

Polyhydramnios: Excess of liquor favours free movement of the fetus.

Placenta previa: The placenta in the lower segment favours malpresentations.

Fetal anomalies: A fetus with hydrocephalus is more likely to present as breech, as the voluminous head cannot be accommodated in the lower pole of the uterus.

Multiple pregnancy: The likelihood of breech presentation is high in multiple pregnancy, in the first, second or both fetuses.

Breech Presentation

Breech presentation is common remote from term pregnancy. But the presentation is unstable because the volume of liquor is more and the fetus spontaneously turns to cephalic presentation. However, in about 3% to 4% of singleton pregnancies, the presentation continues to remain as breech. The type of breech, as illustrated in **Fig. 28.1**, influences its management and has been classified as follows.

Classification

Breech with extended knees: It is also called **frank breech**. The thighs are flexed on the fetal abdomen. The presenting part is well defined.

Breech with flexed lower limbs: In this type of breech, the fetus is in an attitude of universal flexion, the legs and the thighs being flexed. The presenting part is bulky and consists of the buttocks, external genitalia and both feet.

Footling and knee presentations: The terms are self-descriptive: footling, if the feet are below the buttocks, and knee, if they are the lowest part of the breech.

A breech presentation is said to be **complicated** if there are associated obstetric complications like preeclampsia, previous cesarean section and elderly gravida.

Complications

In breech delivery, the frequency of operative intervention is high and therefore the mother is subjected to a greater risk. For the baby, the risk of

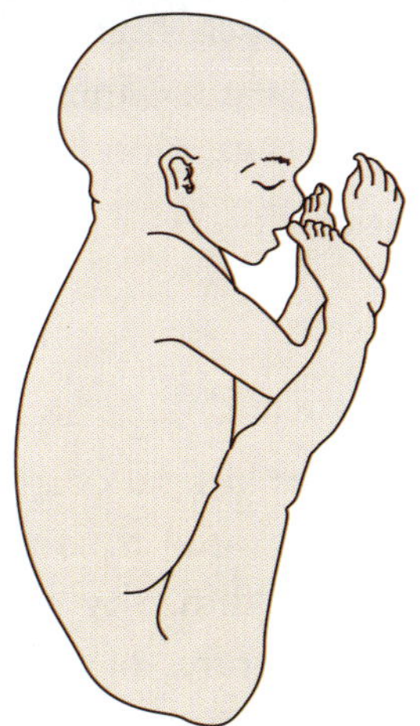

Frank or extended

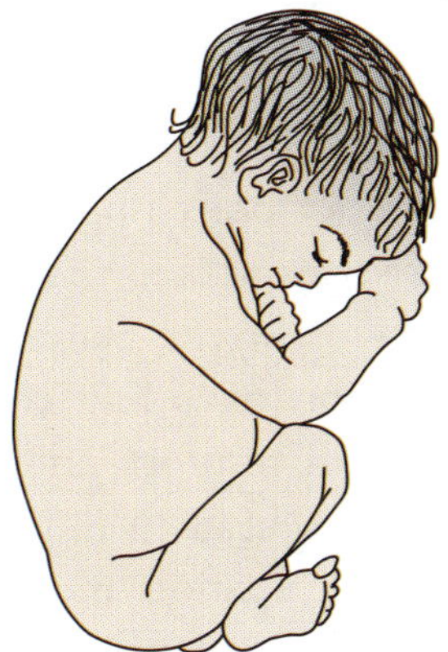

Flexed

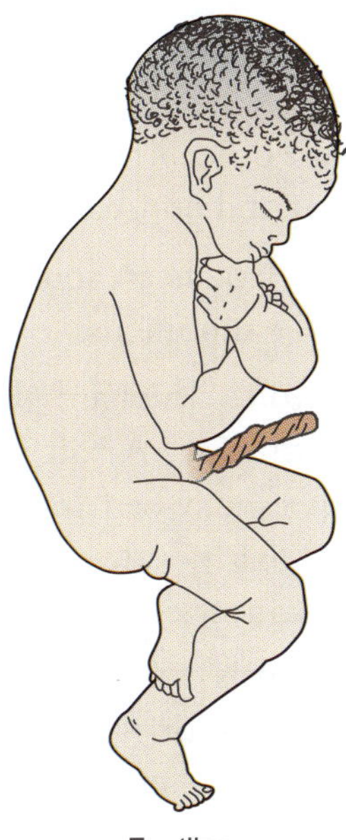

Footling

Fig. 28.1 Types of breech presentation.

injury and death is much higher than in cephalic presentation. The factors influencing perinatal outcome in breech presentation include:

- period of gestation
- type of breech
- size of the fetus
- skill of the obstetrician.

The principal causes of fetal death are intracranial hemorrhage due to tentorial tears and asphyxia due to cord prolapse and difficulty in delivery. Large babies are prone to fractures of the femur, humerus and clavicle. These dangers can be reduced by careful selection of the mode of delivery; an obstetrician experienced in conducting breech delivery should be in charge.

Diagnosis

Since the mortality for breech presentation is nearly 3–4 times that of vertex, it is important to detect the presentation by 34–36 weeks. Rarely does a woman with this presentation have any complaint. There may be occasional discomfort under the ribs due to the presence of the head in the upper pole. The diagnosis is made by palpation; medical imaging like ultrasonography is used to confirm the diagnosis and to plan the mode of delivery.

Palpation: On fundal grip, a well-defined, hard, globular, ballotable mass is felt. On lateral grip, the lie is noted to be longitudinal, with the back on one side and the limbs on the other. The lower pole is occupied by a broad, irregular and non-ballotable mass.

Auscultation: The fetal heart sounds are heard at or above the level of the umbilicus.

Vaginal examination: The hard globular head that is normally felt is missing. A soft broad buttock or irregular feet or knees may be felt.

Imaging, particularly ultrasonography is an extremely useful diagnostic tool as it helps to:

- confirm the diagnosis
- detect fetal malformation
- find out the type of breech and the attitude of the head
- estimate fetal weight
- assess the quantity of amniotic fluid
- localise the placenta
- detect uterine anomalies.

Management in pregnancy

Once a breech presentation is diagnosed at 34 weeks or beyond, the case must be evaluated to find out if there are any associated obstetric complications like PIH, placenta previa or contracted pelvis. If none exist and the breech is of the flexed type, a biophysical profile must be performed. If the fetal status is good, external cephalic version should be attempted. The version must be performed gently, preferably without anesthesia. If the procedure is successful, vaginal delivery can be anticipated.

External cephalic version: This is the procedure by which the transverse lie or podalic presentation is changed to cephalic presentation by external manipulation on the abdomen. An NST is performed before and after the procedure to ensure fetal wellbeing. The contraindications for external version are as follows:

- complicated breech
- large baby
- previous uterine scar
- polyhydramnios or oligohydramnios
- preeclampsia
- antepartum hemorrhage
- malformed or dead fetus
- contracted pelvis.

The complications of version are:

- preterm labour
- PROM
- abruption
- Rh isoimmunisation
- cord accidents.

Mechanism of labour

In a cephalic presentation, the most voluminous and hard part of the fetus, the head, is delivered first, followed automatically by the shoulders and the buttocks. In case of a breech presentation, there is an increased risk of fetal morbidity/mortality because there are three important stages in the delivery of the fetus: the buttocks, the shoulders and the head. Unless the fetus is very large, the

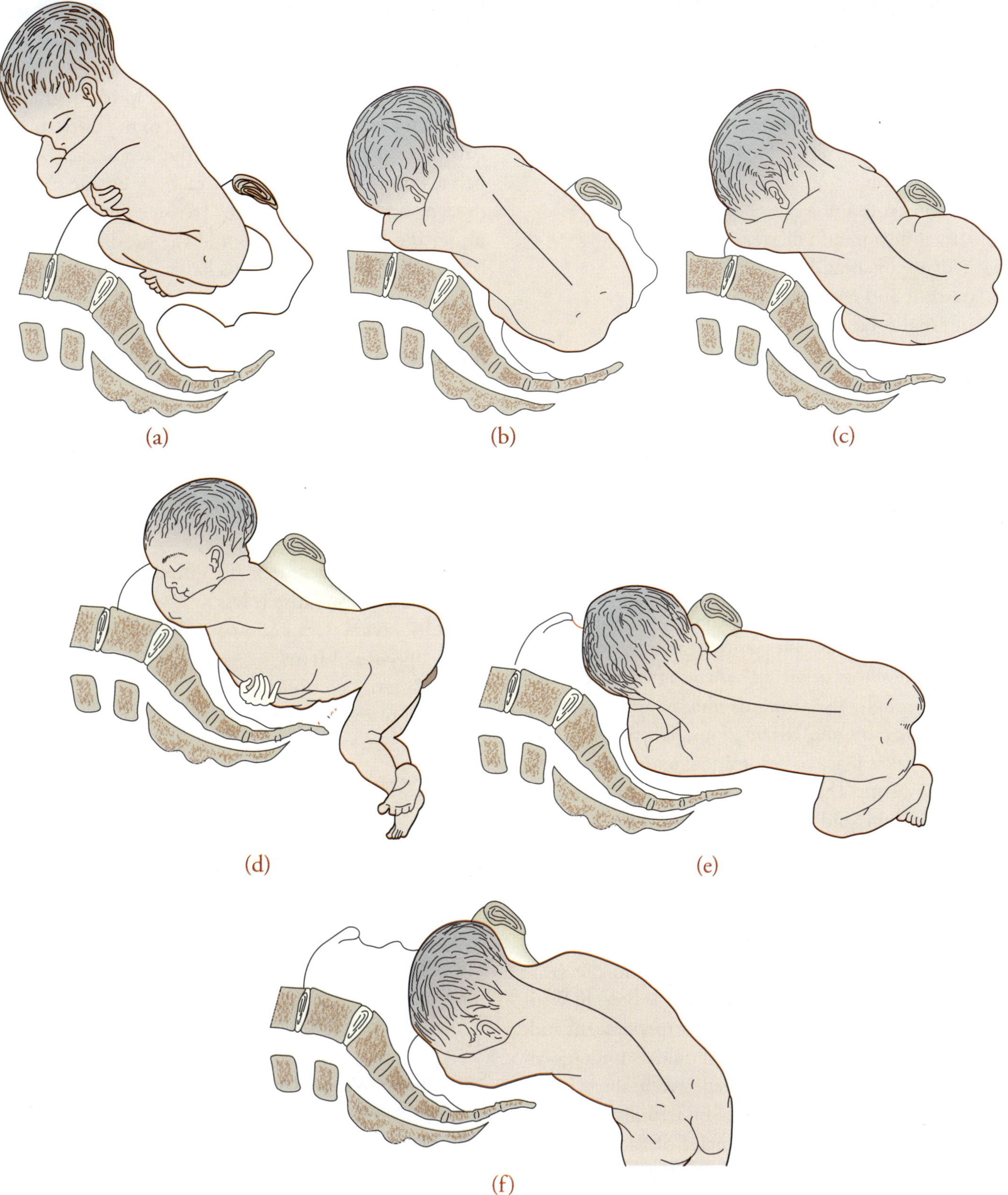

Fig. 28.2 a: Engagement of breech b: The bitrochanteric diameter in the antero-posterior diameter of the pelvis c: Lateral flexion d: Birth of breech and engagement of shoulder e: Delivery of anterior shoulder f: Delivery of posterior shoulder and engagement of head.

buttocks and the shoulders deliver easily; the delivery of the head is usually difficult because it is the least compressible.

The following cardinal movements occur in the mechanism of breech delivery (**Fig. 28.2**):

1. descent
2. compaction
3. internal rotation
4. lateral flexion and delivery of buttock
5. delivery of shoulder
6. descent and engagement of head
7. internal rotation of head
8. flexion and delivery of head.

Delivery of the breech: In breech presentation, **the sacrum is the denominator** and hence the positions are designated as: left sacro-anterior/posterior (LSA, LSP) or right sacro-anterior/posterior (RSA, RSP). The engaging diameter in breech is the bitrochanteric diameter.

In the anterior position, the breech enters the pelvis with the **bitrochanteric diameter** in the oblique diameter of the pelvis and gets engaged. With good uterine contractions, the fetus descends; when the fetus touches the pelvic floor, the anterior buttock rotates through 45°, towards the symphysis pubis. With further uterine contractions, lateral flexion of the trunk takes place to accommodate the fetus to the pelvic curvature. The anterior buttock then passes the symphysis pubis and is born, followed by the posterior buttock. The breech then undergoes external rotation by 45° and lies in the transverse diameter of the outlet. If the breech is flexed, the feet drop out.

Delivery of the shoulders: The shoulders enter the pelvis with the bisacromial diameter in the same oblique diameter of the pelvic brim as the breech. With good uterine contractions, there is further descent and, on reaching the pelvic floor, the shoulders undergo an internal rotation of 45°; this is reflected in the external rotation of the breech. Now the bisacromial diameter lies in the anteroposterior diameter of the outlet. At the same time, the head enters the pelvic brim in the opposite oblique diameter. The body then flexes anteriorly so that the anterior shoulder is delivered from behind the symphysis pubis. Next, the posterior shoulder is delivered by anterior flexion of the body.

Delivery of the head: The head engages in the pelvic brim as the shoulders rotate anteriorly at the level of the pelvic floor. Descent takes place with further flexion of the head; the suboccipito-bregmatic diameter of the fetal head is applied to the birth canal. An internal rotation occurs as the head reaches the pelvic floor. Good uterine contractions ensure further descent and further flexion. The occiput is hitched under the symphysis pubis and the head is delivered by flexion. This course of mechanism must be kept in mind while assisting the delivery of the head.

Management of breech delivery

Whenever a breech presentation is seen, the woman must be examined thoroughly and evaluated ultrasonologically. A pelvic assessment is made to rule out any element of contraction. Currently, vaginal delivery is considered only when the following conditions are fulfilled:

- frank breech because it fits into the pelvis and the risk of cord prolapse is less
- multigravida with good past obstetric record
- average size of fetus
- no obstetric complications
- skilled obstetrician present.

It is best to await spontaneous labour. There is almost no place for induction of labour. The labour is on a 'trial' basis and the woman must be prepared for a CS at any point of time during labour.

First stage of labour: A vaginal examination is performed to confirm the breech presentation and to assess the pelvic capacity. A second vaginal examination is done when membranes rupture to exclude cord prolapse. Maternal and fetal monitoring and other elements of management are as for a normal delivery.

Second stage: Once the cervix is fully dilated, the level of breech is assessed. If the breech has not reached the lower pelvis an hour after full cervical dilatation, the case must be reassessed. When the perineum is distended and the anterior buttock is seen at the vulva, the woman is placed in the lithotomy position.

Delivery of the baby: In breech presentation, vaginal delivery can take place by three methods:

Spontaneous vaginal delivery: It occurs occasionally when the fetus is very small and is expelled spontaneously.

Assisted breech delivery: If there is onset of spontaneous labour, this can help to deliver the buttocks, shoulders and head safely.

Breech extraction: This allows complete extraction of the buttocks, shoulders and head under anesthesia. This mode of delivery is rarely practised as fetal mortality is unacceptable.

Assisted breech delivery

At this juncture, the obstetrician must ensure the presence of an assistant, an anesthetist and a neonatologist. He must keep long forceps available, should the need arise to help out the head and arrange for management of neonatal asphyxia.

Delivery of the breech: As discussed earlier, when the woman is in the second stage of labour, she is put in the lithotomy position, the obstetrician gowned and gloved, preferably gives a pudendal block, if epidural anesthesia has not already been administered. He then performs a mediolateral episiotomy. During the next few contractions, the buttocks descend further; if the breech is of the flexed type, the buttocks are delivered, followed by the feet. Sometimes minimum traction on the groin during uterine contractions expels the buttocks (**Fig. 28.3**). If the legs are extended, they are released by applying pressure on the popliteal fossa so as to flex and abduct the knees (**Pinard's maneuver**) (**Fig. 28.4**). Once the buttocks are delivered, a loop of cord is brought down to prevent compression, and the obstetrician must make sure that the baby's back is anterior. The baby is covered with a warm towel to avoid external stimuli which may trigger premature inspiration. The rest of the delivery is conducted slowly over five minutes.

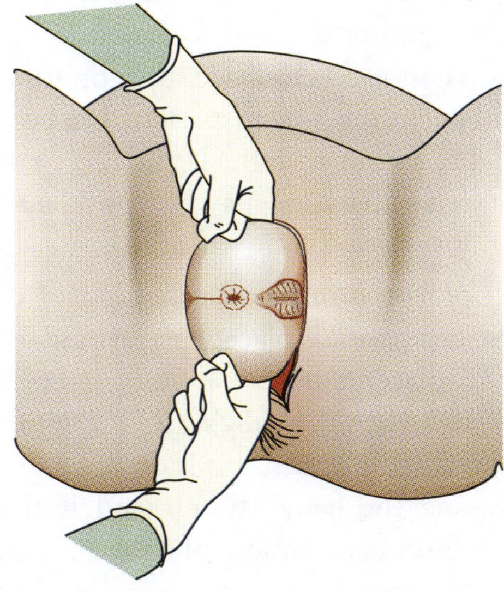

Fig. 28.3 Groin traction.

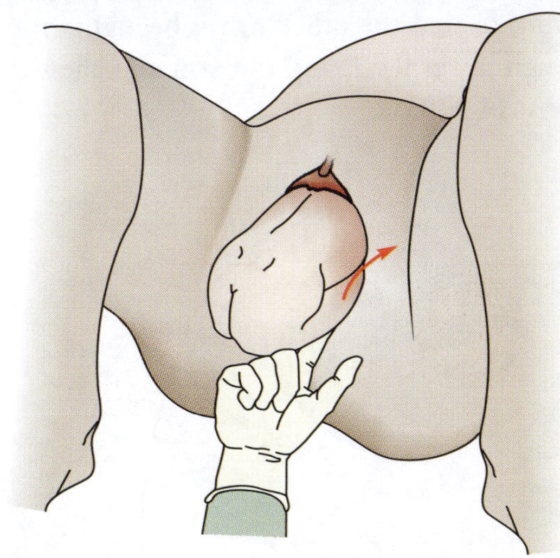

Fig. 28.4 Flexion and abduction to deliver the anterior extended leg.

Delivery of shoulders: Next, the obstetrician must support the baby by holding the feet, but should not exert any traction. With further contractions, the trunk descends; one must wait till the baby's axillary folds/lower end of scapula appears. Most often, the arms are flexed across the chest and the posterior arm is born first, followed by the anterior arm. If this does not happen, one may hook down the arms or use **Lovset's rotation method**, which is particularly useful when the arms are extended or in the nuchal postion. This maneuver is based on the fact that the posterior shoulder enters the brim first due to pelvic inclination and hence is at a lower level. The baby's body is held gently and rotated with slight traction through 180 degrees, so that the posterior shoulder comes to lie anteriorly just under the symphysis pubis and can deliver spontaneously, or the arm can be hooked out since it is accessible. The baby's body is now rotated through 180 degrees in the opposite direction, so that the other arm is brought anteriorly at a much lower level, and the arm and the shoulder are born (**Fig.28.5**).

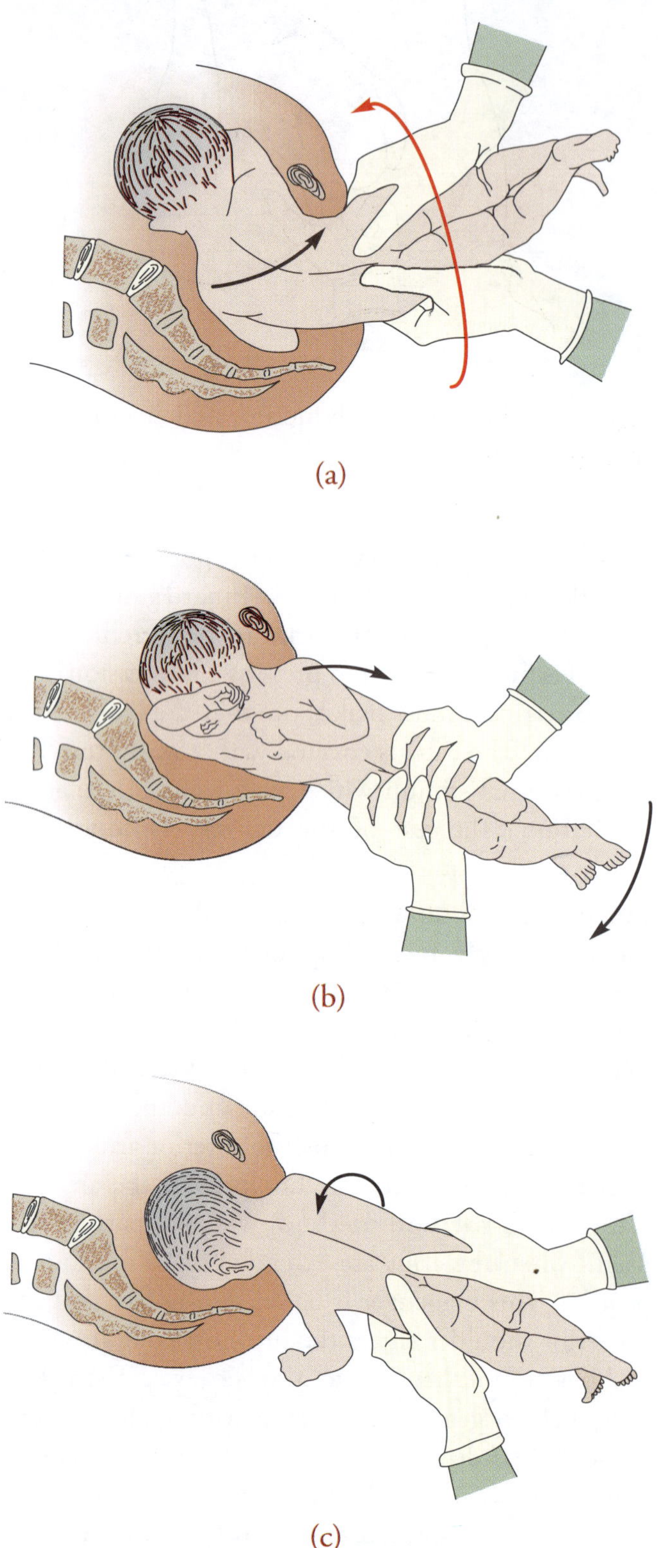

Fig. 28.5 Lovset's maneuver.

Delivery of the head: This is the most crucial part of breech delivery as the most voluminous, least compressible and vital part is delivered last. Throughout the conduct of breech delivery it is important to keep the baby's head in a flexed position by ensuring good uterine contractions and suprapubic pressure. The baby should hang by its own weight, while the feet are held for support, till the nape of the neck appears at the subpubic angle. In case it does not appear, continued suprapubic pressure is applied downwards and backwards. The obstetrician then swings the baby in an arc, towards the mother's abdomen while suprapubic pressure is maintained and the head is born. This method of delivering the head is known as the **Burns–Marshall technique** (Fig. 28.6).

An alternative method is the **Mauriceau–Smellie–Veit technique** or the 'jaw-flexion and shoulder traction' method. The middle finger of one pronated hand is placed on the baby's suboccipital region, the index and ring fingers are placed on the shoulders. The baby lies astride on the supinated hand; the index and middle fingers of the supinated hand are placed on the malar eminences of the baby. The pronated hand maintains flexion, as two hands apply traction to the baby in the pelvic axis (**Fig. 28.7**). Some obstetricians may opt to routinely apply Piper's forceps to the aftercoming head (**Fig. 28.8**).

Complications of breech delivery

Arrest of breech: This complication is suspected if the breech does not descend for one hour after full cervical dilatation. Fetopelvic disproportion or a contracted pelvis must be suspected. The best option is CS, if the station is high. If the breech is at the outlet, breech extraction may be considered, if the attending obstetrician is experienced.

Extension of the arms: Full extension of the arms above the head, or displacement behind the neck (**nuchal displacement**) is a rare complication. It is suspected when the baby's trunk is not delivered beyond the costal margin; this is detected by passing a finger along the baby's thorax and if the elbow cannot be found, extension of arms is diagnosed. One may attempt Lovset maneuver to deliver the arms. Alternatively, the baby is held by the pelvic

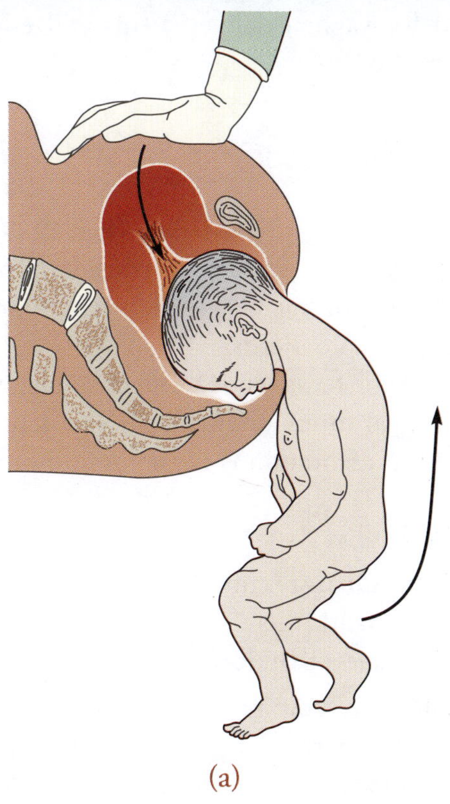

(a)

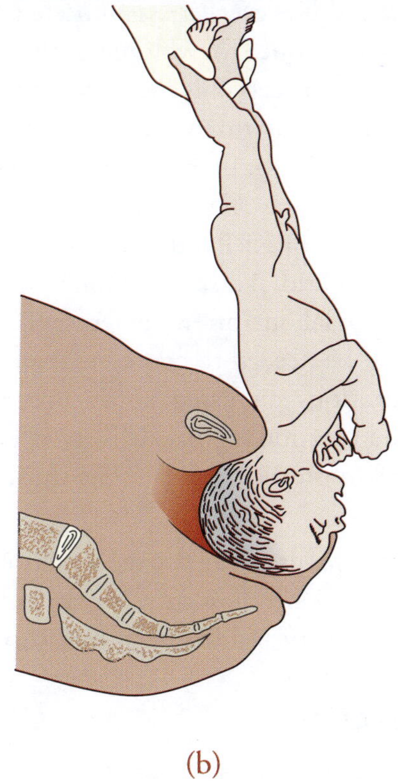

(b)

Fig. 28.6 Burns–Marshall technique.

girdle and a downward traction is applied to bring the anterior scapula in view. Then the baby's body is swung upwards, a hand is introduced along the sacral hollow to reach the elbow of the posterior arm, the antecubital fossa is recognised and with firm pressure on the humerus, made to flex the arm across the baby's thorax.

Arrest of the aftercoming head: The head may get arrested at the pelvic brim, in the cavity or at the outlet. The causes could be a deflexed head, hydrocephalus, cephalopelvic disproportion, a contracted pelvis or an incompletely dilated cervix. The intervention depends on the cause of the arrest. With the availability of USG, hydrocephalus is rarely

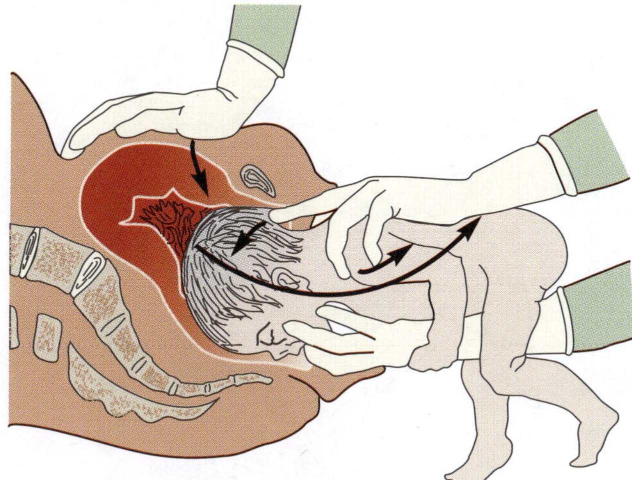

Fig. 28.7 Mauriceau–Smellie–Veit maneuver.

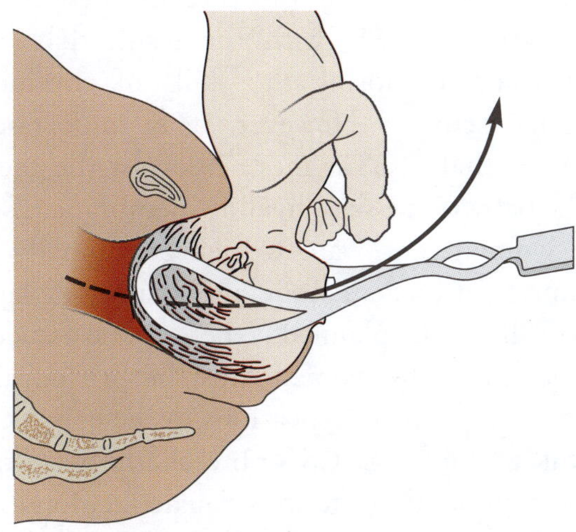

Fig. 28.8 Delivery of the head using forceps.

seen at this stage; however, if encountered, efforts should be made to reduce the volume of the head by cephalocentesis. If the cervix is incompletely dilated, the cervix is incised at three locations (2 o'clock, 6 o'clock and 10 o'clock); then the head is delivered. In other situations, the Mauriceau—Smellie—Veit technique or Piper's or Kielland's forceps are used to try and deliver the head. If disproportion is discovered at this late stage of labour, often the fetus will die and craniotomy may be needed to complete the delivery.

The complications discussed above occur rarely, especially if the case for vaginal delivery is carefully selected and an obstetrician is present through out labour.

Cord prolapse: This is an anticipated complication of breech delivery. When it occurs, it is an indication for immediate delivery and CS must be resorted to.

Cesarean section

If there are complications such as contracted pelvis or fetopelvic disproportion, a cesarean section (CS) must be performed. The operation is also indicated if there are associated obstetric complications like PIH, placenta previa and previous CS.

There is a trend these days to perform a CS for all breech presentations. If the baby weighs less than 2,000 g, the risk of birth trauma to the fetus is greater in vaginal delivery than in CS. When babies are larger than 3,500 g, vaginal delivery is difficult and fractures of the femur and humerus are common. For these reasons, most breech presentations are delivered by CS, with the result that many obstetricians are losing the skills of conducting a vaginal delivery. However, it is important to remember that a CS is more risky for the mother and the baby is at risk of hyaline membrane disease. Some women may want to deliver vaginally, and they must not be denied the opportunity. A vaginal delivery should be planned if there are no associated complications: the woman must be briefed about the unanticipated complications to the baby.

While performing a CS for breech, the obstetrician must remember to make an adequate incision on the lower segment, and the method of delivering the baby through the uterine incision is similar to that described for vaginal delivery. This will ensure safe delivery of the baby.

Shoulder Presentation

Whenever shoulder presentation (**Fig. 28.9**) is seen in a primigravida, one must consider underlying pathology like contracted pelvis, placenta previa and bicornuate/arcuate uterus.

The lie of the fetus tends to be unstable; it may be oblique, and at times longitudinal. The denominator in shoulder presentation is the acromion process.

Diagnosis

Inspection: On inspection, the abdominal distension is transverse, and therefore it seems that uterine enlargement is less than for the period of gestation.

Palpation: The symphysiofundal height is less than normal for the period of gestation. On fundal grip, limbs or the back may be felt depending on whether the baby's back is anterior or posterior. On lateral grip, the head is felt on one side and the breech on the opposite side. Sometimes, the head/breech could be in one of the iliac fossa. The lower pole of the uterus feels 'empty' on pelvic grips.

Auscultation: The fetal heart sounds are best heard around the umbilicus.

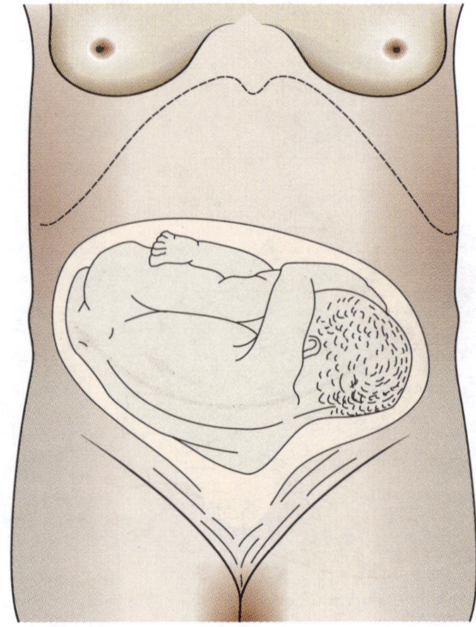

Fig. 28.9 Transverse lie.

Vaginal examination: This examination confirms the absence of head or breech as presenting parts. When the woman is in labour and the cervix is dilated, hand, elbow, the shoulders or the ribs are felt, giving a 'grid-iron' feel. If the membranes rupture, the likelihood of cord and hand prolapse must be checked for.

Management during pregnancy

Once a diagnosis is made clinically, it is essential to evaluate the pregnancy by using medical imaging. With ultrasonography, one can detect uterine malformations, localise the placenta and detect the presence of any fetal abnormalities.

After 34–36 weeks of gestation, transverse lie, unlike breech, continues to be unstable. The chances of a spontaneous version to cephalic/breech presentation are good, particularly if the lie happens to be oblique. An external cephalic version can be performed at any time till early labour provided the membranes are intact. If the external cephalic version is successful after 37–38 weeks, the head is fixed and an artificial rupture of membranes is done to facilitate the descent of the head into the pelvis and labour induced.

When the baby is of average size, vaginal delivery is mechanically impossible. Therefore, if external cephalic version fails, or is contraindicated, it is best to perform a CS.

Management in labour

Average baby and average pelvis: As stated above, when both the maternal pelvis and the baby are of average size, vaginal delivery is impossible. If the woman goes in to labour, she is likely to have premature rupture of membranes, followed by cord and hand prolapse. A CS must be performed in the interests of the mother and her baby.

Late in labour: When labour continues and the fetus is arrested without further progress, the labour is said to be **obstructed.** The condition is labelled 'neglected shoulder presentation' and has detrimental effects on both the mother and the child. If no intervention is instituted, the upper segment contracts and the lower segment continues to stretch, and ultimately the uterus may rupture. In order to prevent this, a CS must be resorted to.

Dead baby: If the baby is dead and small, the cervix is fully dilated and membranes have recently ruptured, an internal podalic version (a procedure that brings down a foot), followed by breech extraction may be tried under general anesthesia. The other interventions are destructive operations like decapitation or embryotomy that reduce the bulk and extract the baby in parts. However, these procedures must never be undertaken if there are signs of threatened rupture of uterus: thinned-out lower segment, presence of Bandl's ring and suprapubic tenderness.

Transverse lie in the second of twins: One may encounter a transverse lie in the second baby of a twin pregnancy. After the delivery of the first baby, if the second baby is found to be in the transverse lie, an external cephalic version, followed by the rupture of membranes of the second sac may achieve vaginal delivery. However, if this method fails and there is cord prolapse, internal podalic version and breech extraction would help deliver the baby. This is the only indication for internal podalic version in modern obstetrics.

Prognosis

For the mother: If shoulder presentation is not diagnosed during pregnancy and early labour, the mother may have an obstructed labour and suffer its sequelae, such as rupture of the uterus.

For the baby: The extent of fetal loss depends on the time of intervention. An increased risk of cord and hand prolapse, asphyxia and birth injuries due to prolonged and obstructed labour contribute to poor fetal outcome.

KEY POINTS

- Breech presentation complicates 3% of all deliveries.
- Breech and shoulder presentations are associated with prematurity, fetal and uterine malformations, placenta previa and contracted pelvis.
- Perinatal mortality and morbidity and maternal morbidity are increased in these conditions.
- Ultrasound is invaluable in the assessment of these women.
- Labour is more difficult in breech presentation because the most difficult part, the head, is delivered last.
- In a few women, vaginal delivery is permissible in breech presentation provided other factors are taken into consideration.
- Transverse lie is an uncommon condition.
- External cephalic version may be performed in both breech and shoulder presentations.
- Normally, vaginal delivery is not possible if the baby is in the transverse lie.

QUESTIONS

Select the single most appropriate answer:

1. Breech presentation is commonly associated with
   a. anthropoid type of pelvis
   b. fibroid uterus
   c. uterine malformation
   d. android type of pelvis
2. The most frequent cause of fetal death in vaginal breech delivery is
   a. asphyxia
   b. tentorial tears
   c. injury to liver
   d. fetal anomalies
3. In a case of breech presentation, all of the following are contraindications for external cephalic version *except*
   a. type II placenta previa
   b. twin pregnancy
   c. previous cesarean section
   d. flexed type of breech
4. The most common method of delivering the aftercoming head in assisted breech delivery is
   a. Burns–Marshall technique
   b. Mauriceau–Smellie–Veit trechnique
   c. use of Piper's forceps
   d. use of Kielland's forceps
5. The most common reason for arrest of the aftercoming head in breech delivery is
   a. cephalopelvic disproportion
   b. incompletely dilated cervix
   c. extended head
   d. mutliple loops of cord around the neck

In the following questions, there are two statements. Select the appropriate answer using the following key:

a. if both statements are true and causally related
b. if both statements are true but not causally related
c. if the first statement is true and the second is false
d. if the first statement is false and the second is true
e. if both statements are false

6. External cephalic version can be performed in all types of breech presentation *because*
   If external cephalic version is successful, a normal delivery is possible.
7. Cesarean section is recommended for breech presentation when the baby weighs less than 2,000 g *because*
   A baby weighing less than 2,000 g can easily be delivered vaginally.

Select the appropriate answer using the following key:

a. if only responses 1, 2 and 3 are correct
b. if only 1 and 3 are correct
c. if only 2 and 4 are correct
d. if only 4 is correct
e. if all are correct

8. Perinatal outcome in breech delivery depends on
   1. period of gestation
   2. type of breech
   3. skill of the obstetrician
   4. age of the mother
9. In case of transverse lie, an external cephalic version may be performed if
   1. there is no scar on the uterus
   2. there is a history of bleeding
   3. the membranes are intact
   4. there is a history of fetal loss
10. If transverse lie is not diagnosed at the onset of labour, the consequences could be
    1. obstructed labour
    2. increased risk of cord prolapse
    3. increased risk of hand prolapse
    4. injuries to the baby

29

Mutiple Pregnancy

Lakshmi Seshadri

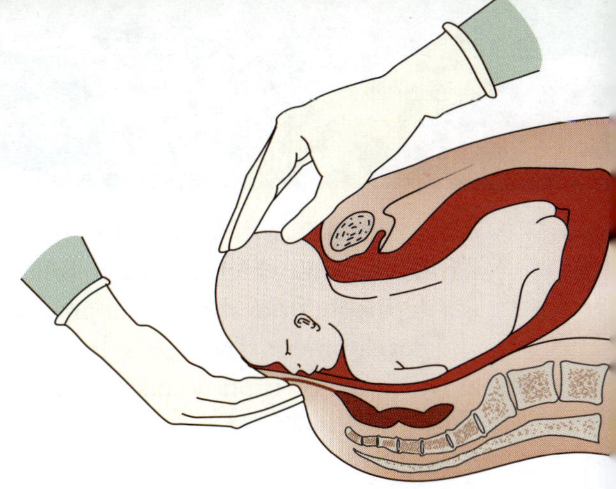

LEARNING OBJECTIVES

At the end of this chapter, the reader should be able to:

- explain the etiology of multiple pregnancy
- list the clinical features of multiple pregnancy
- list the maternal and fetal complications
- diagnose complications early
- provide antenatal care for women with multiple pregnancy
- refer at the appropriate time
- outline the management of labour
- provide appropriate counselling

Introduction

The term multiple pregnancy refers to a pregnancy in which there are two or more fetuses. In general, 1%–2% of all pregnancies are multiple. The number and rate of multiple pregnancies have increased all over the world in the past decade due to assisted reproductive techniques (ART). The incidence also varies in different ethnic groups and populations. Twins are the most common and triplets, quadruplets and higher order pregnancies are seen with decreasing frequency. The condition is of concern to the obstetrician because perinatal mortality and maternal morbidity and mortality are increased. Recent advances in diagnosis and management have changed many aspects of care in multiple pregnancy. Since triplets and higher order multifetal pregnancies are uncommon, this chapter deals essentially with twin pregnancy.

Twin Pregnancy

Pathogenesis and embryology

The most common multiple pregnancy is twin pregnancy. This may result from a single ovum (monozygotic) or from two ova (dizygotic).

Dizygotic twins: These are caused by the fertilisation of two eggs and are a duplication of the normal process of conception and further development.

- Each fetus has its own chorion and amnion.
- The two placentae may be separate or fused.
- Fetuses can be of the same or different sex.
- Genetic constitution is different.
- Blood groups are different.

Incidence of dizygotic twinning increases with age, hereditary predisposition, assisted reproduction and induction of ovulation.

Monozygotic twins: These arise from a single fertilised ovum which divides to result in twins. This is a departure from the normal process of conception and development. The type is determined by the time at which the division occurs; the earlier it occurs, the better the chance of two separate fetuses with their own membranes (**Fig. 29.1**).

- If splitting occurs **within three days** of fertilisation, two separate blastocysts form and it results in **dichorionic, diamniotic twins.**
- If cleavage occurs **4–7 days** after fertilisation, there is a single blastocyst and single chorion. Two amniotic cavities are present (**monochorionic, diamniotic**)
- If division occurs **8–12 days** after fertilisation, a single amnion arises (**monochorionic, monoamniotic**). This is rare.
- Division **13 days after** fertilisation results in **conjoined** twins.

Whenever the chorion is single, vascular anastomoses between arteries, veins or artery to vein may develop.

The following characteristics have been observed regarding monozygotic twins:

- may have two chorions and amnions or a common chorion and amnion
- have a single placenta
- are of the same sex
- are genetically identical and immunologically compatible
- have the same blood group
- incidence remains unchanged geographically.

Incidence

Incidence of monozygotic twins is 3–4 per 1,000 live births the world over. The incidence of dizygotic twins is variable. **Figure 29.2** shows the placenta and the membranes in twin pregnancies.

Etiology

Monozygotic twinning is a random event. However, the incidence of dizygotic twinning is on the increase. The factors known to be associated with dizygotic twinning are:

Age: Increasing age at conception and increasing parity are associated with a higher risk. Incidence is 1.5% in women under 20 years but 4% in women above 30 years.

Assisted reproductive techniques: Induction of ovulation with clomiphene, gonadotrophins and, in vitro fertilisation are all associated with an increase in multifetal pregnancies including twins, triplets and quadruplets. About 25%–30% of all pregnancies resulting from ART are twins, 5% are triplets.

Race: Twin pregnancies are more common in the African and Caucasian races.

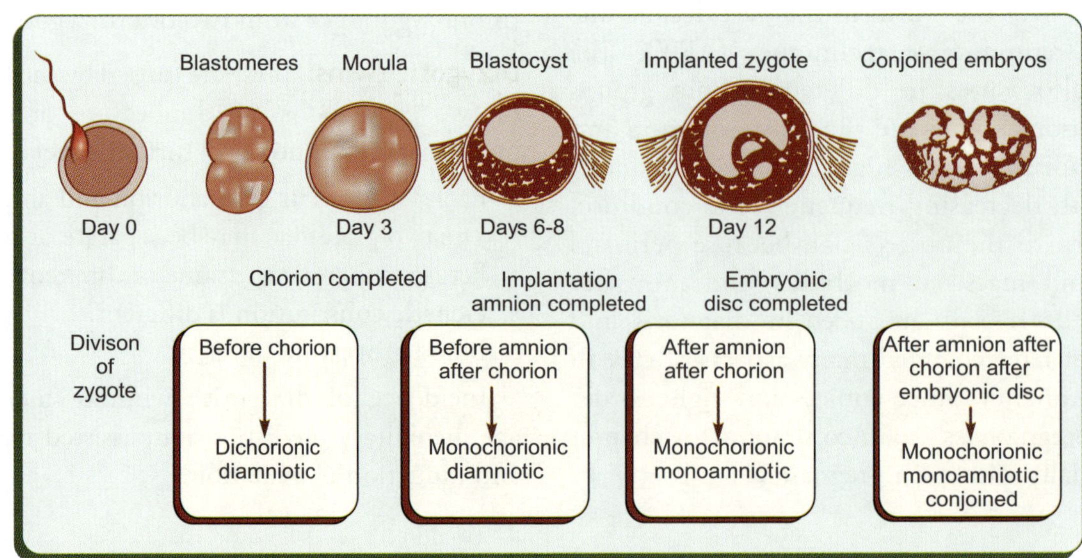

Fig. 29.1 Monozygous twinning.

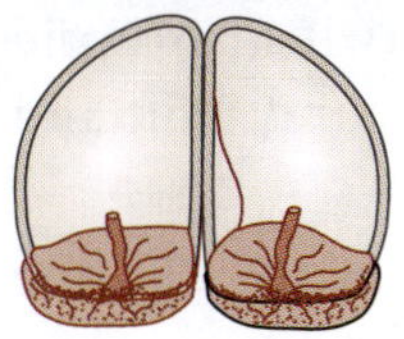

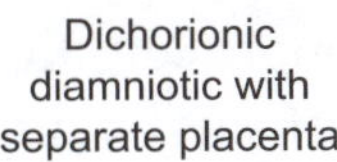

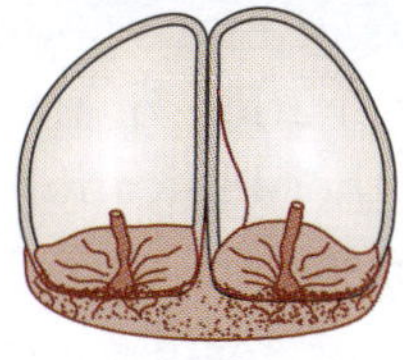

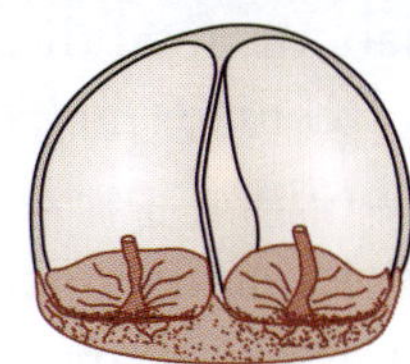

Fig. 29.2 Placenta and membranes in twin pregnancies.

Heredity: Family history of the mother is more important than that of the father. Women who were one of twins have an increased risk of having twins.

Nutritional status: Chances of multifetal pregnancy are higher in well-nourished women.

Maternal adaptation

All the physiologic changes that take place in pregnancy are exaggerated in multifetal pregnancy. Blood volume expansion, increase in red cell mass and cardiac output are greater. Cardiac output increases 20% more than in singletons and is due to an increase in stroke volume and heart rate, the mid-trimester fall and third trimester rise in blood pressure are also more marked.

The uterus is larger and can lead to displacement of the diaphragm and abdominal viscera leading to respiratory and gastrointestinal discomfort. Pressure on the vena cava can lead to pedal edema.

Complications of Multiple Pregnancy

Due to the physiological changes, increased levels of placental hormones, placental insufficiency and large size of the uterus, several maternal and fetal complications occur.

Maternal complications

First trimester

Abortion: Spontaneous abortion is more common and is often seen in monozygotic twins.

Hyperemesis gravidarum: Almost 50% of women experience nausea and vomiting. Hyperemesis is also seen more commonly and is attributed to the increase in the levels of human chorionic gonadotropin.

Second trimester

Anemia: There is increased demand for iron and folate leading to iron deficiency anemia or dimorphic anemia. Physiological hemodilution is also exaggerated.

Cardiovascular risks: The increase in blood volume and cardiac output is normally tolerated well but in women with valvular disease, cardiac failure and acute pulmonary edema may occur.

Gestational diabetes: It is known to be the effect of diabetogenic hormones of pregnancy, especially human placental lactogen. The levels of this hormone are higher in multifetal pregnancy, increasing the incidence of gestational diabetes threefold. Fasting plasma glucose levels are lower and postprandial levels are higher than in singletons.

Urinary tract infections: Due to increased stasis in the urinary tract, cystitis is common.

Gestational hypertension/preeclampsia: Early onset and more severe hypertension are seen in multiple gestations. The incidence increases from 7% in singletons to 14% in twins. Women with hypertension are also more prone to volume overload and pulmonary edema.

Third trimester

Preterm labour: This is by far the most important complication of multiple pregnancy. The risk of preterm labour increases corresponding to the number of fetuses. The incidence ranges from 20% to 40%. It is attributed to the overdistended uterus since contractions occur at a critical degree of stretching of the myometrium. The etiology is probably more complex.

Antepartum hemorrhage: Abruptio placentae is the main cause of antepartum hemorrhage in multiple pregnancy. Even when there is no hypertension, the incidence increases threefold. Premature detachment of the placenta of the second twin after delivery of the first twin also occurs. Incidence of placenta previa may be increased because of the large placental size.

Polyhydramnios: This occurs in 2% to 5% of twin pregnancies. It is more common with monozygotic twins. This may be associated with twin-to-twin transfusion. Acute hydramnios with respiratory embarrassment can also occur.

Preterm premature rupture of membranes: This complicates about 14% of twin pregnancies and may be caused by overdistension of the uterus or polyhydramnios. Following rupture of membranes, labour ensues earlier in twin pregnancies compared to singletons.

Intrapartum complications

Malpresentations: They are common in the first and second twin. A non-vertex presentation of the first twin is associated with greater risk of premature rupture of membranes and cord prolapse. Presentation of the second twin can change after the delivery of the first twin. Therefore, the presentation should be ascertained after the first twin is delivered. The increased incidence of malpresentations increases the chance of cesarean section, intrauterine manipulations and operative vaginal deliveries.

Prolonged labour: The first stage of labour is more likely to be prolonged in multiple pregnancies. This could be due to the overdistended uterus and the resultant uterine contractile dysfunction. Augmentation with oxytocin is often required.

Prolapse of the umbilical cord: Polyhydramnios, malpresentations and premature rupture of membranes may be associated with cord prolapse. This increases the mortality in twins.

Operative vaginal delivery: The incidence of operative vaginal delivery for the first twin is increased compared to singletons. After the delivery of the first twin, external cephalic version, assisted breech delivery, internal podalic version, breech extraction and forceps or ventouse delivery are common.

Cesarean section: The incidence of cesarean section in twin pregnancies is on the increase. Elective section is recommended when the first twin presents by breech or is in the transverse lie. Maternal complications like gestational hypertension or eclampsia are also indications. Poor progress in labour, fetal distress of one or both twins, abruptio placentae, malpresentation of the second twin and cord prolapse are other indications.

Postpartum hemorrhage: Overdistension causing uterine atony is the main cause of postpartum hemorrhage. Retained placenta is also more common for the same reason. Retained placental tissue, obesity, multiparity and tocolytics used for preterm labour contribute to postpartum hemorrhage.

Postpartum complications: Complications like subinvolution, sepsis and lactation difficulties are more common in multiple pregnancy.

Fetal complications

Vanishing twin syndrome: This occurs commonly in the first trimester. Between 20% and 50% of multiple fetuses identified by ultrasonogram in early pregnancy are lost. The fetus dies and is reabsorbed. This may be associated with vaginal bleeding.

Congenital anomalies: The incidence of congenital anomalies is considerably greater. Major anomalies are seen in 2% and minor malformations in 4% of twins. The majority of malformations occur in monozygotic twins. There could be an 'acardiac' fetus where one or more of the fetuses have no heart at all or only a rudimentary cardiac tissue and associated with other multiple anomalies. Conjoint twins are also seen in monozygotic twinning. Chromosomal abnormalities are seen more often in twins. Maternal age-related chromosomal anomalies are seen in dizygotic twins. Down syndrome occurs at an earlier maternal age in twin pregnancies.

Intrauterine growth restriction: This is one of the important causes of perinatal mortality and morbidity in twin pregnancy. If normal singleton standards of weight are used, 20%–25% of twins are small for gestational age. The average growth begins to slacken in the third trimester. Since fetal growth in multiple gestations is different from growth in singletons, different growth charts must be used. In dizygotic twins, marked discordance may result from unequal placentation. The degree of growth restriction in monozygotic twins is greater because of vascular anastomoses and unequal distribution of nutrients and oxygen.

Growth discordance: Discordant growth is common in multifetal pregnancy. It is not always due to TTTS (twin-to-twin transfusion syndrome). Compensated vascular anastomoses may be a contributing factor in monozygotic twins. Defective placentation of one twin can cause growth restriction in one fetus in dizygotic twins. As long as each fetus follows its own growth curve, there is no need for early intervention.

Prematurity: This is the leading cause of perinatal mortality in multifetal pregnancy. The morbidity increases if the babies are also discordant. All neonatal complications of prematurity, namely respiratory distress syndrome, pulmonary hemorrhage and necrotising enterocolitis, can cause mortality.

Twin-to-twin transfusion syndrome: This is a serious complication seen in monozygotic/monochorionic twins. Vascular connections between two placentae are found in most monochorionic placentae. These can be artery to artery, vein to vein or artery to vein. When they are hemodynamically balanced, they are of no significance. But when there are uncompensated arteriovenous shunts, TTTS can occur. This complicates about 5% of monochorionic gestations. The arterial donor twin is generally anemic, hypotensive, growth retarded and oligohydramniotic. The recipient twin is polycythemic, hypervolemic and polyhydramniotic and may develop cardiac failure due to fluid overload. TTTS is diagnosed by ultrasound examination. The mortality is higher in the recipient twin.

Death of one fetus in utero: This happens in all types of twins. It could be due to maternal complications like hypertension, fetal anomaly, cord accidents or vascular connections. There is increased risk to the surviving twin and therefore the pregnancy should be closely followed. Maternal coagulation defects may occur.

Mortality and morbidity: Perinatal mortality in twin pregnancies is three- to tenfold higher than that in singletons. The most important etiological factor is prematurity. Intrauterine growth restriction (IUGR), congenital anomalies, vascular complications, infections, abruptio placentae and maternal complications with resultant placental insufficiency are contributing factors.

Management

Management consists of (**Table 29.1**):

- diagnosis of multifetal pregnancy
- determination of chorionicity
- prevention and early identification of maternal complications
- prevention of prematurity
- antepartum fetal surveillance
- appropriate intrapartum management
- expert neonatal care.

Diagnosis: Multifetal pregnancies should be suspected whenever the uterus is large-for-date and/or when the woman presents with symptoms like hyperemesis or severe anemia. With the increasing use of ultrasound in the first trimester, multiple pregnancies are diagnosed early. All women who conceive following assisted reproductive techniques and those with high risk factors for multifetal pregnancies should undergo an ultrasound scan in the first trimester.

Determination of chorionicity: Since the risk of complications depends on whether the placenta is monochorionic or dichorionic, it is important to determine the chorionicity. This is determined ultrasonographically in the first half of pregnancy (12–18 weeks) since fetuses are smaller and visualisation of membranes and placenta is better.

Number of placentae: If two separate placentae are visualised, it indicates dichorionicity.

Examination of the dividing membrane:

- Thickness of more than 2 mm indicates dichorionicity.
- **Number of layers in the membrane:** Two layers are seen in monochorionic diamniotic placentae and 3 or 4 layers in dichorionic placentae. Three layers indicate fused chorion.
- Assessment of the junction of the membrane with the placenta for 'twin peak' sign or 'lambda' sign. This is a triangular projection of placental tissue from the chorionic plate into the cleft between the layers of the intervening membrane. When present, it indicates dichorionic placenta. In monochorionic placenta, the junction of the intervening membrane with placenta is at right

Table 29.1 Antenatal management of twin pregnancy

Antenatal visits are scheduled once in four weeks till 24 weeks. Thereafter, the visits should be more frequent in order to be able to detect any of the complications mentioned earlier. Hospitalisation is required if the mother develops any complications. Routine hospitalisation has not been found to be beneficial in improving fetal outcome.

First trimester
- History and clinical examination
- Ultrasound scan: number of fetuses
- Number of sacs
- Inter-twin septum
- Routine blood tests
- Folic acid 1 mg daily

Second trimester

12–14 weeks
- Scan for chorionicity
- Vanishing twin

18–20 weeks
- Scan for fetal morphology, chorionicity
- Cervical length
- Iron 60 mg daily, folic acid 1 mg daily and calcium 1.5 g daily

24–26 weeks
- BP, proteinuria
- Glucose tolerance test

Third trimester

28 weeks
- Hemoglobin
- Hypertension, proteinuria
- Fetal biometry
- USG for discordance

32 weeks
- Hospitalisation
- Hemoglobin
- Hypertension, proteinuria
- Scan for fetal growth

36 weeks
- Fetal growth assessed
- Maternal complications assessed

38 weeks
- Presentation of both fetuses
- Estimated weight of fetuses
- Delivery planned

angles, with no placental tissue in between, called the 'T' sign.

Fetal sex: If the fetuses are of different sex, dichorionicity is confirmed. But fetuses of the same sex can be mono- or dichorionic.

Diagnosis of anomalies: The first trimester scan for nuchal translucency is performed to exclude Down syndrome. An ultrasound scan at 18–20 weeks, gestation is mandatory in all multifetal pregnancies for the detection of fetal anomalies. Diagnosis of congenital anomalies, assessment of gestational age, measurement of the length of the cervix and confirmation of chorionicity are performed.

Diet: The requirements of calories, protein, minerals, vitamins, iron and folic acid are all increased. Calorie consumption should be increased by 300 kcal/day and protein intake should be 100 g/day. Recommended weight gain is about 12–15 kg. Supplementation with iron and folic acid is required. Calcium supplementation of 1.5 g/day is beneficial.

Prevention of prematurity

Bed rest: Though hospitalisation for the purpose of bed rest has not been shown to be beneficial, restriction of activity and increased rest are associated with decreased uterine activity and increase in birth weight.

Predictors of preterm labour like measurement of cervical length and fetal fibronectin in cervicovaginal secretions have been found to be useful.

Tocolytic therapy: Prophylactic tocolysis is not routinely recommended. Once preterm labour sets in, tocolysis is useful. Even short term prolongation of pregnancy by 48–72 hours is beneficial since it allows time for transfer to a tertiary care centre and to administer steroids for the enhancement of pulmonary maturity. It should be remembered that a combination of β-mimetics and steroids can lead to pulmonary edema.

Preterm labour in multifetal pregnancy can occur any time in the late second trimester or early third trimester. Once the diagnosis is made, treatment is as for singletons, using tocolytic agents like beta sympathomimetics, calcium channel blockers and magnesium sulphate. Cervical cerclage may be useful when the length of the cervix is less than 2.5 cm before 26 weeks.

Antenatal steroids: They are found to be beneficial from 24 weeks to 34 weeks for acceleration of pulmonary maturity. Routine use of steroids is not indicated in uncomplicated twin pregnancy but should be given to all women where preterm labour is suspected.

Antepartum fetal surveillance: Since IUGR, growth discordance and polyhydramnios are common, fetal surveillance is essential.

- Serial ultrasonography from 28 weeks is performed to assess biometry, discordance, amniotic fluid and IUGR
- Doppler velocimetry of the umbilical and cerebral arteries, if indicated
- Non-stress test from 32 weeks, repeated weekly and more often if fetal growth is abnormal

Prevention/early identification of maternal complications: Since iron and folic acid deficiency anemia are common, supplementation with 60–100 mg of iron and 1 mg of folic acid daily is required throughout pregnancy. Hemoglobin should be checked at booking and at 28 and 34 weeks. Women with severe anemia should be identified and treated immediately, with blood transfusion if required, since preterm labour is common and there may not be sufficient time for hemoglobin levels to improve with iron therapy.

Antenatal visits should be more frequent. At each visit, blood pressure should be measured. Urinalysis for proteinuria should be performed. Glucose tolerance test should be done at 26–28 weeks. Advice regarding adequate rest, lifestyle modification, symptoms of preterm labour and preterm premature rupture of membranes should be given. Usually these women are admitted at 32–34 weeks because of the risk of preterm delivery, so that immediate neonatal care can be given.

Timing of delivery

Twin fetuses are said to mature earlier than singletons and features of postmaturity appear by 40 weeks. Perinatal mortality in twins is lowest when fetuses are delivered at 37–38 weeks. Elective cesarean section, when indicated, can be performed at 38 weeks. Induction of labour is recommended by 39–40 weeks. In those with maternal or fetal complications, induction must be initiated earlier.

Intrapartum management

Since several complications like uterine dysfunction, malpresentation, cord prolapse, premature separation of the placenta and postpartum hemorrhage may occur, special precautions are required when delivering twins.

- Appropriately trained obstetrician and assistant should be present.
- Trained neonatologist should be available.
- Blood or blood products should be readily available.
- Intravenous infusion systems for delivering IV fluids and oxytocics should be in place.
- Electronic fetal monitoring of both fetuses is recommended, if available.
- Obstetric forceps and ventouse should be kept ready.
- Oxytocin, ergometrine and carboprost should be readily available.

Mode of delivery depends on the presentation of the first twin. Various combinations are possible but in general they are classified as vertex–vertex, vertex–non-vertex and first twin–non-vertex.

Vertex–vertex: This is the most common and is seen in about 40%–45% of twin pregnancies. Vaginal delivery is possible and is recommended. After delivery of the first twin, the cord is clamped and the placenta left in situ. The lie and presentation of the second twin should be reconfirmed. Careful oxytocin augmentation can be used if contractions are not adequate after waiting for 10 minutes. Membranes of the second twin are ruptured artificially and delivery is proceeded with. Prophylactic methyl ergometrine 0.2 mg intravenously or carboprost 125 μg intramuscularly is given at the time of delivery of the shoulder of the second twin. Two clamps are applied to the placental side of the umbilical cord. Twenty units of oxytocin should be added to the infusion at this point. The placenta is now delivered.

The uterus should be massaged to ensure that it is well contracted.

The placenta should be examined carefully to check for missing cotyledons. The inter-twin membrane must be examined to see if there are two, three or four layers and the chorionicity confirmed.

Vertex—non-vertex: This is seen in 35%–40% of twins. The first twin is delivered vaginally as usual. The lie and presentation of the second twin must be confirmed after the delivery of the first twin; if non-vertex, an external cephalic version is attempted. If the version is successful, membranes are ruptured and delivery of the second twin is conducted in the usual manner. If the version is not successful and the second presentation is breech, the membranes are ruptured and assisted breech delivery performed. If the second twin is in the transverse lie and external version is unsuccessful, internal podalic version and breech extraction are done. In the presence of premature separation of placenta or fetal heart rate abnormalities of the second twin, cesarean section is recommended.

First twin—non-vertex: This occurs in about 20 % of twin pregnancies. If the first twin is in the transverse lie, the delivery is by cesarean section. If the first twin presents as breech, vaginal delivery is possible but most obstetricians will prefer cesarean section.

Higher-order Multiple Pregnancies

Perinatal mortality and morbidity and maternal complications associated with triplets and quadruplets are high. Extreme prematurity is the leading cause of mortality. Congenital anomalies are common. Cesarean section is advisable if the fetuses are of salvageable gestational age.

KEY POINTS

- In multifetal pregnancy, there are two or more fetuses; twins are the most common.
- The incidence of multifetal pregnancy is 1%–2% of all deliveries.
- Twin pregnancy is of two types: dizygotic and monozygotic.
- The incidence of dizygotic twin pregnancy has increased due to the advent of assisted reproductive techniques, but the incidence of monozygotic twins has remained unchanged.
- Ultrasound in early pregnancy is useful in determining the type of twins.
- A woman with twin pregnancy is at a higher risk of developing complications like anemia, PIH, gestational diabetes mellitus, preterm labour and PPH.
- Antepartum fetal surveillance is invaluable in the management of twin pregnancy.
- The risk of operative intervention is increased.
- Perinatal morbidity and mortality are high and are attributed to prematurity, IUGR and maternal complications like PIH.
- A woman with twin pregnancy should be advised to deliver in an institution with facilities for expert neonatal care.

QUESTIONS

Select the single most appropriate answer:

1. Which one of the following statements about dizygotic twin pregnancy is false?
   a. blood groups of fetuses are different
   b. each fetus has its own chorion and amnion
   c. the incidence is unchanged geographically
   d. the two placenta may be separate or fused
2. The incidence of monozygotic twins per 1,000 live births is
   a. 1–2 b. 3–4 c. 5–6 d. 7–8
3. The most common complication of multiple pregnancy is
   a. antepartum hemorrhage c. hyperemesis gravidarum
   b. anemia d. preterm labour
4. What percentage of twin pregnancies is complicated by premature rupture of membranes?
   a. 10% b. 12% c. 14% d. 16%
5. Which statement about monozygotic twins is *not* correct?
   a. if the fertilised ovum splits within three days, the twins are dichorionic and diamniotic
   b. the incidence remains unchanged geographically
   c. when cleavage occurs within 4–7 days, the result is monochorionic and monoamniotic twins
   d. monochorionic twins are of the same sex

In the following questions, there are two statements. Select the appropriate answer using the following key:

a. if both statements are true and causally related
b. if both statements are true but not causally related
c. if the first statement is true and the second is false
d. if the first statement is false and the second is true
e. if both statements are false

6. There is a rise in the incidence of dizygotic twins *because*
   There is a rise in assisted reproductive techniques.
7. Vascular anastomosis between arteries and veins is seen in dizygotic twins *because*
   The placenta can be fused in dizygotic twins.
8. Internal podalic version can be performed on the second of twins *because*
   The baby is small and the uterine cavity is large.

Select the appropriate answer using the following key:

a. if only responses 1, 2 and 3 are correct
b. if only 1 and 3 are correct
c. if only 2 and 4 are correct
d. if only 4 is correct
e. if all are correct

9. As compared to singleton pregnancy, multiple pregnancy is frequently associated with which of the following?
   1. antepartum hemorrhage
   2. anemia
   3. polyhydramnios
   4. normal fetal presentation
10. Elective cesarean section is indicated most frequently in twin pregnancy if
    1. fetal distress is present
    2. first baby presents as breech
    3. placental abruption occurs
    4. both babies present as transverse lie

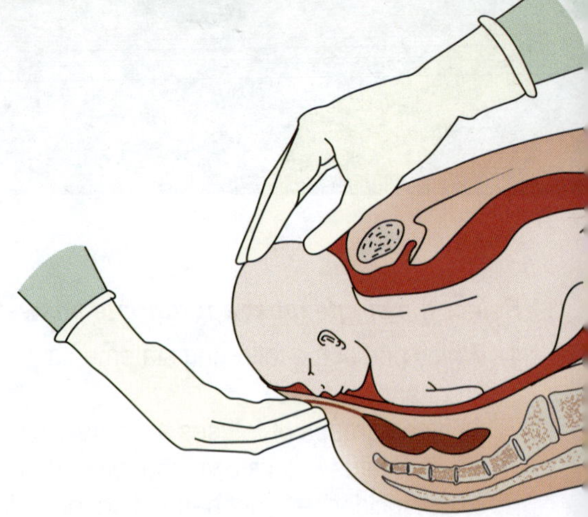

30

Induction of Labour

Manorama Purwar

LEARNING OBJECTIVES

At the end of this chapter, the reader should be able to:

- define induction of labour
- appreciate the principles that govern induction of labour
- enumerate the indications
- enumerate the contraindications
- define 'cervical ripening'
- describe the assessment of cervical status
- enumerate the methods for cervical ripening and induction of labour
- describe how the mother and fetus are monitored
- enumerate the complications of induction of labour

Introduction

Termination of pregnancy after the period of viability may be necessary in the interests of the fetus, the mother or both. It may be carried out before term (before 37 weeks), at term (37 weeks to 42 weeks) or after term (after the completion of 42 weeks). The method selected for termination will depend on the urgency for the delivery, the status of the cervix and the presenting part. If there is an indication to terminate a pregnancy immediately (without delay), the fetus has an unengaged head and an unfavourable cervix for induction of labour, cesarean section is the best method. Otherwise, one may decide to induce labour using interventions to produce uterine contractions as in normal labour in anticipation of vaginal delivery. In general, the aim is to deliver vaginally provided there is no risk to the mother or the fetus.

Definition

Induction of labour is defined as the artificial initiation of uterine contractions before spontaneous onset of contractions after week 28 of gestation with an aim to secure delivery by the vaginal route.

The ideal method of induction of labour should combine the following factors:

- safety for the mother and fetus
- short induction–delivery interval
- minimal side effects

Indications

Labour is induced for the benefit of the fetus, the mother and sometimes, in the interest of both.

Fetal indications

Post-maturity: There is evidence that prolonging the pregnancy beyond 42 weeks adds significantly to the risk for the fetus. The baby grows larger, the skull is more ossified and the risk of intrauterine death is increased. Therefore, after ascertaining the period of gestation, labour is induced when the pregnancy continues beyond 41 weeks.

Diabetes mellitus complicating pregnancy: The risk of sudden intrauterine death increases with the period of gestation. In all women suffering from diabetes mellitus, labour may have to be induced at term or a few weeks before term if indicated.

Rhesus isoimmunisation: In this condition, the antibodies cause hemolysis in the fetus leading to fetal anemia, cardiac failure and hydrops fetalis. If pregnancy is near term, labour is induced to salvage the fetus.

Intrauterine Fetal Growth Restriction (IUGR): In some cases of fetal growth restriction, labour is induced to avoid intrauterine fetal death.

Intrauterine fetal death: Once the fetus is dead, it is expelled spontaneously in 3 to 5 weeks. In some cases, disseminated intravascular coagulation may complicate the pregnancy: in such cases, labour needs to be induced. Another reason is that psychologically the mother may feel upset to know that she is carrying a dead fetus.

Fetal malformations: Once fetal malformations like anencephaly, hydrocephalus or achondroplasia are diagnosed, labour is induced for the benefit of the mother.

Maternal and fetal indications

Pregnancy-induced hypertension: Preeclampsia and eclampsia are the most common indications for induction of labour. Once the pregnancy reaches 37 weeks, induction of labour is indicated in the interests of the mother and her child.

Premature rupture of membranes and chorioamnionitis: After the membranes rupture, the majority of women will go into labour within 24 hours. If that does not happen, infection is likely to set in, leading to chorioamnionitis which adversely affects not only the mother but also the fetus. In developing countries where the risk of infection is high, labour is usually induced 4–6 hours after membranes have ruptured.

Antepartum hemorrhage: Bleeding from placental abruption or placenta previa is detrimental to both the mother and the fetus. Artificial rupture of membranes followed by oxytocin prevents further bleeding in case of placental abruption and minor degrees of placenta previa.

Maternal indications

Maternal medical illnesses: Labour may have to be induced when the mother is suffering from progressively worsening conditions like renal or hepatic disorders, autoimmune diseases and cancer.

Elective Induction

It refers to the induction of labour in a woman whose pregnancy is uncomplicated. The reason for induction is the convenience of the woman and her obstetrician. There is evidence that elective induction is associated with a higher incidence of dystocia, fetal distress and a two- to threefold increase in the risk of cesarean section. For these reasons, elective induction is not recommended.

Contraindications

Under some conditions, it may be detrimental to both the woman and her child if labour is induced. Therefore, one must rule out these clinical conditions prior to inducing labour. The contraindications may be absolute and relative.

Absolute contraindications

The primary contraindication is the absence of an indication:

- cephalopelvic disproportion
- transverse/oblique lie
- malpresentations
- cord presentation
- major degree placenta previa
- scar on the upper segment of the uterus
- woman is HIV-positive
- active genital herpes
- pelvic tumours
- invasive carcinoma cervix.

Relative contraindications

- multiple gestation
- fetal macrosomia (>4,500 g)
- unstable fetal lie
- previous lower segment CS.

Prerequisites for induction of labour

For induction of labour to be successful with minimal adverse effects on the mother and her child, certain conditions must be fulfilled. First of all, like for any intervention, there must be a genuine/legitimate indication for the induction, and the presentation must be cephalic, vertex or mento-anterior. Cephalopelvic disproportion must necessarily be ruled out. When pregnancy is to be terminated before term, tests for fetal maturity must be carried out to plan neonatal care.

A careful clinical evaluation of the mother and the fetus is mandatory. The risks and benefits of induction should be explained to the mother and her relatives and an informed consent must be obtained.

Pre-induction cervical scoring

Before the onset of labour, the cervix is softened, shortened and sometimes dilated a little. These changes are referred to as the '**ripening of cervix**' or '**favourable cervix**'. These changes result in decreased resistance for dilatation of the cervix during labour and provide a basis for the **standardised numeric cervical scoring system**. The success of induction depends largely on the degree of ripening of the cervix at the time of induction.

Bishop was the first to introduce a clinically acceptable numeric scoring system to evaluate the cervix. This scoring system is based on predetermined factors, and each factor is given a score of 0, 1 or 2 depending on the condition of the concerned factor. This is illustrated in **Table 30.1**.

The Bishop score ranges from 0 to 13. A score of 7 or above is indicative of a favourable cervix and induction of labour is anticipated to be successful. A score of 4 or less identifies an unfavourable cervix and requires ripening of the cervix prior to induction of labour.

Table 30.1 Bishop score

Factor	Points			
	0	1	2	3
Dilatation of cervix (cm)	<1	1–2	2–4	>4
Effacement (%)	0–30	40–50	60–70	>80
Consistency of cervix	Firm	Average	Soft	
Position of cervix in the vagina	Posterior	Mid/ Anterior		
Station (relative to ischial spine)	-3	-2	-1/0	+1/+2

Methods of cervical ripening

Medical and mechanical methods are available for ripening of the cervix before induction of labour. In some cases, it may be necessary to use both. Prostaglandins are currently used for this purpose.

Medical methods: Prostaglandins (PG) are derivatives of prostanoic acid and are widely distributed in the tissues. Prostaglandins E and F stimulate myometrial contractions during pregnancy.

Prostaglandin E_2, dinoprostone, is used for ripening of the cervix as it is more effective and less toxic compared to PGF_2. In addition to ripening of the cervix, prostaglandins lead to an increase in myometrial activity and an enhanced response to oxytocin. PGE_2 is available as a gel for intracervical application or as vaginal pessaries. The response to intracervical application is predictable and therefore safer to use. The gel contains 0.5 mg dinoprostone and is supplied in a prefilled, specially designed and ready-to-use disposable syringe with a catheter for local application. For vaginal application, the dose is 2–5 mg (**Fig. 30.1**).

Prostaglandins should be administered in or near the delivery suite, where uterine activity and fetal heart rate can be monitored.

A good protocol for cervical ripening is to insert the PGE_2 gel (endocervical/vaginal) the night before the induction is planned. The cervical score should be reassessed 6–8 hours after application; if found unfavourable, a second application may be considered.

When the cervix is favourable, an amniotomy may be performed and if uterine contractions are not established, an oxytocin infusion should be started. There should be an interval of at least 6 hours between application of the PGE_2 gel and starting the infusion of oxytocin.

Mechanical methods: The mechanical methods comprise sweeping of the membranes, use of

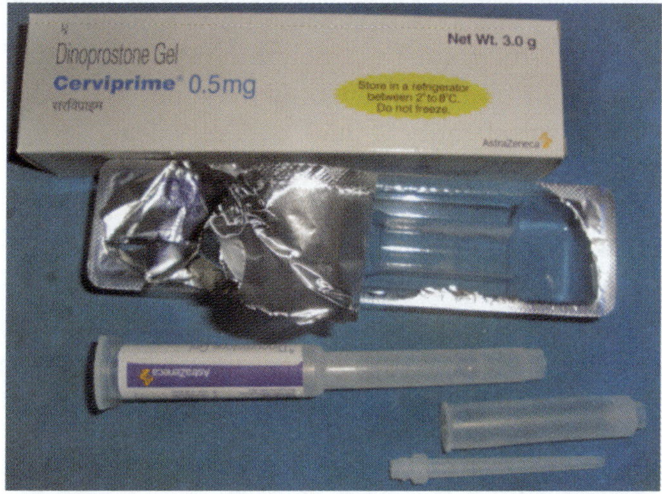

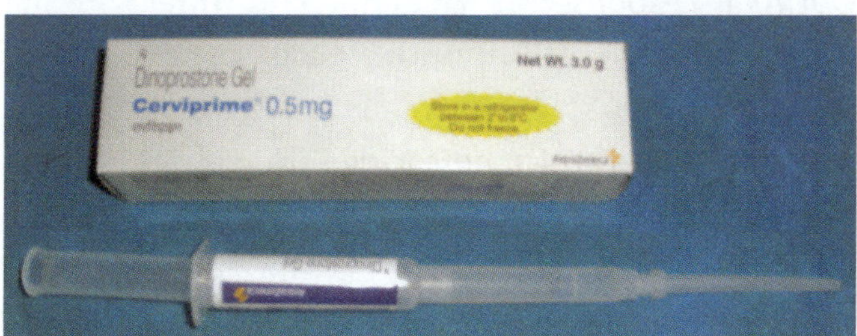

Fig. 30.1 Device for administering PGE_2 gel.

hygroscopic agents and insertion of catheters in the cervical canal.

Sweeping of membranes: In this method, digital separation of the membranes from the lower uterine segment results in prostaglandin surge. This simple procedure may be carried out in the outpatient department without any increased risk of maternal or fetal infection.

Insertion of Foley's catheter: A 20 or 22 size Foley catheter may be inserted through the cervical os and the bulb inflated with 50–75 ml of saline. The catheter is strapped to the thigh of the patient. In about 12 hours, the cervix ripens and the catheter may be expelled or removed.

Methods of induction of labour

Historically, a wide variety of mechanical and medical methods have been used for the induction of labour. In modern obstetrics, however, oxytocics are extensively used preceded or followed by amniotomy.

Sweeping of membranes: This procedure has been described above and is widely used for induction of labour at term.

Amniotomy/artificial rupture of membranes: It is an irreversible method and calls for a firm commitment to delivery. When combined with intravenous oxytocin infusion, it reduces the induction–delivery interval. The main disadvantage of amniotomy is maternal and fetal infection. Amniotomy has a therapeutic role in accidental hemorrhage and is contraindicated in intrauterine fetal death.

Technique: After explaining the procedure to the patient and her relatives, informed consent is obtained. The woman is placed in the lithotomy position; under aseptic precautions, vaginal examination is performed. With a finger between the cervix and the bag of waters, the membranes are swept while maintaining fundal pressure. Kocher's forceps is introduced along the palmar aspect of the fingers, with the tip closed. The tip is opened and membranes are torn with twisting movements leading to the escape of the amniotic fluid (**Fig. 30.2**).

Points to be noted after amniotomy: Once an amniotomy is performed, one must particularly check for the following:

- presence of cord
- colour of amniotic fluid
- bleeding, if any
- station of the presenting part
- fetal heart rate.

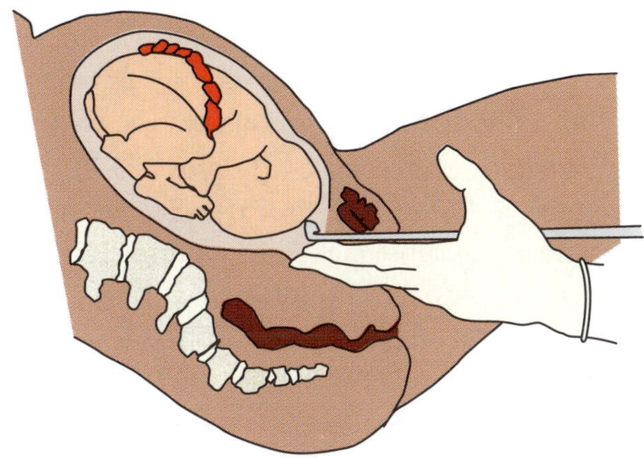

Fig. 30.2 Technique of amniotomy.

Complications:
- cord prolapse
- injury to cervix
- rarely, injury to the fetal scalp
- maternal and/or fetal infection
- accidental hemorrhage (due to sudden decompression of the uterus, fluid)
- tearing of vasa previa leading to fetal blood loss
- failure of induction.

Hind water amniotomy: In women with polyhydramnios, rupture of membranes involves the risk of cord prolopse and abruptio placentae. Hence, controlled rupture of hind waters is carried out with a Drew–Smythe catheter. It is rarely used in modern obstetrics. The claimed advantages are: reduced risk of infection and cord prolapse due to controlled release of the amniotic fluid. The procedure may cause damage to the fetus, placenta and maternal genital tract.

Oxytocin

It was introduced as an intravenous infusion in 1940 and has become the most widely used agent for induction of labour.

Turnbull and Anderson (1968) recognised the wide difference in the response of the pregnant uterus to oxytocin and introduced the concept of 'titration' of oxytocin dos in response to uterine contractions.

Routes of administration: Currently, intravenous oxytocin infusion is the universal method for induction of labour though the buccal and nasal routes are also available.

Another route of administration is the pulsatile oxytocin delivery system; it mimics the pituitary release of oxytocin during spontaneous labour. This system significantly reduces the amount of oxytocin and fluid administered but it is not readily available.

Dose schedule and vehicle of infusion: The aim of oxytocin infusion is to initiate effective uterine contractions and subsequently maintain them.

The dose of oxytocin infusion is 2–10 units oxytocin per 500 ml of Ringer lactate (RL). Oxytocin infusion is better expressed as mU/min rather than drops/minute. The starting dose is 2–4 mU/min and the dose is subsequently escalated every 30 minutes till optimal response is achieved (**Table 30.2**). The maximum dose of oxytocin infusion should not exceed 40 mU/min.The amount of oxytocin infused is best controlled using an infusion pump; its use also restricts the quantity of fluid used as vehicle.

It is worth noting that RL is the best vehicle for administration as its use avoids water intoxication. To avoid fluid overload due to the antidiuretic action of oxytocin, the amount of fluid infused in 24 hours should not exceed one litre. It is better to increase the concentration of oxytocin rather than increasing the amount of fluid infused. This point must be borne in mind in conditions like preeclampsia associated with fluid retention.

Optimal response: It is defined as three uterine contractions in 10 minutes, each lasting for 45 seconds or more.

Maternal and fetal monitoring: This monitoring is best done using a partogram.

- maternal pulse and blood pressure, hourly
- frequency, intensity and duration of uterine contractions, half-hourly
- fetal heart rate, half-hourly.

Continuous cardiotocographic monitoring is preferred, where possible. During oxytocin infusion, if uterine hyperstimulation occurs, the infusion should be stopped immediately. If there is no response, tocolysis with 0.25 mg of terbutaline SC should be given.

Contraindications

Absolute contraindications:
- grand multipara
- scar in the upper segment of the uterus (classical CS/myomectomy)
- placenta previa major.

Relative contraindications:
- previous lower segment cesarean section
- multiple pregnancy

Table 30.2 Oxytocin infusion

Oxytocin units in 500 ml	(drops/min) 15 (mU/min)	30 (mU/min)	60 (mU/min)
2	4	8	16
5	10	20	40

- placenta previa minor: oxytocin infusion should be given after rupturing the membranes.

Prostaglandins

Prostaglandins $F_2\alpha$ and E_2 have been used for induction of labour by various routes. Oral $PGF_2\alpha$ is less effective and has more gastrointestinal side effects compared to oral PGE_2; hence, oral $PGF_2\alpha$ is not recommended. Intravenous prostaglandins have not found wide clinical acceptance because of gastrointestinal side effects and local phlebitis. PGE_2 is administered by the oral or vaginal route.

PGE_2 marketed as dinoprostone tablet containing 0.5 mg dinoprostone, is used for induction of labour. An initial dose of 0.5 mg (1 tablet) is used and subsequently 1 mg (2 tablets) is repeated hourly till labour is well established. A single dose of dinoprostone should not exceed 1.5 mg. The maximum dose which may be given is 5 mg (10 tablets). Oral PGE_2 is more convenient and acceptable, as the mobility of the patient is not restricted, but the onset and maintenance of contractions is less predictable and reversible.

The dose for vaginal administration is a 3 mg dinoprostone tablet inserted in the posterior fornix. Labour usually starts within 6–8 hours of insertion. The dose may be repeated after 4–6 hours but the maximum dose should not exceed 6 mg.

Misoprostol: It is an analogue of PGE_1 and has recently been used for induction of labour. It is available as 25 μg and 200 μg tablets. The most accepted regimen is 25 μg vaginally every 4–6 hours. It has been observed that in patients with ruptured membranes, misoprostol appears to be more effective in induction of labour compared to vaginal PGE_2 and intravenous oxytocin. It is inexpensive, can be stored at room temperature and is easy to administer.

Risks of induction of labour

Each method of induction carries its inherent risks.

Maternal risks:

- failed induction
- increased rate of cesarean section
- uterine hyperstimulation
- antepartum hemorrhage
- postpartum hemorrhage
- placental site retraction
- genital tract infection
- amniotic fluid embolism.

Fetal risks:

- iatrogenic prematurity
- asphyxia
- prolapsed umbilical cord
- fetal infection
- neonatal jaundice.

It must be understood that induction of labour should be done with the objective of achieving normal vaginal delivery. If the selection of the patient is appropriate and the prerequisites for induction are met, induction of labour is likely to be most successful.

KEY POINTS

- Induction of labour is defined as the artificial initiation of uterine contractions before their spontaneous onset after week 28 of gestation with an aim to secure delivery per vias naturalis.
- No method of induction can be absolutely certain and safe.
- There should be a legitimate indication for induction of labour.
- All the prerequisites must be fulfilled before inducing labour.
- Successful induction depends on the preinduction cervical score.
- Endocervical PGE_2 gel application is the most effective method of 'ripening' the cervix.
- Amniotomy has a therapeutic role in accidental hemorrhage and it is contraindicated in intrauterine fetal death.
- Intravenous oxytocin infusion is the universal method for induction.
- For oxytocin infusion, Ringer lactate is the preferred vehicle.
- Maternal and fetal monitoring using a partogram is mandatory during induction of labour.

QUESTIONS

Select the single most appropriate answer:

1. What is the minimum number of hours after endocervical/vaginal application of PGE_2 gel after which oxytocin infusion should be started?
   a. 4 hours b. 6 hours c. 8 hours c. 10 hours
2. Oxytocin is used for induction of labour by all the following routes *except*
   a. intravenous c. oral tablets
   b. nasal spray d. buccal tablets
3. The maximum possible score for the preinduction assessment of cervical ripening using Bishop's method would be
   a. 13 b. 12 c. 11 d. 9
4. The absolute contraindication for amniotomy in induction of labour is
   a. floating head
   b. intrauterine fetal death
   c. abruptio placenta
   d. preterm labour
5. Infusion of 5 IU of oxytocin in 500 ml of Ringer lactate at the rate of 15 drops/min will amount to
   a. 10 mU/min c. 30 mU/min
   b. 20 mU/min d. 40 mU/min
6. Catheter used for hind water amniotomy is
   a. Foley's catheter
   b. plain rubber catheter
   c. Drew–Smythe catheter
   d. Malecot's catheter
7. The optimal response to oxytocin titration is
   a. 5 contractions in 10 minutes lasting for 30 seconds
   b. 4 contractions in 10 minutes lasting for 1 minute
   c. 3 contractions in 10 minutes lasting for 45 seconds
   d. 3 contractions in 10 minutes lasting for 30 seconds
8. The maximum dose of oxytocin infusion which can be used is
   a. 10 mU/min c. 30 mU/min
   b. 20 mU/min d. 40 mU/min
9. What is the amount of dinoprostone in the PGE_2 gel?
   a. 0.25 mg c. 1.0 mg
   b. 0.5 mg d. 1.5 mg
10. The preferred vehicle for the administration of intravenous oxytocin infusion is
    a. normal saline c. dextrose saline
    b. 5% dextrose d. Ringer lactate

31

Vaginal Operative Deliveries

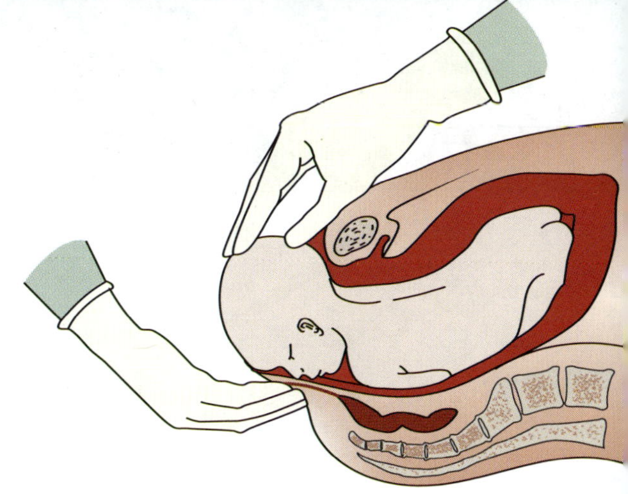

S Habeebullah

LEARNING OBJECTIVES

At the end of this chapter, the reader should be able to:

- enumerate the vaginal operative deliveries
- describe the structure of forceps
- enlist the indications for forceps delivery
- enumerate the prerequisites for the application of outlet and low forceps
- describe the criteria for the correct application of the instruments
- enumerate the steps of outlet and low forceps delivery, including anesthesia
- describe the direction of traction
- enumerate the complications of forceps delivery in the mother and the baby
- describe the structure and function of the vacuum extractor (ventouse)
- list the indications for the use of the vacuum extractor
- describe the steps of vacuum extraction
- enumerate the advantages of vacuum extraction over forceps delivery
- enumerate the complications in the mother and the baby
- describe the principle underlying destructive operations
- list the types of destructive operations

Introduction

Under certain conditions, the delivery of the baby needs to be completed by vaginal operations like obstetric forceps delivery and vacuum extraction. In certain situations, vaginal operative delivery is the most appropriate method, and when performed carefully, the maternal and perinatal outcome are not adversely affected.

In some cases of obstructed labour, where the baby is dead, one may resort to destructive procedures: these deliver the baby after reducing the bulk.

Obstetric Forceps

It is an instrument designed to extract the fetal head. The history of forceps dates back to the 17th century when members of the Chamberlain family in London first used it to deliver live babies. Since then, innumerable types of forceps have been designed, the most commonly used among them being Wrigley's (**Fig. 31.1**), Simpson's (**Fig. 31.2**), Das', Kielland's (**Fig. 31.3**) and Piper's forceps.

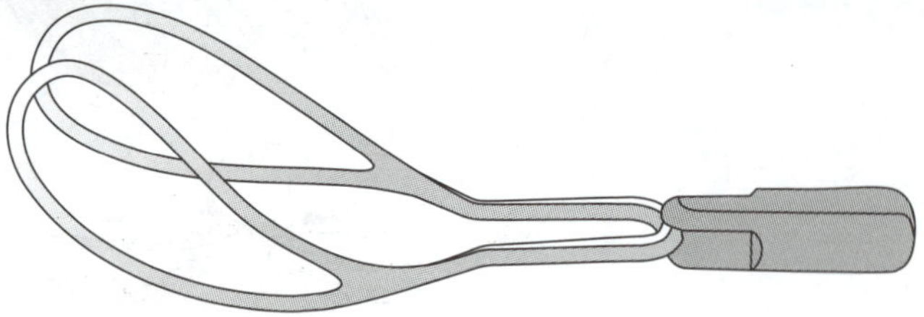

Fig. 31.1 Wrigley's forceps.

Parts of forceps

The forceps consists of a pair of branches, right and left. Each branch consists of the following parts (**Fig. 31.2**):

Blade: This is fenestrated and has cephalic and pelvic curves. The cephalic curve conforms to the shape of the fetal head and the pelvic curve to the maternal birth canal. Kielland's forceps does not have a pelvic curve.

Shank: This connects the blade to the handle and adds to the length of the forceps.

Lock: Both the blades join at the lock. This fixes the instrument. The socket type of lock seen in Wrigley's forceps is known as the British type. The screw type of lock seen in Tarnier's forceps is of the French type. Kielland's forceps has a sliding lock.

Handle: This provides grip during traction.

Functions of forceps

Forceps are mainly used for **traction** and sometimes for **rotation**. Some amount of **compression** of the head (about 4 mm) also occurs. However, if compression is excessive (as in faulty application), it may result in trauma to the head. It also **protects** (acts like a cage) in cases of preterm head.

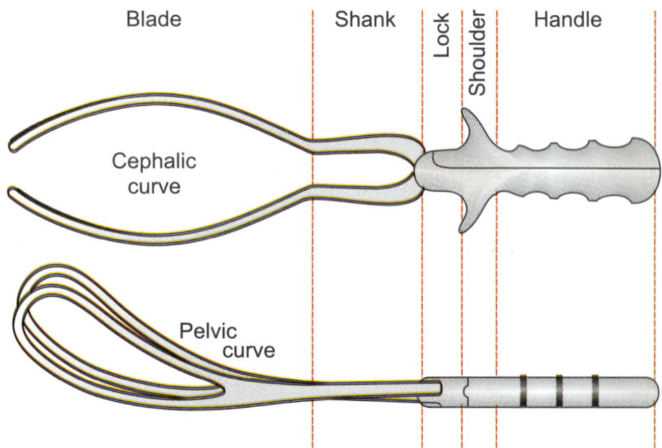

Fig. 31.2 Simpson's forceps.

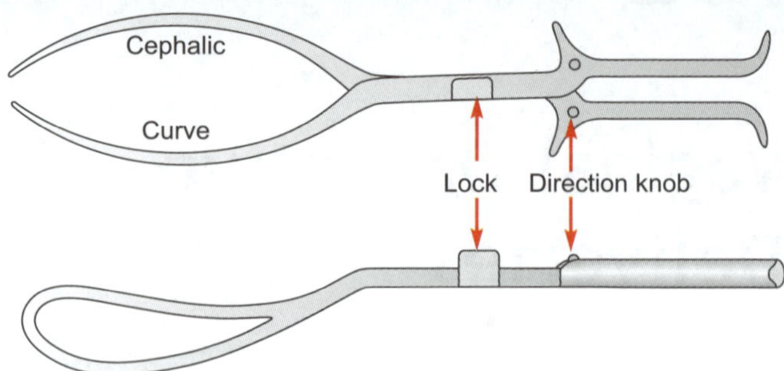

Fig. 31.3 Kielland's forceps.

Classification of forceps delivery

In modern obstetrics, midforceps deliveries are rarely performed. A few experienced obstetricians still use Kielland's forceps for rotation and delivery of the fetal head. The criteria for forceps application as recommended by the American College of Obstetricians and Gynecologists (ACOG) are listed in **Table 31.1**.

Indications for forceps delivery

Forceps are mainly used to cut short the second stage of labour for the benefit of the mother and the fetus (**Table 31.2**).

Table 31.1 Criteria for forceps application recommended by the American College of Obstetricians and Gynecologists (ACOG)

Outlet forceps	Scalp visible at introitus without separating the labia Fetal skull has reached the pelvic floor Sagittal suture is in the AP diameter or right or left occipito-anterior or posterior position Fetal head is at or on the perineum Rotation does not exceed 45°
Low forceps	Leading bony point of fetal skull at ≥+2 station and not pelvic floor Rotation is 45° or less
Midcavity forceps	Station above +2 but head engaged Rotation >45°

Table 31.2 Indications for forceps delivery

Maternal indications	Fetal indications
Conditions that worsen with maternal efforts, such as heart disease, preeclampsia/ eclampsia, respiratory diseases, intrapartum infection Failure of maternal power Prolonged second stage	Fetal distress as evidenced by fetal heart abnormalities on CTG or due to cord compression or prolapse of cord and abruptio placentae (as in the second of twins) Preterm delivery Aftercoming head in breech delivery

Contraindications

In order to avoid detrimental effects on the mother and the fetus, a forceps delivery should never be contemplated under the following conditions:

- cephalopelvic disproportion
- unfulfilled prerequisites

Prophylactic (elective) forceps: There is no definite indication for forceps except that damage to the maternal perineum is anticipated if the fetal head lies there for a long time. This concept was advocated by DeLee. Only an outlet forceps should be applied in this situation.

Prerequisites

The following conditions should be fulfilled for forceps delivery:

- The cervical os should be fully dilated.
- The membranes must be ruptured.
- CPD should be ruled out.
- The head must be engaged. It is imperative to ensure that no part of the head is palpable on abdominal examination, because in the presence of severe moulding, the leading bony point could be below +2 station, while the head is palpable abdominally. The presence of caput may also result in error in assessing the 'station'.
- The presentation should be suitable, for example, vertex, mento-anterior face, aftercoming head in breech.
- An informed consent is obtained.

The technique

Occipito-anterior position: The conditions mentioned above should be fulfilled. The woman is brought to the edge of the table and placed in the dorsal lithotomy position. The bladder is emptied; the perineum is cleaned and draped. Usually, a pudendal block with perineal infiltration of lignocaine is used for anesthesia.

The correct position of the head is ascertained and both blades are assembled. After lubricating the blades with antiseptic lubricant, the left blade, held with the left hand and with the two fingers of the right hand guiding it, is inserted to the left side of the maternal pelvis. The handle presses towards the perineum and is held by an assistant. Similarly, the right blade is applied (**Fig. 31.4**). If applied correctly, both blades lock easily; the sagittal suture is equidistant from the margins of both blades. Ideally, the cephalic and pelvic applications should coincide. However, in unrotated head, cephalic application is performed.

Traction: After locking the blades, the handles are held and traction is applied during contractions after doing an episiotomy:

- the direction of the traction outlet forceps is forward and upwards
- for low forceps, the direction of traction is downwards and forward and then upwards (**Fig. 31.5**).

After the head is delivered, the blades are removed, oropharyngeal suction performed and the rest of the baby is delivered slowly. After the delivery of the placenta, the vagina and cervix are inspected for any tears. The episiotomy wound is then repaired.

Occipito-posterior position: In the occipito-posterior position, after application of the forceps, the direction of traction is horizontal till the root of the nose is under the symphysis; then the traction is directed forward to flex the head so that the occiput is delivered. Thereafter, the nose, face and chin are delivered by extension, with the traction directed downwards. The risk of complete perineal tear is increased in a face-to-pubis delivery and therefore a liberal mediolateral episiotomy is recommended.

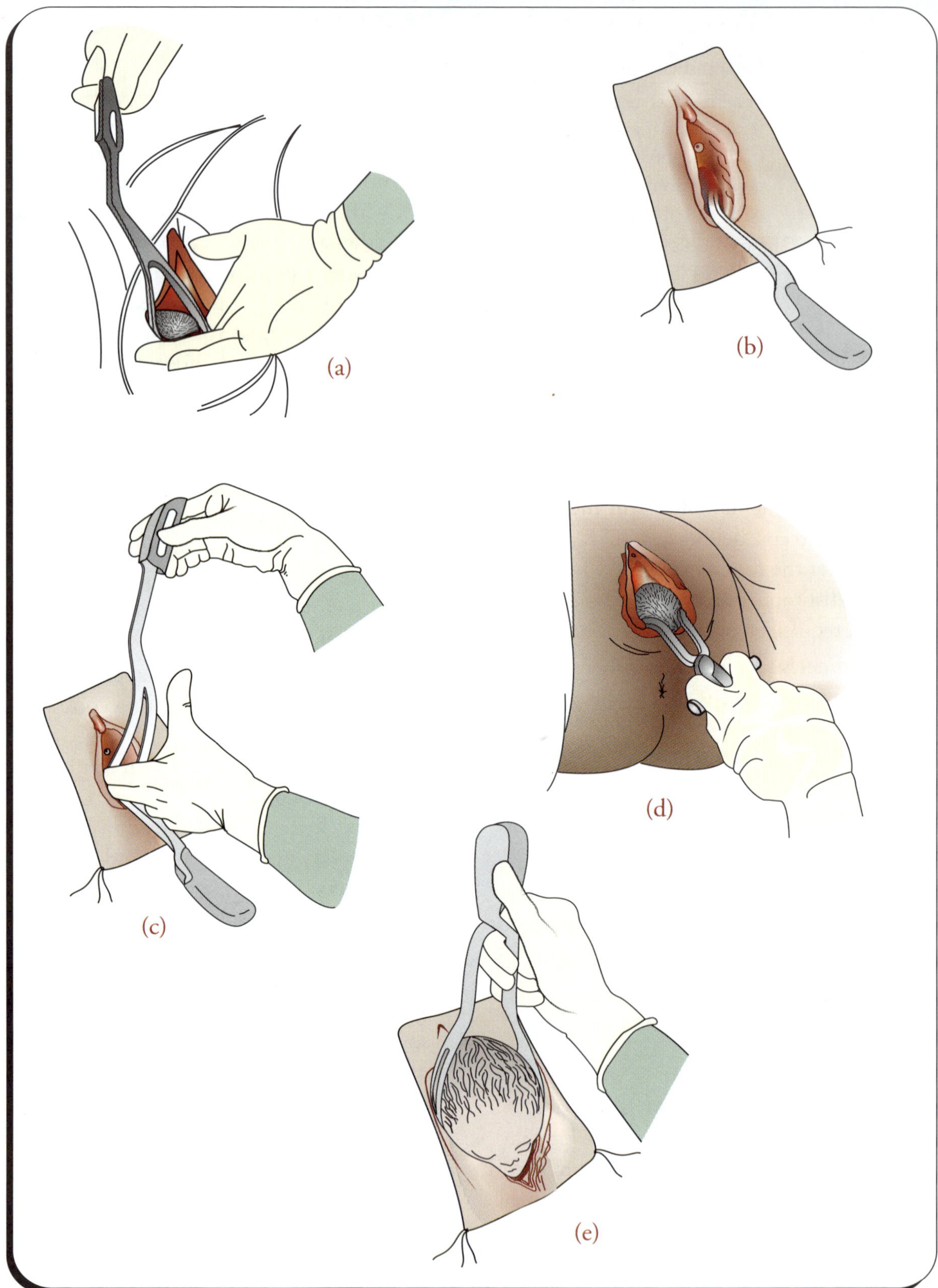

Fig. 31.4 Method of application of forceps.

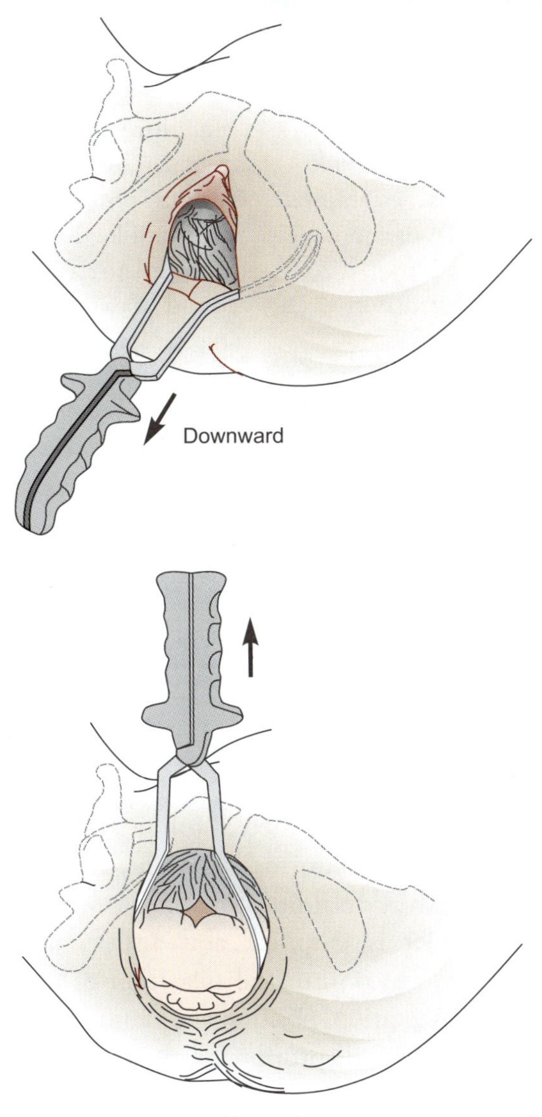

Fig. 31.5 Direction of traction in low forceps.

Delivery of the aftercoming head in breech: Piper's forceps has been specially devised to deliver the aftercoming head. However, a long curved forceps (such as Simpson's) can also be used for this purpose. The technique is described under breech delivery (**Fig. 28.8**).

Nowadays, only experienced obstetricians use Kielland's forceps for the rotation and extraction of the fetal head from the level of the midcavity. The procedure is best performed under general or regional anesthesia. If an unskilled person uses it, serious complications like vaginal lacerations, rupture of the uterus and fetal injuries may result.

Trial forceps

Trial forceps refers to a situation where one anticipates an unsuccessful forceps delivery. It is attempted in the operation theatre, keeping everything ready for cesarean section. In case there is difficulty in locking, or delivery of the baby is not achieved after 2–3 tentative pulls, the procedure is abandoned and a cesarean section is performed.

Failed forceps

The procedure refers to a situation where, despite all efforts, delivery of the baby by forceps is not accomplished. The causes of failed forceps are undiagnosed CPD, occipito-posterior position and wrong application of blades and at a higher station of the fetal head. Maternal and perinatal complications are high in such cases. Careful selection of cases is, therefore, important.

Complications

If one resorts to 'easy' forceps delivery, most of the complications can be avoided (**Table 31.3**).

Vacuum Extraction (Ventouse)

The principle underlying this procedure is to apply negative pressure to the fetal head and effect delivery by traction. Ventouse delivery was introduced and popularised by Malmstrom of Sweden in 1954. Many modifications have taken place; the most important one is by Bird (1969) who separated the traction

Table 31.3 Complications of forceps delivery

Maternal	Fetal
Injury to maternal soft tissues for example, vaginal and cervical lacerations, complete perineal tear, colporrhexis and rupture uterus may occur and cause traumatic PPH. Rarely, broad ligament and paravaginal hematomas form, leading to shock. Traumatic shock can result, especially when proper anesthesia is not used.	Cephalhematoma Lacerations of the scalp and face Facial palsy Intracranial hemorrhage Skull fractures

chain from the tubing that created the suction.

The basic components of the instrument are (**Fig. 31.6**):

- a cup which needs to be applied to the fetal head
- a glass bottle connected to the cup by a plate and chain in tubing
- a pump to create negative pressure connected to the bottle; the pump can be manual or electric. There is a manometer to indicate the negative pressure.

Basically two types of cups are available: metal and silastic. The **metal cups** made of stainless steel are available in three sizes, 40, 50 and 60 mm. The edges are inverted. Usually 50 or 60 mm cups are used as they give a better grip. Metal cups give firmer grip and are used in unrotated head and in occipito-posterior position but are more traumatic. The **silastic cups (soft cups)** are less traumatic but the chances of slippage are greater. They are best suited for a well rotated head at a lower station.

Indications

Table 31.4 gives the maternal and fetal indications for vacuum extraction.

Contraindications

No attempt should be made to deliver the baby by vacuum extraction under the following circumstances:

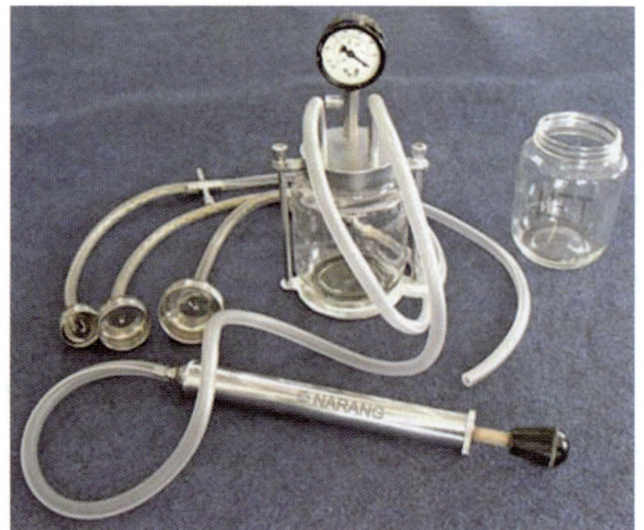

Fig. 31.6 Vacuum extraction equipment.

Table 31.4 Indications for vacuum extraction

Maternal	Fetal
Prolonged second stage Maternal conditions like cardiac disease, eclampsia/preeclampsia, previous cesarean section Maternal exhaustion in second stage	Fetal distress with unrotated head Occipito-posterior position (like deep transverse arrest) Second of twins even with a higher station of head: +2 and above

- cephalopelvic disproportion
- preterm head (<34 weeks)
- non-vertex presentation (face, aftercoming head in breech)
- fetal coagulopathy
- following fetal scalp blood sampling
- vertex above 'zero' station.

The procedure

The procedure is performed as follows (**Fig. 31.7**):

1. After obtaining informed consent, the woman is placed in the dorsal lithotomy position.
2. The bladder is emptied, and an examination is performed to confirm full dilatation of the cervix, vertex presentation, position and station of the head.
3. Cephalopelvic disproportion is ruled out. The cervix should be fully or nearly fully dilated.
4. Pudendal block and perineal infiltration is preferred.
5. The largest available cup (50 or 60 mm) is selected and applied on the flexion point of the fetal head, which is 1.5 cm anterior to the edge of the posterior fontanelle or 6 cm posterior to the centre of the anterior fontanelle in the midline. This helps in flexion of the head during traction.
6. Vacuum 0.2 kg/cm^2 is created and care is taken to ensure that soft parts like the cervix and vagina are not included. Now, vacuum is increased step-wise every 2 minutes to a maximum of 0.8 kg/cm^2. This results in the formation of a large caput called chignon.
7. With each uterine contraction, traction is applied at right angles to the cup, applying counterpressure with two fingers of the left hand. The direction of pull is in the axis of the birth canal, as in the case of forceps (**Fig. 31.8**).

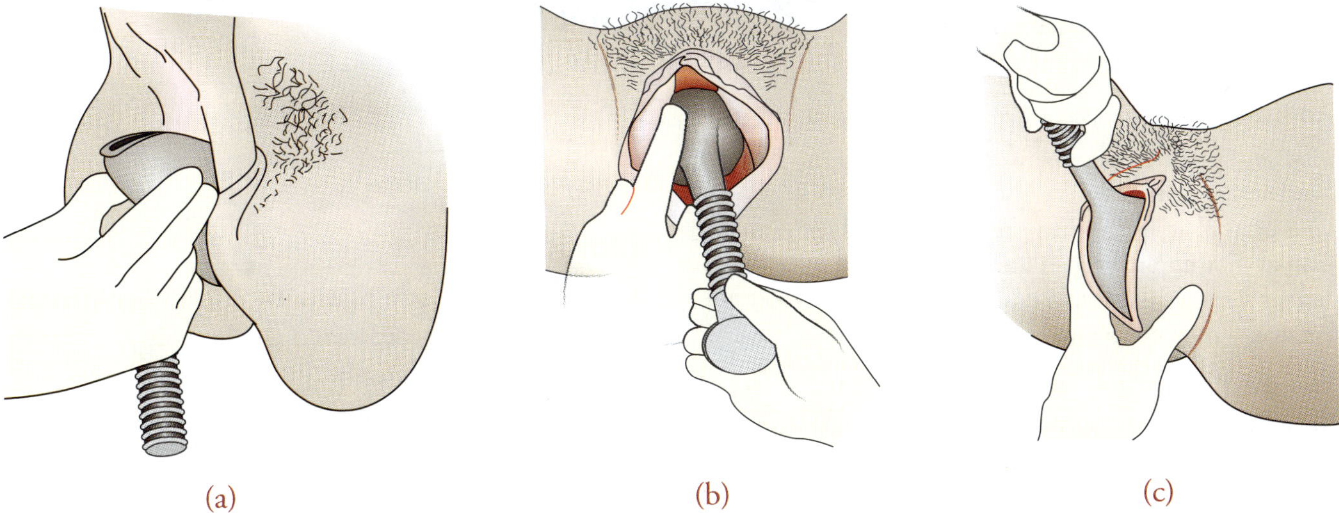

Fig. 31.7 Sil-cup ventouse delivery.

8. If descent occurs with each pull, delivery is usually completed with three pulls in about 15 minutes. After the head is fully delivered, suction is released and the rest of the delivery completed. If the cup slips, it can be reapplied once more. If it slips, twice, the procedure should be abandoned. Sometimes, the cup slips after the rotation is complete and the head is on the perineum: in that case, delivery can be completed using outlet forceps. In case vacuum delivery fails, one should not resort to forceps as this causes increased morbidity.

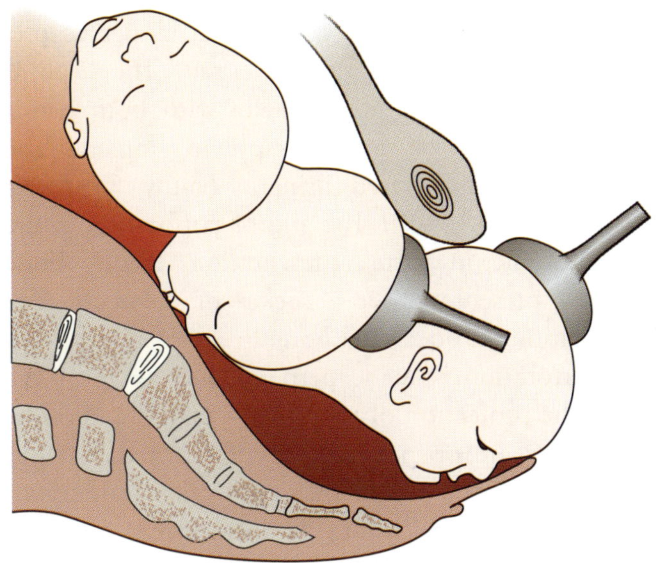

Fig. 31.8 Traction down the pelvic axis.

Complications

Vacuum extraction like forceps delivery may be associated with complications for the mother and the baby.

- Maternal injuries such as lacerations of the vagina and cervix occur; rarely, an annular detachment of cervix has been recorded. Long-term effects may include incompetent os and uterine prolapse, especially if applied before full dilatation of the cervix.
- Fetal complications are scalp lacerations and necrosis, cephalhematoma, intracranial hemorrhage, subgaleal hematoma, retinal and subconjunctival hemorrhage, neonatal jaundice, convulsions and birth asphyxia.
- These complications are associated with a prolonged application of ventouse.

The advantages and disadvantages of vacuum extraction are summarised in **Table 31.5**.

Destructive Operations

Destructive operations refer to procedures where the bulk of the fetus is reduced and then delivered vaginally. The objective is to avoid a cesarean section in case of a dead or grossly malformed fetus. As a result of improved obstetric care and increased safety of cesarean section, destructive operations are rarely performed; however, in developing countries, cesarean section continues to be unsafe and the risk

Table 31.5 Advantages and disadvantages of vacuum extraction

Advantages
Does not require space between the side of the fetal head and the pelvic wall
Can be applied even when the cervix is 8–9 cm dilated
Can also be applied on an unrotated head at relatively higher station (as in second of twins)
Analgesia may not be necessary
Disadvantages
Takes time to create vacuum and therefore cannot be used in acute fetal distress; however, a soft cup ventouse may be used as vacuum is created rapidly in 1–2 minutes
High risk of injury to both the mother and the fetus
Cannot be applied in non-vertex presentations
Cannot be applied in the presence of large caput
Cannot be applied in preterm head (<34 weeks)
Requires maternal effort, and hence not suitable when mother cannot bear down
Greater risk of cephalhematoma

of subsequent scar rupture is high; hence, the need to perform destructive operations.

Types of operations

- cleidotomy
- craniotomy
- decapitation
- evisceration
- spondylotomy

Indications

- shoulder dystocia
- obstructed labour where the baby is dead
- gross hydrocephalus

Contraindications

- live fetus
- threatened/suspected uterine rupture
- major degree placenta previa
- grossly contracted pelvis
- pelvic tumours like fibroids obstructing the passage

Complications

- bladder and rectal injury
- vaginal and cervical lacerations
- rupture of uterus
- vesico-vaginal fistula

Cleidotomy

It is performed as a last resort in case of shoulder dystocia, encountered when the fetus is macrosomic (diabetic women, post-term pregnancy). This is the only destructive operation which can be undertaken in a live fetus. One or both the clavicles are cut with cleidotomy scissors. This results in reduction of the bisacromial diameter, thus reducing the bulk of the fetus and resulting in vaginal delivery.

Craniotomy

In this condition, the fetal skull is perforated and the intracranial contents are evacuated, thus reducing the size of the fetal skull and effecting an easy vaginal delivery.

The indications are:

- dead fetus with CPD/obstructed labour
- gross hydrocephalus

Procedure

Craniotomy: It is performed under general anesthesia. A meticulous examination is performed to rule out impending rupture of the uterus. Presentation, position and station are confirmed. Under aseptic measures, the bladder is catheterised. The head is fixed by an assistant abdominally with both hands or the same can be done by applying forceps. The fetal skull is perforated using a handy Simpson's perforator (**Fig. 31.9**). The site of perforation is the parietal bone in vertex presentation, frontal bone in brow presentation, eye socket or palate in face presentation and occipital bone in aftercoming head. The perforation is made perpendicular to the bone under the protection of two fingers placed anteriorly. The blades are opened and closed, turned 90° and again opened and closed making a cruciate incision. A blunt flushing curette is introduced into the cranial cavity; the brain matter is churned and flushed out, thus reducing the size of the head. If forceps is

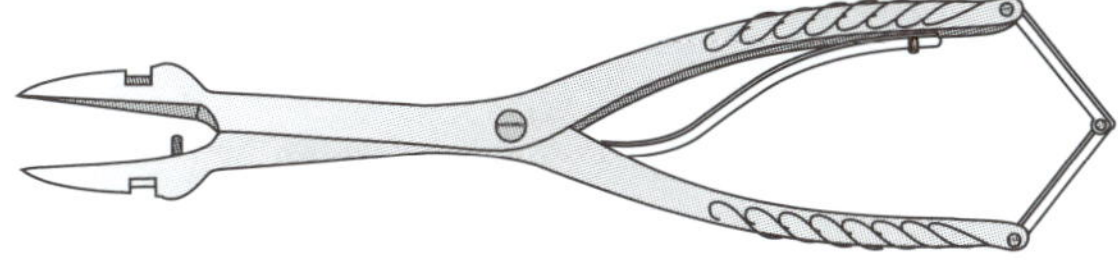

Fig. 31.9 Simpson's perforator.

already applied, delivery can be completed. Otherwise, the decompressed head can be held with vulsellum or cranioclast and delivered. The vagina, cervix and uterus should be checked for signs of trauma.

In hydrocephalus, instead of using a perforator, a thick-bore needle (14–16G) may be used to drain the CSF, resulting in collapse of the head.

Decapitation: This procedure is sometimes performed in cases of neglected shoulder presentation with dead fetus where the neck is accessible. Under general anesthesia, taking all the precautions listed above, the fetus is severed into two by cutting the neck and delivering the trunk followed by head. The neck can be cut using **Jardine's hook** with a knife or the Blond–Heidler **decapitation saw** taking care to avoid injury to the bladder. The prolapsed hand can be pulled to deliver the trunk. The head is grasped with fingers or crochet and delivered. Soft tissues are explored for any damage.

Evisceration and spondylotomy: This operation is performed on a dead fetus in the transverse lie where the fetal abdomen is accessible or in the presence of abdominal tumours. A long pair of scissors known as **evisceration scissors** is used to incise the abdomen and remove the contents. Thoracic contents can also be removed if necessary to further debulk the fetus. The spine can be divided (spondylotomy) and the fetus is delivered in two parts.

Postoperative care

After performing any destructive operation, the patient should be observed for traumatic/atonic PPH. In prolonged/obstructed labour, antibiotics should be used and the bladder should be drained for a week to prevent the development of vesico-vaginal fistula.

KEY POINTS

- Operative vaginal delivery is used in about 10% of deliveries.
- The most common indications are: prolonged second stage and fetal distress in second stage and maternal medical disorders like cardiac disease.
- 'Easy' forceps delivery (low and outlet forceps with fully rotated/short of rotation) is safe.
- Proper evaluation, following the prerequisites and adequate analgesia are the key factors for successful outcome.
- Ventouse has the advantage of less fetomaternal trauma, especially when the obstetrician is not very experienced, though it cannot be applied in non-vertex presentations.
- Repeated 'pop offs' are associated with increased morbidity; so also the use of vacuum followed by forceps.
- Destructive operations are rarely performed; the most common are craniotomy and cleidotomy.
- Careful selection of cases and expertise in these operations can reduce the complications. This in turn prevents the complications associated with second-stage cesarean section.

QUESTIONS

Select the single most appropriate answer:

1. Piper's forceps is specially designed for
   a. delivery of the aftercoming head
   b. rotation of the fetal head
   c. delivery in face presentation
   d. face-to-pubis delivery
2. All of the following are favourable for the application of outlet forceps *except*
   a. os fully dilated
   b. head engaged
   c. rotation of head <45°
   d. vertex at +3 station
3. Which one of the following regarding vacuum delivery is *not* correct?
   a. can be applied when os is not fully dilated
   b. can be applied in unrotated head
   c. can be applied at +1 station
   d. can be applied to the preterm head
4. The negative pressure applied for ventouse delivery is
   a. 1 kg/cm^2
   b. 0.8 kg/cm^2
   c. 0.6 kg/cm^2
   d. 0.4 kg/cm^2
5. Which of the following is the most important prerequisite to be met for application of forceps?
   a. cervix should be fully dilated
   b. vertex should be at +3 station
   c. there should be an indication
   d. there should be uterine contractions

32

Cesarean Section

Sunesh Kumar

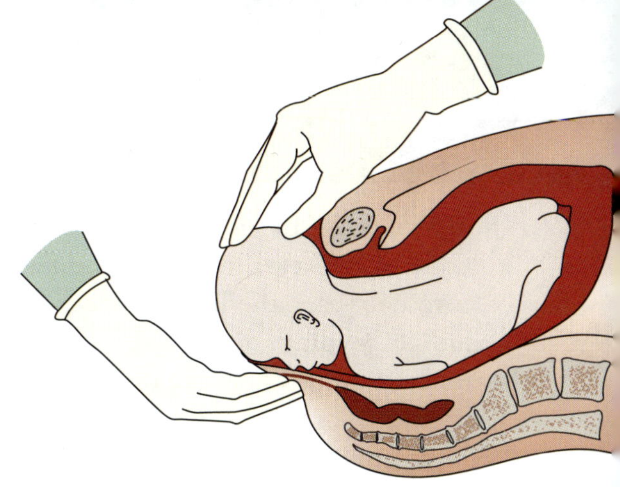

LEARNING OBJECTIVES

At the end of this chapter, the reader should be able to:

- define cesarean section (CS)
- enumerate the types of cesarean section
- list the indications for this operation
- describe preoperative care
- enumerate the steps of lower segment cesarean section (LSCS)
- state how classical CS differs from LSCS
- list the complications of cesarean section
- describe postoperative care
- appreciate that vaginal delivery is safer than CS
- enumerate the reasons for the rising rates of CS
- appreciate the need to contain the rates of CS
- outline the management of previous CS

Introduction

Cesarean section (CS) is a surgical procedure by which the fetus is delivered after incising the abdominal wall and the uterus. The term cesarean section should not be used if a fetus is removed from the peritoneal cavity in case of rupture of the uterus or abdominal pregnancy. The origin of the term cesarean section is debatable. However, there are three explanations: (a) Julius Cesar was born by cesarean section, (b) during the reign of Cesar, by law the operation had to be performed to save the child when the mother was in her last few weeks of pregnancy and (c) the word may be derived from the Latin word 'cedere' which means 'to cut'. The last one seems to be the most plausible explanation.

Cesarean section is the most common major operation carried out in obstetric practice. It is indicated for a number of fetal and maternal conditions. An appropriately performed CS can help save the life of the mother and of her child. It is estimated that 5%–25% of all deliveries are by CS. The technological advances in the administration of anesthesia, blood transfusion and antibiotics have made CS a safe operation, leading to rising rates of this operation. However, it is documented that it associated with higher maternal morbidity and mortality as compared to vaginal delivery. The high rates of CS have not contributed to a reduction in perinatal mortality in developing countries.

Indications

In obstetric practice, there is a need to perform CS for several conditions that affect the mother and her unborn child. In some circumstances, CS is the only mode of delivery; in others, the need is debatable. In recent years, the list of indications has expanded due to medical, legal and personal reasons. The indications for CS can be classified as maternal, fetal or both. Note that a number of diseases that affect the mother also affect the fetus.

The list of indications for CS in the order of frequency is given below.

Maternal indications

Cephalopelvic disproportion and contracted pelvis: Disproportion between the size of the fetal head and pelvis is the most common indication. Diagnosis of cephalopelvic disproportion (CPD) can be made at 37–38 weeks, when a pelvic examination is done to assess the pelvis. Whereas gross CPD (major-degree CPD) can be easily identified, borderline disproportion between the pelvis and fetal head size may be difficult to detect. However, the diagnosis of CPD is made more definitely during labour when the fetal head fails to descend into the pelvis in spite of good uterine contractions as documented by the partogram.

Associated obstetric complications: Cesarean section may be necessary in the following conditions.

Placenta previa: Cesarean section must be performed in case of major degree placenta previa: type II posterior, type III and type IV.

Accidental hemorrhage (abruptio placentae): Most cases of accidental hemorrhage deliver vaginally following artificial rupture of membranes and oxytocin infusion. However, cesarean section may be required if the patient fails to deliver within 6–8 hours, or when the pregnancy is near term and the fetus is alive.

Preeclampsia and eclampsia: In severe preeclampsia or eclampsia, a CS is indicated when the pregnancy has to be terminated rapidly and the cervix is unfavourable.

Maternal diseases: When the woman suffers from medical or surgical disorders, a CS may be required under some circumstances.

Diabetes mellitus: Cesarean section for a diabetic may be indicated to avoid possible sudden intrauterine death.

Maternal HIV infection: A CS is recommended in order to reduce the risk of transmission of infection to the child.

Cancer of the uterine cervix: A classical or upper segment CS should be performed to avoid hemorrhage and dissemination of the disease associated with vaginal delivery.

Previous cesarean section: Under the following conditions, a repeat CS is indicated when the woman has had her previous delivery by CS:

- two or more lower segment cesarean sections (LSCS)
- classical CS
- one LSCS with postoperative infection, uncertain scar integrity, or there is an obstetric complication.

Other operations on the uterus: The scars of the following operations carry a greater risk of rupture of the uterus, and therefore a CS is recommended:

- hysterotomy
- repair of rent consequent to rupture of the uterus
- myomectomy where the endometrial cavity had been opened.

Soft tissue obstruction: Pelvic tumours like fibroids or ovarian cysts and stenosis of the vagina and cervix can obstruct labour. Hence, a CS is the best method of delivery.

Uterine dysfunction: A CS is indicated when medical intervention fails and labour gets prolonged abnormally with adverse effects on the mother and the fetus.

Fetal indications

Fetal distress: Changes in fetal heart rate; fall in fetal heart rate below 100 beats/minute or persistent rise above 160 beats/minute, non-reassuring fetal heart rate patterns, especially persistent late deceleration, and passage of meconium point to fetal hypoxia; in such cases, a CS is indicated if rapid delivery by the vaginal route is not possible.

Cord prolapse: When the umbilical cord prolapses with an incompletely dilated cervix and the fetus is alive, the best way to salvage the fetus is by CS.

Malpresentations: In the following malpresentations, CS is performed.

Breech presentation: Breech vaginal delivery may be associated with complications in up to 10% of cases. In order to ensure safe delivery of the fetus, one may have to consider CS if breech presentation is associated with (i) big baby (weight >3.5 kg) (ii) even slightest degree of contracted pelvis, (iii) complicated breech or (iv) flexed breech. Some obstetricians advocate cesarean section for all breech presentations; others prefer a CS for breech in all primigravida.

Transverse lie: Cesarean section should be performed when the fetus is in the transverse lie during labour or in cases where external cephalic version has failed.

Face and brow presentation: A vaginal delivery should be anticipated if the position is mento-anterior. Face presentation, where the chin is posterior (mento-posterior), or brow presentation require CS.

Malpositions: A CS is indicated in the occipito-posterior position when there is incomplete or failure of rotation of the head leading to 'deep transverse arrest' or 'persistent occipito-posterior', and instrumental vaginal delivery is contraindicated.

Recurrent pregnancy loss: Some women have a history of stillbirths, early neonatal deaths following difficult deliveries and repeated abortions. An elective CS may be needed in such cases.

Elective cesarean section

This is a planned CS carried out before the onset of labour at a pre-fixed date and time. A woman posted for an elective CS undergoes proper preoperative evaluation and preparation like an empty stomach and ensuring availability of blood. The presence of an anesthesiologist, neonatologist and other staff is ensured. The intra- and postoperative complications are much fewer than in an emergency CS. The only disadvantage is the possible delivery of a preterm baby, due to incorrect assessment of the period of gestation.

Emergency cesarean section

When a CS is carried out for an indication which arises suddenly during pregnancy or labour, it is termed an emergency CS. Since there is no time for preparation, the woman may suffer from serious complications like Mendelson syndrome, which is associated with high mortality.

Procedure for Lower Segment Cesarean Section

Preoperative care

- The pregnant woman and a responsible relative are briefed about the need for CS, and informed consent is obtained.
- A thorough clinical evaluation and relevant laboratory investigations are performed.
- Blood is cross-matched and kept available.
- In case of emergency CS, oral antacids or IV H_2 blockers are administered.
- Hair over the lower abdomen is clipped.
- A catheter is inserted in the bladder.
- Anesthesia is administered.

Operative procedure

Abdominal incision

- Transverse incision, also known as Pfannensteil incision, is made above the symphysis pubis. The rectus sheath is cut transversely and separated from the underlying recti muscles. The muscles are separated in the midline to expose the peritoneum, which is then cut vertically. The postoperative discomfort is less, healing and cosmetic results are excellent and the risk of hernia is negligible.
- Vertical incision could be midline or right paramedian. It is faster and can be extended easily, if necessary. This incision is indicated if the fetus has to be delivered very rapidly, if pregnancy is complicated by tumours or in situations where classical CS is planned.

Technique of LSCS: The steps of LSCS are shown in **Fig. 32.1**.

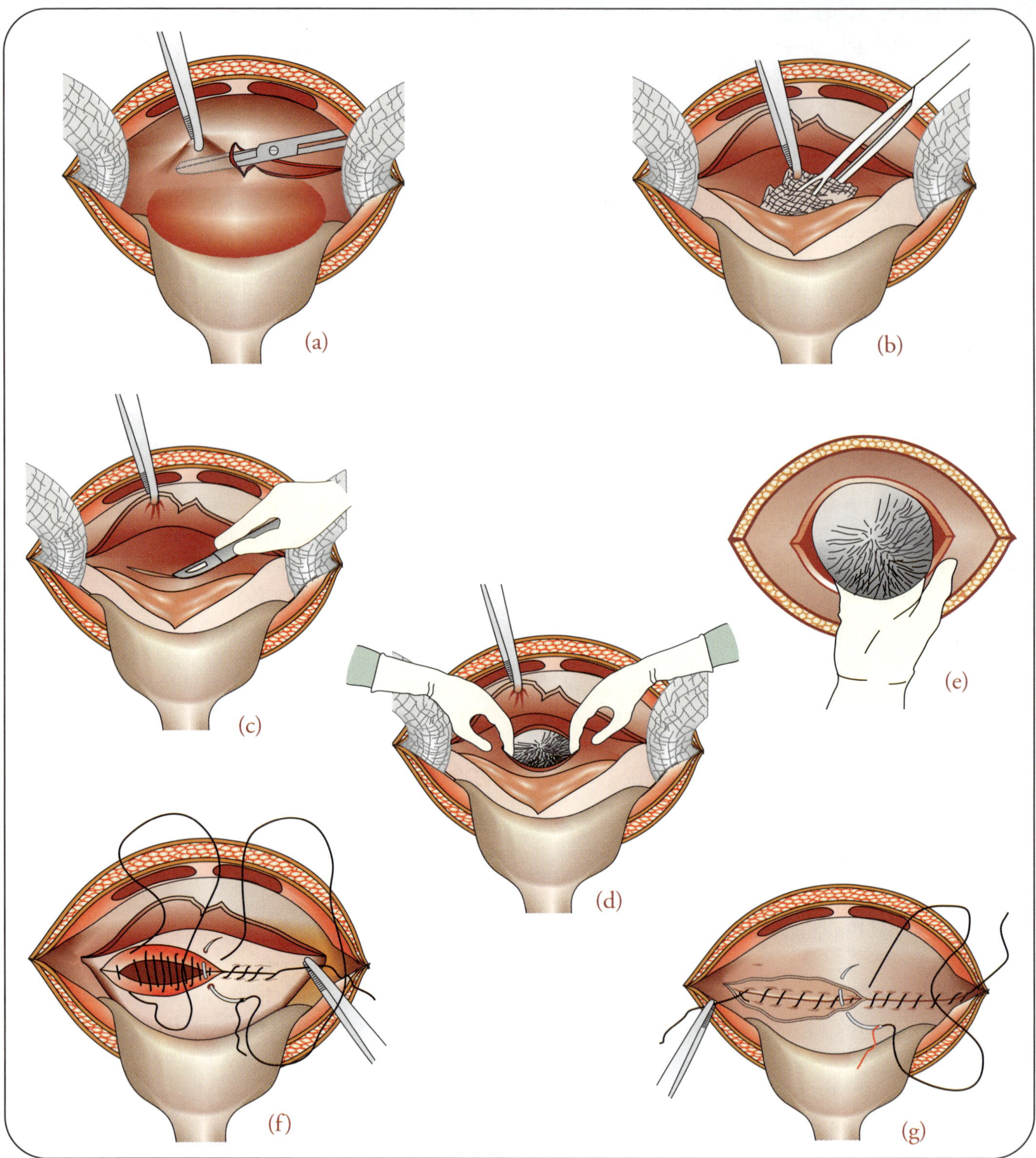

Fig. 32.1 Steps of LSCS a: Incision of utero-vesical peritoneum b: Mobilising the urinary bladder c: Incising the lower uterine segment d: The incision is extended laterally with fingers or scissors e: Delivery of fetal head through uterine incision f: Suturing of uterine incision g: Peritoneal suturing.

1. **Centralisation** of the uterus is recommended as the uterus is generally dextrorotated.
2. The **lower segment is identified.** The loose fold of uterovesical peritoneum is identified, cut and the bladder pushed down.
3. *Incision of lower segment:* A Doyen's retractor is placed at the lower edge of the incision to keep the bladder out of the operating field. A 2 cm incision is made on the lower segment, 1 cm below the upper margin of the reflected peritoneum; it may be placed higher in women with near-full dilatation of the cervix to minimise lateral extension of the incision. The incision is then extended with scissors or stretched with fingers and should be large enough to allow the delivery of the fetus. If the placenta is encountered in the line of incision, it is either cut or separated; in such cases, the fetus must be delivered rapidly and the cord clamped to prevent fetal hemorrhage.
4. *Delivery of the fetus:* In cephalic presentation, a hand is inserted between the head and the symphysis pubis and the head is levered out gently using the fingers and palm through the incision, keeping it flexed, aided by gentle fundal pressure. In order to prevent aspiration of blood or liquor by the fetus, the mouth and nares are sucked out. Then the shoulders and the trunk are delivered slowly, the umbilical cord is divided between clamps and the baby is handed over to the neonatologist. The anesthesiologist is requested to administer the antibiotic and start slow infusion of 10 units of oxytocin with the delivery of the anterior shoulder to ensure uterine contractions. The angles of the uterine incision and any bleeding points on the edges of the wound are held with Green–Armytage hemostatic clamps.
5. *Delivery of placenta:* Within 1–5 minutes of the delivery of the baby, the placenta separates: gentle traction on the cord will be sufficient to deliver the placenta. In case it does not separate, one should check if the uterus is contracted; if the uterus is not contracted, an additional dose of oxytocin is infused or 0.2 mg of methyl ergometrine is injected intravenously and the placenta removed manually. Care is taken to remove the membranes entirely.
6. *Closure of uterine incision:* It is generally closed in two layers using either a delayed absorbable suture like polyglycolic acid 1/0 or chromic catgut No. 1. The first layer is closed by continuous suture including the inner two-thirds of the myometrium. The suture should begin and end beyond the angles of the incision. The second layer includes the remaining one-third of the myometrium and the sutures are taken so as to bury the the first layer (**Lembert sutures**). Any individual bleeding vessels are best ligated separately. It is essential to ensure hemostasis. The incision can also be closed in a single layer using delayed absorbable suture. It has been found to be as good as double layer closure.

   Exteriorising the uterus through the incision has the advantage that the uterine incision can be inspected thoroughly and it also permits early recognition of uterine relaxation. It also helps to recognise conditions like fibroid and inspect the adnexae.

   The visceral peritoneum over the lower uterine incision is closed with loosely placed continuous suture using 1/0 chromic catgut. It can also be left unsutured with no adverse effects on healing. The abdominal packs, if any, are removed and the peritoneal cavity is cleaned. The surgeon must ensure that no pack or instrument is left in the peritoneal cavity.
7. *Closure of abdominal wall:* It is closed in layers. Parietal peritoneum closure is optional. The rectus sheath is closed with a nonabsorbable suture. The subcutaneous layer is closed with 2/0 chromic catgut if it is more than 2 cm thick. After ensuring hemostasis, skin edges are approximated with cotton sutures. Alternatively, subcuticular closure can be done with 3/0 polyglycolic acid suture. A dressing is applied over the wound.
8. *Vaginal toilet:* The vagina is gently cleaned to remove all blood clots. Urinary catheter may be removed or left in situ for a variable period as decided by the surgeon.

Classical cesarean section

In some situations it may be necessary to perform a classical CS. Those indications are listed below:

- the lower segment cannot be exposed due to extensive adhesion of the bladder or the presence of a fibroid
- a classical CS reduces the risk of excessive bleeding and dissemination of cervical carcinoma
- some cases of transverse lie with a large fetus and anterior implantation of the placenta previa.

The uterine incision in the upper segment is begun in the midline with a scalpel above the level of attachment of the bladder and extended above for 12 to 15 cm with scissors to obtain enough space. The fetus is delivered as breech, getting hold of its foot. The placenta is removed as described earlier. The upper segment is much thicker and more vascular than the lower segment and it involutes actively during puerperium. So, healing of the classical incision is not as good as with a lower segment incision.

Postoperative care

Monitoring of vital signs: The vital signs are monitored carefully and excessive vaginal bleeding checked for; the fundus of the uterus is palpated to assess the status of the uterus. Urine output is measured.

Intravenous fluids: Most cases of cesarean section are kept nil orally for about 12 hours and intravenous fluids are administered. The decision to discontinue intravenous fluids is based on the return of bowel sounds. For a woman who undergoes CS under regional anesthesia, oral fluids may be given earlier.

Antibiotics: Surgical antibiotic prophylaxis with one dose with clamping of the umbilical cord is adequate for most cases. However, for those who are operated following prolonged rupture of membranes or those at increased risk of infection, it is advisable to continue antibiotics.

Bladder and bowel care: The catheter may be removed the morning after surgery or once oral fluids are started. She can start taking a soft diet after she passes flatus.

Early ambulation: The woman is encouraged to move out of bed early, preferably within 24 hours.

Breastfeeding: The baby is put to breast as early as possible.

Discharge from hospital: After an uncomplicated CS, most women are discharged on the third or fourth day after delivery. If the skin sutures need to be removed, she may return on the eighth postoperative day.

Intraoperative complications

Injury to other organs: The urinary bladder is at risk of being injured, particularly if it is distended, edematous or adherent due to previous surgery. Bowel injury may rarely occur while opening the abdomen if there are extensive adhesions.

Extension of the angle of uterine incision: In cesarean sections done when the head is deeply engaged as in advanced labour or if dextrorotation is not corrected, the angle of the uterine incision may extend and involve the uterine vessels, resulting in profuse bleeding.

Postoperative complications

Excessive bleeding: This is often due to uterine atony and usually responds to oxytocics; blood should be transfused. If the uterus continues to be relaxed, or the bleeding continues from a well-contracted uterus, the woman must be taken up for exploratory laparotomy to institute surgical measures to control the bleeding.

Febrile morbidity: When it occurs, it points to a focus of infection. Identify the site and nature of organisms responsible for the infection and administer appropriate antibiotics. Check for the presence of thrombophlebitis.

Wound infection: The risk of wound sepsis is high in a woman who undergoes CS as there is a wound on the uterus and the abdominal wall, besides the placental site. However, it is more common among women who had prolonged rupture of membranes, who had several vaginal examinations or in whom there is a focus of infection elsewhere in the body.

Urinary tract infection is basically related to catheterisation. Great care must be taken to exercise aseptic and antiseptic precautions while inserting a bladder catheter. Infection is also related to the duration of catheterisation.

Paralytic ileus: This may occur due to infection and sometimes due to hypokalemia. Both of these conditions are seen in women who have had prolonged labour. Gastric aspiration, witholding oral feeds, restoration of fluid and electrolyte balance are the mainstay of treatment.

Maternal morbidity and mortality

Delivery by CS requires anesthesia; it is also associated with greater blood loss (1,000 ml) as compared to a vaginal delivery. It is well documented that the risk of both maternal morbidity and mortality are significantly higher in CS. It may be argued that the risk is higher when there are associated complications. However, like any other surgery, CS should not be performed in the absence of an indication.

Measures to contain cesarean rates

There is universal concern about the rising rates of cesarean section and attempts are being made to contain it. One of the reasons for the high rates of CS is repeat CS. The measures to reduce the rates of CS are to:

- exercise greater discrimination in performing the first CS
- seek a second opinion
- consider vaginal delivery when possible in post-cesarean pregnancies

Post-cesarean Pregnancy

The management of a pregnant woman who has had a CS earlier calls for a thorough evaluation before planning the mode of delivery. Successful vaginal delivery is possible if there is only a small risk of scar rupture. For a woman with previous LSCS, the chances of successful vaginal delivery are 40%–60% or more, and the risk of scar rupture during delivery is 0.3%–2%. Therefore, an evaluation is made keeping in mind the following points:

Indication for previous CS: If the indication was contracted pelvis, it is a recurrent indication. Non-recurrent indications like fetal distress or transverse lie are favourable for vaginal delivery.

Type of scar: A woman with a scar in the upper segment or with a T-shaped scar which is prone to rupture should never be considered for vaginal delivery.

Number of previous CSs: The risk of scar rupture increases with the number of cesarean sections performed in the past. If the woman has undergone two or more LSCSs, the condition is unfavourable for vaginal delivery.

Prior vaginal delivery: If there has been a normal delivery after or before a CS, it greatly improves the chances of vaginal delivery.

Complications during the previous section: Extension of angle and/or postoperative sepsis increase the risk and suggest repeat section.

Maternal complications: Presence of any maternal complications is a contraindication for vaginal delivery

Size of the fetus and maternal pelvis: The fetus should be of average size and should be presenting by vertex. The pelvis should be adequately wide.

Management during labour

In a woman with previous LSCS, the delivery must be in a well-equipped hospital. A unit of blood is cross-matched and kept readily available. The woman is permitted a fluid diet. She is monitored very closely for pulse and fetal heart sounds. Maternal tachycardia, fetal heart abnormalities, tenderness in the suprapubic region, blood-stained urine and bleeding per vaginum are indicative of impending scar rupture: the woman must be taken up for CS.

If the progress of labour is satisfactory, the second stage of labour should be cut short using outlet forceps. The placenta and the membranes are delivered. There is no need to routinely explore the lower segment for scar rupture. This may be done if there is any sign of scar rupture. The uterus is explored and a laparotomy is indicated if the blood loss is excessive or scar rupture is detected.

As an operation, CS has become safe with the availability of antibiotics, blood transfusion and safe anesthesia. It is less safe than a vaginal delivery and the operation should be used only when indicated.

KEY POINTS

- Cesarean section (CS) is a surgical procedure where the baby is delivered after making an incision in the abdominal wall and the uterus.
- It is the most frequently performed major obstetric operation.
- The operation is associated with all the complications of surgery and anesthesia.
- The maternal mortality in CS is seven times higher than in vaginal delivery, and morbidity is several folds higher.
- The woman must be given proper pre- and postoperative care.
- In order to reduce the risk of postoperative infection, a single dose of antibiotic should be given intravenously with clamping of the umbilical cord.
- Increasing the rate of CS has not contributed to reduction in perinatal mortality.

QUESTIONS

Select the single most appropriate answer:

1. The commonest indication for cesarean section is
   a. fetal distress
   b. placenta previa
   c. cephalopelvic disproportion
   d. breech presentation
2. In which one of the following conditions is cesarean section performed to prevent obstructed labour?
   a. placental abruption c. contracted pelvis
   b. fetal distress d. diabetes mellitus
3. A woman presents at term pregnancy with a previous cesarean section. For which condition should she undergo an elective cesarean section for her current pregnancy?
   a. first cesarean section was done for fetal distress
   b. she had wound infection after the first cesarean section
   c. there was no extension of the angle of the uterine incision
   d. the woman was in labour when the first cesarean section was performed
4. The average blood loss during a lower segment cesarean section is
   a. 400 ml c. 800 ml
   b. 600 ml d. 1,000 ml

Select the appropriate answer using the following key:

a. if only responses 1, 2 and 3 are correct
b. if only 1 and 3 are correct
c. if only 2 and 4 are correct
d. if only 4 is correct
e. if all are correct

5. In a woman with breech presentation and no element of pelvic contraction, elective cesarean section is recommended if
   1. the estimated weight of the baby is 2,500 g
   2. the woman has preeclampsia
   3. the estimated weight of the baby is 3,000 g
   4. the estimated weight of the baby is 3,500 g
6. A classical cesarean section should be performed in a pregnant woman with cancer of the uterine cervix in order to
   1. avoid excessive bleeding
   2. prevent obstructed labour
   3. prevent dissemination of the cancer
   4. be able to administer radiotherapy

In the following questions, there are two statements. Select the appropriate answer using the following key:

a. if both statements are true and causally related
b. if both statements are true but not causally related
c. if the first statement is true and the second is false
d. if the first statement is false and the second is true
e. if both statements are false

7. A lower segment cesarean section is preferred over classical cesarean section *because*
   A lower segment cesarean section has significantly lower risk of scar rupture in a subsequent pregnancy.
8. It is not desirable to perform a large number of cesarean sections *because*
   An increased number of cesarean sections does not necessarily reduce the perinatal mortality rate.

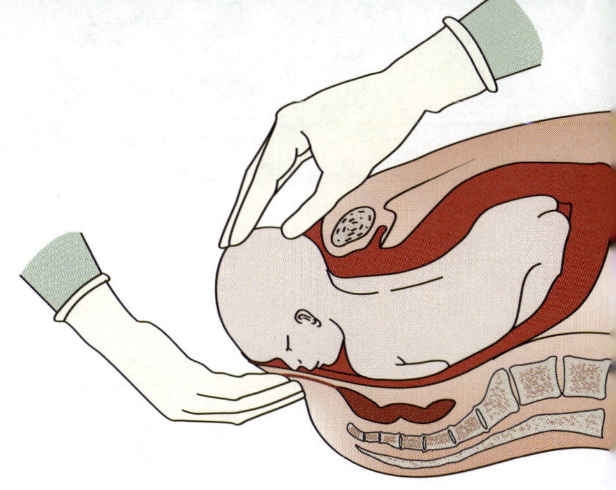

33

Complications of the Third Stage of Labour

N Sundari

LEARNING OBJECTIVES

At the end of this chapter, the reader should be able to:

- define the third stage of labour
- recapitulate the physiology of the third stage of labour
- enumerate the complications of the third stage of labour
- define postpartum hemorrhage (PPH)
- enumerate the causes of PPH and the predisposing factors
- list the clinical features of PPH
- assess the hemodynamic changes in the mother
- describe immediate management and refer appropriately
- enumerate the measures that can prevent PPH
- outline the management of the complications
- appreciate that hemorrhage due to complications of the third stage account for significant maternal mortality and morbidity

Introduction

The third stage of labour extends from the delivery of the fetus till the complete delivery of the placenta. This stage is associated with more complications than the first two stages. The complications that arise during this period are postpartum hemorrhage (PPH), retained placenta and inversion of the uterus. The obstetrician is often caught unawares as these complications can occur suddenly. Therefore, the third stage of labour is believed to be the most treacherous; a successful delivery can turn into a disaster within minutes. Along with other causes of hemorrhage in obstetrics, the third stage complications account for 25% of maternal deaths in India.

Physiology of the third stage of labour

After the delivery of the fetus, the uterus contracts and retracts leading to separation of the placenta and its expulsion. There is kinking of the stretched uterine vessels. Further, the vessels are occluded as they pass between the uterine muscle fibres, which act as 'living ligatures'; this phenomenon effectively prevents blood flow and promotes thrombosis of the vessels (**Fig. 33.1**).

Primary Postpartum Hemorrhage

Definition

Primary postpartum hemorrhage is defined as blood loss of more than 500 ml occurring within 24 hours

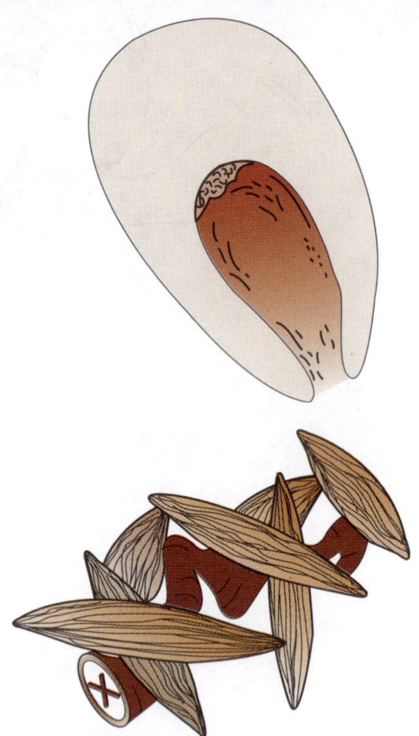

Fig. 33.1 Living ligatures.

of delivery. It includes blood loss from the placental site, due to retained placenta and membranes and injury to the genital tract.

Women who are anemic are likely to be adversely affected even with hemorrhage of less than 500 ml. It is also difficult to assess the amount of bleeding accurately, especially if it occurs as a continuous trickle or the blood is collected in the uterine cavity. Hence, one must go by the general condition of the woman rather than the quantity of blood loss.

Etiology

In 80% of cases, primary PPH is due to uterine atony, where the uterus fails to contract and occlude the blood vessels in the placental bed. In others, retention of the placenta and membranes, lacerations of the genital tract including rupture of the uterus and blood dyscrasias are responsible.

Predisposing factors: Primary PPH can occur unexpectedly, but there are several conditions that make a woman prone to uterine atony. Check for these in every woman who seeks obstetric care to prevent the hemorrhage or deal with it early and effectively when it occurs. The following factors predispose a woman to PPH:

History: Multiparity, occurrence of PPH in previous deliveries or blood dyscrasias

Overdistension of the uterus: This due to multiple pregnancy, large baby and polyhydramnios. In all these conditions, the uterine muscle fibres are overstretched and fail to respond to endogenous oxytocin. The placental area is large with an increase in the number of blood vessels in case of multiple pregnancy and a large baby.

Prolonged labour: The element of uterine inefficiency may continue through the third stage of labour.

Precipitate labour: Since various events of labour occur in rapid succession, there is insufficient time for the uterus to contract and retract, resulting in atony and bleeding.

Antepartum hemorrhage: Fibroids and uterine malformations interfere with effective uterine contractions.

Oxytocin use for induction or augmentation: If oxytocin has been used for induction or augmentation of labour, it should be continued for at least 1–2 hours after delivery to prevent uterine atony.

Drugs: Magnesium sulphate, anesthetic agents like halothane and ether can interfere with uterine contractions.

Mismanaged third stage of labour: Attempts to deliver the placenta before it is separated, massaging or squeezing the uterus, undue cord traction, non-use of prophylactic oxytocics can cause PPH.

Clinical features

The diagnosis is obvious in most cases, except when the blood is collected in the uterine cavity which gets distended; whenever there is a contraction, blood is expelled. The loss is usually intermittent.

The general condition of the woman will depend on the amount of blood loss. The pulse rate, blood pressure and urine output should be carefully monitored. When a woman bleeds after delivery, a hand on the uterus will reveal whether PPH is atonic or traumatic; a flabby uterus indicates atony and if the uterus is well contracted, it suggests traumatic PPH.

Management of Postpartum Hemorrhage

Since PPH can unexpectedly complicate even normal deliveries, the attending physician should anticipate and be prepared to prevent and treat the condition.

Preventive measures

Prevention begins during the antenatal period. Every effort must be made to detect and treat anemia. Women who are prone to develop PPH must be advised to deliver in institutions equipped to deal with emergencies.

During labour, the possibility of PPH must be anticipated in women at risk. Blood should be cross-matched and kept available. After the delivery of the baby, one must watch for signs of placental separation before attempting to deliver the placenta.

Active management of the third stage of labour (AMTSL) and avoidance of unnecessary handling of the uterus reduce postpartum blood loss. Active management consists of:

1. Administration of prophylactic oxytocic, 0.2 mg of methergin intravenously or carboprost 125 µg intramuscularly with the delivery of the anterior shoulder, or oxytocin 5–10 units IM after the delivery of the baby. Misoprostol 400 µg can be administered orally or rectally. It is particularly useful in peripheral health facilities as it is heat stable, relatively cheap and easy to administer.
2. Early clamping of the umbilical cord.
3. Delivery of the placenta by controlled cord traction (Brandt–Andrews' technique). A downward traction is applied to the cord and the uterus is pushed upwards and backwards.

Curative measures

The objectives of treatment of PPH are mainly to:

- arrest the bleeding
- replace the blood

Whenever there is excessive bleeding after delivery of the baby, it is most often due to uterine atony. Therefore, it is prudent to administer an oxytocic immediately. Intravenous access should be obtained with a large bore cannula. Blood should be collected for cross-matching, estimation of hemoglobin and, if indicated, for the evaluation of serum electrolytes. Until blood is available, crystalloids are used to restore the fluid volume; the best crystalloid for replacement is Ringer lactate. An indwelling catheter is inserted in the urinary bladder to empty it as a full bladder can interfere with uterine contractions; it is also useful in monitoring urine output. The woman's pulse, respiration and blood pressure should be monitored continuously. In order to allay anxiety, the woman should be briefed about the hemorrhage and reassured that all efforts are being made to arrest it; she should be injected with 15 mg of morphine IM or 100 mg of pethidine. The woman's relatives must be kept informed about her condition.

Further management will depend on whether the placenta has been delivered or not.

Third stage bleeding

If hemorrhage occurs before expulsion of the placenta, the uterus must be massaged gently to produce contractions; controlled cord traction must be performed to deliver the placenta, if it has separated. If these measures fail, further intervention is advised depending on the place of delivery. If facilities for anesthesia are not available, a second dose of methergin/oxytocin is administered and the woman is referred to a better-equipped hospital for further management.

PPH after delivery of the placenta

Hemorrhage that starts or persists after the expulsion of the placenta is referred to as **true PPH** as it occurs after all the stages of labour are completed. Immediate measures must be instituted, as discussed earlier. If not already given, 0.2 mg of methergin must be injected intravenously; the fundus of the uterus is massaged. The placenta is examined to check for missing cotyledons; if missing, the uterine cavity must be explored and the remnants removed. Meanwhile, if the uterus tends to relax, 20 units of oxytocin is added to 500 ml of Ringer lactate or 5% dextrose and administered at a rate that maintains the contracted state. More than 80% of cases of atonic PPH respond well to methyl ergometrine or oxytocin; the former has a wide margin of safety and can be repeated, 3–4 times if necessary. If these measures fail to produce uterine contractions, carboprost 250 μg should be administered intramuscularly.

Bimanual compression of the uterus is useful. The clenched fist of one hand is introduced in the anterior fornix while the other hand is placed on the abdomen, behind the fundus, bringing the uterus over the fist in the vagina: the uterus is compressed between both the hands (**Fig. 33.2**).

If all the above measures fail, surgical intervention must be considered. The procedure of choice is uterine artery ligation. Another intervention to arrest the hemorrhage effectively is the use of the B-Lynch suture. The procedure consists of oversewing the uterus with a polyglycolic suture passing through the anterior and posterior walls which is then tightened so as to compress the walls together (**Fig. 33.3**). Ligation of the anterior trunk of the internal iliac artery is a good method to arrest bleeding. Very rarely, hysterectomy may be required.

Another method to arrest hemorrhage is embolisation of the internal iliac artery or uterine artery. Attempts have been made to control uterine hemorrhage using a Foley's catheter with a 30 ml balloon. The tip of the catheter is guided into the uterine cavity and the balloon is inflated with 60–80 ml of saline and kept in situ for 12–24 hours. Blood from the uterine cavity drains through the open tip continuously.

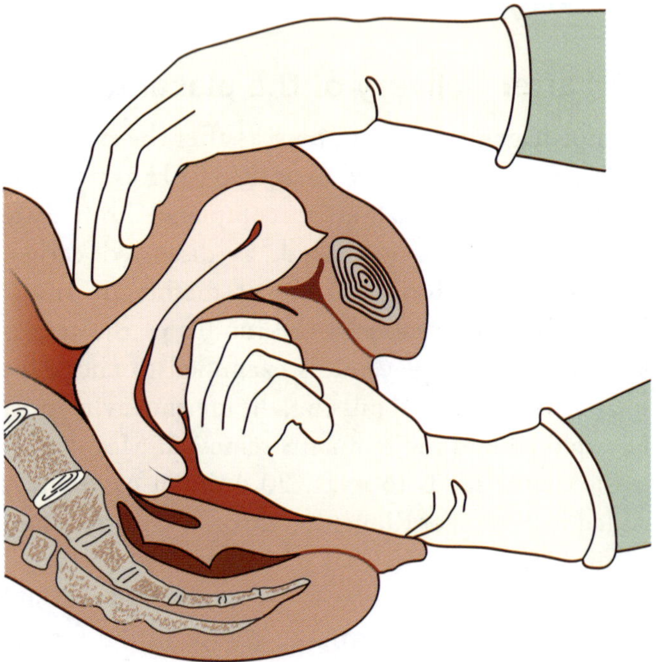

Fig. 33.2 Bimanual compression of the uterus.

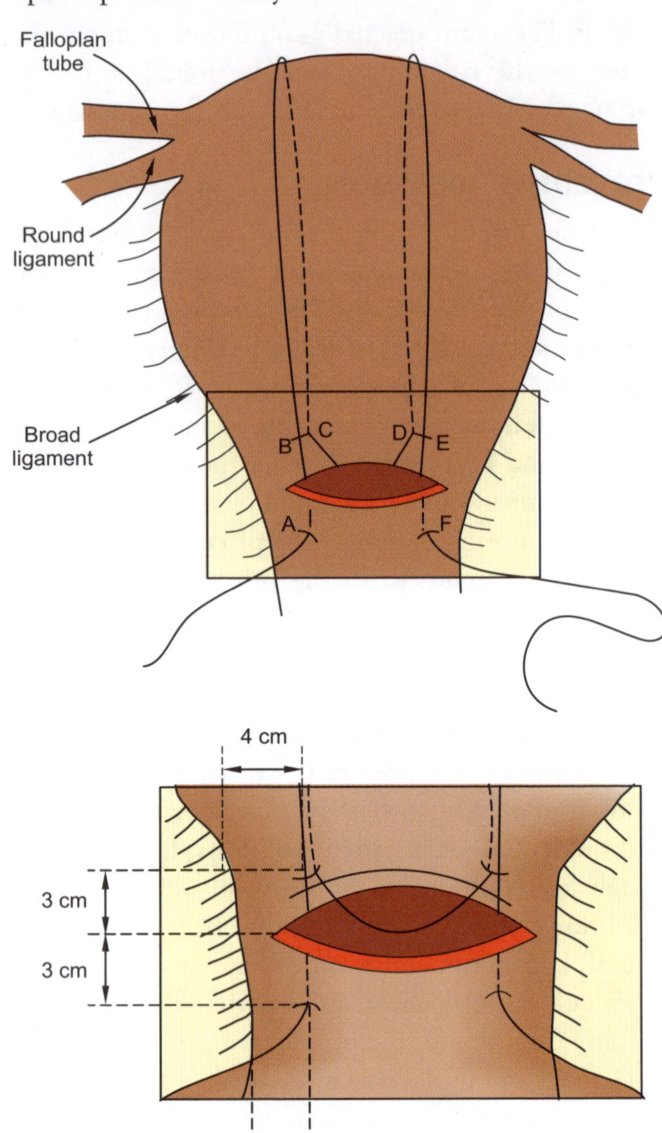

Fig. 33.3 Technique of B-Lynch suture for compression of uterus. The letters indicate the sequence in which the needle passes through the uterus A: The needle pierces the lower segment below the incision to enter the uterine cavity B: The needle comes out of the cavity above the incision C: The suture loops over the fundus and enters on the posterior surface of the uterus D: The needle exits on the opposite side and then loops over to the anterior aspect of the uterus E: The needle enters the cavity above the upper margin of the incision F: The needle exits below the lower margin of the incision.

The woman's blood volume must be restored adequately and early, particularly if she is anemic, the blood loss exceeds 1,000 ml or there is deterioration of the condition. If hypovolemia persists, central venous pressure is monitored to avoid overtransfusion. Evaluation of blood biochemistry is essential to avoid metabolic acidosis and respiratory alkalosis.

Traumatic PPH

Bleeding in spite of a contracted uterus points to traumatic PPH. The common sites of injury are the vulva, perineum, vagina and cervix. Instrumental deliveries increase the risk of injury. Even a delay in repairing an episiotomy may result in significant blood loss. Rarely, rupture of the uterus may be the cause of bleeding.

The essence of management lies in identifying the site of trauma and immediate repair, in addition to the general measures.

Retained Placenta

Definition: The placenta normally gets separated and is expelled soon after the delivery of the baby. The placenta is said to be retained if it is not expelled at the end of 30 minutes.The longer the placenta remains in the uterus, the greater is the risk to the mother of hemorrhage, shock and sepsis.

Etiology: A full bladder may cause the placenta to be retained. Uterine atony is an important cause of retained placenta, others being incarceration of a separated placenta by a constriction ring and adherent type placenta.

Management: Interventions like emptying the bladder and administration of an oxytocic are usually sufficient. If these measures fail, and even if there is no hemorrhage, the placenta must be manually removed (see under management of third stage hemorrhage).

Manual removal of the placenta: Under general anesthesia, the woman is placed in the lithotomy position; the perineum is cleaned and draped. A gloved hand is lubricated and introduced into the uterine cavity in a cone-shaped manner and the edge of the placenta is identified by following the cord. Keeping the palm facing the uterine cavity, the placenta is separated from its bed by a 'slicing' movement (**Fig. 33.4**). The other hand steadies the fundus during the maneuver. Once the placenta lies freely in the cavity, it is brought out and 0.2 mg of methergin is injected intravenously. The placenta is inspected to ensure completeness; if there is any doubt, it is best to explore the uterine cavity.

Adherent Placenta

Definition: Adherent placenta occurs when the trophoblast penetrates to a variable degree through the decidua up to the myometrium. It is labelled **placenta accreta** when the placental villi are attached to the myometrium, and known as **placenta increta** or **percreta** in more advanced forms. In the last type, the trophoblast invades through the full thickness of the myometrium.

Etiology: Adherent placenta may be the result of previous infection following manual removal of placenta or repeated curettage.

Clinical features: The condition is suspected when the placenta is retained despite a contracted uterus and there is no bleeding, or occasionally while attempting manual removal.

Management: It is difficult to remove the placenta completely; if there is hemorrhage, oxytocics could be used. As some placental tissue may remain, one must anticipate complications like hemorrhage, infection and formation of placental polyp.

Inversion of Uterus

Definition: Inversion of the uterus is a very rare condition in which the uterus turns inside out. It is classified as partial when the fundus of the uterus is seen at the cervix and complete when whole uterus appears outside the vulva (**Fig. 33.5**).

Etiology: Following delivery, the cervix is well dilated. Traction on the cord before placental separation, fundal attachment or adherent placenta, pressure on the fundus and a flaccid uterus can precipitate inversion.

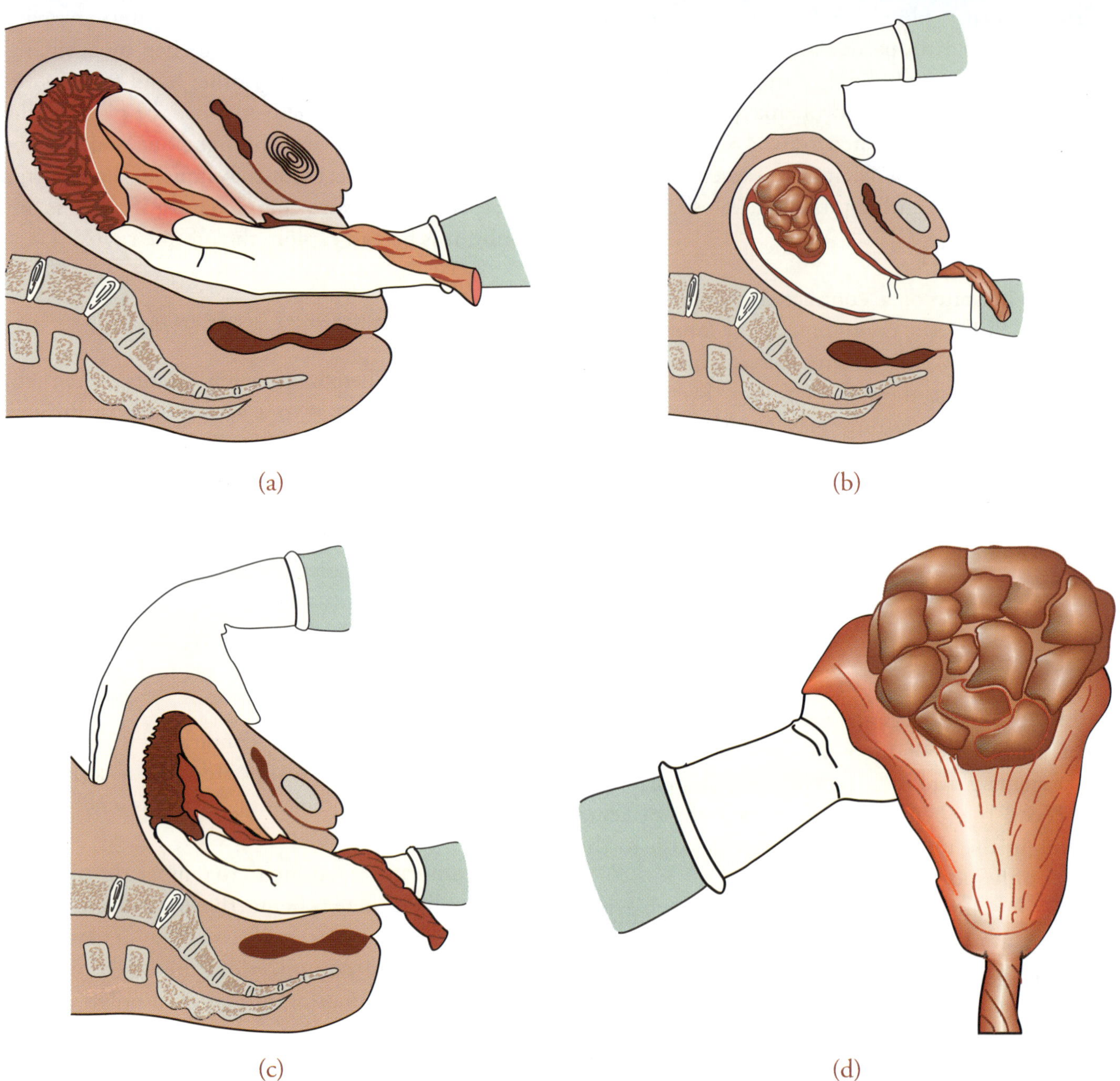

Fig. 33.4 Manual removal of the placenta.

Clinical features: The woman may complain of severe pain. Shock follows a little later, particularly if the inversion is complete, and it may be neurogenic or hypovolemic. On abdominal examination, the uterus is not palpable. On inspection of the vulva, a reddish mass is seen; on vaginal examination, the cervical rim is felt around the mass.

Treatment: Injection of morphine 15 mg will help in relieving pain. If the inversion is partial and the woman is not in shock, the placenta is removed and manual replacement is attempted under anesthesia. When the woman is in shock, the shock is treated and then the uterus is replaced.

Secondary Postpartum Hemorrhage

Definition: **Secondary postpartum hemorrhage** is defined as excessive bleeding occurring more than 24 hours after delivery, and within six weeks postpartum. However, it generally occurs between days 5 and 15 postpartum.

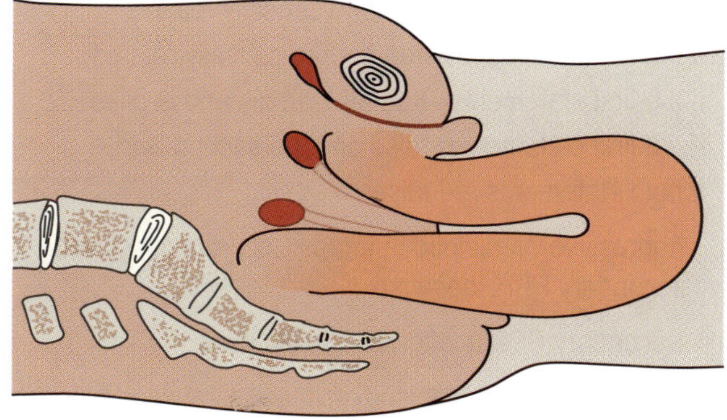

Fig. 33.5 Inversion of the uterus.

Etiology: Secondary PPH is often due to retained products and/or infection causing delayed epithelialisation of the placental site. Other causes are placental polyp, a submucous fibroid and, rarely, choriocarcinoma.

Management: Besides bleeding, the woman may complain of fever and malaise especially in the presence of infection. Ultrasonography helps detect retained products. Aggressive antibiotic therapy is effective in most cases. If there are retained products, they should be removed under anesthesia by curetting the cavity. Blood loss is replaced, if needed.

KEY POINTS

- Complications of the third stage of labour contribute significantly to maternal mortality and morbidity.
- Primary PPH is the commonest complication and is defined as blood loss of more than 500 ml after the delivery of the baby and within the first 24 hours.
- Secondary PPH refers to abnormal bleeding 24 hours after delivery and within six weeks.
- Primary PPH is most frequently due to uterine atony and responds well to oxytocics.
- Identification of risk factors and active management of the third stage of labour reduce the occurrence of PPH.
- If the hemorrhage is not arrested with the initial treatment, the woman should be referred to an institution where blood transfusion and operation theatre facilities are available.
- The other complications of the third stage of labour are retained placenta, adherent placenta and inversion of the uterus.
- The consequences of complications of the third stage of labour can be minimised by correcting anemia during the antenatal period and judicious management of labour.

QUESTIONS

Select the single most appropriate answer:

1. The most common complication of the third stage of labour is
   a. acute inversion of the uterus
   b. amniotic fluid embolism
   c. postpartum hemorrhage
   d. obstetric shock
2. The normal duration of the third stage of labour is
   a. 15 minutes c. 45 minutes
   b. 30 minutes d. 60 minutes
3. Postpartum hemorrhage is defined as blood loss of more than
   a. 500 ml c. 900 ml
   b. 700 ml d. 1,100 ml
4. Active management of the third stage of labour includes all of the following *except*
   a. controlled cord traction
   b. administration of an oxytocic

c. massaging of the uterus
d. early clamping of the cord

5. The most common cause of postpartum hemorrhage is
a. uterine atony
b. injury to the genital tract
c. coagulation disorders
d. fibroid polyp

6. The most common cause of acute uterine inversion is
a. pedunculated fibroid
b. fundal pressure given during delivery
c. failure to administer an oxytocic
d. credes technique used for the delivery of the placenta

7. The placenta is said to be retained when it is not delivered after how many minutes of the delivery of the baby?
a. 20 minutes
b. 30 minutes
c. 40 minutes
d. 50 minutes

8. When a woman continues to bleed after delivery and the uterus is well contracted, one must
a. administer methergin
b. examine the placenta for completeness
c. look for coagulation failure
d. look for genital tract injury

In the following questions, there are two statements. Select the appropriate answer using the following key:

a. if both statements are true and causally related
b. if both statements are true but not causally related
c. if the first statement is true and the second is false
d. if the first statement is false and the second is true
e. if both statements are false

9. Aggressive antibiotic therapy is recommended for secondary PPH *because*

Secondary PPH is often due to infection.

10. When there is no bleeding in case of retained placenta, it need not be removed *because*

Retained placenta is unlikely to result in any complication.

34

Care of the Newborn

S Mahadevan

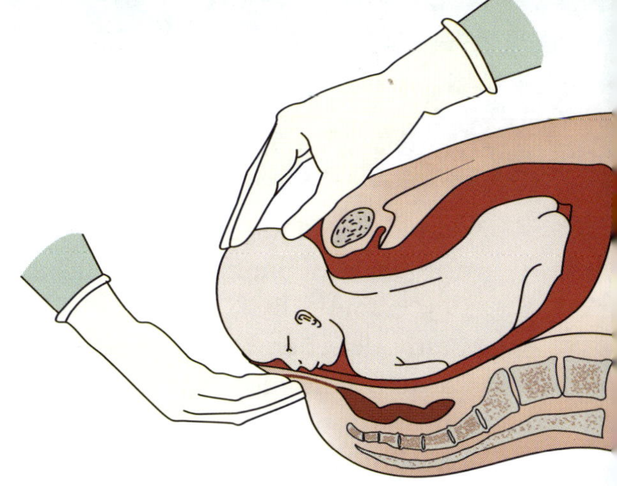

LEARNING OBJECTIVES

At the end of this chapter, the reader should be able to:

- appreciate the importance of neonatal care
- list the objectives of neonatal care
- enumerate the steps to be taken while attending to a newborn at birth
- follow the guidelines for cutting and taking care of the umbilical cord
- enumerate the various measurements to be taken in a newborn
- outline the basic examination of the newborn
- identify and manage common problems in the newborn

Introduction

The first week of life is a period of great vulnerability for the newborn because adaptation to a separate existence must occur rapidly and successfully. It depends largely on fetal health. The most frequent problems of the first three days are related to the establishment of cardio-respiratory functions, although inadequacy of other systems may also cause symptoms and signs (often vague and nonspecific). Most congenital abnormalities can be detected during the first week. The remaining three weeks of the neonatal period carry the common and serious hazards of infection and failure of satisfactory nutrition. Much more rarely, congenital heart or renal disease is responsible for serious morbidity and mortality.

At this time, the mother is also undergoing a process of physical and mental adaptation, establishment of lactation, development of a satisfactory mother–child relationship and adjustment to the return to normal family life.

While it may be best to have a pediatrician/neonatologist to attend to a newborn, this is often not practicable. Hence, the obstetrician or doctor attending to the parturient woman should be able to provide basic care to the newborn.

As serious problems may afflict infants in the first month, all personnel responsible for their care should be able to detect early signs of deviation from normal and know how to prevent malnutrition and infection: the two most important problems.

Objectives of Newborn Care

In order to impart optimum care, the following objectives should be achieved.

Adaptation from fetus to independent existence:

- initial clinical examination with further planned examinations at the intervals necessary for assessment of progress
- establishment and maintenance of respiration
- maintenance of body temperature by suitable ambient temperature and clothing
- establishment of a satisfactory feeding regime

- avoidance of infection and administration of such prophylactic immunisation as may be indicated, for example, BCG
- early detection and treatment of congenital and acquired disorders, especially infection
- it must be ensured that the baby remains healthy and that the mother is given adequate instruction on the general care and nutrition of her baby.

Follow-up care:

- close supervision of all babies, wherever they are born, by nursing/midwifery and other suitably trained personnel either at home or at health facilities
- organising special clinics by pediatricians, either at the hospital or health centre, for certain categories of babies who are at risk of sequelae of early neonatal problems.

Immediate care of the newborn at birth

The following procedures can be recommended for regular practice.

- The persons attending on the newborn should wash their hands, wear a clean gown and mask or at least clean clothes.
- As soon as the baby's head is born, the eyelids are wiped from the inner to the outer canthus with dry sterile swabs; the nostrils are also cleaned with a sterile swab.
- As soon as the baby is born and before the cord is cut, it is lifted by the ankles, head down, holding the ankles with the left hand, supporting the head with the right hand to facilitate drainage of any secretions. At this stage, the baby is shown to the mother so that she sees the sex of the baby. The air passages are cleared by suction. Swabs and fingers should not be used for this purpose as there is a risk of damage to the mucosa and infection. The Apgar score is recorded, and the baby is kept in a horizontal position (**Table 34.1**).
- The baby is wrapped in a clean towel on the bed or across the mother's chest or abdomen to maintain body heat.
- The baby is labelled with a name-tape or band on the left wrist.

Table 34.1 Constituents of the Apgar score

		0	1	2
A	Appearance or colour	Pale	Blue	Pink
P	Pulse rate	Absent	<100	≥100
G	Grimace	Nil	Grimace	Cry and cough
A	Activity (tone)	Limp	Some flexion	Well flexed
R	Respiratory effort	Absent	Gasping or irregular	Strong cry

- As soon as the cord has ceased pulsating, it is cut and the baby is separated from the mother.

Care of the umbilical cord

Procedure for cutting the cord: The cord is covered with the hand or gauze before cutting to prevent blood splashing; it is cut with sterile scissors or scalpel. The cord is tied with a sterile thread 2.5 cm from the skin or clamped with a plastic clamp. A sterile rubber band may be applied instead of a plastic clamp or thread ligature by holding the cord with artery forceps and stretching the band and twisting it around the cord until it is tight. The end of the cord is dabbed on a sterile gauze swab to remove blood and adequate ligation of cord can be ensured by checking for bleeding. The umbilical cord contains two arteries and one vein; the presence of a single umbilical artery may be associated with malformations.

Avoidance of hemorrhage: Wharton's jelly is applied on the ligated and severed cord; it shrinks rapidly so that within 2–8 hours of birth, ligatures may become slack and bleeding can occur from the cord vessels. This risk can be minimised if a correctly applied rubber band or plastic disposable clamp is used. The rubber band is cheap, easy to sterilise and widely available. Plastic disposable clamps are easy to use but may occasionally slip off; the disadvantages are cost and lack of availability. The cord **must be inspected** for bleeding every 2–6 hours.

Separation of the cord: The cord dries, shrivels up and separates by aseptic necrosis from the enfolded umbilical skin in 5–8 days; thereafter, the moist area around the base rapidly heals and is epithelialised. The application of sterile zinc and starch powder, dressing or certain paints and sprays assist this drying process.

Prevention of infection: Infection introduced while cutting the cord, or before the cord dries and the vessels are effectively sealed, causes bacteremia, septicemia or portal pyelophlebitis. The risk of sepsis, particularly tetanus, is increased when deliveries are conducted in unclean surroundings and aseptic precautions are not followed.

Infection delays necrosis and separation of the cord. Until the umbilicus is completely healed, bacterial colonisation in this area is considerably greater than elsewhere on the surface of the body. Pathogenic organisms, especially *Staphylococcus aureus,* hemolytic streptococci, *E coli* and *Pseudomonas pyocyaneus* can be found around the base of the cord at the end of 48 hours in a considerable proportion of infants. This reservoir of bacterial colonisation may cause lesions elsewhere on the body and act as a source of infection for other babies, particularly in hospitals.

To reduce the risk of infection, an effective antiseptic preparation (such as povidone iodine, chlorhexidine, hexachlorophane in zinc and starch powder or triple dye in alcohol) can be applied on the cord and on the skin of the abdomen: this is the most important step for reducing neonatal infection.

Resuscitation of the Newborn

The majority of babies are born normal and cry vigorously at birth when the first breath is taken. In intrauterine life, the lungs are filled with fluid and circulation to the lungs is minimal because of high resistance in pulmonary vessels. The production of fluids in the lungs stops during labour and absorption also begins. Whatever fluid remains is squeezed out of the thorax during labour. When the infant takes the first breath, an air–liquid interface is created which moves down to the alveoli and air enters the alveoli. The resistance in the pulmonary vasculature falls and blood supply increases. This is aided by prostaglandins and nitric oxide.

Infants who have compromised blood supply to the brain (hypoxemia), those with CNS or muscle diseases and those with sepsis may fail to breathe at birth. The Apgar score helps to identify these infants who need resuscitation and dictates the extent of resuscitation. The personnel who attend to the delivery should be able to identify infants who need resuscitation.

- Babies who are pink, breathing and active with a heart rate of ≥100 should be left alone with the mother after cleaning, drying and being wrapped in a towel. Suction is not necessary and may even be harmful in these cases.
- Babies not breathing properly, but with a heart rate of ≥100 and central cyanosis should be wiped dry and placed in a warmer. The stimulation of handling may induce breathing. If the baby does not settle with oropharyngeal suction and oxygen, active resuscitation should begin.
- Babies who are not breathing and have a heart rate of ≤100 and are pale and cyanotic need to be actively resuscitated. Initially, ventilation is done with a mask and some babies will show improvement with this. If the heart rate remains low (around 60 bpm), chest compression should be started, with intubation and assisted ventilation. If the mother has received a narcotic analgesic during labour, naloxone will reverse its respiratory depressive effect.

The **categories** of babies needing different levels of neonatal care are as follows.

Level 1 nursery or postnatal ward: With adequate supervision, babies who need parenteral fluids, tube feeds, phototherapy or monitoring of glucose or bilirubin levels may be treated here.

Level 2 neonatal intensive care unit: Continuous skilled supervision, preferably by medical or trained nursing staff. Examples are babies who need parenteral nutrition, 40%–60% oxygenation, who have arterial lines or chest drains.

Level 3 or maximal neonatal intensive care unit: Here, continuous supervision by qualified and specially trained medical and nursing staff should be available. Babies receiving assisted ventilation including Continuous Positive Airways Pressure (CPAP), those who are born at 28–32 weeks of gestation and who weigh less than 1,000 g are placed here.

Subsequent care of the baby in the labour room

- The baby is placed lying on its right side.
- In order to avoid heat loss, the wet towel is removed, the skin gently mopped dry and the baby wrapped loosely in a clean towel and covered with a blanket.
- The cord is observed for hemorrhage.
- If there is any secretion present in the air passages, it is aspirated with a sterile rubber plastic catheter, bulb or electric suction.
- Rectal or skin temperature is recorded and extra protection provided if it is less than 36 °C.
- The baby is put to breast as early as possible.
- Most babies pass meconium soon after birth. If meconium has not been passed, a soft rubber catheter may be passed through the anus as this may facilitate meconium passage or help diagnose imperforate anus.

Measuring the baby (Anthropometry)

The measurements to be recorded are birth weight, that is, weight recorded within one hour of birth, length from crown to heel, or crown to rump and head circumference. These measurements are recorded in order to:

- assess the baby's size against known standards for the population
- compare the size with the estimated period of gestation
- provide a baseline against which subsequent growth can be monitored.

Birth weight: True birth weight is that recorded within an hour of birth. The naked baby should be placed on a clean scale pan. The sick or premature infant can sometimes be weighed in an incubator using a sling and spring balance. In home delivery, weight should be taken by placing the baby in a sling using a simple spring balance. Babies weighing less than 2.5 kg (low birth weight) and those weighing 4 kg or more will need extra attention.

Length: This need not be measured immediately if the baby's condition requires immediate attention for other reasons, but should be recorded within the first three days. Length can be taken most accurately with a measuring table or board with a fixed head piece on which the infant lies supine with its legs fully extended; it is necessary to press the knees lightly to ensure maximum length. The feet should be kept against the movable footpiece, with the ankles flexed to 90°. Two people are needed to hold the baby correctly and take the measurement. This measuring board may not be available, so improvisation with ruler or tape measure is often necessary. The average length of a term newborn is 50 cm.

Head circumference: This measurement may change slightly during the first three days owing to moulding during labour, scalp edema or bruising and cephalhematoma. It is taken with a tape measure at the maximum circumference of the head in the occipito-frontal diameter at the level of the parietal prominence and supraorbital ridges. At term, the head circumference measures 35 cm.

Examination of the Newborn Infant

The first examination should be made soon after birth and preferably in the delivery room, without undue disturbance to the baby and taking particular care not to expose the baby for too long. If necessary, the examination may be done in a warmer. This examination should be gentle, patient and done with the mother around. The baby is best examined when he/she is asleep or quietly awake. Overall assessment of the newborn is first done and the following points noted:

- establishment of sex
- assessment of maturity
- detection of malformations, especially those requiring urgent treatment
- observing for behaviour and detecting any abnormality of adaptation which may require special care or treatment
- assessment should include posture, cry, colour and movements, muscle tone and certain reflexes, that is, grasp, rooting, tonic neck reflex, Moro's reflex, crossed extension and stepping reflexes

- Vital parameters like heart rate, respiratory rate, temperature and capillary fill time may be recorded wherever possible.

For hospital births, the second examination should be made by a pediatrician, if possible, and within 48 hours of birth. This should be a detailed, systemic examination.

Establishment of sex

Generally, it is easy to assign the sex of the newborn by examining the external genitalia. The rugous scrotum with testes inside, with a penis at least 2.5 cm long is the feature of a male. Typical vulva with closed labia without any rugae and no clitoral enlargement indicates the female sex. In case of any ambiguity or doubt, the assignment of sex should be withheld till an expert opinion is sought.

Assessment of maturity

Maturity should be assessed (particularly in low birth-weight babies) by external physical characteristics, such as skin texture and colour, sole creases, ear cartilage, breast/nipple development, presence of testes in the scrotum and by assessing the scarf sign, popliteal angle and sucking reflex. Absence of sole creases in the posterior part of the sole, scrotum without rugae and testes not in the scrotum, breast nodule less than 5 mm, poor ear cartilage and smooth skin with lanugo hair indicate prematurity.

Detection of malformations

Examination of the following will help to detect malformations and take appropriate action.

Skull: It should be examined for abnormal shape, wide separation of sutures, size of fontanelle (10–30 mm is normal) and presence of abnormal swellings like encephalocele.

Eyes: These should be examined for cataract, iris abnormalities or any corneal abnormality.

Mouth: Look for cleft lip or palate or cysts.

Ears: Presence of ear abnormalities may indicate associated renal malformations.

Skin: Peeling dry skin indicates ichthyosis.

Limbs: The four limbs are examined for the presence of supernumerary digits. The ankles are evaluated for club foot. Joints are examined for hyperextensibility.

Spine: While the presence of a meningo-myelocele will be obvious, a tuft of hair, pigmentation or a small swelling may indicate occult spina bifida.

Abdomen: The newborn abomen is full and the liver and kidneys may be palpable. Gross enlargement of the liver and, spleen may suggest intrauterine infections. If the kidneys are very large, hydronephrosis or tumour should be suspected. Hernial sites and genitalia should be examined for abnormalities. The presence of a scaphoid abdomen indicates diaphragmatic hernia, which requires immediate attention.

Neurological assessment

It is best done by a trained person on the second day of birth. Basic assessment includes symmetrical movements, tone, posture, alertness, cry and neonatal reflexes like the Moro's, sucking and swallowing and, rooting reflexes.

Common Problems in the Newborn

Milia: These are small whitish spots on the face which disappear over time.

Mongolian spots: These are bluish macular lesions, usually appearing over the lower back; they disappear slowly.

Erythema toxicum: This is a rash appearing on the second or third day over the limbs, trunk and face. This does not need treatment and will fade in two or three days.

Transitional stools: Physiological transition from meconium to normal yellow stool may occur over a few days. The stools may be frequent, watery with mucus from the 3rd to about the 10th day. If the mother is anxious, she should be reassured about this.

Vaginal bleeding or discharge: There may be vaginal bleeding in the newborn due to withdrawal of maternal estrogen, which subsides in a few days. The newborn may sometimes have mucoid vaginal discharge which is scanty and self-limiting.

Breast engorgement: Babies of either sex may have nodularity and nipple discharge, which may be due to a maternal hormonal effect. This is transitional and does not require treatment.

Jaundice: Physiological jaundice is the most common cause; it appears on day 2 or 3 and will disappear by days 7 to 10. This is usually mild to moderate and does not need treatment. Other causes of jaundice include incompatibility of ABO group or Rh type; in such cases, jaundice is present at birth and may be more severe. Intrauterine infections, birth trauma including resolving cephalhematoma and G6PD deficiency are other possible causes. High levels of bilirubin (>20 mg/dl) can lead to kernicterus.

Regurgitation of milk: Small amounts of milk regurgitated, particularly soon after feeds, is not a serious cause for concern. The baby must be burped after each feed.

Examination at Discharge

All babies should be examined and weighed on the day of discharge from the hospital in order to:

- determine that nutrition is satisfactory
- detect acquired abnormalities, for example, skin lesions, discharge from the eyes, ears, nose, vagina, oral infection, especially thrush, umbilical sepsis, jaundice, cyanosis and anemia
- test the hip joints for instability
- detect whether visceral abnormality and hernia are present, by inspection and palpation of the abdomen
- detect any abnormality of the heart which may not have been detectable during earlier examinations

The discharge card should contain the gestational age, sex, birth weight, type of delivery, neonatal problems, discharge weight and recommended method of feeding.

KEY POINTS

- The first few minutes after birth are critical in determining the survival and long-term health of the infant.
- The person attending on the newborn should meticulously follow principles of hygiene and cleanliness.
- Appropriate care of the umbilical cord will help prevent hemorrhage and infection.
- The newborn should be assessed from the point of view of establishment of respiration, period of gestation, assignment of sex, anthropological measurements and presence of malformations.
- Breastfeeding should start early and the mother and the baby should be assisted for the establishment of satisfactory breastfeeding.
- Babies that need specialised care should be identified early and appropriately referred.
- Most common minor problems in the newborn are transient and need no intervention.

QUESTIONS

1. The neonatal period includes the
   a. first week of life
   b. first two weeks of life
   c. first four weeks of life
   d. first six weeks of life
2. Immediately after delivery, attention should be paid to all of the following except
   a. respiration of the baby
   b. heart rate
   c. temperature control
   d. polio and BCG vaccination
3. The Apgar score includes all of the following except
   a. passage of meconium
   b. colour
   c. heart rate
   d. respiration
4. Bacterial colonisation is maximum in the newborn in the
   a. oral cavity
   b. umbilical area
   c. anal canal
   d. genitalia

5. Which of the following is *not* a criterion for active neonatal resuscitation?
   a. apneic baby
   b. cyanotic baby
   c. baby with a heart rate of 110 beats/min
   d. pale baby
6. Which of the following babies *does not* require level 3 neonatal intensive care?
   a. baby born at 30 weeks
   b. baby weighing 950 g
   c. baby requiring assisted ventilation
   d. baby that requires phototherapy
7. Which of the following measurements is *not* a part of routine neonatal anthropometry?
   a. midarm circumference
   b. birth weight
   c. head circumference
   d. length
8. The average length of a newborn is
   a. 20 cm b. 30 cm c. 40 cm d. 50 cm
9. The average head circumference of the newborn is
   a. 20 cm b. 25 cm c. 35 cm d. 50 cm
10. Routine initial examination of the newborn should include all of the following *except*
    a. determination of sex
    b. screening for infection
    c. screening for malformations
    d. assessment of maturity
11. In case of doubt about the sex of the baby
    a. it should be declared as male
    b. it should be declared as female
    c. it should be declared as transgender
    d. opinion should be withheld till expert opinion is obtained
12. Which of the following *may not be* considered a minor problem in the neonate?
    a. jaundice at birth
    b. milia
    c. Mongolian spots
    d. transitional stools

Part IV Puerperium

35

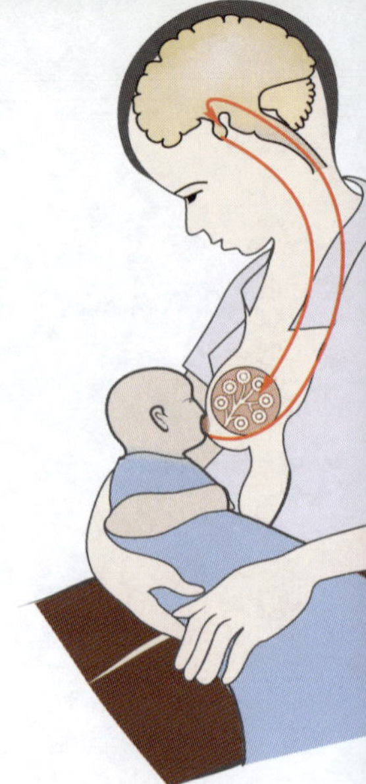

Normal Puerperium

Shyama Kanungo

LEARNING OBJECTIVES

At the end of this chapter, the reader should be able to:

- define normal puerperium
- describe the anatomical changes during puerperium
- describe the physiological changes of puerperium including lactation and the factors controlling it
- counsel the mother on hygiene, breastfeeding, diet, drugs and postnatal exercises
- diagnose and treat minor problems of normal puerperium
- counsel the mother on contraception and utilisation of the nearest health care facilities for immunisation and postnatal services

Introduction

The postpartum period is significant because the parturient and her newborn are still in an 'unusual health mode'. This implies that although puerperium and neonatal periods are both physiological states, the mother and child are vulnerable and can slip easily from 'health' to 'ill-health'. In general, this period tends to receive less attention than the antenatal and intranatal periods. It is important, therefore, to not only understand what changes take place in the normal puerperium along with common disturbances that occur, but also to institute timely and appropriate care to the mother and child.

Definition

Puerperium is the period following completion of the third stage of labour and continues up to six weeks. It is again arbitrarily differentiated into 'immediate' (within 24 hours), 'early' (within seven days; 10 days according to the Government of India guidelines) and 'remote' (from days 7 to 10 till six weeks).

During this period, the pelvic organs return to the prepregnant state, lactation is established and the changes in the metabolic, endocrine, coagulation, cardiovascular, respiratory and urinary systems are reversed. Many of the physiological changes take one to two weeks after delivery to return to normal. Some, however, take much longer.

Anatomical Changes in Puerperium

Changes in the pelvic organs

The process of reversion of the pelvic organs to the normal nonpregnant state is termed **involution**. The entire process takes more than six weeks to be completed and some structures like the cervix do not regain the original (nulliparous) configuration.

Changes in the uterus: Immediately after delivery, the uterus weighs around 1,000 g and extends up to the umbilicus. By the end of the first week, the uterus is felt half way up the umbilicus. At two weeks it is a pelvic organ and by six weeks it is back to the nonpregnant size and weight (50–60 g). The raw placental site is of the size of a palm at delivery. It is 3–4 cm at the end of two weeks. The total number of muscle cells does not decrease; however, individual cells decrease markedly in size. The connective tissue also regresses rapidly. The extrauterine blood vessels immediately return to normal after delivery. Hyaline change obliterates the blood vessels within the uterus.

Placental site involution: Following delivery, the placental bed contracts rapidly; it measures 7.5 cm on the first day. Lymphocytes, macrophages and polymorphs invade the uterine cavity, the space below the placental bed and also the decidua. The re-epethelialisation is complete by day 10, except the placental bed, which by this time is reduced to 2.5 cm and disappears in 4–5 weeks.

Lower uterine segment and perineum: The lower uterine segment, which was large enough to contain the major portion of the fetal head, now involutes to the hardly discernible isthmus of the uterus. The vaginal wall is swollen and bluish due to congestion. The mucosa remains delicate for the first few weeks. The hymen disappears and its remnants are tags called **carunculae myrtiformes**. The perineum regains its normal appearance as early as the fifth day of puerperium.

The cervix usually gets laterally lacerated; it is patulous, bruised and purple; it returns slowly to normal but the external os finally becomes a slit.

Lochia: This refers to the vaginal discharge seen during the first 3–4 weeks of puerperium. It appears red for the first 3–4 days. It contains blood mainly from the placental site. Lochia is serosanguinous from days 5 to 14. A cellular barrier is formed over the raw placental bed. However, it is still vulnerable to infection. It contains blood, leucocytes, decidua and exfoliated pieces of villi covered with trophoblasts shed from the placental site. Thereafter, the lochia becomes turbid white (containing leucocytes and mucus), and stays this way up to 3 to 4 weeks of puerperium.

Sepsis: Inherent vulnerability of the postnatal period for sepsis is due to:

- raw placental bed, which provides a surface for colonisation of bacteria
- alkalinity of the lochia
- lowered general resistance in the puerperium
- devitalised and lacerated tissues of the lower genital tract
- gaping of the introitus for the first few days following delivery.

Physiological Changes

Changes in the vital signs: The pulse rate which had increased by 10–20 beats (80–90 beats/min) during pregnancy comes down to normal in two weeks (60–70 beats/minute). The temperature immediately after delivery may be subnormal. Later, there may be a transient rise from 37 °C to 38 °C as a result of muscle fatigue. However, any persistent rise above 38 °C is abnormal. There is a slight increase in blood pressure for the first five days; the diastolic may be as high as 100 mm Hg.

Changes in the cardiovascular system: There is a decline in all hemodynamic parameters to pre-pregnancy values at 2–3 weeks. Blood volume returns to normal after one week. Cardiac output remains elevated for 48 hours. These changes return to pre-pregnant values at two weeks.

In the immediate puerperium, pulmonary functions do not show much increase except in the residual volume due to reduction in the size of the uterus. The vital capacity may be decreased.

Changes in blood: The red cell mass falls in the immediate puerperium due to normal blood loss at delivery. The reduction continues and returns to prepregnancy levels at the end of six weeks. The leucocyte count increases in early puerperium from the raised count of normal pregnancy. It can go up to 30,000/µl. There is also marked thrombocytosis.

The level of coagulation factors like fibrinogen, and factor VIII falls after two weeks while there is a transient rise in fibrin degradation products. There is increased coagulability of the blood and increased risk of thrombosis in the first two weeks of puerperium. Erythrocyte sedimentation remains high for a week.

Weight changes: After delivery, the mother may lose 5–6 kg because of emptying of the uterine contents as well as normal blood loss through labour. An additional 2–3 kg may be lost due to diuresis.

Endocrine changes: With the delivery of the placenta, the placental hormones are abruptly cut off. Human placental lactogen (hPL) disappears from the system at the end of 24 hours. Human chorionic gonadotropin (hCG) takes 16 days to disappear. Estradiol 17β from the placenta comes down to 10% of the antepartum value three hours after removal of the placenta. Progesterone is also cleared rapidly and by day 3 of puerperium, plasma progesterone falls to <1 ng/ml. The FSH and LH levels remain low, as the pituitary is relatively refractory to GnRH up to four weeks of puerperium.

The ovaries are refractory to gonadotropins. This is independent of circulating prolactin levels, which are erratic after delivery. It rises in spurts only during suckling. Other complex endocrine changes occur with adjustments in the hypothalamo–pituitary–thyroid, and hypothalamo–pituitary–adrenal axes with effects on carbohydrate metabolism as well as thyroid function.

Resumption of menstruation and ovulation is variable and depends on breastfeeding as well as the drugs and contraception used. A normally lactating woman achieves menstruation and ovulation later than a non-lactating woman. Ovulation returns after about four weeks of puerperium in a non-lactating woman and is delayed up to 10 weeks if she is lactating. Hence, by about week 12, a lactating mother ought to adopt a contraceptive.

Changes in the urinary tract: Immediately after delivery, is frequent reflex retention of urine. This is due to suppression of detrusor activity and sphincter spasm due to edema of the bladder base, painful perineum, as well as irritation to the levator ani muscle during labour. There is also a relative insensitivity to intravesical pressure. There is marked diuresis in early puerperium. The mild hydronephrotic and hydroureteric changes that occur in pregnancy reverse by week 6.

Breast changes and lactation: Changes in the breast begin quite early in pregnancy and continue in stages till after delivery. The secretion of colostrum begins in the last few days of pregnancy and is more pronounced in the first few days of puerperium.

Lactogenesis or milk secretion is initiated by prolactin, glucocorticoids and insulin; these initiate milk secretion as levels of estrogen, progesterone and hPL fall after delivery. Maintenance of lactation requires periodic suckling and actual emptying of ducts and alveoli. Prolactin is required for galactopoiesis. Growth hormone, thyroxine, parathyroid hormone, cortisol and insulin have a synergistic effect. Oxytocin plays an important role by increasing the secretion of prolactin. It helps contract myoepithelial cells around the alveoli to eject milk into the lactiferous ducts and sinuses. This is the **milk ejection reflex**. The central nervous system can modulate the release of oxytocin through supraoptic and paraventricular neurons. This explains how factors related to nursing, crying of an infant and positive attitudes towards breastfeeding can improve milk yield. This also explains how negative stimuli such as pain, stress, fear, anxiety, insecurity and negative attitudes can inhibit lactation.

Postnatal Care

The components of postnatal care are:

- A thorough general examination with focus on pulse, BP, temperature and respiration is performed.
- Rest is advised for the first 2–3 hours as she is in a state of fatigue. She may be given a hot stimulating drink. On subsequent days, 8–10 hours of sleep is advised.
- Diet on the first day should be light. Subsequently, normal balanced meals may be eaten. A lactating mother needs 550 calories in excess of normal requirements. The total requirement should be no more than 2,600–2,800 kcal/day (see Chapter 11)
- The bladder tends to get atonic with poor voiding. Frequent voiding should be advised and if retention occurs, warm water bags, posture changes and, standing near a running tap may be advised. Catheterisation should be the last resort and may be used for 48–72 hours from the time of insertion.

- Perineal wounds should be dressed daily with antiseptic solution. Pain management includes warm fomentation and analgesics like paracetamol and ibuprofen. A sterile pad should be used. This is important for the prevention of puerperal sepsis. She should wash with soap and water after every voiding of urine or defecation.
- Care of the bowel may be required as there is a tendency for constipation due to mild ileus and pain in the perineal region. Roughage in diet and mild laxatives are mostly sufficient.
- Care of the breasts includes cleaning of the nipples and areola with clean water, drying the area and instituting early breastfeeding. The baby should be put to breast as soon after delivery as possible. She should be properly positioned, with the head supported on the mother's forearm, the other arm being free to guide it to the breast. The nipple should touch the soft palate of the baby and both its lips should grip the areola.
- Care of the neonate includes keeping it warm and, clean and handling it with clean hands.
- Handling of the baby should be minimal.
- Drugs required in the early puerperium are analgesics, antispasmodics for 'after-pains' or pain in the episiotomy wound. Daily iron (100 mg salt with 30 mg elemental iron) and calcium (1.2 g) should be continued as long as the mother is breastfeeding (see also Chapter 12).
- Postpartum immunisation of the mother is needed for the prevention of Rh isoimmunisation in Rh-negative mothers with Rh-positive babies. Anti-D gammaglobulin 300 μg should be administered intramuscularly to the non-immunised mother within 72 hours of birth to destroy the Rh-positive cells of the fetus, which have entered maternal circulation.
- According to the Government of India guidelines, the first postnatal check-up should be performed within two days and the second one at 42 days.
- Postnatal exercises have several benefits. They help tone up the muscles and ligaments which had stretched during pregnancy and labour, and improve the diminished pulmonary function. Exercises reduce the risk of thromboembolism; release of endorphins helps reduce myalgia and cramps and ward off postpartum blues.

Minor ailments

After-pains: These are common, especially during breastfeeding, and relieved by analgesics or antispasmodics.

Retention of urine: This can be dealt with as described earlier. In case of cystitis, a urine culture specimen is collected and antibiotics given.

Pain: In the perineal wound, it warrants careful examination to exclude hematoma. If there is no hematoma, a cold sitz bath and ibuprofen 400 mg twice or thrice a day should be given after food. Local wound infection or cellulitis requires the administration of antibiotics and a warm compress.

Engorgement of the breast: Frequent feeding of the baby prevents this. Warm fomentation and gentle massage from the periphery towards the areola helps express some of the milk and thus provides some relief. In extreme cases, an analgesic may be required.

Postpartum blues: Also called 'puerperal blues' or 'maternity blues' it occurs in 50%–70% of women 3–5 days after childbirth and usually settles by day 10 of the puerperium. It is characterised by tearfulness, anxiety, irritation and restlessness. Reassurance and 'tender loving care' help the parturient. Tranquilisers like diazepam 5 mg or alprazolam 0.25 mg at bedtime may be administered.

The mother should be counselled regarding contraception options at the earliest and informed that she starts ovulating about 12 weeks after delivery (earlier if she is not lactating). Information should be given on child care and continuation of the immunisation schedule and feeding practices. The mother should also be advised to come in for early consultation in case of difficulties in the neonatal period.

KEY POINTS

- Puerperium is a period of six weeks after completion of the third stage of labour.
- During this period, the uterus and cervix involute to near nonpregnant state.
- Diuresis occurs and about 2 to 3 litres of fluid are lost; the blood volume returns to normal by the end of two weeks.
- The placental site in the uterine is a raw surface and is prone to infection.
- The lochia is the discharge from the raw placental site. It is red to start with, then gradually becomes white.
- It is imperative to watch out for symptoms and signs of infection like fever and foul-smelling lochia.
- The mother should be instructed to breastfeed the baby at the earliest.
- Counselling regarding care of the baby, contraception and continuation of breastfeeding and immunisation of the baby is essential.
- In the postnatal period, the woman may suffer from minor ailments like after-pains, engorged breasts and excessive fatigue.

QUESTIONS

Select the single most appropriate answer:

1. Puerperium begins with the end of the third stage of labour and extends up to
   a. 4 weeks
   b. 6 weeks
   c. 8 weeks
   d. 12 weeks
2. The uterus involutes to become a pelvic organ how many weeks after delivery?
   a. 1 week b. 2 weeks c. 3 weeks d. 4 weeks
3. The most important reason for vulnerability to infection during puerperium is
   a. alkalinity of lochia
   b. lowered general resistance
   c. raw placental area
   d. gaping of introitus
4. The changes that occurred during pregnancy in the cardiovascular system return to those of the nonpregnant status by the end of
   a. 8 weeks
   b. 6 weeks
   c. 4 weeks
   d. 2 weeks
5. If a woman complains of abdominal pain during puerperium, it is most often due to
   a. distended bladder
   b. constipation
   c. after-pains
   d. pelvic infection
6. How many days after delivery does the hCG disappear?
   a. 4 days b. 8 days c. 12 days d. 16 days

In the following questions, there are two statements. Select the appropriate answer using the following key:

a. if both statements are true and causally related
b. if both statements are true but not causally related
c. if the first statement is true and the second is false
d. if the first statement is false and the second is true
e. if both statements are false

7. In a non-lactating mother, ovulation is likely to occur by the end of four weeks *because*

   The ovaries are refractory to FSH and LH for four weeks after delivery.
8. Lactogenesis is initiated by prolactin, glucocorticoids and insulin *because*

   Lactogenesis is not influenced by levels of hPL, estrogen and progesterone.

36

Lactation and Breastfeeding

N Sundari

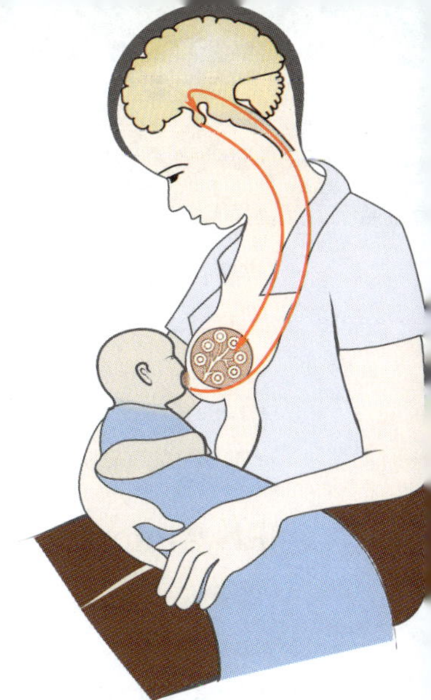

LEARNING OBJECTIVES

At the end of this chapter, the reader should be able to:

- describe the anatomy of the breast
- describe briefly the physiology of lactation
- list the constituents of breast milk
- list the advantages of breast milk to the baby
- list the benefits of breastfeeding to the mother
- explain how breastfeeding acts as a contraceptive
- outline the steps in helping the mother to breastfeed
- list the drugs that are secreted in breast milk
- list the contraindications for breastfeeding
- list the likely complications in the breast

Introduction

Breastfeeding the baby is usually a natural sequel to childbirth. However, the availability of commercial substitutes for breast milk has led to a decline in breastfeeding in the last few decades. Research findings have reemphasised the advantages of breastfeeding to both the mother and her infant. Therefore, all those concerned with maternal and child health should advocate breastfeeding.

Changes in the breast during pregnancy

Anatomy: The breast consists of 15 to 25 lobes, arranged in a radial manner, separated from one another by fat. Each lobe consists of several lobules, and each lobule in turn is made up of a number of alveoli. The small ducts from the alveoli join together to form one large duct, in each lobe. These lactiferous ducts open separately on the nipple. The myoepithelial cells that surround the alveoli respond to a reflex initiated by suckling; the milk is propelled through the ducts.

Preparation of the breast: During pregnancy, breasts develop consequent to increased levels of estrogen, progesterone and human placental lactogen (hPL). Estrogen is responsible for the increase in the size of the breasts and the number of the collecting ducts. Progesterone appears to increase the number of alveolar cells, and hPL stimulates the development of the cells lining the alveoli; it also stimulates the synthesis of casein, lactalbumin and lactoglobulin. Under the influence both estrogen and progesterone, a large amount of fat is deposited around the lobules, thus increasing the size of the breasts.

Prolactin levels rise considerably during pregnancy. The function of prolactin is to induce the alveolar cells to secrete milk. The absence of lactation during pregnancy may be attributed to high levels of estrogen and progesterone.

Physiology of lactation

Within three days of delivery, the levels of estrogen and progesterone fall considerably and permit prolactin to act on the alveoli to initiate lactation.

Colostrum: It is the initial secretion from the breasts following delivery. It is a thick yellow fluid which (compared to mature milk) contains more minerals and protein, and less sugar and fat. It has been described as 'a high-density and low-volume feed'. Antibodies are present in colostrum; immunoglobulin A offers protection to the newborn against enteric pathogens. It contains a number of other immunoglobulins and host resistance factors, also found in mature milk. Colostrum is rich in both vitamins A and K; one of the measures to prevent vitamin K deficiency in the infant is to ensure that the newborn gets colostrum early.

Milk: Colostrum is gradually converted to 'mature milk'. As the baby grows, the mother's milk increases in volume and changes its composition to meet the baby's changing needs. In the mature milk, protein accounts for 0.8%–0.9% of the milk volume. Lactose, the major carbohydrate, provides 40% of the energy in a breast milk feed, while fat coming late in the feed provides up to 50% of the energy. Long-chain polyunsaturated fatty acids such as docosahexanoic acid (DHA) are present in large quantities in breast milk and promote the development of the nervous system. Breast milk also has large amounts of interleukin-6, the maximum being present in colostrum. All the vitamins are present in human milk except vitamin K. The concentration of iron is very low, but it is extremely bioavailable. A lactating mother secretes about 600 ml of milk per day.

Maintenance of lactation

Whenever the mother suckles her child, there is secretion and release of prolactin, which helps maintain lactation (**Fig. 36.1a**). During lactation, the levels of FSH are elevated and those of LH are low, and the release of GnRH is reduced. For maintenance of lactation, levels of ACTH, thyroid hormone, insulin and growth hormone are also essential.

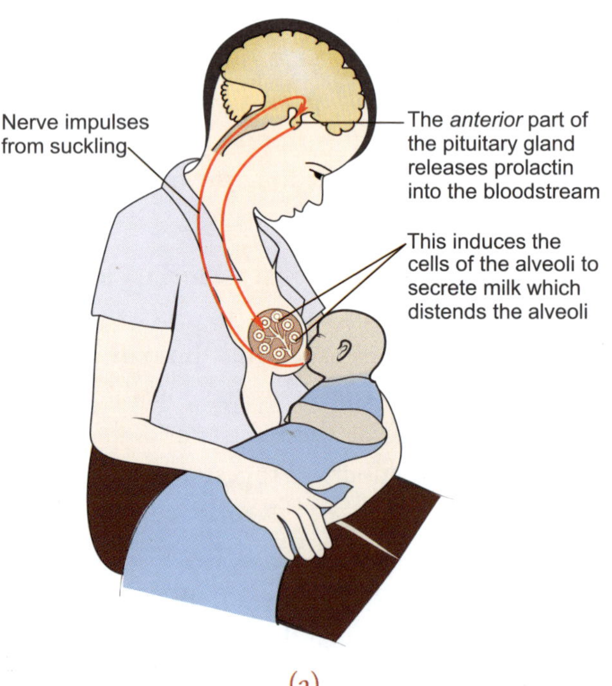

(a)

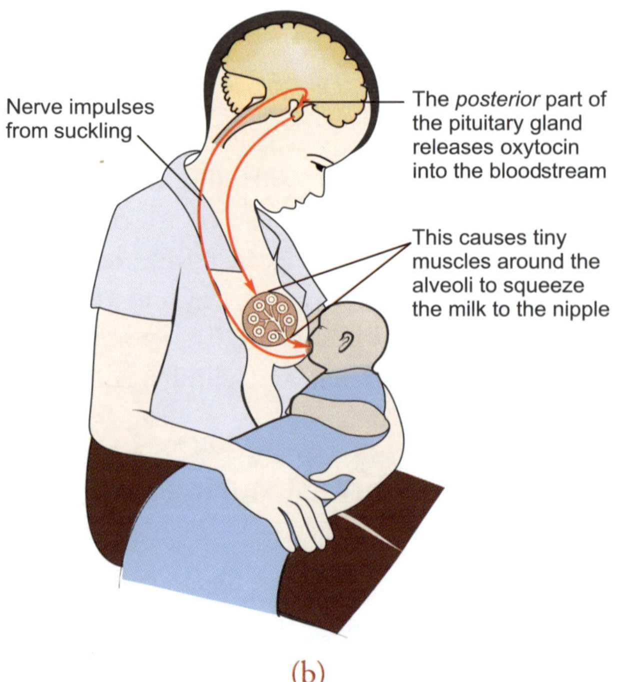

(b)

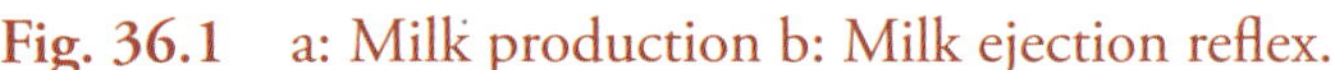

Fig. 36.1 a: Milk production b: Milk ejection reflex.

Ejection of milk

The myoepithelial fibres that surround the alveoli respond to a reflex initiated by suckling. The milk secreted by the alveoli is propelled along the ducts and is stored in lactiferous sinuses (small reservoirs) under the areola. The milk ejection reflex is of the neuroendocrine type, and is mediated via the hypothalamus and the neurohypophysis which ultimately releases oxytocin that is responsible for the contraction of myoepthelial fibres (**Fig. 36.1b**). The secreted milk is thus ejected from the alveoli. The reflex stimulates further secretion of prolactin and suppresses the release of prolactin inhibiting factor from the hypothalamus, and contributes to maintenance of lactation.

Factors affecting lactation

Both physical and emotional stress can adversely affect lactation. However, the most important factor in, maintenance of lactation is regular suckling the where the prolactin reflex and the ejection reflex have a positive influence. No medications seem to increase milk secretion except metoclopromide (given as 10 mg three times a day for 10–14 days).

Drugs secreted in breast milk

Most drugs are secreted in small quantities in breast milk; the drugs do not have a significant effect on the baby. However, it is advisable to be cautious while prescribing drugs to a lactating mother (see Chapter 12).

Advantages of Breastfeeding

Breastfeeding is a secure and safe source of food for the baby. It has both health and economic advantages.

Benefits to the baby

Nutrition: Breastfeeding offers every baby optimal nutrition and is specially adapted to the baby's changing needs. No substitute food can do this. Also, most vitamins and minerals, and polyunsaturated fatty acids are available in breast milk.

Protection: Colostrum protects the immature organs of the newborn, particularly the kidneys, from fluid overload. Besides nutrition, it provides antibodies that protect the infant against acute and chronic diseases. Acute respiratory infections and diarrheas are rarely encountered in babies who are exclusively breastfed for six months. Other infections like those of the middle ear and lower respiratory tract are reduced three- to fourfold in breastfed infants. There is data to show that the risk and severity of chronic diseases is increased among children who were not breastfed.

Benefits to the mother

- Emotional bonding between the mother and her baby is greater when she has breastfed her infant.
- For every month of breastfeeding, the mother reduces her risk of breast cancer. Risk of ovarian cancer is also reduced.
- **Contraception:** When a mother is exclusively breastfeeding, the levels of prolactin remain high and she is amenorrheic. Endocrine studies have shown that the FSH levels are high and LH levels are low, but there is no pulsatile activity (that is, GnRH is reduced). Estrogen levels are low because of lack of follicular development. However, one must remember that once the baby starts other feeds, the chances of ovulation increases. In such cases, the mother should use contraceptives.
- Food security and economic considerations are important, especially in developing countries. Breastfeeding provides food security not only for the baby, but also to other members of the family for whom money, fuel and time are saved. The use of commercial baby foods are a burden on the scarce resources of the family. The risk of infection is increased if the bottle and teat are not washed properly, or the water used to prepare the food is unsafe for drinking. The resulting illness further increases the financial burden on the family.

Helping the mother to breastfeed

- **Preparation for breastfeeding** should start during the antenatal period. At every visit, the health care provider should discuss breastfeeding in the sociocultural context of the woman. In many societies, breastfeeding is considered essential; this concept needs to be reinforced by citing the benefits that have been scientifically proven. Some mothers may not want to breastfeed. These women should be counselled effectively by presenting the advantages to them as well as to their babies.

Every health care provider must examine the breasts of the woman at the first antenatal visit, with special focus on the nipples. The objective is to determine if the nipples are flat or retracted; the woman is advised to gently pull out the nipple using a lubricant. If the nipple does not become protractile, there may be some adhesions which may anchor the nipple to the tissues under the areola. Exercises should be started in the second half of pregnancy to break these adhesions. The woman is instructed to place her thumbs on either side of the nipples at the areolar margins, first in the horizontal plane and then in the vertical plane. The use of a nipple shield under the brassiere is also useful.

Nipple care is very important during pregnancy. They should be washed with soap and water to remove any crust. If there are any abrasions, the same are treated with creams containing anhydrous lanolin. After delivery, the mother must be encouraged to put the baby to breast at the earliest. This helps in establishing lactation, as suckling operates through the milk ejection reflex by maintaining high levels of prolactin and also by bringing about contraction of the myoepithelial cells, which in turn propel the milk along the ducts. Practices like separating the baby and the mother, giving water or glucose water or the routine of feeding the baby at fixed intervals must be avoided.

For successful establishment of lactation and breastfeeding, the mother and her baby must 'bond' as soon as possible after birth; they must continue to room in together and the baby must be put to breast frequently. Once the milk flow is established, the baby may be fed on demand.

The mother should be told about the advantages of colostrum and how with frequent suckling the mature milk will flow in 3–4 days. She should be instructed to sit comfortably with a back rest in a chair, ensure that the nipple is well within the baby's mouth and that the act of feeding would take time and that she should not be in a hurry. One must remember that lactation can be influenced by emotions and therefore it is very important to help the mother to adopt a positive attitude to breastfeeding.

Maternal complications during lactation

A mother may suffer from some problems during lactation. The following complications may be encountered:

- **Breast engorgement** occurs when the infant is unable to suck and there is milk stasis. The breasts are distended, tender and hard; these features are often associated with pyrexia. Treatment consists in providing good breast support and analgesics. The milk should be expressed manually or using a breast pump, followed by a binder.
- **Mastitis** is the infection of the breast parenchyma and is commonly seen during puerperium. The breast is hard, tender and reddish; the involvement is mostly unilateral. Constitutional symptoms of infections like general malaise and fever are present. The offending organism is *Staphylococcus aureus*. The penicillin group of antibiotics should be prescribed unless the woman is allergic, in which case erythromycin may be given. Testing for culture and sensitivity should be done, if possible. Antibiotics should be continued for 7–10 days. The affected breast should be emptied gently. Breastfeeding should be continued from the normal beast.
- **Breast abscess** should be suspected when mastitis does not resolve. One should look for fluctuation and confirm it by ultrasound examination if necessary. While continuing antibiotics, surgical drainage must be performed under general anesthesia and a drain left in place.

Problems in breastfeeding

Breastfeeding is contraindicated if the mother has AIDS, and uses hard drugs or alcohol.

Inhibition or suppression of lactation may be necessary if the baby is born dead or if the woman decides not to breastfeed her child. The drug of choice is cabergolin 1 mg as a single dose. When lactation is established and needs to be suppressed,

0.25 mg cabergolin is given 12 hourly for two days. Alternatively, bromocriptine 2.5 mg twice a day for 14 days is used.

Failure of lactation is often due to an emotional disturbance in the mother, when she is severely ill or has had severe PPH.

KEY POINTS

- Breastfeeding establishes within a few hours of delivery.
- Colostrum, secreted initially, is important for the baby.
- Lactation is helped by suckling and when the mother is positively inclined to breastfeeding.
- Breastfeeding has many benefits for both the mother and the baby.
- Breastfeeding has a contraceptive effect.
- The common problems associated with lactation are preventable and easily treatable.

QUESTIONS

Select the single most appropriate answer:

1. How soon after birth should a mother ideally start breastfeeding her baby?
   a. 1 hour c. 12 hours
   b. 6 hours d. 24 hours
2. Which of the two hormones is essential for the maintenance of lactation?
   a. oxytocin and progesterone
   b. oxytocin and estrogen
   c. estrogen and progesterone
   d. oxytocin and prolactin
3. A mother who breastfeeds her child has a significantly reduced risk of
   a. cancer of the uterine cervix
   b. cancer of the breast
   c. cancer of the liver
   d. cancer of the endometrium
4. Which hormone is responsible for an increase in the number of alveolar cells during pregnancy?
   a. estrogen c. progesterone
   b. hPL d. hCG
5. Breast milk contains all of the following *except*
   a. docosahexanoic acid c. immunoglobulins
   b. vitamin K d. vitamin A
6. Infants who are breastfed are protected against all of the following *except*
   a. dermatitis c. middle ear infection
   b. respiratory infections d. measles
7. In breast abscess, the mainstay of treatment is
   a. administration of antibiotics
   b. provision of breast support
   c. incision and drainage
   d. stopping breastfeeding

In the following questions, there are two statements. Select the appropriate answer using the following key:

a. if both statements are true and causally related
b. if both statements are true but not causally related
c. if the first statement is true and the second is false
d. if the first statement is false and the second is true
e. if both statements are false

8. Lactogenesis is initiated by prolactin, glucocorticoids and insulin *because*

   Lactogenesis is not influenced by levels of hPL, estrogen and progesterone.
9. The development of the nervous system is good in breastfed babies *because*

   Breast milk contains large quantities of docohexanoic acid.
10. In developing countries, breastfeeding does not provide food security to the family *because*

    Commercially available baby foods are expensive.

37

Abnormal Puerperium

SN Tripathy

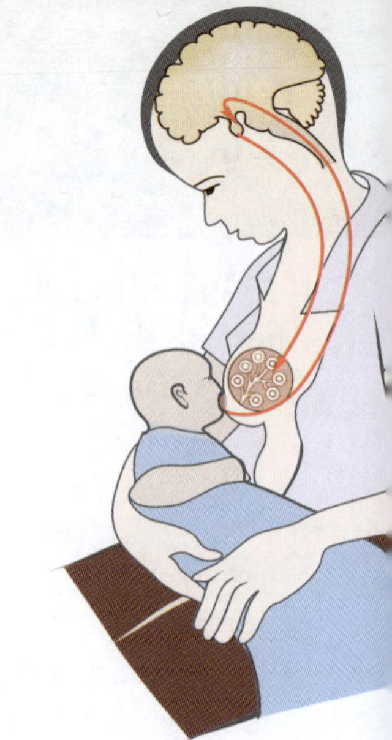

LEARNING OBJECTIVES

At the end of this chapter, the reader should be able to:

- define puerperal pyrexia and puerperal infection
- explain why a woman is prone to infection during puerperium
- enumerate the differential diagnosis of puerperal fever
- describe the pathology of uterine infection
- list the factors that predispose to puerperal infection and the strategies to prevent it
- list the bacteria responsible for the infection
- plan the laboratory investigations that help in its management
- outline the treatment of puerperal infections
- enumerate the complications of infections of the genital tract
- list the other problems that occur during puerperium

Introduction

The postnatal period is a time of physiological resolution and emotional satisfaction. Conventionally, puerperium is the period that starts from the completion of the third stage of labour and extends up to six weeks after delivery. Although the most important event of pregnancy is over, one should remember that even after a normal delivery, the placental site is a 'wound' like elsewhere in the body that can get infected or may bleed. Besides infection, the resolving anatomical and physiological changes of pregnancy continue to contribute to the occurrence of several other complications: it has been documented that most maternal deaths occur in the postnatal period. It is, therefore, important to be aware of these complications, anticipate them to prevent them, or detect them early to institute appropriate treatment.

Puerperal Infection

Infection during the puerperium was recognised as a communicable disease by Semmelweiss and Holmes in the 1840s. The former introduced the concept of asepsis and 'begged' the midwives to wash their hands in chlorine water before conducting a delivery. Lister advocated the use of carbolic acid, which was an antiseptic. These measures brought down the incidence of puerperal infection. Though there is a steady decline in puerperal sepsis, it is still responsible for a significant number of maternal deaths in India.

Puerperal infection or sepsis is defined as an infection of the genital tract occurring at any time till the 42nd day postpartum in which two or more of the following are present:

- pelvic pain
- fever
- purulent vaginal discharge
- subinvolution of the uterus.

Since the rise in temperature in the puerperium is largely attributed to an infection of the genital tract, fever after childbirth is a reliable index of its frequency or incidence.

Puerperal pyrexia is defined as a temperation recording of 38 °C or more on any two occasions in the first 10 days postpartum, excluding the first 24 hours. The temperature must be recorded using an oral thermometer by a standard technique, at least four times a day.

Differential diagnosis of fever

If a temperature of 38 °C is recorded in the postpartum period, the woman must be investigated thoroughly, as the fever could be caused by infection outside the genital tract. However, **most fevers after delivery are due to an infection of the genital tract.**

Urinary tract infections: The changes in the urinary tract predispose a woman to urinary tract infections (UTI). After delivery, loss of bladder tone, reflex retention due to a painful perineal wound and catheterisation of the bladder contribute to the occurrence of UTI. Acute renal infections like pyelonephritis may mimic an acute pelvic infection. The condition is characterised by spiking fever, bacteriuria, pyuria and costovertebral tenderness (see also Chapter 51).

Breast conditions: The most frequent cause of fever is breast engorgement. The rise in temperature is noted in the first few days. In case of mastitis and breast abscess, the fever appears later.

Uterine infection: The postpartum infection of the uterus is generally referred to as **endometritis**; it is called **metritis** and **parametritis** when the infection involves the myometrium and the parametrium. However, uterine infections are rare following an uncomplicated vaginal delivery, but are a significant problem in women who undergo CS.

Thrombosis and thrombophlebitis: Pregnancy is a hypercoagulable state and thrombosis of deep veins may complicate the puerperium. The fever is low grade in deep vein thrombosis, but thrombophlebitis often presents with higher grades of fever.

Respiratory infection: This and other intercurrent illnesses like enteric fever, malaria and filariasis may also be responsible for puerperal fever.

Predisposing factors for puerperal infection

Any woman, even after an uncomplicated vaginal delivery, is potentially at risk of developing puerperal infection. However, some factors predispose a woman to infection in the postnatal period. These factors operate during the antenatal or intranatal period, or both (**Table 37.1**).

General risk factors: Certain patient characteristics favour the occurrence of postpartum pelvic infection.

Nutrition: The general debility associated with malnutrition and anemia often encountered in women of poor socioeconomic status predisposes them to puerperal infection.

Table 37.1 Predisposing factors for puerperal infection

Antenatal	Intranatal
Anemia and malnutrition	Repeated PV examination
Sexual intercourse	Prolonged rupture of membranes
Antenatal intrauterine infection	Prolonged labour
Immunocompromised state	Instrumental delivery
Lower genital tract infection	Cesarean section
URTI/septic focus	Home delivery
Three or more courses of betamethasone (given in women at risk of preterm labour)	Delivery by untrained traditional birth attendant (TBA)
Prolonged induction of labour, cervical encerclage	Manual removal of placenta
Preterm labour	**Postnatal**
Premature rupture of membranes	Retained products of conception (RPOC)
Preeclampsia	Trauma/devitalised tissue
Retained placenta	Hematoma
Large placental area like multiple pregnancy, hydramnios	

Infections: When present elsewhere in the body, these are important risk factors. Women below the age of 18 years, malnourished women, those with multiple pregnancies and those suffering from diabetes mellitus are more prone to infection.

Bacterial flora: Colonisation of the lower genital tract with by pathogenic bacteria is a causative factor.

Disregard for aseptic and antiseptic techniques: Neglect of aseptic and antiseptic techniques contributes immensely to postpartum infection.

Route of delivery: This is the single most significant independent risk factor.

Vaginal delivery: The incidence of postpartum infection after a vaginal delivery is much lower than that after CS. However, when a woman has risk factors like prolonged interval between rupture of membranes and delivery, multiple vaginal examinations, prolonged labour, instrumental vaginal delivery, chorioamnionitis, home delivery and unskilled attendant at birth, the incidence increases many times.

Cesarean section: Following CS, the risk of metritis is significantly higher (10–15 times) compared to that for vaginal delivery. Other risk factors are the same as discussed in the previous section.

Causative organisms in puerperal sepsis

The normal vagina is colonised by bacterial flora comprising predominantly nonpathogenic lactobacilli and diptheroids; however, other organisms are invariably present and generally cause no symptoms in the non-puerperal women. The bacteria commonly responsible for female genital tract infections are aerobes and anerobes:

Aerobes: Gram-positive cocci like Streptococci A, B (Beta-hemolytic streptoccoci of Group A causes the most serious type of infection), *Enterococcus* and *Staphylococus aureus*. Gram-negative bacteria like *Escherichia coli, Klebsiella pneumoniae, Proteus mirabilis* and *Pseudomonas aeruginosa*.

Anerobes: Peptococcus species, Peptostreptococcus species, *Bacteroides fragilis* group, Clostridium species and Fusobacterium species,

Occasionally, other bacteria such as Mycobacterium species, *Chlamydia trachomatis* and *Neisseria gonorrheae* are recovered.

Mode of transmission

Puerperal infection is acquired in several ways:

Nosocomial: The pathogenic organisms in the hospital environment cause the infection.

Exogenous: The organisms from the respiratory tract of the attendants (often doctors and nurses), infected/contaminated linen, blankets and non-sterile instruments could cause the infection. The infection may be from droplets or be dust-borne. Infections from *Staphylococcus aureus* and *Streptococcus beta hemolyticus* are also common.

Endogenous: The normal bacterial flora present in the genital tract before delivery become pathogenic in the presence of predisposing factors, and can cause puerperal sepsis, for example, anerobic Streptococcus.

Autogenous: The organisms present elsewhere in the body migrate to the genital organ through the bloodstream, by droplet infection or direct contamination. *Streptococcus beta hemolyticus* and Staphylococcus may migrate from septic throat or skin infection and *E coli* from the feces.

Pathogenesis

The site of placental attachment, which is a raw area in the uterine cavity is most vulnerable to infection. Besides, wounds like an episiotomy, laceration/tears in the cervix and vagina and a cesarean wound can also get infected.

Uterus: It is the most common site of puerperal infection. The remnants of the decidua, especially over the placental area of separation, contribute to the infection. The uterine infection is of two types:

- In putrid endometritis, the decidua gets infected and becomes necrosed and may slough off, but the infection to the deep myometrium is prevented by a zone of leucocytic barrier. Causative organisms are *E coli,* Gram-negative anerobic organisms, staphylococci, chlamydia and mycoplasma.
- In septic endometritis, the infection becomes very severe. There is no leucocytic barrier. This favours local invasion to the myometrium and spread to other sites like the peritoneum, tubes, ovaries and pelvic cellular tissue. The organisms responsible are β-hemolytic streptococci.

Cervix and vagina: These are most often infected following tears and lacerations. They may be infected directly or from a perineal infection; the mucosa is swollen and hyperemic, resulting in necrosis and sloughing. Rarely, a forgotten swab may be the source of infection.

Perineum: After infection, the wound edge becomes red and swollen; there may be a collection of seropurulent discharge or pus which results in complete disruption of the episiotomy wound.

Spread of infection: Infection from the uterus may spread directly, by the bloodstream or via the lymphatics.

Salpingitis: The fallopian tubes are commonly affected when the infection from the uterine cavity spreads upwards. The affected tubes become swollen and congested, and ovaries may be involved leading to the formation of tubo-ovarian masses.

Pelvic cellulitis: Infection from the lower uterine cavity and cervix spreads laterally through the uterine wall to involve the connective tissues of the uterine ligaments, leading to pelvic cellulitis. The infection starts insidiously, but may become severe if treatment for uterine infection is not started early.

Pelvic peritonitis: The infection spreads directly through the fallopian tubes or via the lymphatics, resulting in localised peritonitis, which may resolve completely or become localised to form a pelvic abscess. In severe infection, peritonitis may become generalised.

Clinical features

Fever: When present in the postpartum period, fever must be considered to be due to puerperal infection. The rise in temperature is generally proportional to the severity of infection. Chills and rigor associated with fever point to bacteremia; the possibility of malaria must be kept in mind.

Abdominal pain: Once uterine infection sets in, the woman complains of abdominal pain. The **uterus could be subinvoluted and tender**. On bimanual examination, tenderness is elicited in the parametrial region, indicating a spread of infection. In peritonitis, paralytic ileus develops resulting in abdominal distension.

Abnormal lochia: If there is uterine infection, the woman is likely to complain of foul-smelling lochia. In severe cases, it could be purulent. Scanty, odourless lochia is characteristic of group A β-hemolytic streptococci.

Secondary postpartum hemorrhage: Frank bleeding is due to infection and non-epethelialisation of the placental wound.

Wound infections: The woman may complain of pain and discharge from the episiotomy or abdominal wound following CS. The edges of the wounds may be red and indurated with purulent discharge; check for wound dehiscence.

Investigations

Every case of puerperal fever is considered to be due to puerperal infection unless proven otherwise. A meticulous history and a thorough clinical examination will help locate the infection. The laboratory investigations are directed at assessing the general condition of the woman and to confirm the diagnosis and detect any complication.

The basic investigations include the following:

- hemoglobin, total and differential leucocyte, counts
- midstream urine checked for pus cells, culture and sensitivity.
- high vaginal and endocervical swabs for culture and antibiotic sensitivity test
- pus from the wounds for culture and sensitivity
- blood is taken at the peak of temperature for culture and sensitivity; also checked for malarial parasites and microfilaria
- liver and renal function tests, if indicated
- coagulation profile if Gram-negative septicemia is suspected
- USG of the pelvis may help to detect retained products of conception, foreign body inside the uterus, pelvic abscess and peritonitis.

Treatment

General treatment: The following measures must be instituted:

- Record of pulse, blood pressure and temperature is maintained.

- Plenty of oral fluids with vitamins and minerals should be added. Parenteral fluids and electrolytes are administered only if the woman is unable to retain oral fluids or if the dehydration is severe.
- Blood transfusion is indicated if the woman is severely anemic.
- Symptomatic treatment with antipyretics or tepid sponging are recommended as needed

Specific treatment: It consists essentially of antibiotic administration and surgical intervention when indicated.

Antimicrobial therapy: Antibiotics are the mainstay of treatment of puerperal sepsis: start with oral amoxycillin 500 mg 6 hourly and metronidazole 400 mg 8 hourly. At the end of 48 hours, the response must be assessed. If satisfactory, the same antibiotics may be continued for seven days; if not, antibiotics should be changed according to the organisms isolated and their sensitivity. In moderate to severe infection, the most accepted antibiotic regimen is a combination of ampicillin, metronidazole and gentamicin.

Alternatively, administer intravenously cefotaxime 1 g 12 hourly or cefuroxime 750 mg 8 hourly. Intravenous administration of ampicillin with clavulinic acid 500 mg 12 hourly and metronidazole 500 mg, 8 hourly are effective in anerobic infections.

Surgical treatment: It is required if there is accumulation of pus or retained products of conception in the uterine cavity, or a visceral injury.

Infected perineal wound: Stitches should be removed to facilitate drainage of pus.

Uterine cavity: Retained products of conception if present, should be removed; pyometra must be drained.

Pelvic abscess: It is drained by posterior colpotomy. Exploratory laparotomy must be performed if there is evidence of pus in the peritoneal cavity, recurrent uterine hemorrhage and suspicion of uterine injury.

Prevention

Puerperal infection is largely preventable. During the antenatal period, anemia must be corrected and any infection must be treated. **The guidelines for asepsis and antisepsis must be meticulously adhered to during every delivery.** In the postnatal period, one must monitor the mother closely so as to detect and treat any infection at the earliest.

Breast-related complications

Some breast complications may be encountered during the puerperium. Examination of the breasts during antenatal care and correction of retracted nipples can reduce the incidence of complications.

Sore and cracked nipple: This is a common complication among lactating mothers. Fissures occur in the duct openings of nipples as a result of vigorous sucking when the breasts are engorged or if secretion is inadequate. The nipples are very painful, and if infected can lead to mastitis.

The woman must be advised to clean the breasts after feeding, and to apply chlorhexidine or hexachlorophane cream and wash before the next feed.

Breast engorgement: Once milk secretion is established, the breasts become distended, nodular and tender. If the baby is unable to feed because of flat or retracted nipples, the breasts become swollen, heavy and painful; engorgement of the breasts is associated with a rise in temperature. Treatment includes breast support with a binder/brassiere, cold compress and analgesics. The breasts should be thoroughly emptied manually or by using a pump. This is a painful procedure and it is best to prevent breast engorgement.

Lactation may need to be suppressed if the baby is dead or the mother is too sick to feed it. Traditionally, pyridoxine 100 mg thrice a day for 7–10 days is given. Cabergoline, a newer drug, in doses of 0.25 mg twice a day for two days is more effective and faster in action.

Mastitis and breast abscess: Mastitis is an infection of the parenchymal tissue of the breast. The condition is often preceded by breast engorgement. The infection is usually unilateral with erythema, tenderness, induration and rise in local temperature. Constitutional symptoms of mastitis and breast abscess tend to be severe. It occurs within 2–4 weeks of puerperium. The most common infecting organism is *Staphylococcus aureus.* Treatment consists of providing breast support, administering antibiotics like erythromycin and ampicillin; most importantly, milk must be expressed. Breastfeeding can be continued from the other breast.

Breast abscess occurs in 10% of women who are treated for mastitis. Signs and symptoms are the same as for mastitis with the addition of a fluctuant area. The abscess should be drained under general anesthesia, with an incision along the skin line. Aspiration of pus under ultrasound guidance is the a current option.

Failing lactation: When the mother cannot provide an adequate quantity of milk for an adequate time, it is termed failing lactation. There is no definite reason assigned, but failing lactation has been observed when the mother is very ill, is reluctant to breastfeed the baby, or is in a state of depression. The woman must be instructed to take plenty of fluids and consume a nutritious diet; above all she must be reassured. If these measures fail, metoclopromide 10 mg three times a day for 10–14 days may be useful.

Complications of the urinary tract

The most common urinary complication in the puerperium is infection; however, urinary retention or urinary incontinence may also cause problems.

Urinary tract infection: It is one of the common causes of puerperal pyrexia; the incidence is 1%–5% of all deliveries. The factors that predispose to urinary tract infection (UTI) during pregnancy and puerperium have been discussed in Chapter 51.

Besides fever, the woman may complain of frequency, urgency and dysuria. The urine may be cloudy and have an offensive odour. A rise in temperature is associated with rigor; pain and tenderness in the renal angle is characteristic of pyelonephritis.

Management consists of urinalysis including culture and sensitivity and the use of antibiotics. Cystoscopy and intravenous pyelography are indicated in recurrent UTI.

Urinary retention: Bruising around the bladder base, episiotomy wound and epidural anesthesia predispose to retention of urine following delivery. The condition must be treated with an indwelling catheter for 48–72 hours.

Incontinence of urine: Urinary fistulae consequent to obstructed labour could cause urinary incontinence; they are rare but may be encountered in areas where obstetric care is poor. There may also be aureteric injury during lower segment CS. Small fistulae may heal with continuous bladder drainage (for 2–3 weeks). If this measure fails, it may be surgically repaired three months after delivery.

Venous complications

During pregnancy, there is a significant increase in plasma fibrinogen, platelets and factors VII, VIII and X, and a decrease in fibrinolytic activity. These alterations in the blood predispose a woman to thrombosis during pregnancy and puerperium. As compared to spontaneous vaginal delivery, the incidence of thrombosis is 20 times greater after CS. Superficial venous thrombosis is the commonest form of thrombosis during the puerperium, and occurs in preexisting varicose veins. Treatment includes the application of compression bandage, elevation of the leg and early mobilisation. Anticoagulants are withheld unless the deep veins are involved.

Deep vein thrombosis (DVT): This usually occurs during the puerperium, especially among obese women or those who have undergone CS. The thrombotic process involves the veins of the calf, and may extend to the femoral and pelvic veins. The risk of pulmonary embolism is high, if the pelvic veins are involved.

Clinical signs of DVT are not very characteristic. Low grade pyrexia, tachycardia and a feeling of uneasiness must make one suspect DVT. Local examination of the leg may reveal tenderness on firm pressure on the calf muscles. Elicitation of tenderness on dorsiflexion of the foot (Homan sign) is not always reliable. At present, real-time ultrasonography with duplex and colour Doppler is advocated to detect proximal DVT.

It is important to anticipate and institute measures to prevent DVT. Early ambulation prevents stasis of blood due to immobility. The woman must be instructed to carry out deep-breathing exercises. Prophylactic anticoagulant therapy should be started for women with varicose veins and also for obese women undergoing operative delivery. The most common prophylactic is low-dose heparin. It is given 5000 IU SC before surgery and 8–12 hours thereafter till the woman is fully ambulatory. This treatment results in a 50%–75% reduction in post-cesarean thromboembolism.

Curative treatment of DVT includes anticoagulants, bed rest, elevation of the foot and analgesics. The initial anticoagulation is with heparin or fractionated heparin (low molecular heparin) during pregnancy and puerperium. However, in the postpartum period, both intravenous heparin and oral warfarin may be started; after five days, heparin can be safely stopped. The intravenous loading dose of heparin is minimum 5000 units, followed by an infusion. Alternatively, DVT can be treated with the subcutaneous administration of heparin, adjusted to maintain accelerated partial thromboplastin time (aPTT) at 1.5 times the control value.

The main complications of using heparin are hemorrhage from different sites, wound hematoma, thrombocytopenia and osteopenia. Gentle movement on the bed is allowed when pain subsides (usually at the end of the first week). After edema subsides, she should be allowed out of bed with an elastic bandage on the affected leg.

Pulmonary embolism: Pulmonary embolism is not common during pregnancy and puerperium. The most common symptoms are breathlessness, chest pain, cough, hemoptysis and syncope. The salient clinical features are tachycardia, dyspnea and hemoptysis. Ventilation-perfusion scintigraphy or angiography are used to diagnose the condition. Treatment consists of an initial intravenous bolus of 10,000 units of heparin; subsequent doses are adjusted to maintain a PTT at twice the control. Heparin may also be given SC, 10,000 units every 8 hours/12 hours; the daily dose is 25,000 to 40,000 units.

Thrombophlebitis: Septic thrombus on the placental site may involve the ovarian vein; sometimes, the uterine veins are involved and it may spread through the inferior vena cava. The infected thrombus may dislodge as septic emboli to occlude the microcirculation of vital organs like the lungs, kidney, brain and heart causing life-threatening complications.

Obstetric palsy

Occasionally, the roots of the sciatic or obturator nerves in the pelvis may be injured by pressure during the second stage of labour. There may be loss of sensation, loss of muscle power and muscular wasting. The 4th and 5th sacral nerves are the most commonly affected. Foot drop is a common symptom. Recovery is slow, but almost invariably complete. Physiotherapy is necessary.

Psychiatric problems during the puerperium may range from mood disorders to severe psychosis (see Chapter 55).

KEY POINTS

- Puerperal pyrexia is defined as a rise in temperature to 38 °C or more, on two occasions after the first 24 hours of delivery, recorded by a standard technique.
- Infection of the genital tract is the most frequent complication during puerperium, and contributes to 10%–15% of maternal deaths in India.
- Fever in the postpartum period could also be due to UTI, respiratory tract infections and communicable diseases like malaria.
- Breast engorgement may manifest as puerperal pyrexia. Treatment consists of analgesics and, breast support with binder/brassiere.
- Secondary postpartum hemorrhage is attributed to an infection of the placental site. The mainstay of therapy is antibiotics.
- Venous complications, though uncommon, may often occur in persons with preexisting varicose veins. Treatment must be instituted early to avoid fatal complications.
- Most of the complications in the postpartum period can be prevented by managing predisposing factors in the antenatal period, strict adherence to surgical asepsis and antisepsis during delivery and careful monitoring in the postpartum period.

QUESTIONS

Select the single most appropriate answer:

1. Puerperal pyrexia is defined as an increase in temperature to more than
   a. 37 °C b. 38 °C c. 38.5 °C d. 39 °C
2. Severe endometritis is characterised by all of the following *except*
   a. fever with chills and rigors
   b. foul-smelling vaginal discharge
   c. tachycardia out of proportion with the temperature rise
   d. an involuted uterus
3. In the initial therapy of puerperal infection, the choice of antibiotics should ideally be
   a. amoxycillin + cefotaxime
   b. amoxycillin + cefuroxime
   c. amoxycillin + gentamicin
   d. amoxycillin + metronidazole
4. All of the following are common causes of secondary postpartum hemorrhage *except*
   a. retained placenta c. delayed involution
   b. infection d. choriocarcinoma
5. Urinary tract infection in puerperium is due to
   a. physiological changes leading to urinary stasis
   b. catheterisation
   c. previous asymptomatic bacteriuria
   d. all of the above
6. Which organism is most frequently responsible for severe endometritis?
   a. beta-hemolytic streptococci of group A
   b. chlamydia
   c. staphylococus
   d. bacteroides
7. Treatment of subinvolution of the uterus is not required when the patient
   a. is asymptomatic
   b. has features of infection
   c. complains of prolonged lochial discharge
   d. complains of excessive bleeding
8. The drug of choice to treat deep vein thrombosis during puerperium is
   a. heparin c. antibiotics
   a. warfarin d. streptokinase

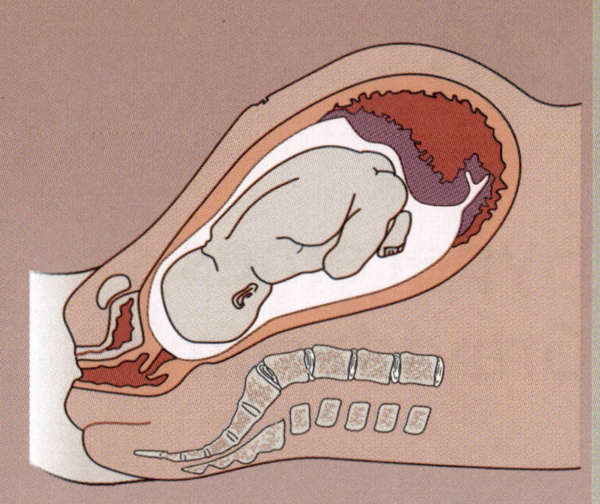

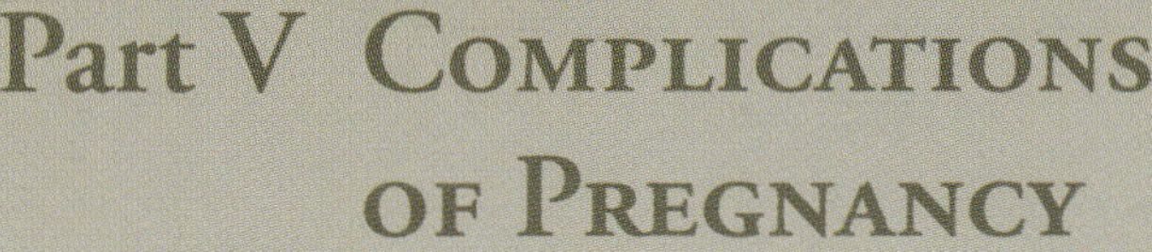

Part V Complications of Pregnancy

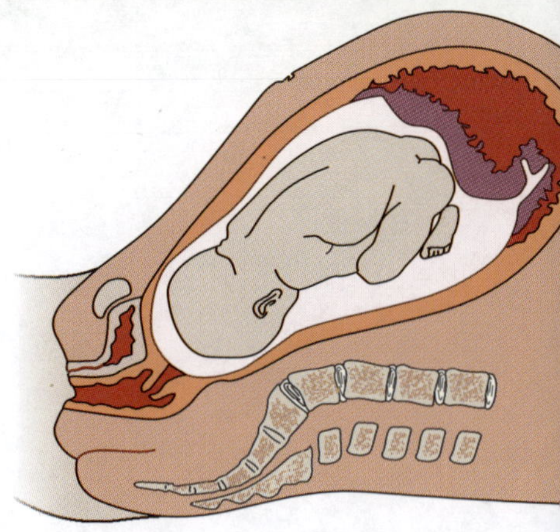

38

Hyperemesis Gravidarum

V Mathini

LEARNING OBJECTIVES

At the end of this chapter, the reader should be able to:

- define hyperemesis gravidarum
- enumerate the theories related to the causes of vomiting
- diagnose the condition
- consider other causes of vomiting
- select appropriate investigations
- outline the management of the mother
- enumerate the complications of hyperemesis gravidarum

Introduction

Nausea and vomiting are common symptoms of early pregnancy and occur in 70% of all pregnant women who generally respond to diet changes and reassurance; antiemetics are rarely required. The symptoms start a few days after the missed period, peak at 8–12 weeks and resolve by 20 weeks. Hyperemesis gravidarum is a severe and intractable form of nausea and vomiting of pregnancy, resulting in dehydration, weight loss, nutritional deficiencies, abnormal fluid and electrolyte and acid–base balance; the liver and brain may be involved in very severe and persistent hyperemesis.

Etiology

The etiology of nausea and vomiting during pregnancy is unknown. Several theories have been postulated based on the physiological changes.

- Rapidly increasing levels of human chorionic gonadotrophin (hCG) seem a plausible cause as vomiting coincides with peak levels of hCG in a normal pregnancy. In case of molar and multiple pregnancies, the vomiting is more severe and persists through later pregnancy, since the levels of hCG are high.
- Chronic infection with *Helicobacter pylori*, the agent causing peptic ulcer disease, has been suggested as contributing to hyperemesis gravidarum.
- There may be a genetic predisposition since women with hyperemesis report that their mother and/or sisters suffered from hyperemesis.
- Women younger than 30 years seem more prone to vomiting.
- Women with pregestational diabetes, migraine and motion sickness are more likely to suffer from hyperemesis.
- Psychological factors influence the severity of vomiting. This theory has been substantiated by the fact that women improve when removed from their surroundings.

Complications

In mild to moderate vomiting, there is hardly any morbidity for the mother or to the fetus. In hyperemesis gravidarum, morbidities like Wernicke's encephalopathy, Mallory–Weiss syndrome and esophageal rupture and renal tubular necrosis may occur. Termination of pregnancy is rarely indicated and maternal mortality has not been recorded when vomiting is controlled and the fluid–electrolyte balance is restored.

Clinical features

Symptoms: The woman presents early in pregnancy, essentially with vomiting; other symptoms are due to dehydration, starvation and subsequent deficiency of thiamine.

- excessive vomiting in hyperemesis gravidarum may be severe enough to prevent the woman from even drinking water
- oliguria
- epigastric pain
- dizziness, weakness, cramps
- symptoms of complications:
  - insomnia, blindness, convulsions or coma in Wernicke's encephalopathy due to thiamine deficiency
  - mental confusion with amnesia for recent events: Korsakoff's psychosis
  - blurring of vision, diplopia
  - peripheral neuritis

The symptoms listed above are very rare if nausea and vomiting of pregnancy can be effectively managed at presentation.

Signs: Pregnancy must be confirmed by physical examination or laboratory tests as it will rule out other conditions responsible for excessive vomiting. The patient appears anxious and has the following features:

- sunken eyes
- dry tongue
- loss of skin turgor
- tachycardia
- hypotension
- breath with ketotic odour
- icterus (in severe cases when the liver is affected)
- tenderness in the epigastrium is often present; there could be other conditions like gastritis, peptic ulcer and pancreatitis.

Differential diagnosis

There are a few other conditions in which the woman may present with excessive vomiting and its complications. These are:

- acute appendicitis
- acute cholecystitis
- hepatitis
- urinary tract infection, especially pyelonephritis
- pseudotumor cerebri.

Investigations

Laboratory investigations can help assess the severity of hyperemesis and rule out or confirm the presence of conditions considered for differential diagnosis.

- urine analysis for albumin, sugar, acetone, pus cells and casts, bile salts and bile pigments
- urine culture and sensitivity if more than 10 pus cells are seen in one high-power field
- serum electrolytes
- blood urea
- serum creatinine
- liver function tests (LFT)
- hematocrit
- fundus examination for retinal hemorrhage or detachment
- ECG to detect hypokalemia
- ultrasonological examination for confirmation of singleton or multiple pregnancy or H.mole.

Management

Early management of nausea and vomiting of pregnancy can prevent progress to hyperemesis. The first line of management consists of reassurance, small, frequent, easily digestible meals high in protein and avoidance of stimuli that act as a trigger. Antiemetics like doxylamine are added as second-line management. If vomiting persists, the following measures must be instituted:

- The patient should be admitted to the hospital and intravenous fluids started in order to replace fluid and electrolyte loss; antiemetics should also be given. Intravenous fluids like Ringer lactate and normal saline or dextrose saline are infused. Further addition of electrolytes is planned according to the serum levels. Addition of dextrose is said to prevent fat breakdown. Administration of pyridoxine and thiamine are useful. The patient should be instructed not to take anything orally for 24–48 hours till the vomiting stops completely.

- Anitemetics like pyridoxine (Vitamin B_6) given orally in a dose of 25 mg, 2–3 times a day is effective in controlling nausea and vomiting. Doxylamine 10 mg reduces vomiting among 70% of pregnant women, especially in combination with pyridoxine. The drug does not increase the risk of congenital anomalies. Metoclopromide can be given orally as a tablet 10 mg, 2–3 times a day or as an injection intramuscularly and intravenously. Promethazine and prochlorperazine are good second-line drugs.
- Corticosteroids have been tried parenterally in severe cases of hyperemesis gravidarum with varying results.
- Oral alimentation can be started once the acute phase is over. Small, frequent, fat-free, bland feeds are recommended.
- Other measures: Ginger, particularly in the powdered form, has been known to control hyperemesis gravidarum. Acupuncture has been tried with some success.

Termination of pregnancy should be considered only if all the above measures fail to control hyperemesis and the patient's condition deteriorates. However, such a situation hardly arises in the current scenario.

KEY POINTS

- Nausea and vomiting occur in 70% of pregnant women.
- Severe intractable vomiting in pregnancy associated with dehydration and electrolyte imbalance is termed hyperemesis gravidarum.
- Molar pregnancy and multiple pregnancy must be considered when hyperemesis gravidarum persists through the second trimester.
- Other causes associated with vomiting like acute abdomen, pyelonephritis and hepatitis must be kept in mind.
- The patient must be examined and monitored very closely to avoid complications of hyperemesis gravidarum.
- Most cases of hyperemesis respond well to therapeutic intervention with antiemetics and correction of fluid and electrolyte imbalance.

QUESTIONS

Select the single most appropriate answer:

1. Nausea and vomiting of pregnancy start after a few days of pregnancy and definitely resolve by
   a. 8 weeks
   b. 12 weeks
   c. 16 weeks
   d. 20 weeks
2. Which of the following is the most well-established cause of hyperemesis?
   a. infection with *Helicobacter pylori*
   b. high levels of progesterone
   c. high levels of hCG
   d. overdistension of the uterus
3. When a woman presents with excessive vomiting, she should be
   a. reassured
   b. advised small frequent meals
   c. prescribed antiemetics
   d. all of the above

In the following questions, there are two statements. Select the appropriate answer using the following key:

a. if both statements are true and causally related
b. if both statements are true but not causally related

c. if the first statement is true and the second is false
d. if the first statement is false and the second is true
e. if both statements are false

4. It is necessary to counsel a woman with severe hyperemesis *because*
   Psychological factors strongly influence the severity of hyperemesis.
5. Medical termination of pregnancy is rarely indicated in severe hyperemesis *because*
   Severe hyperemesis can rarely result in life-threatening renal tubular necrosis.

39

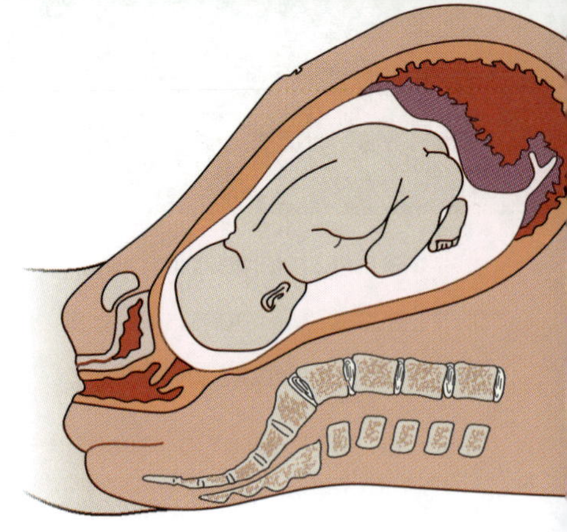

Hypertensive Disorders

S Habeebullah

LEARNING OBJECTIVES

At the end of this chapter, the reader should be able to:

- define hypertension in pregnancy
- classify hypertensive disorders in pregnancy
- list the factors that indicate a woman as prone to develop preeclampsia
- describe the pathophysiology and pathology of preeclampsia
- enumerate the criteria for the diagnosis of preeclampsia
- list the complications of preeclampsia
- enumerate the essential laboratory investigations
- describe the general management of a woman with preeclampsia
- describe the use of anti-hypertensives
- outline obstetric management in preeclampsia
- enumerate the features of severe preeclampsia
- list the emergency measures to be taken when a woman presents with eclampsia
- describe the magnesium sulphate regimen for the control of eclampsia
- indicate the long-term effects of preeclampsia/eclampsia

Introduction

Hypertensive disorders complicate 5%–15% of all pregnancies; the incidence is higher among primigravidae. They contribute significantly to both maternal and perinatal morbidity and mortality. In India, of all maternal deaths, 12% are caused by hypertensive disorders; thus, they are also the leading cause of perinatal mortality. The disease can be detected early if health care providers are aware of the condition, identify the women prone to develop hypertension, record blood pressure (BP) carefully and interpret it correctly. Thereafter, appropriate interventions can prevent complications and minimise morbidity and mortality.

Hypertension in Pregnancy

Definition

Hypertension in pregnancy is defined as systolic blood pressure (SBP) ≥140 mm Hg and diastolic blood pressure (DBP) ≥90 mm Hg recorded on two occasions at least six hours apart. Mean arterial pressure (MAP) ≥105 mm Hg or increase in MAP by 20 mm Hg also indicates hypertension. Mean arterial pressure is derived by the formula:

$$[SBP + (DBP \times 2)] \div 3$$

Severe hypertension is diagnosed when blood pressure (BP) is ≥160/110 or MAP is >126 mm Hg.

Classification

Hypertensive disorders complicating pregnancy can be classified into the following types:

Gestational hypertension: BP ≥140/90 mm Hg for the first time during pregnancy, absence of proteinuria and BP returning to normal within 12 weeks postpartum.

Preeclampsia: BP ≥140/90 mm Hg after 20 weeks of gestation, proteinuria ≥300 mg/24 hours or ≥1+ dipstick. Preeclampsia is severe if the pressure is ≥160/110 mm Hg, proteinuria ≥5 g/24 hours and/or 2+ dipstick.

Eclampsia: Preeclampsia with convulsions not attributable to any other cause.

Chronic hypertension: Preexisting hypertension or hypertension detected before 20 weeks, but not attributable to trophoblastic disease.

Preeclampsia/eclampsia **superimposed on** chronic hypertension.

Gestational hypertension/preeclampsia usually occurs in the third trimester of pregnancy. However, in some women, it may occur before 32 weeks. This is termed **early onset preeclampsia** and is associated with higher maternal morbidity and poor perinatal outcome.

PREECLAMPSIA

Predisposing factors

The exact cause of preeclampsia is not known. However, in the presence of the following factors, there is a higher risk of developing preeclampsia.

- **Genetic predisposition:** If the mother or sister has had hypertension during pregnancy, the risk is eight times higher.
- Primigravidae are 15 times more prone than parous women.
- Women who suffered from preeclampsia in the first pregnancy are more likely to suffer from the condition in subsequent pregnancies.
- Age below 18 years and over 35 years
- Socially disadvantaged women
- Women with BMI ≥35
- Multiple pregnancy, molar pregnancy, hydramnios and hydrops fetalis
- Essential hypertension, diabetes mellitus, obesity, renal disease and connective tissue diseases like systemic lupus erythematosus and antiphospholipid antibody syndrome. Thrombophilias are associated with early onset preeclampsia and recur in subsequent pregnancies.

Pathogenesis

Gestational hypertension and preeclampsia are unique to human pregnancy and are relieved after delivery. The basic factor seems to be defective placentation. In early pregnancy, normally, the decidual spiral arterioles are invaded by the cytotrophoblast. The musculoelastic tissue of these vessels is replaced by fibrinoid tissue, leading to dilatation of these vessels and thus reducing the resistance to blood flow.

In a normal pregnancy, a second trophoblastic invasion of the myometrial radial arteries occurs at about 18 weeks, further reducing vascular resistance and increasing placental blood flow. Failure of this secondary invasion results in increased vascular resistance and decreased uteroplacental flow.

The basic pathology causing the multiple organ systems to be involved in preeclampsia is vasospasm and endothelial damage. Prostacyclin (PGI_2) is a vasodilator and prevents platelet aggregation in vessels, whereas thromboxane A_2 (TXA_2) has the opposite effect. In preeclampsia, there is an imbalance between PGI_2 and TXA_2; the relatively high levels of TXA_2 cause vasoconstriction and platelet aggregation.

Nitric oxide, a potent vasodilator, maintains the low pressure state of fetoplacental perfusion in normal pregnancy. Preeclampsia is associated with a reduction in nitric oxide synthesis. The endothelium, when damaged, secretes substances which promote coagulation and increase vascular sensitivity; it also allows leakage of platelets and fibrinogen, which deposit subendothelially.

Pathophysiology

Cardiovascular changes: In normal pregnancy, cardiac output is increased by 40%–50% but peripheral resistance is reduced by 25%. However, in preeclampsia, in addition to elevated cardiac output, peripheral resistance is also increased due to **generalised vasospasm**. The other major abnormality, **endothelial injury,** leads to the extravascular leakage of plasma. These result in **reduction of intravascular volume**. These patients are abnormally sensitive to even normal blood loss at the time of delivery and are prone to develop fluid overload with intravenous fluid administration.

Hematological changes: In normal pregnancy, the blood volume is increased by 50% with more of plasma than red cell mass, and an attendant fall in hematocrit. In preeclampsia, this expansion of blood volume is reduced, leading to hemoconcentration and increased hematocrit. The endothelial injury could cause microangiopathic hemolysis, leading to anemia, thrombocytopenia and fragmentation of red blood cells. Fibrinogen, antithrombin III and factor VIII levels are reduced, whereas fibronectin levels are increased. There is increased fibrinolysis.

Uteroplacental changes: There is decreased uteroplacental perfusion in preeclampsia. This may lead to IUGR and in severe cases, even fetal death.

Pathology

Generalised vasospasm and endothelial damage are responsible for the changes in the various organs.

Kidneys: Glomerular endotheliosis histologically manifests as glomerular epithelial swelling, narrowing of the capillary lumen and subendothelial fibrin deposits.

Liver: Periportal hemorrhagic necrosis, enlargement of the liver and subcapsular hemorrhages are seen in severe disease. Rarely, the liver may rupture.

Brain: In severe cases, cerebral edema, thrombosis, infarcts and hemorrhage may be seen.

Retina: The changes vary from generalised vasospasm to retinal hemorrhages, papilledema and retinal detachment.

Placenta: The placenta is usually small and infarcted with hematoma, proliferative endarteritis and degeneration.

Clinical features

A woman with gestational hypertension/preeclampsia is usually asymptomatic; the diagnosis is made during routine antenatal check-up.

- Prepregnancy BMI ≥ 35 and weight gain of over 0.5 kg/week in the third trimester warrant anticipating preeclampsia. Edema of the lower limbs not relieved by rest and edema in nondependent areas like the face, fingers, abdominal wall and vulva may also herald preeclampsia.
- Oliguria and headache are indicative of severe disease. However, symptoms like persistent frontal headache, blurring of vision, epigastric pain, nausea and vomiting are suggestive of imminent eclampsia.
- In preeclampsia, the hypertension is labile. Therefore, multiple readings (at 4–6 hour intervals) should be taken to assess the severity. Uncontrolled hypertension can lead to complications like eclampsia, cerebral hemorrhage and cardiac failure.
- For recording the blood pressure, the woman rests on a couch or bed on her right with a 15°–30° tilt or sits upright on a chair. The sphygmomanometer is at the level of the eye of the observer with the centre of the cuff over the brachial artery on the upper arm, which is at the level of the heart. A larger cuff is used for obese patients. Diastolic BP is noted when the Korotkoff sounds disappear (phase V).
- Proteinuria is the hallmark of preeclampsia. It is considered significant if there is more than 300 mg protein in urine in 24 hours (≥1+ on dipstick). Proteinuria of ≥2 g/24 hours (2+ or more on dipstick) is a marker of severe preeclampsia.
- Other clinical features like brisk tendon reflexes may be seen in imminent eclampsia.
- Obstetric examination may reveal oligohydramnios and IUGR, especially if the disease is of longer duration and is severe.

Investigations

The investigations are performed mainly to establish the severity of the disease and to assess response to treatment. Since the disease involves multiple organs to varying degrees, a wide range of investigations should be carried out.

- hemoglobin, hematocrit, peripheral smear, platelet count, clotting time, fibrinogen levels, prothrombin time and fibrinogen degradation products
- urinanalysis for the presence of proteins and casts, and bacterial culture
- blood urea, serum creatinine and uric acid
- serum bilirubin, AST, ALT, LDH
- blood glucose
- retinal fundoscopy for evidence of arteriolar spasm, retinal edema, hemorrhages and detachment
- fetal growth is assessed by serial biometry; fetal wellbeing is monitored by daily fetal movement count, NST, biophysical profile and umbilical artery Doppler (if needed).

Criteria for the diagnosis of severe preeclampsia

- SBP ≥160 mm Hg
- DBP ≥110 mm Hg
- proteinuria ≥5 g/24 hours
- oliguria <500 ml/24 hours
- Hepatic dysfunction (LDH >600 IU/ml)
- IUGR/oligohydramnios
- thrombocytopenia (<100,000/mm^3)
- clinical features of imminent eclampsia
- pulmonary edema/cyanosis

Prediction of preeclampsia

The common predictive tests are given below.

Roll-over test: It is performed between weeks 28 and 32. BP is checked first in the left lateral position and then in the supine position. The test is positive if the DBP rises by >20 mm Hg. However, it is important to remember that the test has high false positivity.

Isometric hand grip exercise test: Resting BP is taken; the woman is then asked to press an inflated BP cuff for 30 seconds. She then presses the cuff at 50% of maximal contraction for three minutes. If the rise in DBP is >20 mm Hg, the test is positive. The test takes longer but is more reliable than the roll-over test.

MAP in second trimester: MAP ≥90 mm Hg is predictive of hypertension.

Angiotensin II infusion test: In normal pregnancy, the administration of up to 8 ng/kg body weight of angiotensin does not produce hypertension. If BP rises at <8 ng/kg body weight of infusion of angiotensin, the test is positive, indicating that 90% of subjects may subsequently develop hypertension. The test is invasive, time-consuming and is not performed routinely in clinical practice.

Calcium/creatinine ratio: Since in preeclampsia, urinary calcium excretion is reduced, a calcium/creatinine ratio of <0.04 is considered significant. This has a sensitivity of 70%.

Doppler velocimetry: The presence of a diastolic notch in the uterine artery in the second trimester predicts the development of hypertension.

Fetal DNA: The presence of fetal DNA in maternal serum at the time of endothelial activation has been shown to predict the disease earlier in pregnancy.

Elevated fetal fibronectin at about 12 weeks, elevated inhibin A, and corticotropin releasing hormone have not been found to be reliable predictors.

Most of the above tests have good negative predictive value; that is, if the test is negative, the woman may not develop hypertension.

Prevention

A number of pharmacological and non-pharmacological interventions have been advocated for the prevention of preeclampsia, but none has been shown to be of significant benefit.

- In women with dietary deficiency, a daily supplementation of 2 g calcium from week 15 onwards may reduce the risk of developing preeclampsia.
- Administration of low-dose aspirin, 60–75 mg daily has been extensively studied. It is useful in women at risk of preeclampsia (say, those with SLE) or in those who had preeclampsia/eclampsia (especially of the early onset type) in the previous pregnancy. Low-dose aspirin suppresses thromboxane synthesis, resulting in prostacyclin dominance. It should be stopped at 34 weeks of gestation.
- Antioxidants like vitamin C 1,000 mg, vitamin E 400 IU and L-arginine which remove the free radicals, increase nitric oxide and reduce oxidative stress and lipid peroxidation; may be effective.

- Folic acid supplementation may reduce the risk of preeclampsia by lowering homocysteine levels.

Management

The goals of management are:
- prevention of convulsions and other complications in the mother
- carrying the pregnancy to near term
- delivery of a healthy baby.

The definitive treatment of preeclampsia is delivery. However, if the fetus is not mature and the disease is not severe, a conservative approach may be adopted.

General management: It is advisable to initially admit in the hospital all patients with hypertension and assess the severity of the disease through clinical and laboratory evaluation.

- Bed rest in the left lateral position improves uteroplacental perfusion. If the patient is apprehensive, mild sedation (phenobarbitone 60 mg or diazepam 10 mg) is useful.
- Diuretics are not used in preeclampsia as they further reduce the plasma volume leading to decreased placental perfusion. Long-term use of thiazide diuretics may cause hyperuricemia, neonatal hyponatremia, hypokalemia and thrombocytopenia. However, they are used when pulmonary edema and congestive heart failure are present.
- If the disease is mild, in a reliable patient, there is place for outpatient care, preferably in a 'day care' centre where she is assessed twice a week.
- Anti-hypertensives are used when the DBP is ≥100 mm Hg and pregnancy is less than 36 weeks to prevent progression of the disease and its complications like HELLP syndrome, eclampsia and cerebral hemorrhage. They may also improve birth weight and perinatal outcome.
- Assessment of fetal wellbeing is done by daily fetal movement count (DFMC), nonstress test (NST) and ultrasonography (biophysical profile and Doppler studies).
- Delivery is contemplated when:
  i. pregnancy reaches term.
  ii. preeclampsia is severe.
  iii. there is fetal compromise.

Anti-hypertensive management: Women with severe preeclampsia should be hospitalised. After stabilisation, the pregnancy is terminated if the pregnancy has reached term. However, if the pregnancy is at less than 36 weeks, anti-hypertensives are administered under close monitoring. When the diastolic BP is ≥110 mm Hg, sublingual nifedipine 5 mg or injection hydralazine 5–10 mg IV every 30 minutes or injection labetalol 50 mg are administered The aim should be to maintain DBP at around 90 mm Hg.

The commonly used anti-hypertensives are shown in **Table 39.1.**

When there is no response to anti-hypertensives, and especially in the presence of severe IUGR, termination of pregnancy is the best option.

Obstetric management: The objective is to carry the pregnancy to term without maternal or fetal adverse effects. If pregnancy is to be terminated before 34 weeks, injection betamethasone or injection dexamethasone is used to improve fetal lung maturity. If the cervix is favourable, labour is induced by artificial rupture of membranes (ARM) followed by oxytocin drip if necessary. If the cervix is unfavourable, intracervical PGE_2 gel is used followed by ARM and oxytocin. In severe preeclampsia, injection magnesium sulphate administered in a prophylactic dosage will prevent convulsions. Continuous electronic fetal monitoring is preferable with a close watch on the progress of labour. The second stage is cut short by forceps delivery. Cesarean section is performed for obstetric indications, if associated maternal/fetal complications develop, or if the cervix remains unfavourable. To prevent PPH, intraumbilical injection of oxytocin (10 units) is used since **prophylactic methergin should be avoided. The BP should be closely monitored for at least 24 hours after delivery**.

Complications

In preeclampsia, both the mother and her child are likely to suffer from complications, some of which are life-threatening.

Maternal complications: About 2%–5% of women suffering from preeclampsia develop eclampsia. Other

Table 39.1 Anti-hypertensives commonly used in the treatment of preeclampsia

Drug	Action	Dosage	Side effects
1. Alpha methyldopa	Central	250 mg Q 6 up to 2 g/day	Long-term studies have shown it to be safe. Sedation, tiredness, nasal stuffiness
2. Nifedipine	Calcium channel blocker	10 mg Q 8, up to 120 mg/day	Headache, dizziness, mild myocardial depression
3. Labetalol	α, β blocker	50–100 mg BD to 200 mg Q 8, max 2,400 mg/day	Orthostatic hypotension, bradycardia, nasal congestion
4. Atenolol	β blocker	50–200 mg/day in 2 divided doses	Bradycardia, hypotension, hypoglycemia, IUGR

ACE inhibitors are contraindicated in pregnancy as they may cause IUGR, hypokalemia, fetal renal agenesis, oligohydramnios and intrauterine fetal death.

complications include abruptio placentae (5%), renal failure, visual disturbances, cardiac failure, cerebral hemorrhage, increased operative intervention and postpartum collapse. Therefore, the risk of maternal mortality is significantly increased.

Perinatal complications: These are IUGR, prematurity, birth asphyxia and increased perinatal mortality, ranging from 5% to 20% depending on the severity of the disease.

Fulminant preeclampsia: The onset of the disease is acute with rapid deterioration of the condition leading to convulsions or coma. Stabilisation of hypertension, magnesium sulphate therapy and immediate termination of pregnancy can prevent serious complications.

ECLAMPSIA

Eclampsia is preeclampsia with convulsions. In 60%–70% of cases of preeclampsia, eclampsia occurs in the antepartum, in 25% in the intrapartum and in 10%–15% in the postpartum period. It is usually preceded by severe preeclampsia and imminent symptoms; however, in 15%–20%, there may be no evidence of hypertension or proteinuria at the time of convulsions. Maternal mortality is about 2%–6%, but could be higher. The causes of death are cerebral hemorrhage, pulmonary edema, renal failure, hepatic failure, DIC and cardiac failure.

Typically, the eclamptic convulsions are tonic-clonic. The stages of eclamptic convulsions can be described as follows:

Prodromal stage: There may be an aura, followed by rolling and fixation of the eyeballs. Then twitching of the facial muscles begins and lasts for a few seconds to half a minute.

Tonic stage: Arms are flexed, hands clenched, the whole body becomes rigid and respiration stops. This stage lasts for 20–30 seconds.

Clonic stage: This involves jerky convulsions which may throw the woman out of the bed. She is cyanosed and frothy sputum may appear. This stage lasts for about a minute.

Recovery stage: All movements subside. The patient may go into a coma of variable duration. Respiration is rapid and deep.

Differential diagnosis

All patients with convulsions in pregnancy (especially in the third trimester) should be treated for eclampsia until proven otherwise. The other conditions to be considered are epilepsy, meningitis, cerebral malaria, cortical vein thrombosis, poisoning and hypoglycemia.

Management

The management of eclampsia consists of:

General measures: The patient should be nursed in a railed cot, keeping the head to one side with a mouth gag to prevent injuries to the tongue. Intravenous access should be obtained using an 18G needle and IV fluids (Ringer lactate) started. Oxygen should be administered; the patient should be monitored, preferably with pulse oximetry. Throat secretions are sucked out. After control of convulsions, continuous bladder drainage is used and urinary output measured.

Control of convulsions: The drug of choice for the control of convulsions is magnesium sulphate ($MgSO_4$). It can be used in one of the following ways.

Pritchard's regimen: A loading dose of 4 g Mg SO4 (as 20 ml of 20% solution) is given as slow IV over 5 minutes. In addition, 10 g MgSO4 is given IM, 5 g (10 ml of 50%) into each buttock. If convulsions persist, a further 2 g (10 ml of 20%) may be given as IV bolus over 2 minutes. Magnesium sulphate should be continued for 24 hours after delivery or after the last convulsion, whichever is later. Maintenance dose of 5 g MgSO4 every 4 hours IM is given provided:

- respiratory rate is >14/minute,
- knee jerks are present and
- urine output in the previous 4 hours is >100 ml.

If any of the above criteria is not fulfilled, the next dose of $MgSO_4$ is not given.

Sibai regimen: Loading dose is 6 g (30 ml of 20%) over 20 minutes IV; maintenance dose is 2 g/h IV for 24 hours after delivery or last convulsion, whichever is later.

Magnesium sulphate lowers the neuromuscular transmission of acetylcholine esterase. It also causes cerebral cortical depression and cerebral vasodilatation. The serum level of 4–7 mEq/l is considered therapeutic. Loss of patellar reflex indicates early toxicity. Antidote is 10 ml of 10% calcium gluconate which should be kept ready and administered in case of respiratory depression. It does not cause fetal distress.

Other anticonvulsants: **Diazepam** 10 mg IV bolus along with 40 mg in 500 ml of dextrose is given as a drip. If convulsions recur, one more bolus of 10 mg IV can be given. Side effects include neonatal respiratory depression and hypotonia. This can be used in peripheral hospitals where $MgSO_4$ is not available.

Phenytoin sodium is given in the loading dose of 15–25 mg/kg slow IV (not more than 25 mg/min); the next dose of 500 mg IV is given 12 hours later. Maintenance dose is 100 mg IV or IM every 4 hours followed by an oral dose several days postpartum.

For rapid control of BP, nifedipine 5 mg is administered sublingually. Alternatively, 5 mg of hydralazine is administered as IV bolus every 20 to 30 minute till BP is stabilised. Parenteral labetalol may also be used. Maintaining fluid and electrolyte balance is essential. Fluid management is best done by central venous pressure monitoring.

Status eclampticus is managed in an ICU set-up with the help of an anesthetist using thiopentone, muscle relaxants and intubation.

Anti-hypertensive management: In women with eclampsia, intravenous administration of labetalol or hydralazine as described above is used for the control of hypertension. Sublingual nifedipine may be difficult to administer in a convulsing patient.

Obstetric management: Obstetric management consists of prompt delivery. If the patient is already in labour or if the cervix is favourable, an ARM is done, followed by oxytocin augmentation. If the cervix is unfavourable, cervical ripening is achieved using PGE_2 gel, followed by ARM. Cesarean section should be reserved for obstetric indications or in a rare case of uncontrolled convulsions.

In most cases, the BP returns to normal after delivery within 48 hours. However, if high BP persists, anti-hypertensives should be continued and BP checked at 6 and 12 weeks postpartum.

Rarely, the convulsions may cease and pregnancy continues for 10 days or more; this is known as **intercurrent eclampsia.**

Long-term sequelae

In 10% of patients, the BP may persist beyond three months postpartum, in which case the condition is labelled **essential hypertension.**

Although preeclampsia is a disease of primigravidae, the risk of recurrence in subsequent pregnancy is 25%–30%. In early onset preeclampsia, the recurrence rate may be as high as 50%–60%. Multiparas with preeclampsia are at risk of recurrence in a subsequent pregnancy.

HELLP Syndrome

HELLP syndrome (Hemolysis, Elevated Liver enzymes and Low Platelet count) occurs in about 5% of cases of severe preeclampsia and eclampsia. Besides the clinical features of severe preeclampsia, peripheral smear shows evidence of microangiopathic hemolysis characterised by burr cells, schistocytes and polychromasia. Serum bilirubin (mostly indirect) may be more than 1.2 mg/dl, LDH more than 600 IU/l and platelet count <100,000/mm^3. Other conditions causing jaundice (viral hepatitis, acute fatty liver, intrahepatic cholestasis, or hyperemesis) should be ruled out.

Management includes careful maternal and fetal evaluation, prevention of convulsions using magnesium sulphate, injection dexamethasone 10 mg IV 12 hourly (continued for 2–3 days after delivery) and packed cell and platelet transfusions. Labour is induced after correcting coagulation abnormalities. Maternal and perinatal mortality rates are high.

Chronic Hypertension in Pregnancy

Hypertension diagnosed prior to pregnancy or before 20 weeks of gestation is defined as chronic hypertension and occurs in about 2% of pregnancies. It is generally idiopathic but in about 20% it may be due to secondary causes. The patients are generally multiparas in their 30s.

The adverse effects on pregnancy are:

- superimposed preeclampsia which is diagnosed by the appearance of proteinuria for the first time or if there is worsening of hypertension or proteinuria or the appearance of thrombocytopenia; the incidence is 20%.
- abruptio placentae (5%–10%)
- other maternal complications like congestive cardiac failure, cerebrovascular accidents, renal failure and malignant hypertension
- fetal complications include IUGR, prematurity and increased perinatal mortality, particularly in superimposed preeclampsia.

Investigations are directed towards detecting secondary causes of hypertension and assessing the severity of the disease. Fetal evaluation should include monitoring for growth and wellbeing.

Management

If a patient presents before pregnancy, she must undergo detailed investigations to establish the primary cause, control of BP with appropriate antihypertensives and counselling regarding lifestyle modification and prognosis. Diuretics and ACE inhibitors should be avoided.

During pregnancy, management mainly includes control of hypertension and, keeping a close watch on the development of the complications mentioned above. In mild and uncomplicated chronic hypertension, pregnancy may be allowed to go to term. In superimposed preeclampsia, the management should be as for preeclampsia.

KEY POINTS

- Preeclampsia/eclampsia are leading causes of maternal and perinatal morbidity and mortality.
- The cause of preeclampsia is unclear though pathophysiology and predisposing factors are known.
- Preeclampsia involves almost all the systems in the body; generalised vasospasm is a classic abnormality.
- The diagnosis of preeclampsia is made in the presence of significant proteinuria with high BP.
- The ultimate cure is delivery of the fetus; if pregnancy is preterm, it may be allowed to go to term if the BP is controlled with anti-hypertensives and the fetus continues to grow.
- Prediction of preeclampsia is unsatisfactory; most tests have good negative predictive value.
- Eclampsia is a serious but preventable complication of preeclampsia. Treatment includes magnesium sulphate, anti-hypertensives and prompt delivery.
- The woman should be counselled regarding recurrence in future pregnancies and given low-dose aspirin.

QUESTIONS

1. Which of the following anti-hypertensives is contraindicated in pregnancy?
   a. captopril
   b. labetalol
   c. metoprolol
   d. nifedipine
2. Which of the following is *not* a feature of severe preeclampsia?
   a. diastolic BP 120 mm Hg
   b. 24-hour proteinuria $\leq$1 g
   c. pulmonary edema
   d. intrauterine growth restriction
3. The risk of recurrence of preeclampsia in a subsequent pregnancy is
   a. 5%
   b. 15%
   c. 25%
   d. 50%
4. The obstetric management of eclampsia presenting at 37 weeks is
   a. termination of pregnancy
   b. continuation of pregnancy till 40 weeks
   c. immediate cesarean section
   d. continuation of pregnancy till 38 weeks
5. All of the following are consistent with HELLP syndrome *except*
   a. schistocytes in peripheral blood smear
   b. lactic dehydrogenase 700 IU/ml
   c. platelet count 1,50,000/mm^3
   d. bilirubin 3 mg%
6. Which of the following statements about eclampsia is *not* correct?
   a. convulsions are controlled with magnesium sulphate
   b. mode of delivery should be cesarean section
   c. fetal mortality is high
   d. there is a possibility of rupture of the liver

40

Antepartum Hemorrhage

C Ambuja

LEARNING OBJECTIVES

At the end of this chapter, the reader should be able to:

- define antepartum hemorrhage (APH)
- enumerate the causes of APH
- describe the pathology of placental abruption
- list the conditions that predispose to placental abruption
- enumerate the clinical features and principles of management of placental abruption
- enumerate the complications in the mother and the fetus
- describe the pathology and clinical features of placenta previa
- clinically differentiate placenta previa from abruptio placentae
- outline the management of placenta previa
- list the complications caused by placenta previa in the mother and fetus

Introduction

Hemorrhage during late pregnancy is an obstetrical emergency associated with significant maternal and fetal morbidity and mortality. The incidence of hemorrhage during pregnancy is approximately 1 in 200 to 1 in 50 deliveries, and contributes to 30% of perinatal mortality and to about one-third of maternal mortality, along with other causes of hemorrhage in obstetrics. The condition needs to be managed with great care for optimal maternal and fetal outcome.

Definition

Antepartum hemorrhage is defined as bleeding from or into the genital tract after the period of viability, that is, 20 weeks of gestation (28 weeks in India), but before the delivery of the baby.

Causes

Vaginal bleeding may be from the placental site or from lesions in the lower genital tract. In a number of cases, no definite cause is established:

- Placental abruption, also known as abruptio placentae or accidental hemorrhage accounts for 30% of cases.
- Placenta previa is noted in 20% of cases.
- Unclassified bleeding is seen in 45% of cases.
- Lower genital tract lesions in 5% of cases; these include cervical polyp, cervical carcinoma, vulvovaginal varices and vaginitis. Very rarely the bleeding could be caused by velamentous insertion of the umbilical cord with hemorrhage from the fetal blood vessels when the membranes rupture.

PLACENTAL ABRUPTION

Definition

The term placental abruption refers to bleeding due to premature separation of a normally implanted placenta in the upper uterine segment, that is, separation of the placenta before delivery of the fetus. The frequency of placental abruption is about 1 in 100 deliveries.

Pathology

Hemorrhage in the decidua basalis begins with placental separation. This leads to splitting of the decidua, although a thin layer of decidua continues to be attached to the myometrium. A decidual hematoma thus formed is responsible for further separation, compression and destruction of the part of the placenta in contact with the hematoma. In some cases, rupture of decidual spiral artery forms a hematoma that separates the placenta. The blood may remain as retroplacental hematoma or extravasate between the uterine musculature. Flowing beyond the placental margins, the blood can separate the membranes and reach the vagina.

The hemorrhage in placental abruption is **concealed** (**Fig. 40.1**) when

- Blood is retained behind the placenta if its margins are intact.
- The whole placenta is separated, but the membranes remain attached to the uterine wall.
- Blood escapes into the amniotic cavity.

The hemorrhage is **revealed** (**Fig. 40.2**) when

- The placental margins separate.
- Membranes are dissected from the uterine wall.

Etiology

It is not known why placental abruption occurs. However, it is associated with certain risk factors:

- advanced maternal age
- increased parity
- previous history of abruption
- preeclampsia
- chronic hypertension
- polyhydramnios
- multiple pregnancy
- prelabour rupture of membranes
- thrombophilias
- uterine fibroids
- cigarette smoking
- use of cocaine.

The most common risk factor is any type of hypertension. The risk increases considerably if the woman suffers from chronic hypertension with preeclampsia and is a smoker. Therefore, control of hypertension is one way to reduce the risk of abruption. External trauma is not a very high risk factor. Some thrombophilias associated with thromboembolic phenomena during pregnancy increase the risk of placental abruption. In case of uterine fibroids, placental abruption may occur if the tumour is behind the site of placental implantation.

Diagnosis

The clinical features are extremely variable. The signs and symptoms may not be consistent with the quantity of external bleeding. The woman could

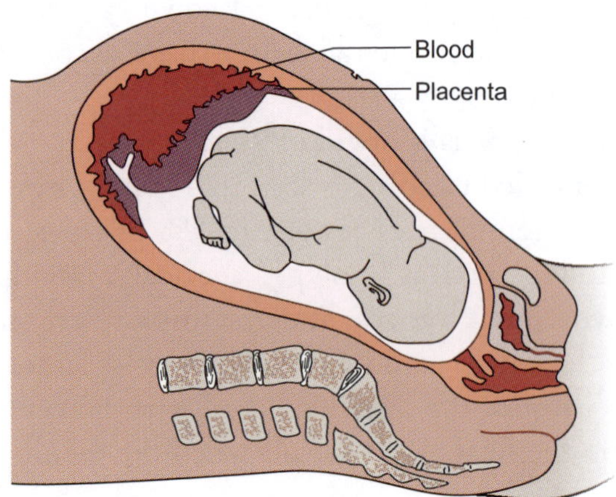

Fig. 40.1 Concealed abruption.

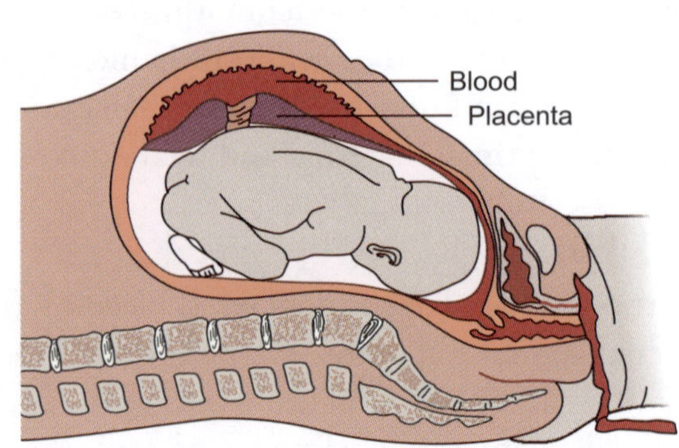

Fig. 40.2 Revealed abruption.

be very pale and even be in shock in the absence of external bleeding but the fetus may be compromised. Placental abruption should be suspected when the following symptoms and signs are noted.

Symptoms

- vaginal bleeding
- abdominal pain
- history of addiction to tobacco/cocaine
- history of hypertensive disorders
- loss of fetal movements

Signs

- pallor, tachycardia and hypotension depending on the blood loss
- tense, tender uterus which may be more than usual for the period of gestation
- fetal parts not easily palpable
- absent fetal heart sounds

Ultrasound: It is useful in the diagnosis of abruption only in the presence of blood or a clot in the retroplacental region. Recent studies show that the clinical diagnosis of abruption was confirmed by ultrasound in only 25% of cases. Thus, a negative finding with ultrasound does not rule out placental abruption.

Differential diagnosis

The main entities to be considered are placenta previa and excessive 'show'. When a woman presents with severe abdominal pain, other causes of acute abdomen must be considered.

Complications

The complications of placental abruption are due to hemorrhage and coagulation failure.

Consumptive coagulopathy or disseminated intravascular coagulation (DIC): The most frequent cause of consumptive coagulopathy is placental abruption. Hypofibrinogenemia, raised levels of fibrinogen-fibrin degradation products and decrease in other coagulation factors and platelets are noted.

Renal failure: Acute renal failure is encountered in placental abruption, particularly when there is a delay in correcting hypovolemia. The frequent association of preeclampsia with placental abruption and massive hemorrhage leads to severe renal failure. Aggressive management of hemorrhage can reduce the severity of renal failure to a considerable extent.

Couvelaire uterus: In this condition the blood extravasates into the uterine musculature. It is also known as uteroplacental apoplexy and was described by Couvelaire in the early 1900s. The effusion of blood in the myometrium rarely interferes with uterine contraction, and thus it is not an indication for hysterectomy.

Postpartum hemorrhage: It is a common complication. It may be due to uterine atony or coagulopathy.

Management

The main aspect of the management of abruption is to expedite delivery in most patients. The focus should be on improving the general condition of the woman and making efforts to salvage the fetus where possible.

The woman's general condition is assessed by both clinical examination and laboratory investigations. The hypovolemia should be corrected using blood, colloids or crystalloids; where indicated, blood components may be administered.

Obstetric management depends on the period of gestation and the severity of placental abruption.

- Cesarean section is preferred when the fetus is alive and salvageable or if there is evidence of fetal distress and labour is likely to be prolonged.
- Vaginal delivery is preferred if the fetus is very premature, malformed or dead, diagnosis of abruption is doubtful or if the woman is in active labour.

The membranes are ruptured and oxytocin is used to expedite delivery. Anticipation of PPH and preparedness to deal with it effectively are crucial in obstetric management.

- Expectant management is occasionally recommended to delay the birth of a premature baby. However, the decision is also guided by the availability of appropriate neonatal care. It must be remembered that abruption can progress very rapidly and fetal death may result; hence, the condition should be carefully considered before resorting to conservative treatment.

Maternal and perinatal outcome

Perinatal morbidity and mortality: Stillbirth occurs due to asphyxia when most of the placenta is separated or there are placental infarcts due to thromboembolism. The other reason for poor perinatal outcome is prematurity and its sequelae.

Maternal morbidity and mortality: Maternal morbidity is essentially due to blood loss, associated conditions like hypertension, consumptive coagulopathy and renal failure. Although maternal outcome has improved with the availability of blood and blood components, placental abruption continues to remain an important cause of maternal mortality in developing countries.

Placenta Previa

Definition

In placenta previa, the placenta is implanted on or very close to the internal os. There are four degrees of placenta previa depending on how close the placenta is to the internal os (**Fig. 40.3**).

- **Total:** Placenta covers the internal os completely (Type IV)
- **Partial:** Placenta covers the internal os partially (Type III)
- **Marginal:** Placenta is at the margin of the internal os (Type II)
- **Low lying placenta:** In this condition, the placenta is situated in the lower segment and is close to the internal os, but the edges of the placenta do not reach the margin of the internal os (Type I)

The first two types and posterior marginal type are of major degree and the others of minor degree. The degree of placenta previa can vary according to the dilatation of the cervix. What is complete at 2 cm of cervical dilatation could become partial when the cervical dilatation is 6 cm. **No attempt should be made to ascertain the degree by vaginal examination as it may precipitate massive hemorrhage.**

The incidence of placenta previa is approximately 1 in 250 deliveries. It depends on the accuracy of documentation; geographical variation is not uncommon.

Etiology

There is no single cause of placenta previa. However, placenta previa is associated with certain conditions:

- advancing maternal age
- multiparity
- previous cesarean section
- prior endometritis
- large placenta, as in multiple pregnancy.

Diagnosis

The clinical presentation in most cases is characteristic. The bleeding is painless, causeless and appears suddenly, stops spontaneously only to recur after a few days or weeks. The initial hemorrhage is of small quantity and has been labelled **warning hemorrhage**. Unlike in placental abruption, association of hypertension is infrequent. Therefore, the bleeding in placenta previa has been described as **painless, causeless and recurrent.**

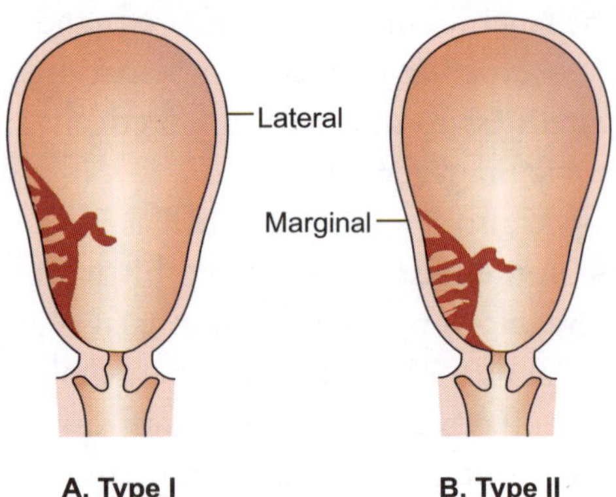

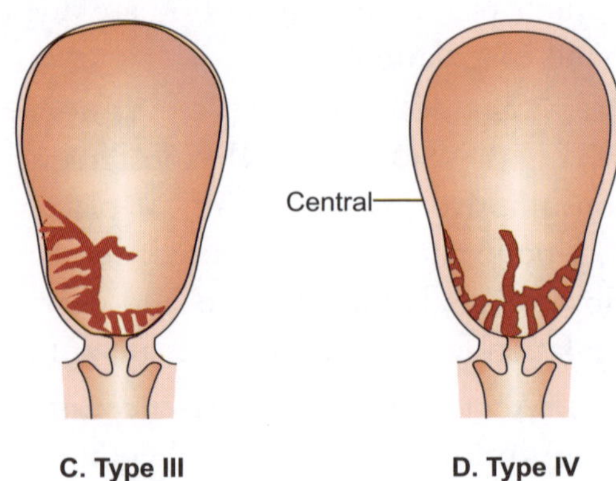

Fig. 40.3 Degrees of placenta previa.

Bleeding is unavoidable in placenta previa; due to the formation of the lower uterine segment and cervical dilatation, the placenta is literally torn away from its attachment. It is further precipitated by the fetal pole exerting downward pressure, while the cervix, as it dilates, is pulled over the presenting part.

Pain could be present if the woman is in labour and the association with hypertension is infrequent. Women with placenta previa are at increased risk of postpartum hemorrhage due to the placenta being implanted over the lower segment which does not contract well. Other complications are due to the massive hemorrhage that may occur in this condition.

On examination, there is usually no hypertension, the abdomen is relaxed and fetal parts are easily palpable; the fetus may present abnormally and fetal heart sounds are present. The differences between placenta previa and abruptio placentae are given in **Table 40.1**.

Ultrasonography: This is extremely useful for localising the placenta. It is precise, simple and easily available/accessible and above all is non-invasive. Abdominal ultrasound localises the placenta accurately (**Fig. 40.4**). However, if a diagnosis of placenta previa is made in the second trimester, the examination should be repeated in the third trimester. In a number of cases, with the enlargement of the uterus and the lower segment, the placenta may be seen to be distant from the internal os. This phenomenon is referred to as **migration of placenta**.

Although other imaging systems are available, ultrasound continues to the best for the diagnosis of placenta previa. A transvaginal ultrasound is more precise and is also safer.

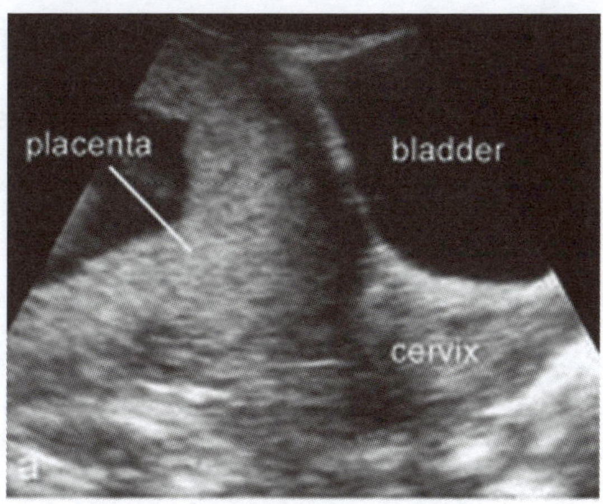

Fig. 40.4 Placenta previa.

Table 40.1 Comparison of clinical features of placenta previa and abruptio placentae

Abruptio placentae	Placenta previa
• May be associated with hypertensive disorders, uterine overdistension, trauma	• Association with hypertensive disorders infrequent
• Abdominal pain and/or backache	• Pain is absent unless the woman is in labour
• Uterine tenderness • Increased uterine tone	• Uterus not tender but relaxed
• Normal fetal presentation	• Malpresentation and/or high presenting part
• Fetal heart beat may be absent	• Fetal heart beat usually normal
• General condition disproportionate to external bleeding	• General condition proportionate to external bleeding

Management

The principles governing management include general measures to treat hypovolemia and blood loss and obstetric management for optimal maternal and fetal outcome.

Expectant management was advocated by McAfee and Johnson in 1945 based on the observation that the bleeding in placenta previa is often scanty and recurrent. It is indicated when the fetus is premature. Under careful supervision, the pregnancy is allowed to continue till 37 weeks, but no further in order to prevent further hemorrhage.

It is best to hospitalise women for expectant management. If hospitalisation is not possible, the risk of sudden hemorrhage must be explained and clear instructions given to transport the woman promptly.

Pregnancy is **terminated** under the following circumstances:

- The fetus is reasonably mature.
- The woman is in labour.
- There is massive hemorrhage.
- The fetus is dead or has severe malformations.

Cesarean section is indicated in all cases of major degree placenta previa. Even if the placenta is situated anteriorly, a transverse incision can be made on the lower uterine segment to deliver the fetus. Maternal or fetal compromise is rare.

Hemorrhage from the placental site should be anticipated as the lower uterine segment contracts poorly. Oversewing of the placental site could be useful in controlling the bleeding. Another complication is adherent placenta; in such cases, hysterectomy may sometimes be necessary.

Vaginal delivery should be considered in marginal and low lying placenta. The membranes are ruptured artificially. This will promote descent of the head which presses on the placenta and prevents further separation of the placenta, thereby preventing hemorrhage. It also helps in initiation of labour. Oxytocin may also be started.

Maternal and perinatal outcome

Maternal mortality due to placenta previa has decreased dramatically since blood transfusion and facilities for cesarean section become available. Perinatal mortality was largely due to prematurity: this too has declined considerably due to expectant management and proper neonatal care.

Vasa previa

In about 1% of singleton and 5% of multiple pregnancies, the umbilical cord inserts into the membranes and the vessels branch out running between the chorion and the amnion before joining the placenta. This is called **velamentous insertion of the cord.** Apart from compression of vessels during labour causing fetal asphyxia, the vessels may be torn during amniotomy leading to fetal exsanguination. Diagnosis is only by colour Doppler ultrasound studies during the antenatal period.

KEY POINTS

- Antepartum hemorrhage is bleeding from the genital tract in late pregnancy; along with other causes of hemorrhage, it accounts for one-third of maternal deaths and 30% of perinatal mortality.
- The main causes of APH are placental abruption, premature separation of a normally situated placenta, placenta previa and separation of a placenta situated on the lower uterine segment.
- Placental abruption is painful and is associated most frequently with hypertensive disorders, a tender uterus, fetal death, coagulation disorders and renal failure.
- Management of abruptio placenta is aimed at correcting hypovolemia and terminating the pregnancy. There is hardly any place for expectant management.
- No attempt should be made whatsoever to confirm the diagnosis of placenta previa or to ascertain the degree by vaginal examination as it may precipitate massive hemorrhage.
- Placenta previa is characterised by painless, causeless and recurrent bleeding; the fetus is usually alive. Ultrasound examination is invaluable for diagnosis.
- Expectant line of management is indicated if the pregnancy is preterm. Pregnancy is terminated if labour sets in, the fetus dies or there is severe hemorrhage.
- Cesarean section is the best mode of delivery in major degree placenta previa.
- Perinatal morbidity and mortality have decreased significantly with the adoption of expectant management.

QUESTIONS

Select the single most appropriate answer:

1. The most common cause of antepartum hemorrhage is
   a. placenta previa c. cervical polyp
   b. placental abruption d. unclassified bleeding
2. Which one of the following is *not* associated with placental abruption?
   a. painless bleeding c. tender uterus
   b. fetus not alive d. hypertension
3. Placenta previa accounts for approximately what percentage of cases of antepartum hemorrhage?
   a. 10% c. 30%
   b 20% d. 40%
4. Placental abruption is associated with all of the following *except*
   a. polyhydramnios c. urinary tract infection
   b. use of cocaine d. multifetal pregnancy
5. For a woman with major degree placenta previa and a grossly malformed baby, the best mode of delivery is
   a. spontaneous vaginal c. cesarean section
   b. application forceps d. vacuum extraction

In the following questions, there are two statements. Select the appropriate answer using the following key:

a. if both statements are true and causally related
b. if both statements are true but not causally related
c. if the first statement is true and the second is false
d. if the first statement is false and the second is true
e. if both statements are false

6. Control of hypertension reduces the risk of placental abruption *because*
   The risk of placental abruption increases considerably if the woman is hypertensive.
7. In a woman with placental abruption at 30 weeks, conservative management is recommended *because*
   Conservative management can help to salvage the fetus.

Select the appropriate answer using the following key:

a. if only responses 1, 2 and 3 are correct
b. if only 1 and 3 are correct
c. if only 2 and 4 are correct
d. if only 4 is correct
e. If all are correct

8. Placenta previa is associated with which of the following?
   1. multiple pregnancy
   2. previous cesarean section
   3. advancing maternal age
   4. use of tobacco
9. Characteristic clinical features of placental abruption are
   1. recurrent bleeding
   2. tender uterus
   3. IUGR
   4. dead fetus
10. In a woman with placenta previa, on conservative management, the pregnancy should be terminated if
    1. there is massive hemorrhage
    2. the woman goes into labour
    3. the fetus is dead
    4. the woman develops preeclampsia

41

Preterm Labour

Lavanya Rai

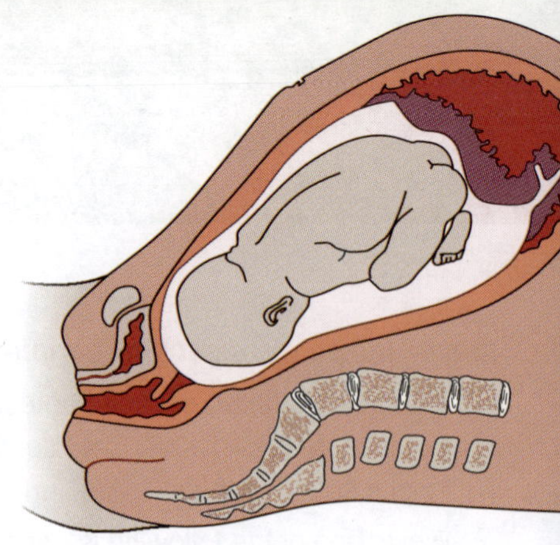

LEARNING OBJECTIVES

At the end of this chapter, the reader should be able to:

- define preterm labour
- list the symptoms and signs of preterm labour
- list the risk factors and markers for screening
- plan the appropriate treatment modality
- enumerate contraindications for tocolysis
- list the commonly used tocolytics and their side effects
- describe other interventions for fetal benefit
- describe the principles of intrapartum management
- list the clinical features and short- and long-term complications of preterm infant
- describe the salient features of neonatal care
- list measures that should be adopted for the prevention of preterm labour

Introduction

Preterm labour is an important cause of perinatal mortality in developing countries, while in the developed countries, it is responsible for considerable short-term and long-term morbidity. The enormous expenditure incurred in caring for these children is a burden even for resource-rich countries. Most of the morbidity and mortality, however, is seen in babies at less than 32 weeks of gestation. Even if they survive the immediate neonatal period, many die in the first year of life, while the survivors are at risk of neurological morbidity and handicap. In many centres, the risk of neonatal mortality/morbidity is so low after 34 weeks that aggressive therapy to suppress labour is no longer used and delivery is allowed. In developing countries, however, this practice is not practicable since neonatal services are not universally available; there is therefore a role for preventing and treating preterm labour.

Definition

Preterm labour is defined as regular contractions that occur **before 37 weeks but after 28 weeks** of gestation and are associated **with changes in the cervix**. The general incidence is 10%–15%. Preterm labour may be spontaneous in onset, and may be induced in case of medical conditions or pregnancy disorders in the mother or her fetus. Prolonging the pregnancy in some cases of spontaneous onset preterm labour may be harmful to the mother/baby and hence it may not be appropriate to arrest all cases of preterm labour.

Risk factors for preterm labour

- Past history of preterm labour remains one of the strongest predictors of recurrent preterm birth.
- Vaginal bleeding in the second or third trimester also increases the risk considerably, by 1.6 to 15 times.

- Previous second trimester loss.
- Premature rupture of membranes contributes to more than 50% of cases.
- Antepartum hemorrhage and preeclampsia may cause spontaneous onset or may be responsible for the majority of induced preterm labour.
- Multiple gestation increases the risk 5–6 times and the incidence of this risk factor will continue to rise with infertility treatment.
- Infections are an important cause.
- Stress increases the release of the corticotrophin releasing factor (CRF) and catecholamines.
- Overdistended uterus as in hydramnios.

Table 41.1 lists the important risk factors for preterm labour.

Table 41.1 Maternal, placental and fetal factors responsible for preterm birth

General	
• Maternal	Low socioeconomic status Occupational stress Idiopathic Teenage pregnancy Age ≥35 years Smoking Psychological stress Recurrent pregnancy loss Low prepregnancy weight Previous preterm delivery Threatened abortion Primigravida Lack of antenatal care
• Placental	Placenta previa Abruptio placentae Circumvallate placenta Chorioamnionitis Hydramnios/oligoamnios
• Fetal	Multiple pregnancy Intrauterine growth restriction Fetal anomalies
Medical/Obstetric	
Preeclampsia Diabetes Anemia Heart disease Other medical disorders: Thyroid, SLE, renal Urinary tract infection High fever Fibroid uterus Uterine anomaly Cervical incompetence Bacterial vaginosis Premature rupture of membranes	

Pathogenesis

Infection may be in the form of bacterial vaginosis, chorioamnionitis, pyelonephritis or periodontitis. Other infections which can cause preterm labour include gonorrhoea, group B streptococcus infections, chlamydiasis, *Ureaplasma urealyticum* and trichomoniasis. Infection induces the cytokine cascade pathway which in turn stimulates prostaglandin release. Bacterial toxins have a stimulatory effect on the uterus. Bacterial products can weaken the membranes leading to rupture of membranes. Periodontitis increases the risk of preterm birth sevenfold. Chorioamnionitis can occur with intact membranes. Amniotic fluid studies have shown positive cultures, leucocyte counts and other biochemical evidence of infection in preterm labour without overt signs of infection.

Screening tests

Over the past decade, several screening tests and risk scoring systems have been devised to predict preterm labour.

- Fetal fibronectin is a glycoprotein which acts as a glue between the membranes and uterine deciduas. Fibronectin is not present in cervicovaginal secretions between 22 and 37 weeks in normal pregnancy. Therefore, it is a predictor of preterm labour, if levels more than 50 ng/ml are present in cervicovaginal secretions.
- Shortening and funnelling of the cervix in asymptomatic patients detected by ultrasound in the early second trimester is useful. The risk of preterm labour increases as cervical length decreases.
- Monitoring uterine activity using an electronic device to identify early signs of preterm labour has been tried.

Maternal salivary estriol is currently being evaluated for the detection of preterm labour.

Symptoms and signs

A detailed history should be taken regarding factors such as infection, antepartum hemorrhage and preecalmpsia. Assess the period of gestation from menstrual history and using ultrasound findings in early pregnancy, before diagnosis.

When **uterine contractions** are present **without any cervical changes**, the labour is considered as **threatened preterm labour**. Early engagement of the head is not always necessary for diagnosis but it may be a warning sign when present.

The criteria to diagnose preterm labour are regular uterine contractions after 28 weeks but before 37 weeks accompanied by one or more of the following:

- cervical effacement of more than 80%
- dilatation of the cervix of more than 2 cm
- progressive change in the cervix.

These clinical criteria are often inaccurate, and over- or underdiagnosis is not uncommon. A cervical length of more than 30 mm reliably excludes preterm labour. In true preterm labour, progressive uterine activity is always associated with cervical changes and progressive descent of the fetal presenting part (Table 41.2).

Management

Investigations are necessary to evaluate suspected underlying factors such as urinary tract infection, gestational diabetes, anemia and cervicovaginal infections. Hematocrit, blood glucose, urine microscopy, culture and sensitivity and endocervical swab culture are routinely performed for preterm labour. Blood counts are necessary when infective etiology such as chorioamnionitis is suspected. Identification of risk factors helps to administer specific therapy.

Ultrasound is essential to rule out fetal anomaly, multiple pregnancies, determine growth and fetal weight, amniotic fluid volume and to evaluate the amniotic fluid and the placenta. Transvaginal ultrasound helps to assess the length of the cervix.

Objectives: These are as follows:

- identification and treatment of etiology
- prophylaxis for fetus
- establishing a plan of management, whether to allow labour to progress or to stop labour.

Protocol: The protocal for the management of preterm labour is given below.

- confirmation of gestational age
- documentation of fetal wellbeing
- search for likely cause
- exclusion of infection
- exclusion of contraindications for tocolysis (Table 41.3)
- prophylaxis for respiratory distress syndrome (RDS) and group B streptococcus (GBS) infection
- tocolysis or continuation of labour
- delivery and care of the preterm infant.

Arrest of labour: The principle behind arresting labour is to allow further intrauterine fetal growth and maturity. Drugs used for arresting labour by inhibiting uterine contractions are called **tocolytics**.

Table 41.2 Symptoms and signs of preterm labour

Symptoms	Signs
Pain with or without perception of contractions	Uterine contractions
Pelvic pressure	Cervical effacement and dilatation
Menstrual-like cramps	Engaged head
Vaginal discharge	
Lower back pain	

Table 41.3 Indications and contraindications for tocolysis

Indications	Contraindications
Normal mother	**Maternal**
Normal baby	Active labour
Not in active labour	Heart disease
Tocolytics not contraindicated	Preeclampsia
	IUGR
	Abruptio placentae
	Severe anemia
	Chorioamnionitis
	Fetal
	Anomalies
	Intrauterine death

Enema is avoided if it has been decided that labour is to be arrested. Though bed rest and sedation are routinely used in the management of preterm labour, their efficacy has not been proven. Bed rest is believed to improve growth and prevent labour while sedation is said to relieve anxiety.

Tocolysis: Tocolytic therapy as such has not proven to be very effective in decreasing fetal morbidity and mortality. However, it helps to prolong the pregnancy by at least 2–7 days which allows time to institute the following interventions to reduce neonatal morbidity.

- steroid prophylaxis for lung maturity
- antibiotic prophylaxis for group B streptococcus infection
- transfer of the mother to a tertiary care centre

Tocolysis needs close monitoring because of possible serious side effects of the drugs used. The duration of therapy should be limited.

- **Beta-mimetics:** Isoxsuprine is the most widely used drug in India. It is used in doses of 20–40 μg/min; the dose is increased gradually till contractions are arrested. Terbutaline 125–250 μg subcutaneously is effective. Ritodrine is a relatively new drug in India and is started with an initial dose of 50 μg/min up to a maximum of 350 μg /min. Pulmonary edema may occur with the use of these drugs.
- **Prostaglandin synthetase inhibitors** decrease prostaglandin production. Indomethacin is the most commonly used drug in preterm labour with hydramnios. The dose is 75 mg rectal suppository followed by 25 mg every 6 hours for 48 hours.
- **Calcium channel blocking drugs** such as nifedipine decrease the amount of free calcium by blocking the entrance of calcium into the myometrial cells. Nifedipine is given in the dose of 10–20 mg every 6–8 hours. Pre-treatment with fluids reduces side effects such as hypotension and reduced uteroplacental perfusion. Nifedipine should not be combined with magnesium sulphate or beta-mimetics, but may be given to diabetics. The incidence of neonatal RDS, necrotising enterocolitis (NEC) and intraventricular hemorrhage (IVH) are said to be low in patients treated with nifedipine. Ease of administration, low maternal side effect profile and low cost are the advantages of this drug.
- **Magnesium sulphate** is widely used for the treatment and prevention of eclampsia. Though it has a relaxant effect on the uterus it is less effective as a tocolytic agent. It is used as a 4–6 g loading dose followed by continuous infusion of 2 g/hour to arrest labour.
- **Nitroglycerine transdermal patches** have been used as tocolytic agents. Nitric oxide is a potent endogenous smooth muscle relaxant.
- Atosiban, an **oxytocin receptor antagonist,** is used in western countries. It has a safe side effect profile compared to other tocolytics though efficacy is not better.
- **Progesterone treatment** is effective in preventing preterm labour in patients with previous preterm deliveries. However, it does not arrest labour once actual contractions have set in. Injection 17-alpha hydroxyprogesterone caproate 500 mg IM weekly or vaginal progesterone 100 mg suppository daily are the two forms in use.

Other useful interventions: Improvement of general nutrition, use of antioxidants, cessation of smoking and abstinence from sexual activity are beneficial.

Antibiotics: As infections play an important role in causing preterm labour, antibiotics are being used liberally in the treatment of urinary tract infections, group B streptococcus infections, bacterial vaginosis, subclinical chorioamnionitis and vaginitis. Bacterial vaginosis is treated with metronidazole or erythromycin. In the absence of active infection, there is no evidence to prove the beneficial effects of prophylactic antibiotics.

Cerclage: Cervical cerclage is advised in patients who have had repeated late abortions or early preterm labour, particularly if features suggestive of incompetent cervical os are present.

Antenatal steroid prophylaxis for respiratory distress syndrome (RDS): Antenatal corticosteroid therapy for women at risk of preterm labour prior to 34 weeks of gestation is given to prevent RDS. It helps reduce neonatal mortality, necrotising enterocolitis and intraventricular hemorrhage besides

RDS. However, it is contraindicated in the presence of systemic infection and chorioamnionitis.

Betamethasone, two doses of 12 mg IM 24 hours apart, or dexamethasone 6 mg, 4 doses IM 12 hours apart, are the standard regimens in use. They increase pulmonary surfactant, which in turn reduces the incidence of RDS by 50%.

Labour management: The objective is the atraumatic birth of a well-oxygenated baby. When tocolysis fails or is contraindicated, delivery is allowed and should be conducted carefully in an institution with facilities for neonatal care to minimise neonatal morbidity and mortality.

First stage: Narcotic drugs like pethidine should be avoided as it may cause respiratory depression. Epidural analgesia is advocated for pain relief. Close monitoring for uterine contractions and fetal heart are mandatory as these babies are unable to withstand even a mild degree of hypoxia. Birth asphyxia aggravates RDS. Artificial rupture of membranes is avoided as the bag of membranes prevents compression of the fetal head and ascending infection.

Second stage: Episiotomy is preferred (even though the baby is small) to facilitate easy delivery without any compression of the head. Prolonged second stage is to be avoided. Outlet forceps is used if a delay is anticipated. However, ventouse is contraindicated for babies at less than 34 weeks of gestation. Early cord clamping, advocated in the past to prevent hypervolemia, is no longer advocated.

Cesarean section is indicated in malpresentations such as breech or for other obstetric indications. If the lower segment is not well formed, a low vertical incision should be made.

Principles of neonatal care

Neonatal intensive care is essential for many preterm neonates that an less than 34 weeks.

- clear airway
- warmer/incubator care/kangaroo mother care for preventing hypothermia
- aseptic handling to prevent infections
- adequate nutrition
- good nursing care
- vitamin K generally administered to prevent intracranial and other bleeding tendencies.

Neonatal prognosis is related to gestational age, associated maternal/fetal problems and the care available.

Clinical features of a preterm baby

Preterm babies have clinical features which indicate their immaturity. Three features depend on the degree of prematurity. The size of the body is small with a relatively large head. Lanugo hair may be present but the vernix is absent or scanty in extreme prematurity. Skin is thin, appears gelatinous and pink. Ear cartilages are deficient. Breast nodules are small and sole creases are absent. The baby has poor general activity and sluggish reflexes. The tone is poor and cry is feeble. In male babies, the scrotum has less rugosity and undescended testis is common. In female babies, the labia majora are poorly developed.

Complications in a preterm baby

This depends on the gestational age of the baby and the etiological factor responsible for the prematurity (**Fig. 41.1**). Neonatal mortality and morbidity is high in preterm labour when it is due to an infection. This is not only due to the infective organism but also the secondary effect of fetal inflammatory response. Immaturity of various organs such as the liver, lungs and kidneys leads to immediate problems in the neonatal period. Nutritional deficiencies are common in the long term, besides neurological deficits. As immunity is low in these babies, septicemia is an important cause of death. Retinopathy of prematurity is an iatrogenic problem due to oxygen therapy.

Prevention of preterm labour

- Regular prenatal care can prevent, detect, treat and improve outcome in preterm labour.
- Identification of risk factors and close monitoring of high-risk pregnancies helps.
- Early engagement of head and cervical changes should serve as warning signs.
- Avoiding physical and psychological stress helps some women. Stress increases catecholamines which in turn cause preterm labour.

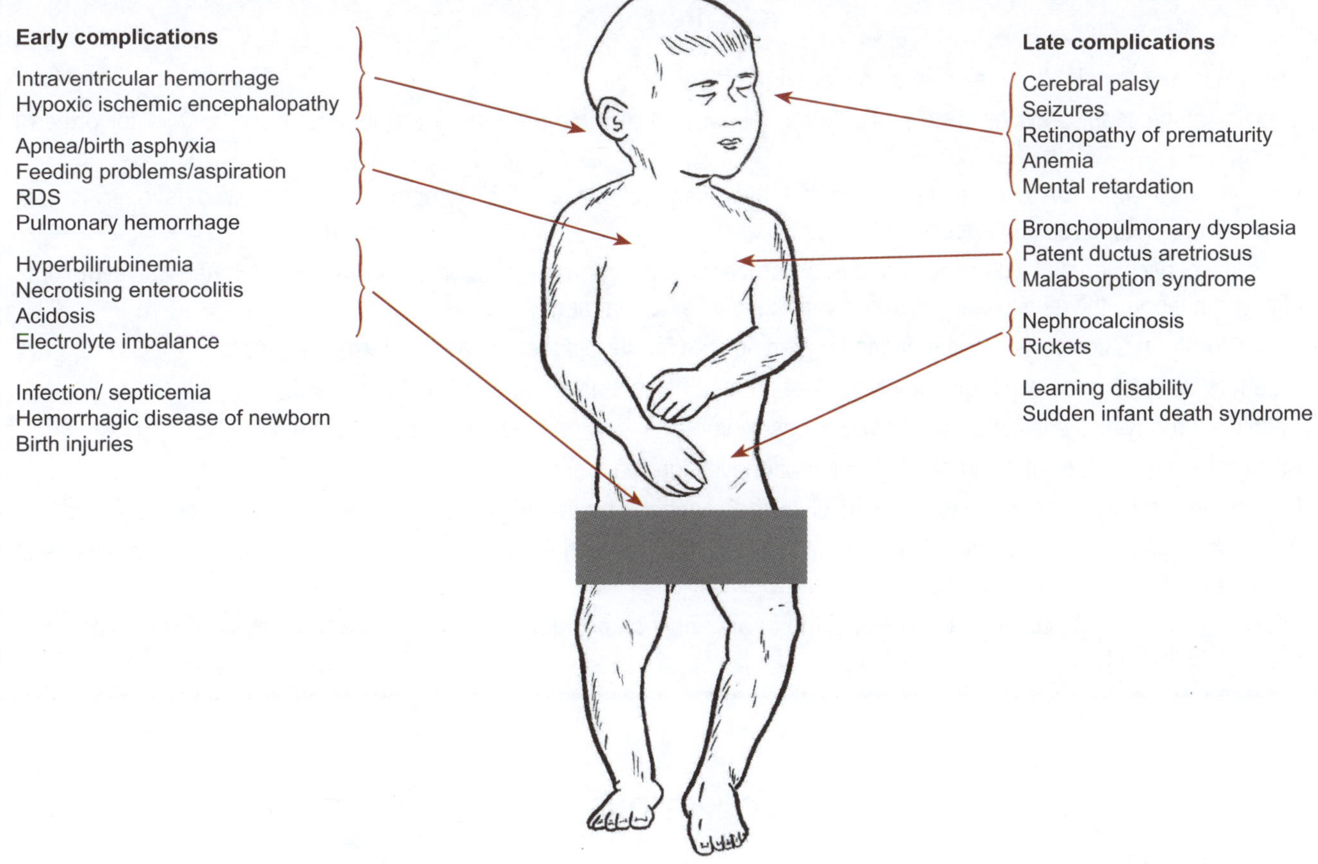

Fig. 41.1 Complications of prematurity.

- Prophylactic cervical encerclage should be offered for women with previous pregnancy loss due to an incompetent cervix.
- Treatment of infections such as urinary tract infections, asymptomatic bacteriuria, vaginitis and bacterial vaginosis, in high-risk cases, prevents preterm labour.
- Coital abstinence and cessation of smoking reduce the risk.
- Progesterone therapy is effective in preventing preterm labour in the high-risk population; it is ineffective once active contractions set in.

KEY POINTS

- Preterm labour contributes to significant perinatal mortality.
- Subclinical infection, previous history of preterm labour and multiple pregnancy are important risk factors for preterm labour.
- Prophylactic therapy like tocolytic drugs, bed rest, hydration and sedation for asymptomatic women who have risk factors for preterm labour is recommended.
- Tests like cervical length by ultrasound and fetal fibronectin have good negative predictive value. In women with symptoms of preterm labour, these are used to avoid overdiagnosis and treatment.
- Only short-term tocolysis is recommended for gaining time for steroid therapy and maternal transport.
- Antenatal steroids decrease the complications of prematurity; a single course is recommended.
- Antibiotic prophylaxis against group B streptococcal infections is given to prevent neonatal infection.
- All tocolytic agents are similar in efficacy and most have significant side effects.
- Maintenance tocolytic therapy after initial tocolysis has not been proven effective and, therefore, is not recommended.
- Atraumatic delivery of an active infant without hypoxia and appropriate neonatal care reduces neonatal morbidity and ensures wellbeing in a preterm baby.
- Lifestyle changes, progesterone therapy and the treatment of some infections may reduce preterm labour in women with significant risk factors.

QUESTIONS

Select the single most appropriate answer:

1. Which of the following is *not* a symptom of preterm labour?
   a. decreased fetal movements
   b. lower back pain
   c. pelvic pressure
   d. vaginal discharge
2. Which is the best criterion for arresting preterm labour?
   a. cervical dilatation >3 cm
   b. fetal growth restriction
   c. no contraindication for tocolytics
   d. presence of chorioamnionitis
3. Which of the following is *not* a tocolytic?
   a. fraxiparine c. ritodrine
   b. isoxsuprine d. terbutaline
4. The drug of choice for tocolysis when the mother has mitral valve prolapse is
   a. isoxsuprine c. magnesium sulphate
   b. indomethacin d. nifedipine
5. A tocolytic which reduces the risk of neonatal RDS is
   a. atosiban c. nifedipine
   b. indomethacin d. nitroglycerine
6. Steroid prophylaxis *does not* reduce the risk of
   a. intraventricular hemorrhage
   b. necrotising enterocolitis
   c. neonatal septicemia
   d. respiratory distress syndrome
7. While conducting the delivery of a preterm baby, avoid the use of
   a. episiotomy c. outlet forceps
   b. epidural analgesia d. ventouse extraction
8. The test with a high false positive rate but a good negative predictive value in predicting preterm labour is
   a. cervical length measurement
   b. fibronectin assay
   c. home uterine activity monitoring
   d. serum progesterone assay
9. A tocolytic with a favourable maternal profile but significant fetal effects is
   a. isoxsuprine c. nifedipine
   b. indomethacin d. nitroglycerine

42

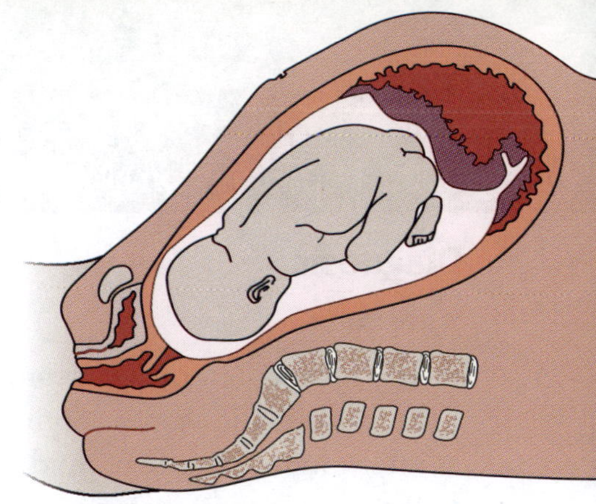

Prelabour Rupture of Membranes

S Soundara Raghavan

LEARNING OBJECTIVES

At the end of this chapter, the reader should be able to:

- define PROM and PPROM
- enumerate the risk factors and etiology of PROM
- list the diagnostic features of PROM
- enumerate the maternal and fetal risks associated with PROM and PPROM
- list the relevant investigations in PROM
- outline the management in a case of PROM and of PPROM

Introduction

Normally, the fetal membranes, made up of the amnion and chorion, rupture during active labour, possibly because of the increasing intrauterine pressure due to contractions and decreasing tensile strength of membranes, a continuous process throughout pregnancy. About 3%–18 % of pregnancies may be complicated by **premature or prelabour rupture of membranes** (PROM), which means spontaneous rupture of membranes before the onset of labour. If the pregnancy is not term (less than 37 weeks), then it is called **preterm premature (or prelabour) rupture of membranes** (PPROM).

PROM and PPROM contribute to significant perinatal mortality and morbidity, maternal morbidity and rarely, maternal mortality.

Premature Rupture of Membranes

Risk factors and etiopathology

Even though PROM can occur without any obvious cause, several risk factors have been identified:

- genital tract infection including chorioamnionitis
- uterine overdistension due to multiple pregnancy or polyhydramnios
- malpresentations
- obstetric maneuvers like version
- trauma
- coitus
- cervical incompetence
- low socioeconomic status
- maternal tobacco use
- connective tissue disorders like Ehlers-Danlos
- second and third trimester bleeding
- nutritional deficiency of copper and ascorbic acid
- maternal gene expression.

There is evidence to suggest that bacterial vaginosis, colonisation of vagina by other organisms like *B fragilis, N gonorrhea,* Chlamydia, Trichomonas and group B streptococci are most commonly associated with PROM. Infection probably decreases the tensile strength of the membranes by the action of metalloproteinases on collagen (collagen is important for maintaining membrane integrity).

Diagnosis

Symptoms

- The most common symptom is a sudden gush of fluid from the vagina. Sometimes, there may be intermittent leakage of fluid and wetness.
- If there is definite infection, the woman may have fever, abdominal pain and sometimes offensive vaginal discharge.
- There may be reduced or absent fetal movements or occasionally transiently increased movements depending on the fetal condition.
- Bleeding per vaginum may indicate placental abruption.
- The woman may complain of the umbilical cord protruding out if there is cord prolapse.

Signs

- Presence of fever is the most reliable indicator of chorioamnionitis. There may also be tachycardia.
- Abdominal examination may reveal the uterus to be smaller than expected for the period of amenorrhea. Uterine tenderness may be elicited if there is sepsis or abruption.
- Auscultation may show fetal tachycardia: another indicator of infection. The fetal heart sounds may be absent if the fetus has died.
- Speculum examination may show fluid leaking through the cervical os or collected in the posterior fornix. If all the liquor has drained out, this may not be appreciated.

It is important to differentiate amniotic fluid from urine (stress incontinence or urge incontinence are common in pregnancy). Excessive vaginal discharge due to trichomonal or gardnerella infection will have to be excluded. If the fluid is due to the presence of excessive cervical mucus, it will be more viscid and mucoid.

Investigations: The investigations to confirm PROM are as follows:

Fern test: A sample of fluid is placed on a glass slide and allowed to dry. When observed under the microscope, a ferning pattern is observed due to the crystallisation of the salts in the amniotic fluid. This may also be seen if the fluid is cervical mucus.

Nitrazine test: Nitrazine paper turns deep blue if the fluid is amniotic fluid (because of its alkalinity). If the fluid is vaginal discharge, the paper stays yellow. Urine, blood, infected discharge and antiseptics may falsify results. A positive nitrazine test with a positive fern test almost always confirms the diagnosis of PROM.

Ultrasound examination: It will show reduced or absent liquor in PROM unless polyhydramnios was present. However, this should not be used as a primary means of diagnosis of PROM, since there are other causes of oligohydramnios. Presence of normal amount of liquor in ultrasound practically rules out PROM. Other aims of performing an ultrasound examination are to assess the period of gestation, fetal weight and wellbeing, ascertain the fetal lie and presentation, rule out malformations and detect placental abruption.

Gram stain: The presence of bacteria or leucocytes on Gram stain of the liquor collected from the posterior fornix is an indicator of infection.

Culture: Cervical or high vaginal swab is useful to identify the organisms and their sensitivity to antibiotics.

Electronic fetal monitoring: It will aid in assessing fetal wellbeing. Nonreactive nonstress test (NST) indicates infection or fetal jeopardy.

Risks associated with PROM

Maternal

- Chorioamniotic infection is the main maternal risk which can complicate the pregnancy of up to 20% of women with PROM. The risk of infection is greater if PROM occurs remote from term. Ureaplasma, Mycoplasma, Bacteroides, Gardnerella, Group B Streptococci, Peptostreptococci, Fusobacterium and, Enterococci are the organisms often found to cause infection. In the hospital setting, Gram-negative organisms like *E coli,* Proteus, Pseudomonas and Klebsiella may be present.
- If there is placental abruption, associated complications like fetal compromise may occur.
- There is also an increased cesarean section rate in PROM, contributing to maternal risk.

Fetal

- Infection is a major risk for the neonate and may take the form of pneumonitis, meningitis or septicemia.
- Prematurity is often associated with PROM. Hyaline membrane disease, intraventricular hemorrhage and necrotising enterocolitis are special problems of prematurity.
- Intrauterine fetal death may occur due to cord prolapse, placental abruption or severe sepsis.
- Pulmonary hypoplasia is a feared risk if PROM occurs before 28 weeks of pregnancy.
- Fetal skeletal deformities of the limbs and skull can also result if PROM occurs before 28 weeks of pregnancy.

Management of PROM

The management of PROM may be:

- **expectant**, waiting for spontaneous onset of labour, which occurs within 24 hours in 80% of women with PROM, or
- **active**, instituting measures to terminate pregnancy immediately

Expectant management is not advised in the presence of any of the following:

- active labour
- fetal malformation
- fetal distress
- abruptio placentae
- cord prolapse
- overt infection
- high-risk conditions for infections like diabetes, and immunosuppressed states
- women with more than 24 hours of PROM

The number of pelvic examinations should be minimised; when performed, strict asepsis and antisepsis should be practised. In the absence of cephalopelvic disproportion and malpresentations, vaginal delivery can be anticipated. The status of the cervix will determine the first step to be taken for labour induction. Intracervical or vaginal prostaglandin E_2 can be used if the cervix is unfavourable. Hypertonic contractions should be watched for. If the cervix is ripe and favourable, oxytocin infusion is used to induce labour. Administration of antibiotics to the mother definitely improves maternal and perinatal outcome.

Management of PPROM

The management of PPROM is not as simple as that of PROM. The decision has to be individualised and the availability of appropriate neonatal services influences the decision. It is to be emphasised that an accurate estimation of the period of gestation is important in planning the management of PPROM.

About 30% of women with PPROM will enter spontaneous labour within three days. **The management strategy is to balance the risk: infection due to conservative management versus prematurity due to immediate delivery.** Most of the contraindications to conservative management listed above also apply to PPROM.

The management depends on the period of gestation at which PPROM occurs, and is planned as follows:

Weeks 32–37: In these women, the risk of infection outweighs the risk of prematurity. Dexamethasone 6 mg IM every 12 hours for 48 hours will decrease the risk of hyaline membrane disease, intraventricular hemorrhage and necrotising enterocolitis. Antibiotics have been found to be useful: ampicillin 500 mg every 6 hours or erythromycin 500 mg every 8 hours. Pregnancy should be terminated following the guidelines given above.

Weeks 28–32: These women are likely to benefit from prolonging the pregnancy because the risk of prematurity is high. Antibiotics and steroids are administered and the mother and the fetus carefully monitored for any evidence of infection. Tocolytic agents have not been found to be beneficial. Pregnancy is terminated if any of the abovementioned conditions is detected. The woman must be referred to a centre with a neonatal intensive care unit (NICU) and where expert neonatal care is available.

Less than 28 weeks: This group has poor perinatal outcome with a perinatal mortality of 60%–90%. About 50% of women will have chorioamnionitis. The fetal outcome is dismal: most neonates develop sepsis, pulmonary hypoplasia, deformities and long-term adverse sequelae. Corticosteroids and antibiotics are administered. The majority of women will deliver within two weeks of PPROM or complications will necessitate termination of pregnancy.

KEY POINTS

- PROM is not an uncommon problem.
- Infection has a cause and effect relationship with PROM.
- It is responsible for significant perinatal mortality, morbidity and maternal morbidity.
- When gestation is 32 weeks or more, it is better to terminate the pregnancy.
- Between 28 and 32 weeks, there is a role for expectant management with careful monitoring.
- Steroids and antibiotics are useful to improve outcome.
- Tocolytics have little role in the management of PROM.
- PPROM before 28 weeks has very poor perinatal outcome.

QUESTIONS

Select the single most appropriate answer:

1. Premature rupture of membranes is defined as rupture of membranes
   a. in the latent phase of labour
   b. before the onset of labour
   c. when the cervix is dilated 2 cm
   d. at 32 weeks of pregnancy
2. When the membranes rupture around 32 weeks, all of the following are advised *except*
   a. antibiotics
   b. corticosteroids
   c. tocolytics
   d. bed rest
3. Premature rupture of membranes is generally associated with
   a. high socioeconomic status
   b. use of cocaine
   c. oligohydramnios
   d. bacterial vaginosis
4. The most frequently noted maternal complication in premature rupture of membranes is
   a. antepartum hemorrhage
   b. postpartum hemorrhage
   c. infection
   d. risk of disseminated intravascular coagulation
5. Most women with premature rupture of membranes at term will go into spontaneous labour within
   a. 6 hours
   b. 12 hours
   c. 18 hours
   d. 24 hours
6. The most reliable indicator of chorioamnionitis is
   a. tachycardia
   b. fever
   c. purulent vaginal discharge
   d. abdominal pain

In the following questions, there are two statements. Select the appropriate answer using the following key:

a. if both statements are true and causally related
b. if both statements are true but not causally related
c. if the first statement is true and the second is false
d. if the first statement is false and the second is true
e. if both statements are false

7. Collagen is essential for the integrity of membranes *because*

   Infection destroys collagen by the action of metalloproteinases.
8. Premature rupture of membranes contributes significantly to perinatal morbidity and mortality *because*

   Preterm labour is often the result of preterm prelabour rupture of membranes.

Select the appropriate answer using the following key:

a. if only responses 1, 2 and 3 are correct
b. if only 1 and 3 are correct
c. if only 2 and 4 are correct
d. if only 4 is correct
e. if all are correct

9. The risk factors associated with premature rupture of membranes are
   1. use of tobacco
   2. connective tissue disorders
   3. deficiency of copper
   4. postmaturity
10. Administration of corticosteroids to women with premature rupture of membranes at 32 to 37 weeks reduces the risk particularly of
    1. neonatal jaundice
    2. hyaline membrane disease
    3. respiratory infection
    4. intraventricular hemorrhage

43

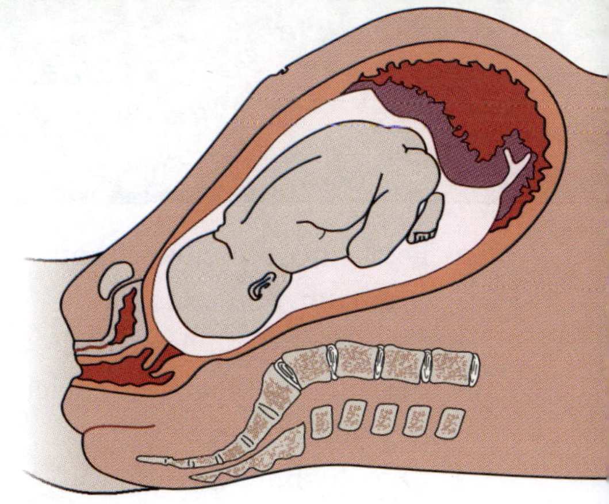

Prolonged Pregnancy

S Soundara Raghavan

LEARNING OBJECTIVES

At the end of this chapter, the reader should be able to:

- define prolonged pregnancy
- list the causes of prolonged pregnancy
- appreciate the need for accurate dating of pregnancy
- explain the pathophysiology of prolonged pregnancy
- enumerate the adverse effects on the mother and fetus
- identify the need for and methods of fetal surveillance
- plan appropriate management

Introduction

A delivery that does not take place even after the expected date calculated by Naegele's rule causes considerable anxiety to both the expectant mother and the attending obstetrician. About 80% of women deliver by 40 weeks and another 10% by 41 weeks. About 10% may not deliver even after 41 weeks of pregnancy. Apart from the anxiety it causes, prolonged pregnancy can have deleterious effects on the health of the mother as well as the fetus.

Definition

Postmaturity indicates a specific appearance of the newborn at birth which occurs only in a small number of babies after prolonged pregnancy.

Postdates may be prolongation of pregnancy by a few days or weeks; this term should be avoided since it is not specific.

Term pregnancy is usually defined as a pregnancy in which the period of gestation is between 37 and 42 completed weeks. The World Health Organization (WHO) defines prolonged pregnancy as 42 weeks or 294 days after the first day of the last menstrual period (LMP). The incidence of prolonged pregnancy is believed to be between 7% and 14%. However, recent perinatal mortality data suggests that prolonged pregnancy should be defined as a gestational age of or over 41 completed weeks.

Causes

- Inaccurate menstrual history is the most common reason for diagnosing prolonged pregnancy.
- In a large number of women, there is no identifiable cause.
- Prolonged pregnancy seems to run in families, particularly the maternal side.
- Past history of prolonged pregnancy causes a 50% chance of recurrence, suggesting a biological determination.
- Prolonged pregnancy is said to be more common in primigravida, elderly or obese women with an affluent lifestyle and sedentary habits.
- The male fetus is often associated with prolonged pregnancy.

- Fetal anencephaly without polyhydramnios and adrenal hypoplasia
- Exposure to ethylene oxide, a sterilising gas
- Placental sulphatase deficiency, a rare sex-linked recessive disorder
- Oligohydramnios seems to have a cause and effect relationship
- Chronic use of NSAIDs.

Diagnosis

Diagnosis of prolonged pregnancy is complicated by the fact that one-third of the women may not be able to accurately recall the first day of the LMP. Even when the dates are known, significant variations in normal menstrual cycles and the occurrence of ovulation earlier or later than expected result in the likelihood of diagnosis of prolonged pregnancy.

There is enough evidence to suggest that clinical estimation of gestational age is less accurate than sonography, particularly early in pregnancy. Hence, the WHO defines 'excellent dates' as estimating the LMP accurately in a woman with regular cycles and a first trimester ultrasound confirming it. Ultrasound assessment of gestational age also suffers from a margin of error of ±7 days in the first trimester, ±14 days in the second trimester and ±21 days in the third trimester. If there is a difference between gestational age by LMP and by ultrasound of more than the above variation, ultrasound estimation should be taken as accurate.

Because of the difficulties mentioned above, all pregnancies judged to be of 42 completed weeks should be managed as abnormally prolonged.

Pathophysiology

Traditionally, it is believed that placental function declines when pregnancy advances after term, even though there are no morphological changes in the placenta to support this hypothesis. The presence of infarcts and calcification in normal term placenta, also make this theory suspect. It has been reported that placental apoptosis is greater at 41–42 weeks than at 36–39 weeks.

It is accepted that the amniotic fluid volume decreases beyond term; this has been attributed to declining placental function. Recent demonstration of abnormal fetal cardiac function in postterm pregnancies raises the possibility of oligohydramnios being secondary to poor renal perfusion primarily due to decreased fetal left ventricular function.

Oligohydramnios results in cord compression and fetal asphyxia. Hence, the fetal movements decrease and fetal cardiotocography (CTG) shows abnormalities like prolonged decelerations, variable decelerations and saltatory patterns. Typically, late deceleration, characteristic of uteroplacental insufficiency, is infrequently seen.

One-third of postterm fetuses have been found to be growth restricted. Perinatal mortality and morbidity are maximum among postterm growth-restricted neonates.

About 10% of postterm neonates have features of 'post maturity syndrome': wrinkled, patchy, peeling skin, long thin body often stained with meconium, wideo-pen, a alert eyes and, worried look. They have long nails and hair. Many fetuses will continue to grow beyond term and may not fall in the birth weight range of intrauterine growth restriction.

In postterm pregnancies, amniotic fluid is often meconium-stained; passage of meconium is normal as pregnancy advances. It has also been suggested that intrauterine hypoxia may lead to increased intestinal peristalsis and sphincter relaxation. Particularly in the presence of oligohydramnios, meconium tends to be thick and viscous. Aspiration of meconium is a complication.

On the whole, the postterm infant suffers from an increased risk of asphyxia, intrauterine, intrapartum as well as postpartum, resulting in increased perinatal mortality and morbidity; these risks may continue in the first two years of life.

Effects of prolonged pregnancy on the fetus

Increased perinatal mortality and morbidity is attributable to events in both the antepartum and intrapartum periods. Most adverse effects occur in the intrapartum period, and contribute to a significant rise in neonatal deaths. Delivery at 38 weeks is associated with the lowest risk of perinatal death.

Effect of prolonged pregnancy on the mother

Most mothers become anxious when delivery does not occur at the expected date of delivery (EDD). The adverse effects of prolonged pregnancy on the mother mainly relate to increased obstetric intervention.

Table 43.1 shows the adverse effects of prolonged pregnancy on the mother and the fetus.

Antepartum fetal surveillance

Fetal surveillance is used in an attempt to decrease perinatal mortality and morbidity and to avoid unnecessary obstetric intervention. The disadvantages of fetal surveillance are false positive tests and the fact that no surveillance can totally eliminate stillbirth. Surveillance should ideally begin at 41 weeks.

The various tests available for antepartum fetal surveillance include fetal kick count, nonstress test (NST), assessment of amniotic fluid volume with ultrasound by measuring amniotic fluid index (AFI), biophysical profile (BPP), modified biophysical profile (MBPP), contraction stress test (CST) and Doppler velocimetry of umbilical vessels. No single test has been found to be superior to another. Doppler studies have not been found to be useful, though absent end diastolic flow is considered dangerous.

It has been shown that adverse pregnancy outcome is more common in oligohydramnios: it is diagnosed when the AFI is less than 5 or there is no vertical fluid pocket measurable and more than 2–3 cm in depth. Fetal surveillance is generally performed twice a week and pregnancy should be terminated if there is fetal compromise or oligohydramnios.

Table 43.1 Adverse effects of prolonged pregnancy

On the fetus
Anoxia, probably due to cord compression, prolonged labour due to cephalopelvic disproportion
Macrosomia
Shoulder dystocia
Growth restriction
Postmaturity syndrome
Birth injury: Brachial plexus, cephalhematoma, fracture of clavicle and humerus
Meconium aspiration syndrome
Birth asphyxia
Neonatal convulsions
Congenital anomalies
Hypothermia
Hypoglycemia
Hypocalcemia
Polycythemia
Sepsis
Need for admission into neonatal intensive care unit (NICU)
On the mother
Maternal anxiety
Induction of labour
Prolonged labour
Increased cesarean section rate
Increased instrumental delivery rate
Perineal injury
Amniotic fluid embolism

Management

The two important alternatives in management are termination of pregnancy and expectant management with fetal surveillance. There is little disagreement about terminating pregnancy at 42 weeks. The factors to be considered to decide the mode of termination include adequacy of the pelvis, size of the fetus, its wellbeing and the presence of other associated complications.

Elective cesarean section is an appropriate choice if the the fetus is estimated to weigh 4.5 kg or more, there is doubt about pelvic capacity or significant fetal compromise (like oligohydramnios) and ominous fetal heart tracings on CTG (like positive CST, prolonged and severe decelerations). Presence of other risk factors like age (elderly primigravida), hypertension and diabetes will tilt the balance in favour of cesarean section.

In the absence of the above factors, induction of labour is the accepted method of management. Routine induction at 41 completed weeks has been found to reduce perinatal mortality. There is no increase in cesarean delivery rate, instrumental delivery, use of analgesia or fetal heart abnormality. There is also reduced maternal anxiety, which is a significant factor.

Some obstetricians prefer not to induce labour at 41 weeks and wait till 42 completed weeks with fetal surveillance. The argument for this is that a percentage of women will go into spontaneous labour; in many others, the cervix will become more favourable, making induction more successful. They also believe that perinatal outcome is not affected as long as surveillance results are reassuring.

Once the decision to induce labour has been made, the status of the cervix must be assessed. If the cervix is favourable, that is, soft, short, anterior, slightly dilated with the vertex at –2 station or below, induction is often successful. Bishop score or its modification has been used to objectively assess the cervical status and a score of 9 or more is considered favourable.

If the cervix is unfavourable, pre-induction cervical ripening may be achieved. The most common method is instillation of prostaglandin E_2 gel (0.5 mg) in the cervical canal. Other methods are misoprostol, Foley catheter, breast stimulation and hygroscopic tents.

Some women may enter labour with pre-induction cervical ripening methods, particularly when prostaglandins are used. If the cervix is favourable, labour is induced with oxytocin infusion. When the cervix is fully effaced and/or dilated 2–3 cm, the membranes can be ruptured artificially with a view to expedite labour.

Intrapartum management

Labour is particularly risky for the fetus in prolonged pregnancy. Hence, the maternal condition, progress of labour and fetal status should be monitored very carefully. A partogram is very useful for this purpose. Fetal bradycardia, prolonged decelerations and post-contraction (late) decelerations indicate fetal distress and cesarean section or instrumental delivery will need to be performed depending on the stage of labour.

There is no consensus on the timing of amniotomy. It helps diagnose thick meconium and favours internal fetal monitoring, where possible. Amnioinfusion through the cervix with Ringer solution or saline has been found to be useful in reducing cesarean rates and NICU admissions. Meconium aspiration syndrome is also believed to be lowered. Nevertheless, amniotomy should be performed at least when the cervix is either fully effaced or dilated to 3 cm.

Most obstetricians will cut short the second stage with ventouse or outlet forceps. Shoulder dystocia should be anticipated; ensure that sufficient expertise and help are available; the presence of a neonatologist is invaluable in such cases.

KEY POINTS

- Prolonged pregnancy is not an uncommon clinical problem.
- There is increased maternal and perinatal adverse outcome in prolonged pregnancy.
- Oligohydramnios and perinatal asphyxia are major problems.
- Fetal surveillance is practised from 41 completed weeks.
- Delivery should be effected if there is oligohydramnios or fetal compromise.
- Labour can be induced at 41 weeks of gestation without any increased risk.
- Cervical ripening is useful in induction of labour when the cervix is unfavourable.

QUESTIONS

Select the single most appropriate answer:

1. According to the WHO, a pregnancy is said to be prolonged if the period of gestation is
   a. 40 weeks b. 41 weeks c. 42 weeks d. 43 weeks
2. Whenever a woman presents with complaints that she has passed her expected date of delivery, the first thing to be done is to
   a. recommend a USG to confirm the period of gestation
   b. do a nonstress test
   c. induce labour
   d. review her menstrual history
3. Approximately what percentage of women deliver by 41 weeks?
   a. 60% b. 70% c. 80% d. 90%
4. If a woman had a prolonged pregnancy in the past, what are the chances of recurrence in a subsequent pregnancy?
   a. 50% b. 40% c. 30% d. 20%
5. It has been observed that if labour is induced at 41 weeks, there is no increase in
   a. cesarean section
   b. fetal heart abnormality
   c. instrumental delivery
   d. all of the above

In the following questions, there are two statements. Select the appropriate answer using the following key:

a. if both statements are true and causally related
b. if both statements are true but not causally related
c. if the first statement is true and the second is false
d. if the first statement is false and the second is true
e. if both statements are false

6. Oligohydramnios occurs in prolonged pregnancy *because*

   In prolonged pregnancy, there is reduced fetal renal perfusion.
7. Meconium stained liquor is seen frequently in postterm pregnancy *because*

   Aspiration of meconium leads to a dangerous complication in the fetus.

44

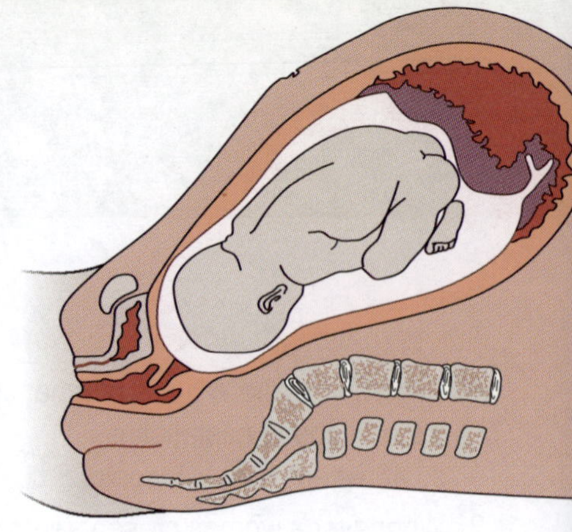

Rhesus Isoimmunisation

Vinita Salvi

LEARNING OBJECTIVES

At the end of this chapter, the reader should be able to:

- explain the pathophysiology of rhesus isoimmunisation
- list the factors that influence the occurrence of Rh isoimmunisation
- enumerate the factors that precipitate fetomaternal hemorrhage
- list the methods used to detect fetomaternal hemorrhage and to identify the immunised pregnant mother
- outline the management of an Rh immunised pregnant mother
- list the principles of management of an affected newborn
- list the measures used to prevent Rh isoimmunisation

Introduction

The clinical condition of erythroblastosis fetalis was described by Ballantyne at the end of the nineteenth century. The etiology was established after the discovery of the Rhesus (Rh) factor by Landsteiner in 1940 and it was then learnt that erythroblastosis fetalis, where the fetus becomes edematous and often dies from severe anemia, is due to maternal isoimmunisation with paternally inherited fetal Rh antigen. Subsequently, it was recognised that spectrophotometry was useful in analysing the amniotic fluid for the severity of hemolysis in the fetus, and that early delivery or intrauterine transfusion could be life-saving. Finally, it was discovered that the administration of anti-D immunoglobulin to the mother at risk would effectively prevent isoimmunisation. This has led to a significant decline in the incidence of Rh isoimmunisation. About 5% of antenatal mothers in India are Rh negative.

Etiopathology

The Rhesus status of an individual is designated as positive or negative depending on the presence or absence of the Rhesus (Rh) antigen on the red blood cells (RBC). The Rh antigen consists of three components: C, D and E. Of these, only the D antigen is of practical importance. These antigens are expressed by the presence of CDE genes and the corresponding alleles cde. Since these CDE genes are dominant, they will phenotypically express in both homozygous and heterozygous states (DD and Dd); the individual is then Rh positive. The presence of dd genes will make the individual Rh negative.

When an Rh-negative woman conceives through an Rh-positive man, the Rh status of the fetus will depend on the zygosity of the man. If he is homozygous (DD), all the offsprings will be Rh positive (Dd); if he is heterozygous (Dd), 50% of the fetuses will be positive (Dd) and 50% will be negative (dd).

When an Rh-negative woman carries an Rh-positive fetus, the mother is exposed to the Rh antigen from the fetus due to fetomaternal hemorrhage during pregnancy and delivery. Once the mother is exposed to the antigen, she becomes sensitised to it and produces antibodies to the D antigen. These ani-bodies are of two types, IgM and IgG. IgM is a macromolecule and does not cross the placenta. IgG can cross the placenta and cause hemolysis in the fetus, resulting in fetal and neonatal anemia and hyperbilirubinemia. Severe hemolysis in utero results in severe anemia and cardiac failure, causing hydrops fetalis.

Hemolysis of fetal cells causes activation of extensive hepatic erythropoiesis, resulting in the distortion and enlargement of the hepatic parenchymal islets of erythropoiesis. This, in turn, causes portal and umbilical venous hypertension and placental edema and trophoblastic hypertrophy. The transplacental transfer of nutrients to the fetus decreases. Ascites appears because of the portal hypertension. Hypoalbuminemia, which is also seen, occurs partly due to distortion of the hepatic cell cords with a resultant decrease in blood flow as well as due to a decrease in the synthesising capacity of the liver. As the hypoproteinemia increases, the ascites worsens and generalised edema appears. Ultimately, anasarca ensues due to extreme hypoproteinemia. Hydrothorax and compression hypoplasia of the lungs and pulmonary edema occur terminally making adequate respiratory exchange impossible after delivery.

Causes of Rh immunisation

Rh immunisation occurs due to exposure of an Rh-negative individual to Rh-positive blood. The Rh-negative individual produces antibodies which can destroy Rh-positive cells. Immunisation may occur due to:

- Transfusion of Rh-positive blood to an Rh-negative person
- Fetomaternal leak from an Rh-positive fetus to an Rh-negative mother under some circumstances such as: abortion (spontaneous or induced) including hydatidiform mole, delivery (normal or operative), ectopic pregnancy, any procedure such as version amniocentesis or manual removal of the placenta

Fetomaternal hemorrhage is also known to occur in pregnancy in the absence of any of the factors mentioned above.

Factors affecting Rh isoimmunisation

The largest amount of fetomaternal hemorrhage occurs at the time of delivery. Transplacental transfer of RBCs occurs only in 5% of women in the first trimester; this incidence increases to 47% by the third trimester. However, this leak is generally small and insufficient to produce a primary immune response. Therefore, primary sensitisation occurs in less than 1% of the first Rh-incompatible pregnancy.

Only 10%–15% of Rh-negative mothers with Rh-positive partners become sensitised after delivery. Three factors affect primary isoimmunisation:

- The size of the inoculum
- Coexistent ABO incompatibility reduces the frequency of isoimmunisation by 50%–75%. When the mother is of group O and the fetus is of group A or B, the fetal cells are cleared rapidly due to ABO incompatibility so that Rh sensitisation is not initiated. Moreover, anti-A and anti-B antibodies in maternal circulation are thought to damage or alter the fetal Rh antigen so that it is no longer immunogenic.
- About 30%–35% of Rh-negative subjects are 'non-responders' and cannot be immunised to the Rh-positive antigen. This ability to respond may be genetically controlled.

It is not clear how long after exposure it takes for the primary immune response to occur, but several weeks can elapse before the first antibodies are detected. The secondary response is a large production of antibodies in response to a small amount of Rh-positive blood. The time of detection of antibody correlates with the severity of the resultant hemolytic disease: the earlier the antibody is detected, the more severe the disease.

Management of an Rh-negative pregnant woman

Identification: At the first antenatal visit, blood grouping and Rh typing is done as a routine investigation for all pregnant mothers if it has not been done earlier.

If the woman is Rh-negative, the partner's blood group and Rh status is determined. If he is Rh-negative, no further investigations are required.

If the man is Rh-positive, the **indirect Coomb's** test is done at the first visit. If there are no anti-Rh antibodies, the test is repeated in the second and third trimesters or whenever there is a risk of fetomaternal transfusion. About one-third of isoimmunised women do not have demonstrable antibody in the first sample. Therefore, all women should have at least two to three samples tested during pregnancy; the last one should be tested in the third trimester. If there are no antibodies at 28 weeks, 300 µg anti-D immune globulin is administered. If antibodies are present, the mother is isoimmunised and requires further management as detailed below.

In a non-immunised pregnancy, at birth, the cord blood is collected for ABO grouping and Rh typing, direct Coomb's test, hemoglobin and bilirubin estimation. If the baby is Rh-positive, the mother should be administered 300 µg anti-D in the postpartum period within 72 hours.

Evaluation of pregnancy in the Rh-isoimmunised woman

In an isoimmunised woman, anti-D antibodies are found in the serum. These are detected by the indirect Coomb's test. This test uses known Rh-positive cells which are treated with the maternal serum, when the antibodies coat the red cells. When an anti-human gammaglobulin (Coomb's reagent) is added to this, the cells clump: this indicates a positive test. This test can also be done semiquantitatively.

Antibody titres: An anti-D antibody titre greater than 1:4 indicates Rh-isoimmunisation. A 'critical titre' is one below which no severe erythroblastosis or perinatal death has been observed; this titre ranges between 1:16 and 1:32. If there is no history of an affected infant or fetal death, and the initial anti-D titre is less than the critical titre, the anti-D titre is estimated once a month from 16–18 weeks onwards. Amniocentesis is performed only if the titre reaches the 'critical' level.

Quantitative estimation of antibodies: Antibody levels are more reliable indicators than titres by indirect Coomb's test. The maternal antibody levels are measured at 2–3 week intervals from week 17 onwards. If the level of antibodies is below 4 IU/ml, fetal hemolysis is mild and the pregnancy can be continued till term and spontaneous labour awaited. If the antibody level is 4–20 IU/ml, there is mild fetal hemolysis; at levels of 20 IU/ml or higher, the disease may be severe and requires further investigation.

Amniocentesis: The first amniocentesis is performed when the indirect Coomb's test reaches the critical level, approximately 10 weeks before the time of the earliest previous fetal death, fetal transfusion or birth of a severely affected baby, but not before gestational week 17–18. The fetal reticuloendothelial system is too immature to cause hemolysis prior to this. The patient scheduled for amniocentesis has a preliminary ultrasound survey. Besides assessing the gestational age, fetal skin edema, pleural and pericardial effusions, ascites, cardiac configuration, amniotic fluid volume and placental size and appearance are noted. Fetal activity and reactivity are noted and an appropriate site selected for amniocentesis. Amniotic fluid bilirubin levels will only indicate the degree of fetal hemolysis and not fetal anemia.

Analysis and interpretation: Amniotic fluid is subjected to spectrophotometry to determine its optical density (OD). The OD of normal amniotic fluid shows a straight line on a graph. On the other hand, amniotic fluid containing bilirubin shows a deviation from the straight line at the optical density of 450 nm (range 250–700). This deviation from the baseline is proportionate to the amount of bilirubin; the deviation is measured and is termed ODD (optical density deviate or Δ OD 450). The ODD is plotted on Liley's chart, which is a graph with the gestational age on the X-axis and ODD on the Y-axis. Liley's chart has three zones (**Fig. 44.1**). The baby's condition is determined by the zone in which the value of the optical density deviate lies:

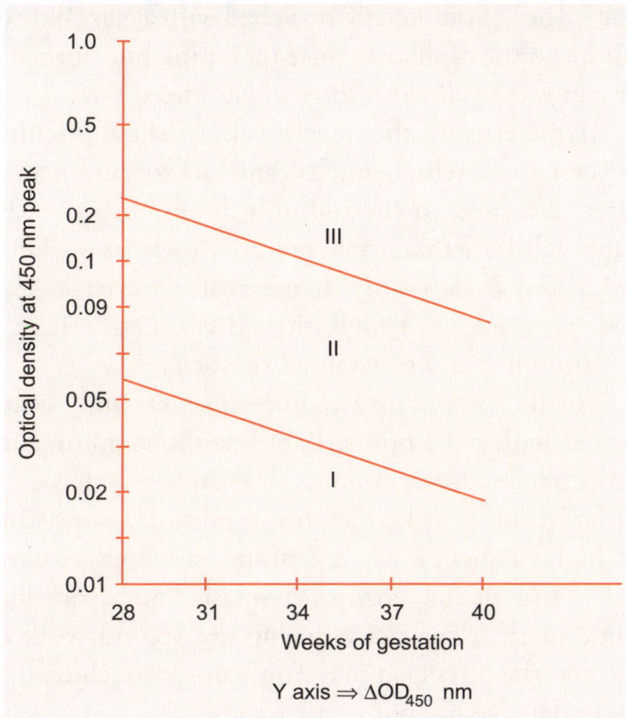

Fig. 44.1 Liley's chart.

Zone I: Baby unaffected and the pregnancy is permitted to continue.

Zone II: Baby is affected and pregnancy may require premature termination.

Zone III: Baby is severely affected and requires intra-uterine transfusion if premature and immediate delivery if mature.

The fetal condition is followed up with serial estimation of ODD.

Fetal blood sampling: Though interpretation of amniotic fluid ODD 450 values are reliable in the third trimester, the most accurate method of assessing the degree of fetal anemia in the second trimester is by fetal blood sampling or cordocentesis. The fetal hematocrit is determined.

Complications of fetal blood sampling include abortion, preterm labour, a marked increase in maternal antibody levels, fetal exsanguination, fetal bradycardia, failure to obtain a sample and cord constriction.

The fetal wellbeing is monitored by various methods. Sinusoidal and decelerative patterns on cardiotocography correlate with severe fetal anemia. Doppler ultrasound measurements of blood velocity in the fetal thoracic aorta and middle cerebral artery are also useful. However, monitoring fetal movements is not very useful since they decline only when the disease is advanced.

Intrauterine fetal transfusion

Indication for transfusion: The decision to start fetal transfusion may be based on ODD 450 values or fetal hematocrit, the primary objective being to allow intrauterine gestation to complete 32–34 weeks. If Liley's charts are being followed, transfusion is performed once the ODD 450 value has reached or is approaching Liley's zone III. Hematocrit levels above 40% at any period of gestation do not require transfusion. They are required if the fetal hematocrit is <25% before 26 weeks, gestation and <30% thereafter. Subsequent transfusions are timed on the basis of both the fetal hematocrit achieved at the end of the previous transfusion and the observation that the fetal hematocrit decreases approximately 1% per day. The fetal hematocrit should be maintained above a third of the normal mean for the period of gestation to prevent the development of hydrops.

Intrauterine transfusion: It is performed by a multidisciplinary team as the mainstay of therapy for severe Rh isoimmunisation; survival rates are 60%–90%. The route of transfusion may be either intravascular or intraperitoneal. The initial enthusiasm for intravascular transfusion has now been tempered by the realisation of the technical skills required and complications such as cord hematoma with tamponade, sudden fetal bradycardia and death. Other complications include fetal thrombocytopenia, leucoencephalopathy and hemorrhage.

Transfusions are performed using continuous real-time ultrasound guidance. The quantity of blood transfused is calculated as 10 ml per week of gestation beyond 20 weeks. In intravascular transfusion, the quantity of blood transfused is determined by the estimated fetoplacental blood volume, the pretransfusion hematocrit and the donor hematocrit. A combination of intravascular and intraperitoneal transfusions with a view to reducing the number of transfusions has also been used.

Termination of pregnancy: Pregnancy should not be allowed to continue beyond 40 weeks in Rh incompatibility. If the Coomb's titres are more than 1:4, but below the critical level, antibody levels are between 4 and 20 IU/ml or amniotic fluid ODD falls in Liley's zone II, pregnancy is terminated at 37–38 weeks. If there is evidence of severe hemolysis, pregnancy is continued at least till 32–34 weeks, with fetal transfusion and antenatal steroid, and then terminated.

Alternative therapies: Other treatment modalities to suppress immune reactions which have been described include the use of promethazine hydrochloride, oral desensitisation with erythrocyte membrane, immunoglobulin therapy and transfusion of marrow stem cells from the Rh-negative mother to the Rh-positive fetus. Oral administration of Rh antigen has been tried in an effort to suppress the secondary immune response. The efficacy of these modalities remains unproven and some of them may even be potentially hazardous.

The Rh-isoimmunised neonate

Clinical features: Classically, these babies present with anemia, jaundice, hepatosplenomegaly and, if untreated, bilirubin encephalopathy (kernicterus). The condition is termed hydrops fetalis if there are features of cardiac failure like anasarca. There is, however, a wide spectrum of presentations, ranging from a barely perceptible hemolysis, jaundice (icterus gravis neonatorum) to death. At birth, most infants are not pale and the cord hemoglobin may be at the lower limit of normal. However, the hemoglobin drops within 24 hours with marked pallor by the second day. Occasionally, the onset of anemia is delayed beyond the immediate neonatal period. However, the hemolytic process is inevitable with severe and sometimes fatal anemia after the second or third week.

Since bilirubin readily crosses the placenta, most infants are not grossly jaundiced at birth. Icterus usually develops in the first 24 hours since placental excretion is lost and the neonatal liver has low levels of glucuronyl transferase. The baby at birth should be examined in daylight or under white fluorescent light. The skin should be blanched with a glass slide to compress the capillaries since their pink hue normally obscures the yellowish tinge of jaundiced skin.

Kernicterus is the macroscopic yellow staining of certain cerebral nuclei and its occurrence is directly related to the bilirubin levels. Initially, the baby will be lethargic, hypotonic, loses its suckling reflex and feeds poorly. It may roll its eyeballs and have an unpleasant high-pitched cry. Later, there is opisthotonus and generalised spasticity.

Usually, respiratory failure occurs and death ensues within 12 hours. Babies without pulmonary disturbance survive months or even years; they may suffer from post-kernicterus syndrome, consisting of high-frequency nerve deafness, athetoid cerebral palsy and dental enamel dysplasia. Survivors lose some of their spasticity during the second week of life and the physician may erroneously conclude that brain damage has not occurred.

Despite exchange transfusion, anemia of delayed onset may occur and the hemoglobin gradually decreases to 5–6 g/dl by 4–6 weeks of life. This anemia is not well understood and may be associated with a persistence of anti-Rh antibodies or a reduced production of RBCs. By the end of the second month, anemia lessens spontaneously and transfusion is rarely necessary. Iron and vitamins are of no value.

Management: The management of the Rh-isoimmunised neonate includes the treatment of anemia and prevention of hyperbilirubinemia. The investigations required at birth are:

- cord blood hemoglobin
- ABO and Rhesus type
- direct Coomb's test
- bilirubin concentration.

Hemoglobin and bilirubin are monitored serially. The management is as follows:

- Double volume exchange transfusions are required in severe hyperbilirubinemia (170 ml per kilogram of body weight at 10–20 ml/minute)
- Phototherapy using blue-green light of wavelength 430–470 nm is useful for the mildly affected neonate or as an adjunct to exchange transfusion. Indirect bilirubin which is toxic is converted to non-toxic, water-soluble isomers that are excreted in urine.

- Phenobarbital 10 mg/kg/24 hours is used to mature the neonatal hepatic glucuronyl transferase enzyme, thereby reducing hyperbilirubinemia.
- Top up transfusions may be required.

Passive immunisation

The use of anti-D immunoglobulin to prevent Rh sensitisation has been one of the landmarks in the management of women with the Rh-negative type. When the mother is administered the anti-D immunoglobulin, it prevents the sensitisation of the mother by destroying the Rh-positive fetal cells.

Anti-D immunoglobulin, in doses of 300 µg, is administered within 72 hours of delivery of an Rh-positive infant. Anti-D antibody administered at the time of delivery prevents about 99% of sensitisations. Antenatal administration of 300 µg of anti-D at 28 weeks, in addition to the postpartum dose will virtually eliminate isoimmunisation, with the incidence dropping to only 0.17%. The time limit of 72 hours for the administration of anti-D is arbitrary and administration even two weeks later will protect as many as 50% of the cases.

Other than the postpartum period, the woman should also be immunised whenever there is a potential risk of fetomaternal hemorrhage, that is, spontaneous and induced abortion, ectopic pregnancy and procedures such as chorion villus biopsy, amniocentesis and external cephalic version. Except for a first trimester abortion, where the dose required is 50 µg, in all other situations, 300 µg of anti-D are indicated. Ideally, a Kleihauer test should be done to determine the number of fetal cells in maternal circulation and the Rh-immune globulin given in a dose of 20 µg per ml of fetal erythrocytes.

KEY POINTS

- About 5%–10% of pregnant mothers may be Rh negative.
- An Rh-negative mother has a 100% chance of carrying a positive fetus if the partner is homozygous positive and 50% chance is he is heterozygous.
- The mother can be exposed to Rh-positive cells by transfusion or fetomaternal bleeding during pregnancy or delivery.
- An exposed mother can get sensitised to the Rh antigen and produce antibodies,which can cross the placenta and produce hemolysis and anemia in the fetus.
- The severity of the disease may vary from mild hemolysis to hydrops fetalis and intrauterine death.
- The condition can be diagnosed by indirect Coomb's test and ultrasound.
- Intrauterine transfusion has improved the survival of the affected fetus.
- Administration of anti-D to the mother protects her from getting immunised.

QUESTIONS

Select the single most appropriate answer:

1. Of the components of Rh antigen which one is of significance in producing isoimmunisation?
   a. component C c. component E
   b. component D d. component D
2. A woman is Rh negative and her husband is heterozygous Rh positive. What percentage of offsprings will be Rh positive?
   a. 20% b. 30% c. 40% d. 50%
3. When is an Rh-negative mother exposed to a leak from an Rh-positive fetus?
   a. ectopic pregnancy c. external cephalic version
   b. normal delivery d. all of the above
4. Which of the following statements about factors causing primary Rh isoimmunisation is false?
   a. the incidence of transplacental transfer of RBCs is 47% in the third trimester

b. the size of the inoculum in the first trimester is large
c. coexistent ABO incompatibility reduces the risk of Rh isoimmunisation
d. about 10% to 35% of women are non-responders

5. In an Rh immunised mother, if the antibody titre is below the 'critical' level and there is no history of fetal death, from week 16 onwards the antibody titre must be measured once every
   a. 8 weeks c. 4 week
   b. 6 weeks d. 2 weeks
6. On quantitative estimation, antibody titre of 20 IU/ml indicates
   a. mild fetal hemolysis
   b. that no intervention is required
   c. severe hemolysis
   d. that estimation must be repeated after 2 weeks

In the following questions, there are two statements. Select the appropriate answer using the following key:

a. If both statements are true and causally related
b. If both statements are true but not causally related
c. If first the statement is true and the second is false
d. If first the statement is false and the second is true
e. If both statements are false

7. Severe hemolysis causes severe anemia and cardiac failure leading to hydrops fetalis *because*
   Hemolysis of fetal cells causes activation of extensive hepatic erythropoiesis.
8. Amniotic fluid is subjected to spectrophotometry to determine its optical density *because*
   The results are useful for further management when plotted on Liley's chart.
9. Intrauterine transfusion is indicated when the ODD 450 value reaches Liley's zone III and fetal hematocrit is ≤25% at 26 weeks of gestation *because*
   Intrauterine transfusion will correct fetal anemia and help to gain maturity of 32 to 34 weeks.

Select the appropriate answer using the following key:

a. If only responses 1, 2 and 3 are correct
b. If only 1 and 3 are correct
c. If only 2 and 4 are correct
d. If only 4 is correct
e. If all are correct

9. If a mother's indirect Coomb's test is negative injection of 300 µg of Anti-D should be given
   1. at 28 weeks of pregnancy
   2. after delivery if the baby is Rh positive
   3. while performing an amniocentesis
   4. during forceps application
10. In a non-immunised mother, which test must be performed on the collected cord blood?
   1. serum bilirubin
   2. direct Coomb's test
   3. hemoglobin
   4. ABO and Rh

45

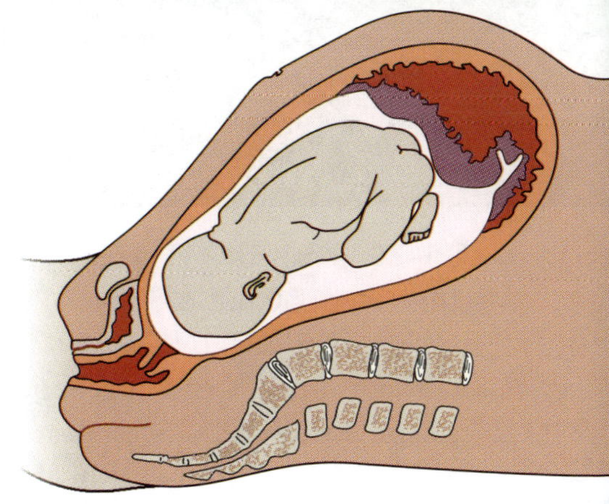

Fetal Growth Restriction

Sunesh Kumar

LEARNING OBJECTIVES

At the end of this chapter, the reader will be able to:

- define IUGR
- appreciate the underlying pathophysiology
- define the types of IUGR
- enlist the causes of IUGR
- enumerate the complications of IUGR
- list the diagnostic criteria of IUGR
- outline the plan of management for IUGR

Introduction

Intrauterine growth restriction (IUGR) is a condition characterised by reduced fetal growth. The birth weight of a newborn is dependent on the gestational age at which it is born. Fetal growth is influenced by genetic factors and the intrauterine environment. About 20% of all newborns in India are of low birth weight; they account for more than 50% of neonatal deaths. The etiology of IUGR is not clear and hence the focus should be on early detection and appropriate management during pregnancy, labour and the neonatal period.

Definition

A fetus which has not attained growth appropriate to the period of gestation is said to be growth restricted. According to conventional international parameters, a baby whose weight at birth is **below the tenth percentile** or less than two standard deviations of range of birth weight for a corresponding period of gestation is said to be **growth restricted**.

The term IUGR should not confused with low birth weight, which includes all babies weighing less than 2,500 g at birth. It is important to differentiate between low birth weight due to fetal growth restriction and that due to prematurity.

Classification

There are two types of IUGR, symmetrical and asymmetrical. **Symmetrical growth restriction** consists of uniform retardation of fetal growth. In **asymmetrical growth restriction**, the whole body, except the head, is growth restricted; the growth of the abdomen lags behind disproportionately, when compared to the head.

Pathophysiology

In the first trimester, fetal growth is due to cellular hyperplasia; in the second trimester, there is both hyperplasia and hypertrophy, followed by only hypertrophy in the third trimester. The weight gain is 5 g/day till 15 weeks of gestation,

15–20 g/day till 24 weeks and then 30–35 g/day from week 30 onwards.

Symmetrical IUGR is most often due to chromosomal and genetic errors, whereas asymmetrical IUGR appears to be caused by a deficiency of nutrients in the placental perfusion. This type of IUGR is associated with maternal diseases like pregnancy-induced hypertension.

Growth hormone, insulin-like growth factor, human placental lactogen and leptin play a crucial role in fetal growth and development: these may be deficient in IUGR. Both types of IUGR are associated with a thrombotic process in the placenta. Further, a prostanoid abnormality in the placenta is responsible for deficient perfusion, leading to reduction in blood flow and fetal malnutrition. The pathological changes in the fetus occur consequent to decreased blood supply to the fetus. This leads to redistribution of blood flow to the vital organs but reduces the blood flow to the splanchnic bed.

- Reduction in the fetal glomerular filtration rate leads to decreased urine output followed by reduction in the volume of amniotic fluid.
- Increase in the number of RBCs causes polycythemia.
- Increased hepatic gluconeogenesis and mobilisation of body fat leads to loss of subcutaneous fat.
- Anerobic glucose metabolism results in the formation of lactic acid and acidosis.

Causes of IUGR

Intrauterine growth restriction may occur due to maternal, placental and fetal causes. In 30%–50% of cases, no obvious cause may be found.

Maternal causes

These factors affect fetal growth in the late second half of pregnancy.

- Women below 17 years and above 35 years are more likely to give birth to smaller babies.
- A mother who has delivered a growth restricted fetus is more prone to delivering a small-for-date baby in subsequent pregnancies.
- Poor nutrition prior to and during pregnancy, pre-pregnancy weight less than 45 kg and height less than 140 cm or constitutionally small build, tend to result in smaller babies. The babies of women from poor socioeconomic status are often growth restricted.
- The babies of women living at high altitude are usually growth restricted.
- There is a definite association between consumption of tobacco and IUGR. Similar observations have been made among mothers addicted to alcohol and hard drugs.
- Hypertension during pregnancy, whether due to pregnancy-induced hypertension (PIH) or chronic or secondary to renal disease, is the most common cause of IUGR. The condition is also seen in diseases like severe anemia, antiphospholipid antibody syndrome, chronic renal disease and major chronic illnesses.

Fetal causes

- Chromosomal and genetic abnormalities are associated with symmetrical IUGR. Trisomy 18 or 21 is associated with variable degree of growth restriction.
- **Fetal malformations:** Fetuses with major anomalies suffer from growth restriction.
- Infections like HIV, malaria, toxoplasmosis, rubella and cytomegalovirus are implicated in IUGR.
- **Ionising radiation and teratogenic drugs:** Exposure to ionising radiation and teratogenic drugs is likely to cause fetal growth restriction.
- **Multiple fetuses:** Fetal growth restriction occurs more frequently in pregnancies with two or more fetuses as compared to a singleton pregnancy.

Placental and other causes: The placenta is the principal organ responsible for blood supply to the fetus. Any lesion in the placenta that decreases blood flow affects fetal growth adversely.

Placental factors: Placental infarction, developmental anomalies like circumvallate placenta and infections such as toxoplasmosis or a low-lying placenta can cause IUGR.

Cord abnormalities: Fetal growth restriction is associated with cord abnormalities like true knots.

Idiopathic causes: In 30%–50% of cases where fetal growth is retarded, no obvious maternal, fetal or placental cause may be evident.

Complications

Babies born with growth restriction are prone to a number of complications. There could be intrauterine death. Other complications of IUGR are birth asphyxia, meconium aspiration syndrome, polycythemia, hypoglycemia, hypocalcemia hypothermia, hyperbilirubinemia, necrotising enterocolitis and convulsions. Later in life they may be found to have low IQ, suffer from chronic ill health, cerebral palsy and convulsions. According to the Barker hypothesis, these babies are more prone to diabetes, hypertension, obesity and coronary artery disease.

Diagnosis

Clinical diagnosis: Intrauterine growth restriction should be detected and managed as early as possible to ensure the best fetal outcome.

Identification of women at risk of IUGR: If a mother has delivered a growth restricted fetus earlier, she has very high chance of delivering a small-for-date baby in subsequent pregnancies.

Risk factors like low socioeconomic status, nutrition, addiction to tobacco and drugs, and medical and obstetric complications should be checked for.

Obstetrical examination: On palpation, IUGR should be suspected if the fundal height lags by four weeks or more for the period of gestation.

Symphysiofundal height: The uterine height measured in centimetres corresponds to the weeks of gestation between 18 and 30 weeks. It is better to use a gravidogram which is a good screening tool for IUGR. If the symphysiofundal height is below the 10th percentile, IUGR is suspected and the woman is referred for further evaluation (see Chapter 10).

Reduced amount of amniotic fluid may indicate IUGR.

Confirmation

Whenever IUGR is suspected clinically, it is confirmed by ultrasonography; fetal wellbeing too can be evaluated by USG. A single ultrasound may not help in the diagnosis of IUGR: serial measurements may be necessary.

Fetal biometry: The measurement of biparietal diameter (BPD), head circumference (HC), abdominal circumference (AC) and femur length (FL) help estimate the period of gestation and the fetal weight. The AC is the most sensitive parameter for the diagnosis of asymmetrical growth restriction. In symmetrical IUGR, all the parameters are reduced, even early in pregnancy.

Evaluation of amniotic fluid volume: It is a very reliable parameter of fetal wellbeing. A reduction in the volume of amniotic fluid has been recognised to be characteristic of IUGR in 95% of women.

Doppler velocimetry: The procedure measures blood flow in fetal vessels and helps detect fetuses with hypoxia due to reduction in blood flow. Absence of diastolic flow (**Fig. 45.1**) and reversal of diastolic blood flow (**Fig. 45.2**) in severe cases of IUGR is indicative of fetal distress.

Management

There is no evidence to suggest that interventions like nutritional supplements and drugs to improve placental blood flow have any benefit. Once IUGR is diagnosed, the objective is to monitor fetal growth and wellbeing serially and decide when continuation of intrauterine existence becomes hazardous to the fetus and plan delivery. This should be balanced against the risk of delivering the fetus prematurely.

Fetal growth and wellbeing are monitored by serially performing the following:

- fetal growth using biometry

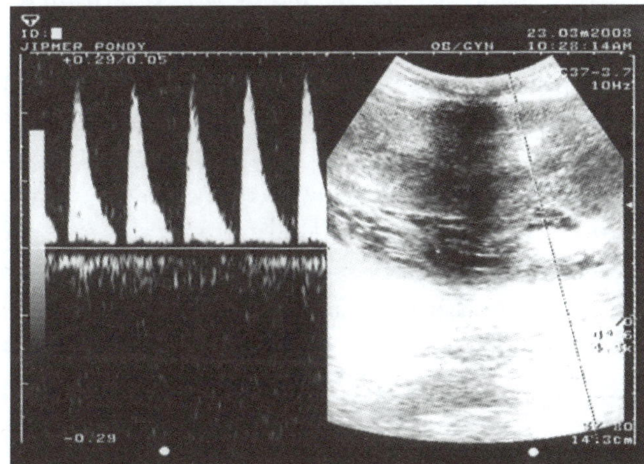

Fig. 45.1 Absent diastolic flow.

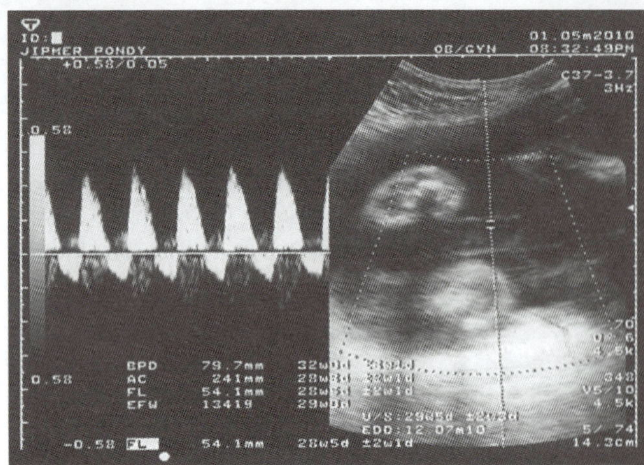

Fig. 45.2 Reversal of diastolic flow.

- maintenance of daily fetal kick count chart
- serial amniotic fluid index
- biophysical profile

Rest: Most obstetricians advise the woman to take adequate rest, particularly in the left lateral position, as it may increase placental blood flow.

Treatment of maternal diseases: It is important to treat maternal diseases like PIH to improve placental blood flow.

Plan for delivery

Time of delivery: If the fetus is growth restricted and, if the duration of pregnancy is 37 weeks or more, the fetus should be delivered, as waiting beyond that period would be detrimental to the fetus and to the mother if she is suffering from PIH or other maternal diseases. The pregnancy is also terminated if there are fetal anomalies incompatible with life. Pregnancies of a gestation of 32–37 weeks are managed conservatively if the tests for wellbeing are reassuring. Steroids for fetal pulmonary maturity are administered, fetal wellbeing carefully monitored and the pregnancy is continued till term. If the tests are not reassuring, delivery should be planned. IUGR in the late second trimester and early third trimester has poor fetal outcome.

Place of delivery: Growth restricted babies are not only small, but also prone to complications in the neonatal period. Therefore, delivery must take place in a hospital with a neonatal intensive care unit. Expert neonatal care in the first few minutes of life will prevent long-term complications.

Mode of delivery: Efforts must be made to deliver vaginally. If the biophysical score indicates the fetus to be doing well, labour is induced. Labour should be monitored very closely to detect any fetal heart rate abnormalities, as preexisting hypoxia can worsen during labour.

Cesarean section: The need for CS is increased in IUGR; however, it should be performed in institutions where expert neonatal care is available. Cesarean section without adequate neonatal support will not help to improve perinatal outcome, and will increase maternal morbidity.

Growth restricted neonate

The newborn with growth restriction has a characteristic appearance, with features like wrinkled, patchy, peeling skin which is thin due to loss of subcutaneous fat. The infant is usually open-eyed, unusually alert and appears old and worried. The nails may be long. These babies are prone to develop hypothermia, hypoglycemia and, hypocalcemia and may be polycythemic (**Fig. 45.3**).

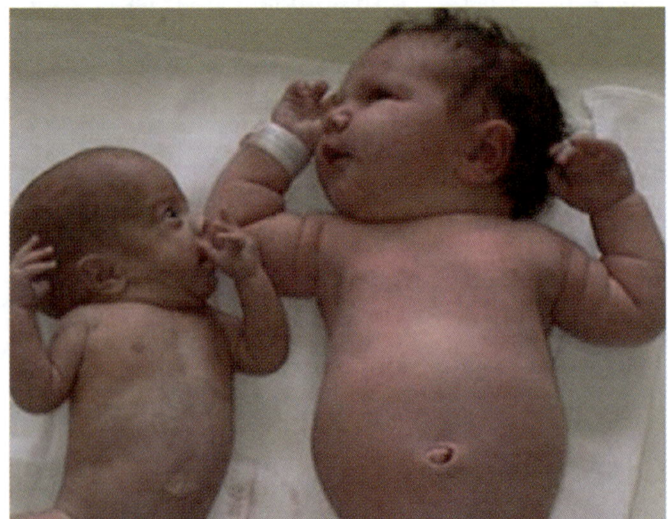

Fig. 45.3 Growth restricted neonate (left) and a normal baby.

KEY POINTS

- A baby whose weight at birth is less than the tenth percentile for a corresponding period of gestation is said to be growth restricted.
- Intrauterine growth restriction (IUGR) is symmetrical if the growth restriction is uniform; it is asymmetrical when vital organs like the brain and heart are spared.
- Symmetrical IUGR is due to fetal causes, while asymmetrical IUGR is affected by maternal, placental and cord factors.
- Intrauterine growth restriction is suspected clinically if the fundal height lags by four weeks or when the symphysiofundal height (measured in cm) is below the tenth percentile on the gravidogram.
- During pregnancy, fetal growth and wellbeing should be monitored clinically and ultrasonologically. Abdominal circumference is the most important parameter for the diagnosis of fetal growth restriction.
- A growth restricted fetus is prone to a number of complications in the neonatal period. Therefore, the mother should preferably be delivered in an institution where a neonatal intensive care unit is available.

QUESTIONS

Select the single most appropriate answer:

1. Which of the following statements is *not* true about IUGR?
   a. it is associated with preeclampsia.
   b. IUGR and prematurity cannot coexist.
   c. gravidogram is a screening tool.
   d. perinatal morbidity increases.
2. From 30 weeks of gestation, the rate of gain in fetal weight is
   a. 10–15 g/day
   b. 20–25 g/day
   c. 30–35 g/day
   d. 40–45 g/day
3. Asymmetrical IUGR is associated with
   a. placenta previa
   b. maternal hypertension
   c. bicornuate uterus
   d. placental abruption
4. On ultrasonological examination, the fetal parameter that is sensitive for detecting IUGR is
   a. head circumference
   b. femur length
   c. abdominal circumference
   d. fetal weight
5. The pathophysiology of IUGR includes all of the following *except*
   a. oligohydramnios
   b. decreased hepatic gluconeogenesis
   c. decreased glomerular filtration
   d. anerobic glucose metabolism
6. Which one of the following is a screening method for IUGR?
   a. obstetric palpation
   b. previous history of IUGR
   c. ultrasound
   d. gravidogram
7. In IUGR, pregnancy should be terminated at
   a. 33 weeks
   b. 35 weeks
   c. 37 weeks
   d. 39 weeks

Select the appropriate answer using the following key:

a. if only responses 1, 2 and 3 are correct
b. if only 1 and 3 are correct
c. if only 2 and 4 are correct
d. if only 4 is correct
e. if all are correct

8. Which of the following are associated with asymmetrical IUGR?
   1. thrombotic process in the placenta
   2. chromosomal abnormalities
   3. diversion of blood from the splanchnic region
   4. Ionising radiation
9. Intrauterine growth restriction occurs because there is a deficiency of
   1. growth hormone
   2. hPL
   3. leptin
   4. progesterone
10. Fetal causes of IUGR include
    1. multiple pregnancy
    2. fetal malformations
    3. fetal infections
    4. trisomy 18

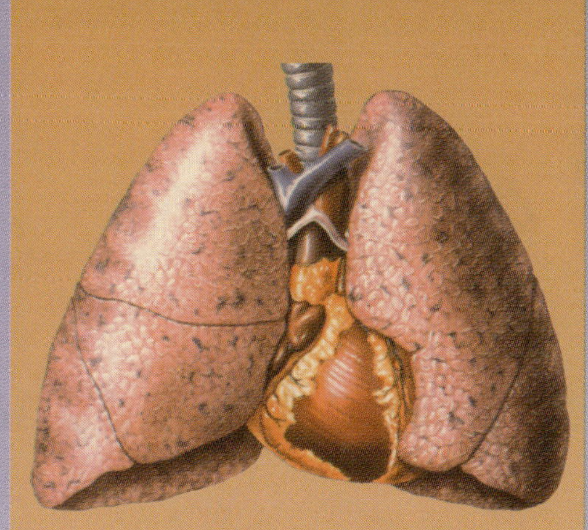

Part VI Medical and Surgical Complications During Pregnancy

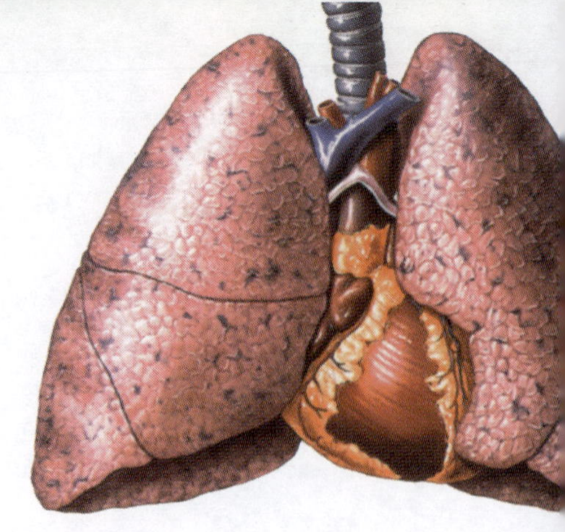

46

Anemia in Pregnancy

C Ambuja

LEARNING OBJECTIVES

At the end of this chapter, the reader should be able to:

- define anemia
- enumerate the hematological changes of pregnancy
- enumerate the common causes of anemia during pregnancy
- describe the clinical features of anemia in pregnancy
- list the appropriate investigations to assess the degree and cause of anemia
- list the deleterious effects on the mother and her child
- outline the management of anemia during pregnancy and labour
- describe the measures to be taken at various levels to prevent anemia
- list the types of non–iron deficiency anemias and outline their management

Introduction

Anemia is the most common medical disorder complicating pregnancy. It is a public health problem all over the world, especially in the developing countries. The WHO reports the prevalence of anemia as 55% among expectant mothers across the world. Severe forms of anemia are seen in developing countries. In India, the incidence varies from 40% to 90%. It accounts for 20% of maternal deaths and significant perinatal loss. Anemia may exist before pregnancy, may become aggravated during pregnancy or may occur for the first time during pregnancy. It is significantly higher in the third trimester than in the first and second trimesters.

Definition

According to the WHO, anemia is defined as a hemoglobin concentration of less than 11 g/dl during pregnancy. Among nonpregnant women, the cut-off is 12 g/dl. It is a pathological condition in which the oxygen carrying capacity of the red cells is insufficient to meet the body's needs.

Table 46.1 shows the classification of anemia according to severity.

Physiological changes in blood during pregnancy

During pregnancy, there is hemodilution due to a disproportionate increase in the plasma volume when compared to red cell volume.

- Plasma volume increases by 40%–50%, starts at six weeks and is maximum at 32 weeks.
- Red cell mass increases by 20%–25%.
- Packed cell volume (PCV) is decreased.
- Mean cell volume (MCV) increases secondary to erythropoiesis.
- Serum iron is decreased and total iron binding capacity is increased.
- Mean corpuscular hemoglobin concentration (MCHC) does not change.

Table 46.1 Classification of anemia depending on its severity

Severity of anemia	ICMR (g/dl)	WHO (g/dl)
Mild	10–11	8–11
Moderate	7–10	6.5–8
Severe	<7	<6.5
Very severe	<4 (decompensated)	

Causes of anemia in pregnancy

Although it may be due to several causes, anemia due to nutritional deficiency is the most common.

- Nutritional anemia is usually caused by dietary deficiency of iron and folic acid. Other causes are deficiency of protein and vitamin B_{12}. It is documented that the presence of phytates in the diet (found in foods like maize, legumes and soya) bind the iron, making it unavailable for absorption.
- Blood loss due to preexisting menorrhagia, hemorrhoids and fissure-in-ano, hookworm infestation and bleeding during pregnancy could be responsible for the anemia.
- Hemolytic anemia may be due to:
  - congenital causes like sickle cell anemia and thalassemia or
  - acquired conditions like malaria and kala azar
- All infections can predispose to anemia; urinary tract infection in particular is associated with iron deficiency anemia and responds poorly to treatment.
- Aplastic anemia may be idiopathic, autoimmune or associated with the prolonged use of drugs like aspirin, indomethacin and zidovudine.

Prevalence of anemia

The reasons for the high prevalence of iron deficiency anemia in India are:

- inadequate intake of calories, protein and iron by pregnant women due to poverty.
- cereal-based foods, habitually consumed by women of the lower socioeconomic strata, reduce bioavailability of dietary iron.

Iron Fact File

The daily iron requirement for an adult nonpregnant woman is about 2 mg. On an average, the Indian diet provides 5–15 mg of elemental iron per day but only 10% of it is absorbed (1–1.5 mg). This is just sufficient to compensate for menstrual loss and other daily losses, with the result that more than 50% of women have deficiency of stored iron. Pregnancy poses an increase in iron requirement. Iron requirements increase from 2.5 mg/day in the first trimester to 7 mg/day in the third trimester.

During pregnancy, an additional 900–1100 mg of iron is needed, which is accounted for as follows:

- 400–500 mg for expansion of maternal red cell volume
- 300–400 mg for the fetus and placenta
- 250 mg for replacement of daily loss
- 200 mg for replacement of blood loss at delivery
- 1 mg/day for lactation

The amount of iron conserved due to amenorrhea is 250–500 mg. Therefore, additional 500–600 mg of iron is required in pregnancy, that is 4–6 mg/day. This quantity of iron cannot be obtained from the diet alone. It is mobilised from iron stores, thus depleting them. Hence, iron supplementation is necessary for all pregnant women in developing countries.

- **Food fads:** In some societies, pregnant women are not allowed to eat certain types of foods. Culturally, some fruits and vegetables are considered detrimental to the health of the mother and her baby, and are therefore forbidden. It is believed by some women that extra nutrition will lead to a large baby and result in a difficult delivery.
- Increased nutritional requirements during adolescence and pregnancy. A significant number of pregnancies continues to occur among adolescent girls in whom the existing nutritional deficiency worsens during pregnancy.
- Pregnancy conditions like multiparity, multiple pregnancy, repeated and closely spaced pregnancies

and, prolonged periods of lactation without iron supplementation play a role in the perpetration of anemia. Lack of iron supplementation also contributes to anemia.

- In intestinal infections like amebiasis and giardiasis iron absorption is defective. Blood loss in infestation with hookworm or schistosomiasis is considerable, amounting to 0.25 ml/worm/day; if 100 worms are present, the loss could be as much as 5 mg of iron per day.

Clinical features

The symptoms and signs are described below.

Symptoms: There may not be any symptoms among the majority of pregnant women. However, some of them may present with tiredness, dizziness, fainting and lethargy. Breathlessness and palpitations are common when the anemia is moderate to severe.

Signs: The most obvious sign is pallor of the conjunctiva and tongue. Signs of deficiency of other nutrients like vitamin B may coexist. A soft systolic murmur can be heard in the mitral area. Edema of the lower limbs when present is due to associated hypoproteinemia. In severe anemia with failure, signs of cardiac failure will be present.

INVESTIGATIONS

A pregnant woman with a hemoglobin level below 10 g/dl is subjected to a full hematological investigation. The objectives of investigations are to find out the degree and type of anemia and the cause.

In order to assess the degree of anemia, the hemoglobin (Hb), total red blood cell (RBC) count and packed cell volume (PCV) must be assessed.

- Hemoglobin value of less than 11 g/dl is considered to be anemia in pregnancy. However, remember that a reduction in Hb is a late manifestation of iron deficiency.
- Packed cell volume is a useful investigation in anemia due to acute blood loss when other parameters are normal.
- **Red cell indices:** A reduction in the MCV to 80 μm^3 and MCHC to less than 32% is characteristic of iron deficiency anemia.

In order to determine the type of anemia, a peripheral smear is done.

- Microcytic hypochromic type is seen in iron deficiency anemia.
- Macrocytic and hypochromic picture is seen in dimorphic anemia which is due to nutritional deficiency or malabsorption leading to both, deficiency of iron and folic acid or vitamin B_{12}.

The following tests will help to establish the cause of anemia:

- Peripheral smear is useful in the detection of cellular abnormalities like fragmentation, anisocytosis and poikilocytosis in hemolytic anemia, sickling in sickle cell anemia, target cells in thalassemia, abnormal cells in leukemias and parasites in infections. In some parts of India, Bangladesh and Sri Lanka where malaria is endemic, screening for anemia and malaria should be a part of routine antenatal testing.
- Stools should be examined to detect helminthic (specially hookworm) infestations and occult blood.
- Urinalysis is performed to exclude urinary tract infection and other renal disorders.
- Bone marrow study is indicated when there are abnormal cells or pancytopenia in the peripheral smear or there is no response to treatment.

Special investigations

- Serum iron and iron binding capacity are optional investigations. Serum iron will be low and iron binding capacity high in iron deficiency anemia.
- Levels of serum ferritin fall in proportion to a decrease in iron stores. It is not affected by pregnancy. A concentration of <12 µg/l is diagnostic of iron deficiency, but it is an expensive method of screening.
- **Serum transferrin receptor**: The level correlates with erythroid precursor proliferation and the adequacy of iron supply to the bone marrow.
- Tests for hemolysis will help to detect conditions like spherocytosis.
- Hemoglobin electrophoresis is done to detect hemoglobinopathies.

Effects of anemia on pregnancy

Anemia has adverse effects on both the mother and the fetus:

- There is increased risk of intercurrent infections and preterm labour.
- Women with significant anemia poorly tolerate even average blood loss of delivery and may collapse.
- During puerperium, there is an increased risk of infection, venous thromboembolic complications, subinvolution and failing lactation.
- An anemic mother has an increased risk of giving birth to a low birth weight baby due to prematurity or intrauterine growth restriction.
- The baby born even to a severely anemic mother is usually not anemic, but draws the iron from the mother, depleting her of her stores.
- The newborn of an anemic mother has poor iron stores and is likely to develop anemia later.

Effects of pregnancy on anemia

- Anemia worsens during pregnancy, both due to the increased demand and the physiological effects.
- In case of severe anemia, congestive cardiac failure is a serious complication. It is most likely to occur at 30–32 weeks of gestation, during labour or following delivery.

Prevention

In developing countries, iron deficiency anemia in pregnancy may be present before and become aggravated during pregnancy. Absorption of iron increases during the last two trimesters of pregnancy to 1–3 mg/day. Even so, an unsupplemented diet cannot provide more than 50% of the normal requirements of pregnancy. Hence, every pregnant woman needs iron supplementation during pregnancy. Iron demand starts in the first trimester but most pregnant women will have nausea and vomiting then. Hence, iron prophylaxis should be started in the second trimester and continued through the third.

The WHO recommends universal supplementation of 60 mg of elemental iron and 0.5 mg of folic acid once daily for six months in pregnancy in countries with a prevalence of anemia of over 40%. An additional supplementation for three months postpartum is recommended in high-prevalence countries. The Reproductive and Child Health Programme of the Ministry of Health and Family Welfare (Government of India) recommends 100 mg of elemental iron with 0.5 mg of folic acid once daily from the second half of pregnancy for a period of at least 100 days.

A realistic balanced diet should be recommended to those in the low socioeconomic group. Iron-rich foods are jaggery, ragi and green leafy vegetables like spinach, mustard leaves and sprouted pulses. Other sources of iron are meat, cereals, seeds, vegetables, milk and eggs. Its absorption can be increased by enhancers like proteins and ascorbic acid and decreased by inhibitors like phytic acid, fibres, calcium, tea (tannins), coffee, chocolate and herbal drinks. Overcooking food also reduces the bioavailability of various nutrients. Concurrent antacid or calcium intake prevents iron absorption.

Adolescents should eat a diet rich in proteins and iron. Besides dietary guidance and iron supplementation, counselling for spacing and limiting the number of pregnancies is very important. Improvement of socioeconomic conditions and health education to create awareness are other interventions which will reduce the prevalence of anemia.

Treatment

Iron therapy, which is the mainstay of treatment, may be administered either orally or parenterally.

Oral iron

It is the treatment of choice in iron deficiency anemia. Ferrous sulfate 200 mg containing 60 mg of elemental iron is given thrice a day until the blood picture becomes normal and is continued for at least 100 days following delivery to replenish iron stores. Vitamin C aids the absorption of iron. Absorption is improved if iron is taken before meals, but gastrointestinal side effects are also greater. Absorption is delayed if taken along with calcium and antacids.

Response to therapy is evidenced by reticulocytosis within 7–10 days, rising PCV and subjective sense of wellbeing. Hemoglobin increases by 0.7 g/dl per week. Side effects include gastrointestinal symptoms like nausea, vomiting, constipation, abdominal cramps and diarrhea. This reduces compliance and tolerance. The strategy in such cases is to reduce the dose or to take the iron tablet just after meals or change to a different preparation like fumarate, succinate, carbonyl iron or hemoglobin preparations.

The reasons for the failure to respond to oral therapy are inaccurate diagnosis, noncompliance, coexisting infections and megaloblastic anemia.

Parenteral iron

Iron deficiency anemia which cannot be managed with oral therapy due to poor compliance, severe gastrointestinal side effects and malabsorption can be managed with parenteral therapy. The main advantage of parenteral therapy is the certainty of administration; the expected rise in hemoglobin levels is similar to that of oral iron.

Estimation of total iron requirement: Elemental iron needed in mg = (Normal Hb in g % – patient's Hb in g %) × weight in kg × 4.4. An additional 50% is to be added for partial replenishment of iron stores. For example, the requirement in a woman weighing 40 kg with Hb% of 8 g/dl is (14–8) × 40 × 4.4 = 1,100 + 550 = 1,650 mg.

Another simple method is multiplying 250 mg of elemental iron with each gram of Hb below normal; to this add 50% for iron stores. In the above case this would be 6 × 250 = 1,500 mg +750 mg.

Routes of parenteral administration

Intramuscular route: Iron dextran and iron sorbitol citric acid complex in dextrin are the preparations available. Intramuscular iron is given on the upper and outer quadrant of the buttock using the Z technique. Oral iron should be stopped before giving iron sorbitol. The initial test dose is given before giving parenteral iron. Adverse reactions are pain, skin discolouration, arthralgia, myalgia, fever, lymphadenopathy and anaphylaxis.

Intravenous route: It is suitable when the patient is unwilling or unable to complete the course of IM injections. The required dose of iron in dextran (1 ml contains 50 mg of elemental iron) mixed with 500 ml of normal saline is infused. If the calculated iron requirement is more than 1,000 mg, it can be administered in two divided doses with a gap of one day between the doses.

Iron–sucrose is currently being used at a dose of 200 mg in 100 ml infused on alternate days. The advantage of this formulation is that hypersensitivity reactions are uncommon and routine sensitivity test is not needed.

Blood transfusion: It is the quickest way of raising the hemoglobin level, but is fraught with risks. Properly grouped, typed and cross-matched packed cell transfusions may be given in anemia due to blood loss, severe anemia, refractory anemia not responding to iron therapy and associated infections. Blood transfusions are given with utmost care to avoid complications like cardiac failure, hemolytic reactions due to mismatch and infections. Partial exchange transfusions may be given in cases of cardiac failure due to anemia to avoid circulatory overload.

Pregnant women are also likely to suffer from anemias other than iron deficiency. Whenever there is a history of anemia in a preexisting pregnancy or there is no response to iron therapy, the woman must be investigated for other types of anemia.

Megaloblastic Anemias

These are caused by impaired DNA synthesis and are relatively rare in pregnancy, accounting for less than 5%. Anemia due to folic acid deficiency is the most common among them.

Folic acid deficiency

During pregnancy, folic acid deficiency anemia occurs in women who do not consume animal protein and green leafy vegetables or cannot absorb due to vomiting. It is also seen in multiple pregnancies and in patients on anticonvulsant therapy. The recommended daily allowance of folic acid in pregnancy is 400 μg as compared to 50–100 μg in the non-pregnant state. The condition can be diagnosed by examining peripheral blood smears showing megloblastic RBCs (resulting in increased MCV) and hypersegmentation of neutrophils. Bone marrow examination reveals megaloblastic erythropoiesis. Serum folic acid levels will be reduced; reduced red cell folate levels are better markers. Even in the presence of severe maternal anemia, the fetus remains non-anemic. Treatment includes diet rich in folates and supplementation of folic acid along with iron.

Vitamin B_{12} Deficiency

This is very rare in pregnancy as those with severe deficiency are usually infertile. It can be seen in women with gastrectomy, Crohn's disease and intestinal parasitic infection. Estimation of serum levels (<80 pg/ml) will confirm the diagnosis. These women may be treated with vitamin B_{12} injection of 1,000 μg weekly for 8 weeks followed by the same once a month.

Hereditary Anemias

Hemoglobinopathies

Hemoglobinopathies are common in certain parts of the world like Mediterranean countries, the Middle East, Africa and Southeast Asia including regions of India. The most common hereditary anemias encountered in pregnancy are thalassemia and sickle cell anemia.

Normal structure of Hb: There are four globin chains associated with the heme complex. Each globin chain is controlled by a separate gene. There are three types of hemoglobins which are normally seen in adults. They are Hb A (α_2 β_2), Hb A2 (α_2 β_2)and Hb F(α_2 β_2). Each contains two pairs of globin chains. About 95% of circulating hemoglobin in adults is HbA.

Prenatal diagnostic tests play a role in these hereditary anemias as termination of pregnancy is mandatory in conditions like Barts disease and thalassemia major.

Thalassemias

These are the most common hemoglobinopathies which occur due to a quantitative abnormality in globin synthesis. The two main forms are α and β thalassemias due to impaired production of α and β peptide chains. The α chain is important for the genetic make-up of normal circulating adult hemoglobin. Absence of synthesis of one or more α chains results in various types of α thalassemia. When two or three normal α genes are present, the condition is α thalassemia trait (α thalassemia minor). They are usually asymptomatic or can have mild anemia. Women with α thalassemia minor usually tolerate pregnancy well.

When only one α gene is present, the condition is known as Hb H. They usually present with moderate degree of anemia. They may also require transfusion. In Hb H disease, the fetus is usually normal **in utero** but develops hemolytic anemia soon after birth. If these children grow up and become pregnant, the condition usually gets worsened during pregnancy.

When there is no functional α gene (**Barts disease**), the fetus usually dies in utero or soon after birth and has features of hydrops.

No abnormal hemoglobin will be detected in blood in α thalassemia and can be diagnosed by the detection of Hb H on electrophoresis or by the detection of 'Hb H inclusions' in supravital stained smears. Usually the condition is diagnosed by DNA analysis using molecular techniques in cases of deletions.

Supplementation of oral iron and folic acid is required throughout pregnancy. Parenteral iron is contraindicated and blood transfusion has to be given whenever necessary.

β thalassemias: There are two forms of β thalassemias: major and minor. Beta thalassemia major is a homozygous state where defective chain is inherited from each parent. The condition is usually fatal within a few years without regular transfusions.

Survival is sometimes possible without regular transfusions but this usually results in severe bone deformities due to massive expansion of marrow tissue. As the anemia is due to increased destruction (hemolytic), it is mandatory to maintain Hb at or above 12 g%.

The heterozygous form is usually asymptomatic, presents after two years of age with features of mild anemia.

Due to advances in medicine, pregnancy is not uncommon in patients with thalassemia minor. But pregnancy is rare with thalassemia major except in those with less iron overload. Increased levels of Hb A_2 of >3.5% is characteristic of β thalassemia minor. Full blood count and Hb indices help in diagnosing β thalassemia along with Hb electrophoresis.

Anemia has to be tackled with iron and folic acid supplementation along with blood transfusion whenever necessary. Parenteral iron is contraindicated. Iron overload can be treated with phlebotomies or with desferioxamine. But complete cure for β thalassemia is only with bone marrow transplantation or stem cell therapy.

If the mother is a carrier of β thalassemia and the father has normal Hb, 50% of offspring will be unaffected and 50% will have β thalassemia minor. If the mother is a carrier and the father is β thalassemia minor, 50% will have β thalassemia minor, 25% will have β thalassemia major and 25% will be normal. Prenatal diagnostic tests help to diagnose such conditions in utero. The couple should be counselled accordingly.

Sickle cell hemoglobinopathies

This qualitative abnormality in globin synthesis is due to the replacement of glutamic acid by valine in the 6th position of the β chain of Hb which results in the production of Hb S. It is more common in African-Americans. This can present either in the homozygous or the heterozygous state. There are various forms of sickle cell hemoglobinopathies like HbSS, HbSA and Hb sickle cell thalassemia. The sickle cell disease and sickle cell β thalassemia are associated with increased maternal and perinatal morbidity and mortality.

Under certain situations like hypoxia, acidosis and dehydration, the abnormal hemoglobin undergoes aggregation, and polymerisation and produces sickling of RBCs. Repeated episodes of such events reduce the lifespan of RBCs resulting in hemolytic anemia. The easily deformable biconcave disc of a normal RBC is transformed into an elongated crescent-shaped non-deformable RBC which is responsible for various presentations of the disease.

The episodes of sickling produce various symptoms known as 'sickling crises', like hemolytic crisis, painful crisis and vasoocclusive crisis. Hemolytic crisis results in anemia, jaundice, fever and leucocytosis. Painful crisis results from the occlusion of small blood vessels by abnormal RBCs. It results in tissue ischemia which produces necrosis and hemolysis. The patient can present with acute joint pain, vomiting, chest pain (acute chest syndrome), hemoptysis and hematuria (due to renal papillary necrosis). Such episodes can cause infarction of various organs like the spleen (auto splenectomy), lungs, and kidneys.

They can present with high output failure due to anemia or shock (either due to infection or infarction). They are prone to various infections because of tissue ischemia.

During pregnancy, they are at risk of developing preeclampsia, asymptomatic bacteriuria and retinopathy, apart from anemia and CCF. The episodes of sequestration are common in late pregnancy, during labour and delivery and early in the puerperal period.

Fetal complications are abortions, IUGR, preterm labour, IUD and stillbirth. These are the consequences of placental infarcts.

Investigations

Hematocrit <25%, increased reticulocyte count (10%–25%), presence of sickle and target cells and increased Hb S on Hb electrophoresis are diagnostic features of sickle cell disease.

Definitive treatment is bone marrow transplantation.

Certain drugs like hydroxyurea are used to increase the level of HbF, because cells containing HbF reverse the process of sickling if the precipitating factor is removed.

Antenatal management

This includes parental counselling, prenatal diagnosis, iron and folic acid supplementation, prophylactic transfusions, pneumococcal vaccine, if necessary, control of infections and screening for bacteriuria.

Labour and delivery

Hypoxia, acidosis, dehydration and stress have to be avoided. Cesarean section should be reserved for obstetric indications.

Contraception: Progestin-only pills, implants and progestin injections are preferred. Combined oral pills are contraindicated. IUCDs are not recommended because of increased risk of infections.

KEY POINTS

- Anemia is the most common medical problem in pregnancy.
- Hemoglobin level below 11 g% in pregnancy is defined as anemia.
- Anemia due to nutritional deficiency is the most common type.
- Tropical infections like malaria and hookworm infestation may cause anemia.
- Anemia has significant adverse effects on pregnancy and contributes to maternal and fetal mortality directly and indirectly.
- Routine iron and folic acid prophylaxis, as recommended in the RCH programme, will prevent anemia in pregnancy.
- Social interventions like alleviation of poverty, health education and adolescent nutrition supplementation will help reduce the prevalence of anemia.
- Measures to space and limit pregnancies will contribute to improve women's health.
- Oral iron therapy is the first line of management.
- Parenteral iron can be given when compliance and tolerance to oral iron are poor.
- Blood transfusion may be required in severe anemia for a quick response.
- Non–iron deficiency anemias are rarely seen in pregnancy. They are due to deficiency of folic acid and vitamin B_{12}, and hemoglobinopathies and Hb electrophoresis clinches the diagnosis.
- Parenteral iron is contraindicated in hemolytic anemias. The mainstay of management is blood transfusion in thalassemia and avoidance of infections and dehydration in sickle cell disease.
- The use of IUCDs and COCs is contraindicated in women with hemolytic anemias.

QUESTIONS

Select the single most appropriate answer:

1. All of the following statements are true regarding anemia *except*
   a. the most common cause of anemia in pregnancy is hemolytic anemia
   b. anemia is the most common medical disorder in pregnancy
   c. it contributes indirectly to maternal mortality
   d. in India, its prevalence is 40%–90%
2. For diagnosing anemia, according to the WHO, the accepted value is hemoglobin less than
   a. 14 g% b. 12 g % c. 11 g% d. 10 g%
3. The most common cause of anemia in pregnancy is
   a. blood loss due to hemorrhoids
   b. nutritional deficiency
   c. hemolytic anemia
   d. urinary tract infection
4. Which of the following predisposes to anemia in pregnancy?
   a. high parity
   b. diet rich in green vegetables
   c. pregnancy after the age of 35 years
   d. high-protein diet
5. All of the following infections/infestations may cause anemia in pregnancy *except*
   a. malaria
   b. intestinal amebiasis
   c. tapeworm infestation
   d. ankylostomiasis
6. Which of the following events of pregnancy has a positive effect on iron balance?

a. food fads of pregnancy c. lactation
b. high calorie diet d. amenorrhea

7. Of the following, the factor that poses a maximum load on iron requirement during pregnancy is
a. fetus and placenta
b. expansion maternal blood volume
c. daily blood loss
d. blood loss at delivery

8. The most likely cause of edema in cases of anemia complicating pregnancy is
a. cardiac failure c. hypoproteinemia
b. preeclampsia d. renal disease

9. The simplest test to determine the type of anemia is
a. hemoglobin estimation c. serum iron level
b. packed cell volume d. peripheral blood smear

10. Bone marrow examination is indicated in anemia complicating pregnancy in all of the following conditions *except*
a. suspected hemolytic anemia
b. abnormal cells in peripheral smear
c. pancytopenia
d. resistance to treatment

11. The factor that is *not* a likely effect of anemia in pregnancy is
a. preterm labour c. intrauterine death
b. infection d. subinvolution

12. In developing countries, anemia in pregnancy can be best prevented by
a. diet rich in carbohydrates
b. mass deworming
c. late marriage
d. routine iron supplementation

13. Parenteral iron is better than oral iron because
a. it has fewer side effects
b. it is cheap
c. it increases hemoglobin faster than oral iron
d. it avoids the problem of compliance and absorption

14. Currently, the most commonly used preparation of parenteral iron is
a. iron dextran c. ferrous ascorbate
b. iron sucrose d. iron sorbitol

15. The most common type of anemia seen in pregnancy is
a. dimorphic anemia c. macrocytic anemia
b. microcytic anemia d. hemolytic anemia

16. Of the following, the micronutrient that should be administered parenterally is
a. iron b. vitamin C c. vitamin B_{12} d. folic acid

17. The most common hemoglobinopathy seen in pregnancy is
a. sickle cell anemia c. congenital spherocytosis
b. Bart's disease d. thalassemia

18. Which of the following interferes with erythropoietin and causes resistant anemia?
a. respiratory infection
b. chronic urinary infection
c. aplastic anemia
d. malabsorption syndrome

19. Which of the following situations is best treated with partial exchange blood transfusion?
a. intolerance to oral iron
b. moderate anemia at term
c. non-compliant patient
d. very severe anemia in pregnancy

47

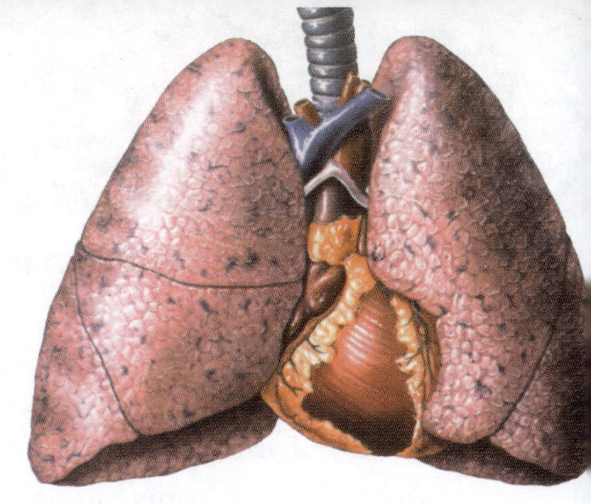

Cardiac Disease

Shyama Kanungo

LEARNING OBJECTIVES

At the end of this chapter, the reader should be able to:

- explain why hemodynamic changes in pregnancy can mimic heart disease
- identify definitive features of cardiac disease
- explain how pregnancy can have an adverse effect on heart disease and vice versa
- classify the cardiac diseases
- outline the management of rheumatic heart disease in pregnancy, labour and puerperium
- select and refer cases where expert intervention is required
- enumerate the indications for medical termination of pregnancy
- help to select appropriate contraceptives

Introduction

The normal heart takes on an extra load in pregnancy. Most heart diseases are progressive in nature and each pregnancy places an additional burden on the heart, thus reducing the life expectancy of the woman. The obstetrician caring for the pregnant woman with a cardiac disease must do so in consultation with a cardiologist to minimise the effects of this strain and prevent serious complications that might be precipitated during pregnancy, labour and puerperium. Previously, rheumatic heart disease was the only heart disease seen in pregnancy. Of late, with advances in diagnostic and surgical techniques, more women with congenital heart disease reach the reproductive age and therefore one encounters pregnancies complicated by these conditions, as well as women who have undergone cardiac surgery.

Physiological changes

Considerable changes occur in the cardiovascular system during pregnancy. There is an increase in bood volume, heart rate, pulse pressure and cardiac output; and a reduction in peripheral resistance and blood pressure. An increase in blood volume and cardiac output result in an increase in the workload of the heart, because of an increase in heart rate and in stroke volume. This additional burden on the heart starts by the eighth week, reaches a peak between weeks 28 and 32, and is then maintained till term (see Chapter 8).

Incidence

The incidence of heart disease complicating pregnancy varies worldwide. It is estimated to be 0.1% to 0.5%. In developed countries, effective control of streptococcal infection and rheumatic fever among children has led to a decline in the incidence of heart disease. However, in India, more than 80% of cardiac diseases among pregnant women are of rheumatic origin, and mostly affect the mitral valves. Other types of cardiac diseases are congenital or due to hypertension.

Difficulties in the diagnosis of heart disease in pregnancy

Some of the symptoms and signs that occur during pregnancy are normal but similar to those present in women with cardiac disease.

Symptoms: The symptoms are breathlessness, easy fatiguability, palpitations, dizziness and swelling of the feet. They may be exaggerated in the presence of anemia, PIH or conditions associated with overdistension of the uterus, like polyhydramnios and multiple pregnancy.

Signs: The signs that mimic those of cardiac disease are edema, tachycardia, hyperdynamic pulse, prominent jugular pulsations, lateral displacement of the apex beat, soft systolic murmur and continuous murmur due to mammary souffle.

Clinical indicators: It is important to look for definitive symptoms and signs of heart disease during pregnancy so that one can confirm the disease earlier in pregnancy and institute appropriate management. These **definitive clinical features** are:

- progressive severe dyspnea
- dyspnea at rest/orthopnea
- paroxysmal nocturnal dyspnea
- angina or syncope with exertion
- hemoptysis.

On clinical examination, some of the signs suggestive of cardiac disease are:

- cyanosis
- persistent jugular venous distension
- loud systolic murmur grade 3/6 or greater, or click with thrill
- diastolic murmur
- cardiomegaly
- parasternal heave
- arrhythmias.

Effect of pregnancy on cardiac disease

The most common cardiac disease is mitral valve disease of rheumatic origin. The normal area of the mitral valve is 4 cm^2. Symptoms develop when the stenosis reduces the area to less than 2.5 cm^2. The cardiovascular changes during pregnancy increase the resting pressure gradient across the mitral valve, leading to ventricular failure and pulmonary edema. Such adverse effects are generally seen between 28 and 32 weeks of gestation and just after delivery.

Effect of cardiac disease on pregnancy

No definite adverse fetal outcome has been noted except in severe disease, where the fetus may be small for date or preterm labour may occur. In cyanotic heart disease, an increased incidence of spontaneous abortion, prematurity and intrauterine growth restriction have been noted. If the maternal cardiac lesion is congenital, the fetus has a 5%–10% chance of a congenital cardiac malformation. Of these, 50% will have the same anomaly as the mother.

Classification according to functional capacity

This classification is useful for the management of heart disease during pregnancy. Irrespective of the anatomical lesion, it is the functional capability of the heart that is most important to determine how the patient will fare. The following is the classification of the New York Heart Association (NYHA):

Class I : Patient has no limitation of physical activity. Ordinary physical activity does not cause undue fatigue, palpitation, dyspnea or anginal pain.

Class II : Patient has slight limitation of physical activity. Ordinary physical activity results in fatigue, palpitation, dyspnea or anginal pain.

Class III : Patient has marked limitation of physical activity. Less than ordinary activity causes fatigue, palpitation, dyspnea or anginal pain.

Class IV : Patient has symptoms of cardiac insufficiency even at rest. She is unable to carry on any physical activity without discomfort.

The majority (80%) of cardiac patients belong to classes I and II. They are likely to deteriorate to classes III and IV due to the additional burden of pregnancy. However, this can be prevented by adequate rest and care during pregnancy, labour and puerperium.

Diagnosis and evaluation

Every pregnant woman must have her heart examined at the first visit, and if there are any suspicious signs, further investigations should be performed, preferably by a cardiologist. Diagnostic modalities must be used with caution during pregnancy. Electrocardiogram, echocardiography and magnetic resonance imaging (MRI) can be safely performed during pregnancy. X-ray examination and cardiac catheterisation are best avoided, especially in early pregnancy, due to the risk of radiation. The echocardiogam is the most useful investigation.

Low-risk cardiac conditions are mitral stenosis classes I and class II, atrial septal defect, ventricular septal defect and patent ductus arteriosus and have a mortality risk of less than 1%. Nonetheless, they require careful monitoring right from the onset of pregnancy up to early puerperium.

High-risk conditions are NYHA classes III and IV, cyanotic disease and pulmonary hypertension.

Prepregnancy counselling

Women with cardiac disease should have a planned pregnancy with proper counselling by a cardiologist. The disease status should be assessed preferably by echocardiography. The functional status should be defined. Should the functional state be of class III or IV and mortality risk >5%, pregnancy should preferably be avoided, at least till definitive treatment to improve the cardiac status is provided. The components of prepregnancy care are:

- a thorough evaluation of the lesion
- optimisation of medical management with avoidance of teratogenic drugs as far as possible
- correction of anemia
- treatment of arrhythmia
- control of hypertension
- corrective cardiac surgery where relevant, to minimise the mortality risk.

Treatment

Antenatal period: Women with cardiac disease require more frequent antenatal visits. Team management will go a long way in improving the outcome.

Two hours of **rest** in the afternoon and 10 hours at night should be ensured.

Weight gain is monitored closely to prevent excessive weight gain. Efforts should be made to detect and manage preeclampsia, as it may precipitate cardiac failure.

Rheumatic prophylaxis with oral penicillin or monthly benzathine penicillin injection is given as in the nonpregnant state.

Vital signs should be closely monitored for cardiac failure: dyspnea at rest, tachycardia, tachypnea, basal crepitations, tender enlarged liver, pedal and dependent edema and sudden weight gain.

Specific preventive measures: In addition to the general ones mentioned above:

- dietary salt restricted to not more than 4–6 g/day
- prophylactic diuretics like frusemide with potassium supplementation
- digoxin which improves myocardial contractility and controls the ventricular rate; the dosage is 0.25 mg daily orally for 5 or 6 days a week

Anticoagulant therapy is advocated in women with valve replacements. Heparin is ideal since it can be withdrawn just 24 hours prior to anticipated onset of labour without having a deleterious effect. Oral anticoagulants, if taken, should be stopped sufficiently ahead of labour and should be substituted with heparin.

Antibiotic prophylaxis for bacterial endocarditis must be given in all risk situations like dental extraction and at the beginning of labour.

Fetal growth is monitored clinically and ultrasonography is used when indicated.

Counselling for contraception is vital for long-term survival as the cardiac disease worsens with each pregnancy.

Admission: The pregnant woman should be advised to deliver in a hospital where facilities are available for the management of cardiac emergencies. Generally, women need to be admitted by 28–32 weeks when the load on the diseased heart reaches its peak.

Management of cardiac failure during pregnancy

- propped up position
- nasal oxygen administration
- intramuscular morphine 7.5 mg
- intravenous frusemide in doses of 40 mg
- intravenous aminophylline, if necessary
- digitalisation

The measures listed above are the mainstay of anti-failure treatment. Primary care prior to immediate referral in such a situation would go a long way in reducing maternal mortality.

Surgical management of valvular heart disease during pregnancy

In women with severe isolated mitral stenosis, sometimes there may be repeated episodes of cardiac failure (pulmonary edema) or cardiac failure may not respond to the usual medical treatment. Such women will benefit from mitral valvotomy performed during pregnancy. The best time to do the valvotomy is in the second trimester; however, it may be done at other times if the situation warrants.

Interventional radiological procedures using cardiac catheter laboratory have reduced the need for open procedures. Balloon mitral valvotomy (BMV) is a very useful procedure in patients with refractory failure.

Other types of cardiac surgery like valve replacement cannot be performed during pregnancy because of the need to use the heart–lung machine and anticoagulation.

Management of labour

The a majority of women with heart disease have an easy vaginal delivery. Adequate **analgesia should be provided to relieve pain and apprehension with a view to prevent tachycardia**. The number of vaginal examinations is kept to a minimum.

Endocarditis prophylaxis should be given IV using ampicillin 2 g and gentamicin 1.5 mg/kg body weight. The mother is propped up throughout the first stage of labour; the supine position should be avoided. Pulse and respiration are monitored very carefully to detect failure at the earliest.

The second stage of labour is cut short using outlet forceps, unless the delivery of the baby is imminent. Pulse and respiratory rates are monitored very carefully as the risk of pulmonary edema is high at this point as there is 'auto-transfusion' of 500–700 ml of blood.

The use of prophylactic methylergometrine is contraindicated. Oxytocin is the drug of choice for the control and prevention of postpartum hemorrhage. The recommended dosage is 10 units given intraumbilically.

In women with heart disease, vaginal delivery is preferred as it is associated with less morbidity. **Cesarean section is performed only for obstetrical indications.**

Care during puerperium

Close monitoring must continue through this period as the woman is prone to cardiac failure for the reasons stated below:

- Burden on the heart in immediate puerperium is increased due to sudden shutting down of uteroplacental circulation, mobilisation of the extracellular fluid and removal of the obstruction of the inferior vena cava caused by the pregnant uterus.
- Puerperal infection predisposes to bacterial endocarditis, especially in valvular lesions.
- Chances of thrombophlebitis and thromboembolic phenomena are increased during early puerperium.
- Peripartum cardiomyopathy occurs mostly during puerperium.
- Associated anemia, preeclampsia, infection and stress can precipitate pulmonary edema.
- Though the normal blood loss during delivery may be beneficial to the woman with heart disease, postpartum hemorrhage is particularly dangerous as the response to sudden hypovolemia and hypoxia is poor in decompensated cardiac disease.

The pulse, blood pressure, temperature and respiration are closely monitored for at least 24 hours.

The patient should be in the hospital for 1–2 weeks, depending on the need. Breastfeeding may be allowed up to class III but not in class IV. Anticoagulants are used when thrombophlebitis or thromboembolic phenomenon is anticipated.

Termination of pregnancy

With advances in the management of cardiac disease, there are very few indications for the termination of pregnancy:

- cases belonging to class III and sometimes class IV after correction of failure
- absolute indications like Eisenmenger syndrome and primary pulmonary hypertension.

If medical termination is necessary, it should be performed before eight weeks of gestation when the risk of anesthesia and surgery are minimal. The procedure must be carried out at a centre well-equipped to deal with cardiac emergencies. Medical abortion may be recommended except in cyanotic disease and primary pulmonary hypertension.

Termination of pregnancy during the second trimester in a woman with heart disease should not be contemplated as it is too risky.

Contraception

Tubectomy is ideally deferred to a time beyond the puerperal period. However, if a woman wants to undergo the procedure while in the hospital, it may be performed 10 days after delivery.

The insertion of an intrauterine device is best done after the first normal period; care must be taken to cut the tail of the device short. Prophylaxis for endocarditis must be administered before any of the above procedures.

In women who prefer oral contraceptive pills, **progestogen-only pills** may be prescribed after puerperium. Barrier methods are also suitable, provided they are correctly used.

KEY POINTS

- The symptoms and signs of normal pregnancy mimic some of those seen in heart disease.
- Cardiac lesions worsen with each pregnancy.
- Cardiac failure may occur at 28–32 weeks; the risk, however, continues throughout labour and early puerperium.
- Functional classification (NYHA) helps to evaluate the functional status and plan the management.
- Prepregnancy counselling for contraception or surgical correction can bring down mortality.
- Surgical correction of the cardiac lesion is best done before pregnancy. With advances in techniques, the correction is performed during pregnancy in selected patients.
- Intelligent antenatal care in consultation with a cardiologist is the essence of management of heart disease complicating pregnancy.
- Most women with heart disease deliver vaginally. They must be monitored carefully to avoid failure and infective endocarditis.
- Women with a cardiac lesion are prone to suffer cardiac failure during puerperium and must therefore be monitored very closely.
- Reliable and relatively safe contraceptive methods are: tubectomy late in puerperium, IUD insertion after a normal period and progestogen-only pills.
- Termination of pregnancy is rarely indicated. However, if required, it must be performed in the first eight weeks of pregnancy in centres equipped to manage cardiac emergencies.

QUESTIONS

Select the single most appropriate answer:

1. The incidence of cardiac disease in pregnancy is
   a. 0.1% to 0.5%
   b. 1.0% to 1.5%
   c. 2.0% to 2.5%
   d. 3.0% to 3.5%

2 Which of the following is *not* a definitive symptom of cardiac disease?
   a. progressive severe dyspnea
   b. easy fatiguability
   c. paroxysmal nocturnal dyspnea
   d. hemoptysis

3. Which of the following is characteristic of cardiac disease in pregnancy?
   a. lateral displacement of the apex beat
   b. prominent jugular pulsations
   c. diastolic murmur
   d. third heart sound and split S1 and S2

4. A pregnant woman with cardiac disease is most likely to go into failure between
   a. 8 and 12 weeks
   b. 14 and 18 weeks
   c. 20 and 26 weeks
   d. 28 and 32 weeks

5. Which is the functional class of heart disease in a pregnant woman if ordinary physical activity causes fatigue?
   a. class I
   b. class II
   c. class III
   d. class IV

6. If a pregnant woman has a congenital heart disease, the chances of the fetus having a congenital cardiac disease is
   a. 1% to 2%
   b. 3% to 4%
   c. 5% to 10%
   d. 11% to 15%

Select the appropriate answer using the following key:

a. if only responses 1, 2 and 3 are correct
b. if only 1 and 3 are correct
c. if only 2 and 4 are correct
d. if only 4 is correct
e. if all are correct

7. During antenatal care, in order to prevent a pregnant woman with mitral stenosis going into failure, particular attention must be paid to control
   1. anemia
   2. diabetes mellitus
   3. pregnancy-induced hypertension
   4. postmaturity

8. In a pregnant woman with mitral stenosis, endocarditis prophylaxis must be instituted
   1. before performing a vaginal examination
   2. at the onset of labour
   3. if the urinary bladder is to be catheterised
   4. at the time of dental extraction

In the following questions, there are two statements. Select the appropriate answer using the following key:

a. if both statements are true and causally related
b. if both statements are true but not causally related
c. if the first statement is true and the second is false
d. if the first statement is false and the second is true
e. if both statements are false

9. In a woman with heart disease, puerperal sterilisation should be performed 10 days after delivery *because*

   After 10 days, the blood volume returns to prepregnant levels and the risk of failure is reduced significantly.

10. A cesarean section should be performed for a pregnant woman with mitral stenosis *because*

    A vaginal delivery may precipitate cardiac failure.

48

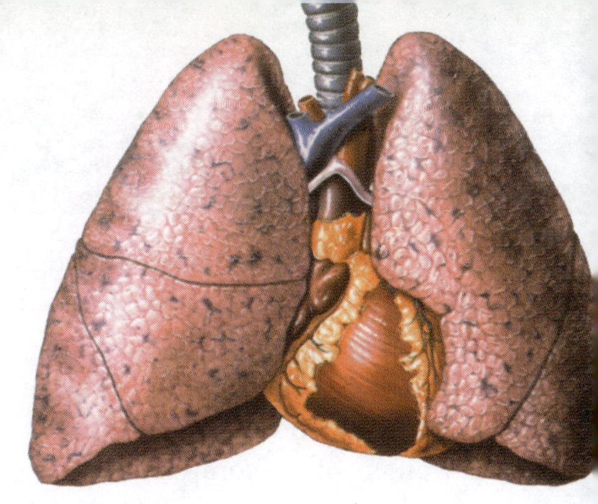

Respiratory Disorders

SN Tripathy

LEARNING OBJECTIVES

At the end of this chapter, the reader should be able to:

- explain the changes in the respiratory system during pregnancy
- list the clinical features of bronchial asthma and pulmonary tuberculosis
- select relevant investigations
- describe the effect of pregnancy on asthma and the effects of asthma on the mother and the fetus
- select appropriate drugs for treatment
- appreciate the risk of transmission of tuberculosis to the child
- list the investigations that can be performed during pregnancy
- outline the management of tuberculosis
- list the effects of antitubercular drugs on the mother and the child
- appreciate the need to refer to a respiratory physician appropriately

Introduction

Pregnancy is associated with both mechanical and biochemical changes that may affect maternal respiratory function and gas exchange. Asthma is becoming more common in the general population, and tuberculosis has remained as before; hence, both the diseases will be seen more frequently in pregnancy. The incidence of pneumonia has declined, but if it occurs during pregnancy, it could prove fatal.

Obstetricians will need to manage more cases of pregnancy complicated by respiratory disorders. Appropriate management is possible with good collaboration between the obstetrician and a respiratory physician.

Changes in the respiratory system

The following changes occur in the respiratory system during pregnancy:

- There is an additional demand for oxygen, an increase of 30%–50% blood volume and cardiac output.
- The enlarging uterus raises the resting position of the diaphragm by 4 cm, reducing the diaphragmatic contribution to breathing; it also changes the configuration of the thorax.
- The raised levels of progesterone make the respiratory system more sensitive to carbon dioxide.
- There is an increase in vital capacity, inspiratory capacity and tidal volume. Expiratory reserve volume and functional residual capacity decrease. The minute ventilatory volume and minute oxygen consumption increase with advancing pregnancy.

Clinical features

The most common symptoms associated with respiratory disorders are dyspnea/breathlessness and cough. The nature of cough and fever will vary depending on the pathology and physical findings.

Dyspnea is defined as an abnormally uncomfortable awareness of breathing whereas normal breathing is an unconscious and automatic act. Pregnant women often complain of dyspnea; 50% do so by midpregnancy and 75% by the beginning of the third trimester. However, the dyspnea of normal pregnancy is relatively mild, does not interfere with routine activities and is uncommon when the woman is at rest. When it is due to a respiratory disorder, the dyspnea is noticed early in pregnancy and interferes with routine activity.

Cough is a common symptom, and is associated with expectoration, depending on the secretions from the respiratory tract. Hemoptysis may be present in pulmonary tuberculosis.

Low-grade fever, especially in the evening, is characteristic of tuberculosis. Bronchial asthma is not normally associated with fever unless there is infection. Fever is more prominent in severe infections like pneumonia.

ASTHMA

Asthma is a common respiratory disease during pregnancy. It is characterised by chronic airway inflammation with increased airway responsiveness to a variety of stimuli, and airway obstruction that is partially or completely reversible with or without treatment. There is limitation of airflow that is more marked during expiration than during inspiration. Asthma is classified as extrinsic or allergic asthma, or intrinsic. Many women develop symptoms in response to infection, pollution, exercise, cold air and emotional stress.

Effects of pregnancy on asthma

The clinical course of the disease remains unchanged in approximately 50%, improves in 30% and worsens in 20%.

Effects of asthma on pregnancy

The overall perinatal outcome is as good as in non-asthmatic women when the disease is managed well during pregnancy. Adverse maternal and fetal outcome (including death) are noted if the woman suffers from prolonged and severe attacks of asthma that are poorly managed.

Pathophysiology

The changes noted in asthma are bronchial inflammation, mucous gland hypertrophy and excessive secretion of mucus, mucosal edema and bronchial smooth muscle contraction.

Clinical features

Asthma may present as an illness, ranging from a mild wheeze to severe bronchoconstriction leading to respiratory failure, severe hypoxia and death. The common physical findings include diffuse rhonchi and, hyperventilation; the presence of pulsus paradoxus and the use of accessory muscles of respiration indicate severe bronchoconstriction.

Differential diagnosis

Conditions like chronic bronchitis, emphysema and, pulmonary eosinophilia mimic asthma. Enquire for a history of asthmatic attacks in the past or in the family.

Investigations

Pulmonary function tests (PFTs) will confirm the diagnosis of asthma and are useful in assessing the respiratory capacity of the woman. The forced expiratory volume, forced vital capacity and pO_2 are decreased during an asthmatic attack. The tests will give an indication of how much the woman will be able to strain in the second stage of labour and her possible risk for general anesthesia.

Management

This is the same as in the nonpregnant state. Medications are administered with the objective of achieving a status that is symptom-free, and optimal pulmonary function. In order to achieve normal fetal umbilical vein pO_2, efforts must be made to maintain maternal pO_2 above 70 mm Hg.

Beta adrenoreceptor agonists produce the greatest bronchodilatation and are the mainstay of the management of asthma. In acute attacks, aerosol preparations such as salbutamol may be used through a nebuliser or terbutaline subcutaneously in doses of 125–250 μg. In severe attacks, corticosteroids like beclomethasone dipropionate (as aerosol), intravenous hydrocortisone and oral prednisolone may be given. Theophylline is given orally as maintenance. The management of an acute attack during pregnancy is similar to that in the nonpregnant asthmatic.

About 10% of asthmatic women may have an attack during labour. It is, therefore, wise to continue medication during labour. Prostaglandin $F_{2\alpha}$ may precipitate bronchospasm and must be avoided. To control postpartum hemorrhage, oxytocin is given.

Only a small quantity of antiasthmatic drugs are secreted in breast milk; the mother may be advised to breastfeed her child.

Tuberculosis

Tuberculosis kills one million women worldwide, many of them in the childbearing age group. The prevalence of tuberculosis during pregnancy is 2%–5%. There is a morbid link between HIV and tuberculosis and the prognosis in such cases is ominous.

Effect of pregnancy on tuberculosis

If the pregnant woman takes regular antitubercular treatment, pregnancy as such does not make the disease worse. The relapse rate is not increased even if the woman becomes pregnant several times.

Effect of tuberculosis on pregnancy

If treated early, there is no adverse effect on the pregnancy. Also, there is no increased risk of congenital anomalies attributable to antitubercular drugs. Occasionally, the fetus may show the primary focus of disease in the lungs or the gut; the lesions are said to be congenital if diagnosed in the first week of life or there is evidence of placental infection.

Clinical features

Cough with expectoration, hemoptysis, weight loss, fever and fatigue are present as in the nonpregnant state. Lymphadenitis is the most common form of extrapulmonary tuberculosis. Physical findings vary with the type of lesion in the lungs and the presence of an extrapulmonary lesion.

Investigations

A skin test with purified protein derivative (PPD) is recommended for women who are infected with HIV, are suffering from diabetes mellitus and those from a low socioeconomic group. In this group of women, the skin test is considered positive if the skin induration measures 5 mm or more. If positive, a radiograph of the chest is done after shielding the abdomen; if the radiograph is suspicious/confirmatory of tuberculosis, three samples of sputum are analysed for the presence of acid-fast bacilli. Gastric aspiration and bronchoscopy are indicated if the results of the first two tests are inconclusive.

Management

This must be in collaboration with a specialist in chest diseases. Short-course chemotherapy is the treatment of choice and the following are accepted protocols: Isoniazid 300 mg, rifampicin 450 mg, ethambutol 800 mg and pyrazinamide 1,200 mg once a day for two months. Then isoniazid 300 mg and rifampicin 450 mg are given three times a week for four months: 2HREZ/4HR3.

The above protocol, popularly known as 2HERZ + 4HR3, is the preferred protocol. None of these drugs have been shown to have teratogenic effects. The mother should be instructed to breastfeed the child before taking the antitubercular drugs to minimise their adverse effect on the newborn.

Streptomycin is ototoxic and is hence contraindicated in pregnancy. Though pyrazinamide is used as the first-line drug in the nonpregnant state, its safety in pregnancy is not established.

HIV and tuberculosis: All pregnant women with tuberculosis must be screened for HIV. Those who test positive for HIV must be put on antiretroviral therapy. Early detection and treatment can reduce the morbidity and mortality due to coexistence of HIV and tuberculosis.

Pneumonia

Pneumonia is not uncommon during pregnancy. It is an acute illness; there is inflammation of the lung parenchyma beyond the larger airways involving the bronchioles and the alveolar units. It causes appreciable loss of ventilatory capacity which is not so well tolerated by the pregnant woman, irrespective of the cause of pneumonia.

Effect on pregnancy

The tolerance to hypoxia and acidosis is poor and the risk of abortion, preterm delivery and intrauterine death is increased. Maternal outcome has improved greatly with the use of potent antibiotics.

The organisms responsible for pneumonia are *Streptococcus pneumoniae, Hemophilus influenza* and influenza viruses A and B of the *Orthomyxoviridae* family. Fungal and parasitic pneumonia is seen most among women suffering from AIDS.

Clinical features

The symptoms of pneumonia are cough with expectoration, hemoptysis, high fever, chest pain and dyspnea, often preceded by mild upper respiratory symptoms. Signs of consolidation of lung tissue are present on physical examination.

Investigations include the examination of Gram-stained sputum for pneumococci or staphylococci and culture. A radiograph of the chest may be helpful in diagnosis.

Management

A pregnant woman suffering from pneumonia must be admitted. Some pregnant women may go into respiratory failure and will require assisted ventilation. Antimicrobial therapy is empirical. Considering that pneumococci and other organisms could be the causative agents, erythromycin appears to be the antibiotic of choice. The intravenous administration of the penicillin group of drugs may be needed in acutely ill patients. However, the antimicrobials should be changed according to clinical response and the sensitivity of the organism to them. Fungal pneumonia is best treated with intravenous amphotericin B and viral pneumonia with amantidine or rimantidine.

KEY POINTS

- Dyspnea is defined as an awareness of breathing; more than 50% of pregnant women complain of dyspnea.
- Asthma is the most common respiratory disease complicating pregnancy. The severity of the disease is unchanged in 50%, improves in 30% and worsens in 20%.
- Asthma has no adverse effects on pregnancy.
- Beta adrenoreceptor agonists and corticosteroids are the drugs of choice.
- Prostaglandin $F_{2\alpha}$ is avoided as it may precpitate an asthmatic attack.
- Pulmonary tuberculosis complicates 2%–5% of pregnancies.
- A chest radiograph must be taken to confirm the diagnosis after shielding the abdomen.
- The antitubercular drugs currently recommended are not teratogenic.
- Breastfeeding should be avoided only if the mother's sputum is positive for acid-fast bacilli.
- Pneumonia may become severe during pregnancy; therefore, the pregnant woman must be hospitalised for proper management.

QUESTIONS

Select the single most appropriate answer:

1. During pregnancy, all the pulmonary function tests are increased *except*
   a. functional residual capacity
   b. vital capacity
   c. tidal volume
   d. inspiratory capacity
2. What should maternal pO_2 be to maintain normal fetal umbilical venous pO_2?
   a. 40–49 mm Hg
   b. 50–59 mm Hg
   c. 60–69 mm Hg
   d. above 70 mm Hg
3. What percentage of pregnant women experience dyspnea by the third trimester?
   a. 55% c. 85%
   b. 75% d. 100%
4. Which of the following statements is not true in asthma complicating pregnancy?
   a. the clinical course is unchanged in 50% of women
   b. the clinical course improves in 30% of women
   c. the course of asthma during successive pregnancies in an individual tends to be similar
   d. labour is associated with worsening of asthma
5. All of the following drugs can be used to treat asthma in pregnancy *except*
   a. beta agonists c. theophylline
   b. inhaled corticosteroids d. oral corticosteroids
6. In an HIV-positive patient, how much induration is considered as a positive tuberculin test?
   a. 5 mm c. 15 mm
   b. 10 mm d. 20 mm
7. The criteria for the diagnosis of congenital tuberculosis are
   a. lesions in the first week of life
   b. primary hepatic complex
   c. tuberculosis infection of the placenta
   d. all of the above
8. The antituberculous drug which *should not be* used during pregnancy is
   a. INH c. streptomycin
   b. rifampicin d. ethambutol

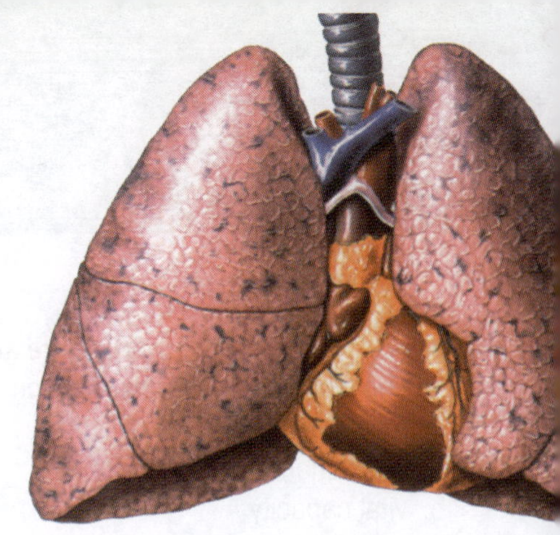

49

Diabetes Mellitus

Lakshmi Seshadri

LEARNING OBJECTIVES

At the end of this chapter, the reader should be able to:

- define and classify diabetes complicating pregnancy
- explain glucose metabolism in pregnancy
- screen for and diagnose diabetes in pregnancy
- advise on the diet for a diabetic patient
- identify and refer pregnant diabetics requiring insulin therapy
- monitor the mother and fetus with a view to obtaining optimal outcome
- plan the intrapartum management of a diabetic woman
- perform preconceptional counselling

Introduction

Diabetes mellitus is a condition of altered glucose metabolism. The prevalence of diabetes is increasing all over the world. Asians, particularly Indians, are at very high risk of diabetes. Its association with obesity, hypertension and metabolic syndrome is well known. It is one of the leading causes of mortality and morbidity. Due to the hormones of pregnancy, pregnant women are more prone to carbohydrate intolerance and diabetes. It occurs in 3%–10% of all pregnant women. This is associated with risks to the fetus and the mother. Perinatal mortality can be reduced drastically if the condition is diagnosed early and managed appropriately. About 50% of women with gestational diabetes develop overt diabetes later in life. Recurrence of gestational diabetes in subsequent pregnancies also occurs in 50% of women.

Definitions and classification

Diabetes in pregnancy can be:

Pregestational diabetes: This is diabetes that is known to exist before pregnancy. This may be of the following two types.

Type 1 or insulin-dependent diabetes mellitus (IDDM): Usually occurs at a younger age and does not respond to oral hypoglycemic agents. They are prone to ketoacidosis, congenital anomalies in the fetus and hypoglycemic episodes. Type 1 diabetes is not commonly encountered in pregnancy.

Type 2 or non-insulin-dependent diabetes mellitus (NIDDM): Occurs at an older age and can be managed by oral drugs. This is the more common type of pregestational diabetes.

Gestational diabetes mellitus (GDM): It is defined as glucose intolerance diagnosed for the first time in pregnancy, irrespective of the need for insulin. If the abnormality persists six weeks after delivery, it may be reclassified as type 2 diabetes. This is more common than pregestational diabetes. More so in India since most women go through pregnancies before the age of 30 years.

Carbohydrate metabolism in pregnancy

The changes in carbohydrate metabolism provide the fetus with a continuous and adequate supply of glucose. The hormones of pregnancy, namely, estrogen, progesterone, cortisol and human placental lactogen (hPL), are diabetogenic. Since their levels increase during the second and third trimesters, gestational diabetes usually manifests after 20 weeks. These hormones increase insulin resistance and shift the principal source of energy for the mother from carbohydrates to ketones and free fatty acids.

Pregnant women have lower plasma glucose levels between meals and during sleep because the fetus continues to draw glucose. The fasting glucose level is, therefore, lower than in the nonpregnant state. With increasing insulin resistance, there is postprandial hyperglycemia. Pancreatic insulin secretion increases and the mother is euglycemic despite these changes.

If the maternal pancreatic reserve is inadequate, the hyperglycemia persists and results in fetal hyperglycemia and hyperinsulinemia. This leads to accelerated growth of the fetus, macrosomia and fat deposition by conversion of excess glucose into fat.

Effect of pregnancy on diabetes

Diabetes worsens during pregnancy. Those who are on diet control will need insulin and those who are on insulin will require higher doses. Women on oral hypoglycemic agents may need to change to insulin to avoid teratogenic effects and to obtain better glycemic control. Women with pregestational diabetes are prone to problems which are different from those seen in women who develop diabetes in pregnancy. Diabetic retinopathy worsens in 50% of women but regression occurs after delivery. Varying degrees of deterioration occur in nephropathy. With increasing renal blood flow and glomerular filtration, proteinuria also increases.

Effect of diabetes on pregnancy

Effect on the mother

Infections: Urinary tract infection is common and asymptomatic bacteriuria should be checked for. Candidal vulvovaginitis is common. Puerperal endometritis and postoperative infection are more common in diabetics.

Diabetic ketoacidosis: This is seen in pregestational diabetics, especially in the first trimester when hyperemesis is present. It can also be precipitated by infection. Ketoacidosis does not occur in gestational diabetics.

Hypertension: Chronic hypertension may be present in pregestational diabetics and can worsen in pregnancy. Hypertension is common in gestational diabetics as well. Early-onset preeclampsia is also known to occur.

Preterm labour: It is more common in women with polyhydramnios and in pregestational diabetics with nephropathy.

Intrapartum problems: Due to the large babies, there are more intrapartum complications:

- prolonged labour
- operative vaginal delivery
- cesarean section
- shoulder dystocia

Effect on the fetus

Almost all the effects on the fetus are due to maternal hyperglycemia. When this is uncontrolled and persistent, fetal hyperglycemia occurs with resultant fetal hyperinsulinemia. The fetal and neonatal complications are direct or indirect effects of these changes.

Spontaneous abortion: This is increased in poorly controlled pregestational diabetics to as high as 50% and is directly related to glycosylated hemoglobin (HbA_1C) levels. The rate comes down to normal with normalisation of blood glucose levels.

Congenital malformations: The incidence is as high as 7%–10% in pregestational diabetics and is again directly related to periconceptional glycemic control. The anomalies mainly involve the central nervous system and cardiovascular system. Embryonic hyperglycemia promotes the release of oxygen-free radicals, which in turn are said to be the cause of malformations. When HbA_1C levels are reduced to less than 7%, the frequency of malformations equals that of the nondiabetic population.

Macrosomia: It is seen in pregestational and gestational diabetics and is an indirect measure of glycemic control. Macrosomia is defined as a birth weight of more than the 90th centile for gestational age or more than 4 kg. Maternal hyperglycemia with resultant fetal hyperglycemia, hyperinsulinemia and increase in growth factors leads to an increase in fat deposition and accelerated growth. Maternal obesity may also be a contributing factor. Incidence is reduced by glycemic control and is an important goal in the management of diabetic pregnancies.

Polyhydramnios: This is also seen in women with poor diabetic control. The increase in amniotic fluid is related to the amniotic fluid glucose levels. Hyperplacentosis and fetal polyuria are other proposed mechanisms.

Prematurity: This may be due to spontaneous preterm labour as seen in women with polyhydramnios or induced preterm labour in women with associated complications.

Late fetal death: This typically occurs in large-for-gestational-age fetuses at 35 weeks or later due to hyperglycemia-mediated chronic aberrations in the transport of oxygen and nutrients to the fetus. Placental insufficiency in pregestational diabetics with vasculopathy and nephropathy, hypertension and preeclampsia also contribute to late fetal deaths.

Intrauterine growth restriction: This is seen in women with diabetic vasculopathy and nephropathy. It occasionally occurs in gestational diabetics with preeclampsia.

Effect on the neonate

Hypoglycemia: The strongest predictor of neonatal hypoglycemia is maternal glucose levels during labour. The complication is usually much milder when maternal diabetes is well controlled during pregnancy and labour. Beta cell hyperplasia of fetal pancreas leads to hyperinsulinemia and this, in the absence of transported glucose from the mother, causes hypoglycemia.

Respiratory distress syndrome: Fetal hyperinsulinemia delays the production of surfactant by the fetal lungs. This was considered to be the cause of respiratory distress in infants of diabetic mothers. But prematurity and cesarean delivery are now said to be the main factors and the incidence of respiratory distress reduces with delay in delivery till 38 weeks.

Hyperbilirubinemia: It occurs in 25% of these infants. Prematurity and polycythemia are the major contributing factors.

Polycythemia: Hyperglycemia is a powerful stimulant of erythropoietin. This causes polycythemia, which can lead to vascular sludging, ischemia and infarction of vital tissues.

Hypocalcemia: The pathophysiology of this condition is not well understood but is attributed to functional hypoparathyroidism. The cut-off level of calcium is <7 mg/dl. Neonatal seizures can occur with hypocalcemia.

Birth injuries: Since babies tend to be larger, shoulder dystocia and resultant brachial plexus injury are often seen. Difficult vaginal delivery and operative vaginal delivery add to the incidence of birth injuries like facial nerve injury and cephalhematoma.

Perinatal mortality and morbidity: Perinatal mortality rates have declined from 50% to under 5% after the advent of insulin, better control of glycemia, fetal monitoring and appropriate timing of delivery. But it is twice as high as in nondiabetic pregnancies. Congenital anomalies are still a major cause of mortality. Prematurity, respiratory distress syndrome and birth asphyxia are other contributory factors.

Diagnosis

For a woman to be considered overt by diabetic, she sould show random plasma glucose of 200 mg/dl and symptoms of diabetes, fasting level of 126 mg/dl or a two-hour postprandial level of 200 mg/dl.

Screening for gestational diabetes: Despite several years of research, there is no consensus regarding screening for gestational diabetes. Since gestational diabetes occurs only in the second trimester, screening is generally recommended between 24 and 28 weeks of gestation. There is controversy regarding universal versus selective screening. Women are generally classified as 'low risk' or 'high risk' for the development of gestational diabetes according to various risk factors. Screening is recommended only for high-risk women according to the American Diabetic Association but the Americans College of Obstetricians and Gynecologists (ACOG) recommends screening for all pregnant women. When the index of suspicion is high, screening must be done at the first prenatal visit (first trimester) and repeated at 24 weeks if negative.

The risk factors for gestational diabetes are:

- age above 30 years
- obesity
- firstdegree relative with diabetes
- previous large baby, congenital anomaly, stillbirth, poor obstetric outcome
- gestational diabetes in previous pregnancy
- glycosuria on more than one occasion.

In addition, a glucose tolerance test must be performed in women whenever signs or symptoms suggestive of gestational diabetes develop in the present pregnancy like candidial vulvovaginitis, recurrent urinary infection, fetal macrosomia, polyhydramnios and early onset hypertension.

Glucose challenge test (GCT): This is used as a screening test in women with no risk factors (low-risk women). Plasma glucose estimation is performed one hour after 50 g oral glucose load without regard to the timing of last meal. The cut-off value of 140 mg/dl is used by most centres. Those with a positive result have to undergo a full three-hour GTT.

Glucose tolerance test (GTT): This is performed in low-risk women when GCT is abnormal and also as primary screening test in high-risk women.

It requires

- three days of normal diet (>150 g carbohydrates)
- overnight fasting
- 100 g oral glucose load
- plasma glucose measured at fasting state, 1 hour, 2 hours and 3 hours after glucose administration
- cut-off values according to the O' Sullivan and Mahan criteria are:

Fasting	95 mg/dl
1 hour	180 mg/dl
2 hour	155 mg/dl
3 hour	140 mg/dl

If two or more values are equal to or exceed the cut-off values, a diagnosis of gestational diabetes is made. If one value is equal to or more than the cut-off, it is categorised as impaired glucose tolerance.

MANAGEMENT

Management of diabetes

The diabetic pregnant woman is best managed by a team of specialists consisting of a dietician, physician, ophthalmologist, anesthesiologist, neonatologist and obstetrician.

The goal is to maintain fasting plasma sugar levels below 90 mg/dl and two-hour postprandial levels of less than 140 mg/dl. Euglycemia throughout pregnancy is essential to prevent all complications. Patient education is therefore essential. The following issues should be addressed:

- understanding the impact of diabetes on pregnancy
- importance of glycemic control
- emphasis on self-care
- emphasis on regular antenatal visits, adherence to diet and insulin
- home glucose monitoring
- self-administration of insulin when required and possible.

Diet: A total of six feeds a day is ideal, consisting of three meals and three snacks. A daily intake of 30–35 kcal/kg of ideal body weight is recommended. Of this, 50% should be carbohydrates and the other 50% should be proteins and fats in equal proportions. Fasting and postprandial plasma glucose should be measured 48–72 hours after the woman starts the diabetic diet.

Exercise: This forms another important part of the management of pregnant diabetics. An exercise regimen appropriate for pregnancy is recommended in consultation with a physiotherapist.

Insulin therapy: If the fasting and/or postprandial sugars are not under control, insulin therapy has to be instituted. About 15% of pregnant women with GDM will need insulin. Aggressive insulin therapy reduces the percentage of macrosomic infants. In general, insulin is required if the fasting plasma glucose is above 105 mg/dl and two-hour postprandial sugar is above 150 mg/dl. With increasing insulin resistance as pregnancy advances, the dose will have to be increased. Multiple doses of insulin are required; generally, twice- or thrice-daily regimens are followed. A mixture of short-acting and intermediate-acting insulin is used to ensure euglycemia throughout the day. Human insulin is advisable since antibody to bovine or porcine insulin will cause increasing resistance and interfere with therapy.

- If fasting plasma sugar is elevated, a combination of short- and intermediate-acting insulin should be administered before dinner.
- If post-breakfast and post-lunch values are high, a combination of short-acting and intermediate-acting insulin should be given before breakfast.
- Short-acting insulin given before breakfast will lower post-breakfast plasma glucose and intermediate-acting insulin will lower post-lunch values.
- A bedtime snack is a must to avoid midnight hypoglycemia.

Glucose monitoring: The best way to monitor glucose levels is to perform a 24-hour glucose profile which includes the estimation of glucose before and after breakfast, lunch and dinner and at 0200 hours. This should be done once in two weeks throughout pregnancy once the levels are stabilised. Home glucose monitoring with a glucometer is convenient and easy.

Preconceptional management

Pregestational diabetics must be seen and counselled prior to pregnancy. Meticulous glycemic control before conception and during early pregnancy is absolutely essential for preventing complications like miscarriage and congenital anomalies. HbA_1C levels must be below 7.5%. Women on oral hypoglycemic agents must be advised to change to insulin. The patient must be advised weight reduction, control of associated hypertension, evaluation of renal function and ophthalmic assessment for retinopathy. Folic acid 4 mg daily should be given to prevent neural tube defects.

Management of pregnancy

First trimester: In women with pregestational diabetes, the following are recommended:

- meticulous control of glycemic status
- advice on diet and insulin
- folic acid supplementation
- watch out for ketoacidosis
- ultrasound assessment for accurate gestational age.

Second trimester: During this trimester, frequent antenatal check-up is advised and investigations are required to assess fetal morphology and to detect maternal complications.

- Maternal serum alpha fetoprotein levels should be measured at 16 weeks in pregestational diabetics to rule out neural tube defects.
- Ultrasonogram at 18–20 weeks is mandatory for fetal morphology in pregestational and gestational diabetics.
- Antenatal check-up should be conducted every two weeks.
- Close watch on blood pressure, test for proteinuria and urinary or genital infections are recommended.
- Fetal echo is recommended at 24 weeks in pregestational diabetics to rule out cardiac anomalies.
- Monitoring of fetal growth should begin at 28 weeks.

Third trimester: Fetal surveillance is the focus during this period since macrosomia, intrauterine death and polyhydramnios occur in the third trimester.

- clinical examination to check blood pressure and fundal height
- urinalysis for proteinuria
- daily fetal movement count
- serial ultrasonogram for growth, macrosomia, fetal weight and, amniotic fluid volume
- nonstress test to assess fetal wellbeing
- fetal biophysical profile
- frequency of the serial evaluation individualised depending on the type of diabetes and the degree of control of plasma glucose
- frequent testing not required for well-controlled gestational diabetics on diet or small doses of insulin.

In general, a baseline scan for the estimation of fetal weight and growth parameters is performed at 28 weeks. Subsequent serial evaluation is mandatory in pregestational diabetics, weekly or biweekly, depending on the severity of diabetes. In women with GDM, if there is no macrosomia or associated complications like hypertension and glycemic control is good, tests for fetal wellbeing can be performed less frequently.

Timing of delivery

The timing of delivery should minimise neonatal mortality and morbidity and maximise the chances of vaginal delivery. Delivery should be as close to term as possible to avoid prematurity, respiratory distress syndrome and failed induction, but should be appropriately timed to avoid stillbirth, macrosomia and shoulder dystocia. In general, postmaturity should be avoided in all diabetics.

- In patients with gestational diabetes and good glycemic control, irrespective of the need for insulin, delivery can be held at 40 weeks.
- Those with associated hypertension or when glycemic control is not good, labour induction at 38 weeks is recommended.
- In uncomplicated pregestational diabetics, delivery is recommended at 38 weeks.
- In the presence of preeclampsia, poor biophysical profile, intrauterine growth restriction or poorly controlled glycemic status, induction may be required earlier.
- If delivery is contemplated before 36 weeks, one should be very sure of the period of gestation.

Mode of delivery

Diabetes is not an indication for cesarean section. However, the incidence of cesarean section is high due to macrosomia, cephalopelvic disproportion and anticipated shoulder dystocia. If the estimated weight of the baby is 4,000 g, elective cesarean section should be considered. Other obstetric indications like fetal distress, failed induction and malpresentations may also necessitate cesarean section. If induction is decided upon, prostaglandins can be used to ripen the cervix.

Intrapartum management

During labour, ketosis can develop. Proper control of plasma glucose in labour minimises the chances of neonatal hypoglycemia and hyperbilirubinemia. Combined infusion of insulin and glucose is used to maintain the plasma glucose value below 140 mg/dl.

- Plasma glucose and urine for ketone bodies are checked every two hours.
- If glycemic control is good, prophylactic antibiotics are not required.
- Artificial rupture of membranes should be performed when in the active phase.
- Electronic fetal monitoring is recommended for all.
- Shoulder dystocia should be anticipated.
- Prolonged labour should be avoided.

Management of the neonate

Early feeding is recommended to avoid hypoglycemia. Blood glucose should be monitored closely. Infusion of intravenous glucose may be required. Serum bilirubin, calcium and magnesium levels should be checked.

Postpartum management

In pregestational diabetics, the insulin requirement falls sharply after delivery. Since the control of glycemia need not be as strict as during pregnancy, the insulin dose can be drastically reduced, plasma glucose monitored and the insulin dose readjusted. Women who were on oral hypoglycemics can be given the same drugs as before. A small percentage of women with GDM may have undiagnosed pregestational diabetes. A two-hour GTT with 75 g glucose load should be performed at the six weeks visit. Counselling about weight reduction, lifestyle changes and chances of developing diabetes later in life should be given.

CONTRACEPTION

Gestational diabetes mellitus is not a contraindication for combined oral contraceptive pills. Well-controlled diabetics can also be given combined OCPs though a progesterone-only pill is preferable. An intrauterine contraceptive device may be inserted in women with GDM and well-controlled diabetics. Early completion of family and restriction of the number of children is advisable in diabetic women.

KEY POINTS

- Diabetes is a condition of altered glucose metabolism. It is pregestational if it precedes pregnancy and gestational if it is recognised during pregnancy.
- Approximately 3%–5% of pregnancies are complicated by diabetes mellitus.
- There is a need to diagnose diabetes early in pregnancy to reduce complications in the mother and her fetus.
- The glucose challenge test has been advocated in low-risk women for screening between 24 and 28 weeks of pregnancy. If it is positive or in high-risk women, a glucose tolerance test is recommended.
- Strict control of diabetes in pregnancy will minimise the adverse effects for the mother and the fetus.
- Oral hypoglycemic drugs are avoided in pregnancy.
- Diet, exercise and insulin form the main components of treatment.
- Careful monitoring of fetal growth and wellbeing are essential in the antenatal period.
- Proper selection of time and mode of delivery is vital to improve outcome.

QUESTIONS

Select the single most appropriate answer:

1. The most common fetal anomaly in pregnancy with diabetes mellitus is
   a. neural tube defects
   b. sacral agenesis
   c. limb defects
   d. cardiac defects
2. Which of the following fetal anomalies is specific to diabetes mellitus complicating pregnancy?
   a. anencephaly
   b. atrial septal defect
   c. sacral agenesis
   d. dysplastic kidney
3. The best method to establish the diagnosis of diabetes mellitus in pregnancy is
   a. random blood glucose
   b. postprandial blood glucose
   c. 24-hour glucose profile
   d. glucose tolerance test
4. The best method to diagnose fetal lung maturity in diabetes complicating pregnancy is
   a. lecithin sphingomyelin ratio
   b. ultrasonography
   c. phosphatidyl glycerol
   d. shake bubble test

In the following questions, there are two statements. Select the appropriate answer using the following key:

a. if both statements are true and causally related
b. if both statements are true but not causally related
c. if the first statement is true and the second is false
d. if the first statement is false and the second is true
e. if both statements are false

5. Diabetes mellitus manifests during pregnancy *because* During pregnancy the levels of hPL and cortisol are elevated.
6. A pregnant mother can never become hypoglycemic *because* The fetus draws on maternal glucose
7. In a diabetic woman, proteinuria increases *because* Renal blood flow and glomerular filtration rate are increased.

Select the appropriate answer using the following key:

a. if only responses 1, 2 and 3 are correct
b. if only 1 and 3 are correct
c. if only 2 and 4 are correct
d. if only 4 is correct
e. if all are correct

8. A pregnant woman with diabetes mellitus is at increased risk of
   1. antepartum hemorrhage
   2. urinary tract infection
   3. postmaturity
   4. preeclampsia
9. In pregnancy complicated by diabetes mellitus, fetal macrosomia is attributed to
   1. maternal hyperglycemia
   2. fetal hyperinsulinemia
   3. increase in growth factors
   4. fetal hyperglycemia
10. The effects of diabetes mellitus on the fetus include
    1. increased risk of spontaneous abortion
    2. increased incidence of congenital anomalies
    3. sudden intrauterine death
    4. increased incidence of oligohydramnios

50

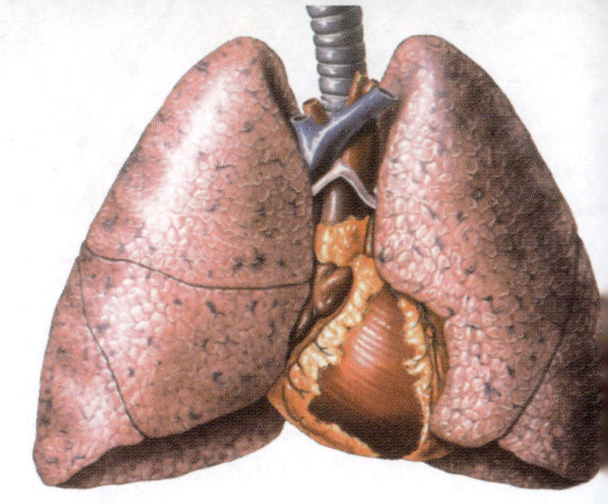

Thyroid Disorders

Asha Oumachigui

LEARNING OBJECTIVES

At the end of this chapter, the reader should be able to:

- describe the changes in thyroid function in the mother
- list the changes in fetal thyroid
- outline the diagnosis of hypothyroidism
- describe the adverse effects of hypothyroidism on the fetus
- describe the principles of management
- outline the diagnosis of hyperthyroidism
- describe the adverse effects of hyperthyroidism on the fetus
- outline the principles of the management of hyperthyroidism
- outline the management of postpartum thyroiditis

Introduction

Thyroid disorders often affect women in the reproductive age group, and are not uncommon during pregnancy. It is estimated that the incidence is approximately 1 in 500 deliveries. Hypothyroidism, hyperthyroidism and postpartum thyroiditis are the most common presentations and are caused by an autoimmune dysfunction. Both the mother and the fetus can suffer from thyroid diseases. Maternal and fetal outcomes are of concern, but can be definitely improved with treatment.

Changes in thyroid function

During pregnancy, the function of the thyroid gland is significantly increased; the production of thyroid hormones is increased to meet maternal and fetal needs.

The changes in the mother result from:

- an estrogen-induced increase in the circulating level of thyroxine binding globulin (TBG) from the liver
- increased urinary excretion of iodine leading to low plasma levels compensated by increased iodine uptake by the thyroid gland
- production of several thyroid stimulatory factors like hCG by the placenta.

These changes lead to enlargement of the thyroid gland due to hyperplasia and increased vascularity.

The level of TBG begins to rise early in pregnancy and reaches its peak by 20 weeks. Serum levels of thyroxine (T4), both free and bound, increase between 6 and 9 weeks; thereafter, the level of free T4 returns to normal. The level of triiodothyronine (T3) rises till week 18 and is stable thereafter. The high levels of hCG in early pregnancy coincide with the raised level of free T4 and low levels of thyrotropin. Despite these changes, the woman remains euthyroid during pregnancy.

In the fetus, the pituitary–thyroid axis is functional by the end of the first trimester. The maternal thyrotropin releasing hormone (TRH) crosses the placenta. At 10–12 weeks, the thyroid gland is able to synthesise the hormone and is autonomous, and the fetus depends on maternal thyroxine mainly in the first 12 weeks, but transfer of maternal thyroxine to fetus continues throughout pregnancy and accounts for 30% at term. Fetal thyroid hormone is essential for the development of all the tissues, particularly the brain.

HYPOTHYROIDISM

Etiology

The most common cause of hypothyroidism in young women is Hashimoto's thyroiditis or autoimmune thyroiditis. The condition is associated with high circulating levels of antibodies to thyroid microsomal antigen (antithyroid peroxidase antibodies).

Diagnosis

Diagnosis of hypothyroidism is confirmed if free T4 levels are low and thyrotropin (TSH) levels are raised. Women suffering from **overt hypothyroidism** are often infertile. Subclinical hypothyroidism is diagnosed when the serum T4 level is normal and TSH is raised in women who are asymptomatic.

Effect on the mother

Hypothyroid women who become pregnant are at a higher risk of preeclampsia, accidental hemorrhage, microcytic anemia, cardiac dysfunction and postpartum hemorrhage.

Effect on the fetus

Fetal outcome in hypothyroid women includes spontaneous abortion, congenital abnormalities, low birth weight baby and stillbirth. The presence of thyroid autoantibodies has been implicated in early pregnancy loss. Maternal hypothyroidism has been associated with poor neuropsychological development of the infant.

Treatment

The condition is treated by replacing thyroxine in a daily dose of 50–100 µg. Response is monitored by measuring serum TSH once in four weeks; the dose of thyroxine is adjusted by 25–50 µg to maintain the level of TSH at or just below normal (2.5–3 mIU/ml). Throughout pregnancy, the serum level of TSH is measured in each trimester. The dose of thyroxine should be increased by 25%–30% once pregnancy is diagnosed.

Adequate intake of iodine is essential for normal fetal thyroid and neurological development. Supplementation of iodine has been recommended for pregnant women from areas where endemic goitre is common because of iodine deficiency. Congenital hypothyroidism in the fetus often leads to abnormal mental development. Hence, universal screening of all neonates is recommended in some countries.

HYPERTHYROIDISM

Etiology

Hyperthyroidism or thyrotoxicosis complicating pregnancy is usually due to Graves' disease. It is the result of an organ-specific autoimmune process associated with thyroid stimulating antibodies.

Diagnosis

It may be difficult to make an early diagnosis clinically, but the presence of the following features could point to hyperthyroidism:

- nervousness
- inability to concentrate
- tachycardia, palpitations
- an abnormally raised sleeping pulse rate
- thyromegaly
- exophthalmos
- weight loss in spite of eating well.

Diagnosis is confirmed by estimating thyroid function which shows an elevated level of T4 and a lowered level of thyrotropin. Thyrotoxicosis is subclinical if the serum thyrotropin level is low and the levels of T4 and T3 are normal.

Effect on the mother and fetus

There are a number of complications if the disease is not controlled. The mother is likely to suffer from preeclampsia and cardiac failure; in severe cases, it may prove fatal.

Perinatal outcome is poor because of increased risk of preterm delivery, intrauterine growth restriction and stillbirth. Transient thyrotoxicosis has been reported in the newborn; the neonate could be hypothyroid or may suffer from goitre. Perinatal mortality is approximately 10%.

Treatment

Treatment of hyperthyroidism during pregnancy is essentially medical. The use of propylthiouracil or methimazole is the mainstay of treatment. Propylthiouracil partially inhibits the conversion of T4 to T3, crosses the placenta less readily than methimazole and is not associated with aplasia cutis, esophageal or choanal atresia (that are associated with methimazole).

Propylthiouracil is administered in doses of 300–400 mg daily and is continued throughout pregnancy; if the drug is discontinued, the risk of neonatal thyrotoxicosis is increased. Good control is achieved within 2–3 weeks. Propylthiouracil is excreted only minimally in breast milk compared to methimazole; however, the thyroid status of the breast-fed infant should be monitored.

Thyroidectomy is best avoided during pregnancy as the increased vascularity of the gland may complicate surgery. Ablation of the thyroid with radioactive iodine is contraindicated.

Thyroid storm is a severe condition; intensive care is needed. The treatment is propylthiouracil, potassium iodide and β blockers.

Postpartum thyroiditis

It is not unusual for women to develop postpartum thyroiditis (PPT). It occurs in three phases: hyperthyroid, hypothyroid and euthyroid. The condition is said to be due to autoimmune thyroiditis. It occurs 1–4 months after delivery and the symptoms are vague; it can be diagnosed only when it is sought carefully.

Thyroiditis appears to be initiated by an inflammation, followed by an autoreaction from the immune system. Autoantibodies (antithyroid peroxidase antibodies) have been detected in women developing PPT, either in early pregnancy or just after delivery.

There are two clinical manifestations of PPT: thyrotoxicosis and hypothyroidism.

- Thyrotoxicosis is transient and is due to excessive release of the preformed hormone due to glandular destruction and not due to excessive production. The woman may complain of fatigue or palpitations and there may be a small goitre. Antithyroid drugs should not be given. If symptoms are severe, a β blocker is useful. Most women return to a euthyroid state; a few may develop hypothyroidism.
- Hypothyroidism manifests 4–8 months after delivery. Some women may have suffered from a thyrotoxic phase of PPT. Fatigue and an inability to concentrate are common symptoms; a goitre may be present. Thyroxine replacement is given for 6–12 months; about one-third of women are likely to become hypothyroid permanently.

KEY POINTS

- Thyroid disorders are seen in 0.2% of all pregnancies.
- The physiological changes of pregnancy affect the interpretation of thyroid function studies.
- High levels of estrogen enhance the synthesis of the thyroid binding globulin. Despite an increase in free and bound T4 and T3, the woman remains euthyroid.
- There is close correlation between maternal and fetal thyroid function.
- Thyroid disorders during pregnancy are hypothyroidism, thyrotoxicosis and PPT and are caused by an autoimmune process.
- Hypothyroidism is associated with infertility, and an increased risk of abortions, preeclampsia and preterm delivery. Thyroxine replacement improves pregnancy outcome.
- Thyrotoxicosis is responsible for an increased risk of preeclampsia, intrauterine growth restriction and stillbirth. The drugs frequently used for its treatment are propylthiouracil and methimazole.
- Postpartum thyroiditis occurs 1–4 months after delivery. An initial phase of thyrotoxicosis is followed by hypothyroidism and then a euthyroid state.

QUESTIONS

Select the single most appropriate answer:

1. Which one of the following is *not true* regarding pregnancy in a woman on treatment for hyperthyroidism?
   a. increased risk of abortions
   b. increased intrauterine growth restriction
   c. neonatal hypothyroidism can occur
   d. radioactive iodine uptake studies can be undertaken in puerperium
2. The thyroxin binding globulin (TBG) rises during pregnancy and reaches a peak by
   a. 10 weeks b. 15 weeks c. 20 weeks d. 25 weeks
3. Which of the following is false regarding thyroid function in pregnancy?
   a. decrease in plasma levels of iodine
   b. decrease in urinary excretion of iodine
   c. increase in the thyroid binding globulin
   d. serum levels of T4 increase by 6–9 weeks

In the following questions, there are two statements. Select the appropriate answer using the following key:

a. if both statements are true and causally related
b. if both statements are true but not causally related
c. if the first statement is true and the second is false
d. if the first statement is false and the second is true
e. if both statements are false

4. The fetus depends on maternal thyroxin only up to 12 weeks *because*

   By 12 weeks, the fetal thyroid gland is able to synthesise the thyroid hormone.
5. Congenital hypothyroidism is associated with impaired neuropsychological development of the infant *because*

   Thyroxin is not required in particular for the development of the brain.

Select the appropriate answer using the following key:

a. if only responses 1, 2 and 3 are correct
b. if only 1 and 3 are correct
c. if only 2 and 4 are correct
d. if only 4 is correct
e. if all are correct

6. A pregnant woman who is hypothyroid is prone to which of the following complications?
   1. placental abruption
   2. cardiac dysfunction
   3. postpartum hemorrhage
   4. adherent placenta
7. Propylthiouracil is better than methimazole for the treatment of hyperthyroidism in pregnancy because it
   1. crosses the placenta less readily
   2. is not associated with aplasia cutis
   3. is not associated with esophageal atresia
   4. has less risk of choanal atresia

51

Urinary Tract Infections

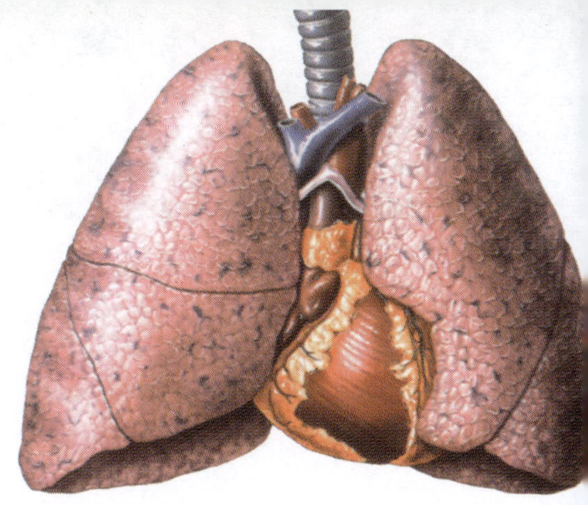

V Mathini

LEARNING OBJECTIVES

At the end of this chapter, the reader should be able to:

- list the changes in pregnancy that predispose to UTI
- list the causative organisms
- define and describe the management of asymptomatic bacteriuria (ASB)
- enumerate the clinical features and laboratory criteria to diagnose cystitis
- outline the management of cystitis
- describe the clinical features of pyelonephritis
- list the conditions in the differential diagnosis of acute pyelonephritis
- outline the management of pyelonephritis
- list the likely adverse pregnancy outcome associated with UTI

Introduction

Urinary tract infections (UTI) are the most common bacterial infections in pregnancy. Symptomatic infection involves the lower urinary tract and manifests as cystitis; involvement of the renal pelvis, calyces and parenchyma manifests as pyelonephritis. If untreated, the infections may lead to adverse pregnancy outcome.

Predisposing factors in pregnancy

Significant changes take place in the urinary tract during normal pregnancy both in structure and function. The increased circulating level of progesterone causes the smooth muscle to relax; this results in dilatation of the renal calyces, pelves and ureter, leading to stasis. After 20 weeks, the ureters are compressed on the pelvic brim by the enlarging uterus and ovarian vein, resulting in further dilatation of the renal calyces and pelves. Progesterone and prostaglandins also cause decreased peristalsis of the ureters. Increased vesicoureteric reflux also predisposes to infection.

Due to the effect of progesterone, there is relaxation of the smooth muscles of the bladder. The displacement of the uterus into the abdomen leads to elongation of the urethra, and incomplete emptying of the bladder leads to an increase in residual urine which predisposes to infection.

Following delivery, especially when there is an episiotomy or the woman was given regional anesthesia, there can be loss of bladder sensation. In such situations, catheterisation for the relief of distension can further contribute to infection.

There is increased excretion of glucose, amino acids and bicarbonates. These changes particularly favour the growth of bacteria, especially *Escherichia coli*.

The commonest organism causing urinary tract infection is *E coli*. Other organisms that may be isolated in culture are the *Klebsiella*, *Hemophilus*, *Acinetobacter* and *Enterobacter* species. *Proteus* and *Pseudomonas* rarely cause urinary infection.

Infections

Most infections are caused by the organisms of the normal perineal/vaginal flora. There are essentially three types of urinary tract infections encounterd in pregnancy:

- asymptomatic bacteriuria
- cystitis
- pyelonephritis

Asymptomatic bacteriuria

Asymptomatic bacteruria (ASB) refers to persistent active multiplication of bacteria in the urinary tract without symptoms. The criterion for diagnosis is the presence of more than 100,000 bacteria per ml in a sample of clean voided urine. The incidence is 2%–11% and depends on parity, race and the socioeconomic status. It is associated with preterm labour and small-for-gestational-age infants. The condition must be treated; if left untreated, 25% of women are likely to develop pyelonephritis.

Women at risk must be screened for ASB, but it is not cost-effective to perform urine culture; less expensive tests like leucocyte esterase, nitrite and dipstick tests may be used.

Women diagnosed with ASB must be treated with any of the available antimicrobial regimens (**Table 51.1**). It is preferable to use an antibiotic to which the organism is sensitive; empirically, however, amoxicillin, ampicillin and cephalosporins can be used safely.

Table 51.1 Antimicrobial regimen used for the treatment of pregnant women with ASB

Single dose	
Amoxicillin	3 g
Ampicillin	2 g
Cephalosporin	2 g
Nitrofurantoin	200 mg*
Sulfonamide	2 g*
Trimethoprim-sulfamethoxazole*	320/1,600 mg
Three-day course	
Amoxicillin 500 mg three times a day	
Ampicillin 250 mg four times a day	
Nitrofurantoin 50–100 mg four times a day or 100 mg twice a day*	
Sulfonamide 500 mg four times a day*	
Other courses	
Nitrofurantoin 100 mg four times a day for 10 days*	
Nitrofurantoin 100 mg at bedtime for 10 days*	
Treatment failure	
Nitrofurantoin 100 mg four times a day for 21 days*	

* Preferably not used in early and late pregnancy

Cystitis

Women with cystitis typically complain of frequency, urgency, dysuria and suprapubic discomfort. Occasionally, pyuria and hematuria may be present. It may be associated with general malaise and fever. On microscopic examination, the presence of more than 10 pus cells per high-power field (hpf) confirms the diagnosis of cystitis. Urine culture helps determine the type of bacteria responsible and their sensitivity to antibiotics. The woman must be treated with a three-day course; if there is no relief, a ten-day course may be given, preferably according to the results of the sensitivity test.

When symptoms of cystitis occur without evidence of bacteriologic infection, they are usually due to urethritis caused by Chlamydia; treatment is with erythromycin.

Acute pyelonephritis

Acute pyelonephritis is a serious medical complication during pregnancy and could lead to septic shock, renal failure and disseminated intravascular coagulation (DIC). It may be preceded by conditions like ASB, urinary tract anomalies, renal calculi and medical conditions like diabetes mellitus and, sickle cell disease or trait.

Onset of the symptoms is abrupt: high fever, chills and rigors, nausea, vomiting, dysuria and pain in the lumbar region. There will be tenderness in the costovertebral angle. Many of the symptoms are due to endotoxemia, especially high spiking fever followed by hypothermia. A serious complication is adult respiratory distress syndrome (ARDS).

Microscopic examination of urine reveals pus cells in clumps and numerous bacteria. Organisms most commonly isolated are *E coli*, *Klebsiella pneumoniae* and Enterobacter. About 15% of the patients are likely to have bacteremia. Serum creatinine must be estimated, as there is a likelihood of decreased glomerular filtration rate in acute pyelonephritis.

It is not difficult to diagnose acute pyelonephritis, but it must be differentiated from other causes of acute abdomen like severe chorioamnionitis, acute appendicitis, placental abruption, torsion of an ovarian cyst and degeneration of a fibroid.

Treatment: The woman should be hospitalised so that her general condition can be monitored closely and any complication dealt with promptly. Intravenous hydration is essential to ensure adequate renal output. It is best to start antibiotics empirically without waiting for urine and blood culture results. The preferred antibiotics are a combination of ampicillin and gentamicin, or cefzolin or ceftriaxone. An outline of the management of acute pyelonephritis is shown in **Table 51.2**. If there is no response to treatment within 72 hours, one should check for urinary stones and, dilatation of the ureters or renal pelves and treat appropriately.

Table 51.2 Management of acute pyelonephritis

- Hospitalisation
- Urine and blood culture
- Hemogram, serum creatinine/blood urea
- Vital signs monitored closely
- Intravenous fluids to ensure urine output of 30 ml/hour
- Intravenous antibiotics
- X-ray chest if needed
- Discharged when afebrile, oral antibiotics for 7–10 days
- Urine culture repeated after two weeks
- Recurrence; if found, must be treated

Acute pyelonephritis can lead to complications like septic shock, DIC, renal failure and adult respiratory distress syndrome in the mother due to the release of endotoxins. Fetal complications are prematurity, intrauterine growth restriction and intrauterine death. Antibiotic prophylaxis is advocated in the following situations to prevent acute pyelonephritis.

Prophylaxis should be considered in pregnant women with urologic complications like ureteral reimplantation, renal transplants and recurrent UTI; treatment is nitrofurantoin 100 mg/day.

In the postpartum period, UTI may occur due to an infection from an indwelling catheter or repeated catheterisation for urinary retention. In such cases, amoxicillin may be given as 500 mg 8 hourly.

KEY POINTS

- Urinary tract infections complicate 2%–11% of pregnancies.
- Asymptomatic bacteriuria, cystitis and acute pyelonephritis must be treated.
- *E coli* and *Klebsiella* are the common infective organisms. The most commonly used antibiotics are ampicillin, nitrofurantoin and cephalosporins.
- A woman with acute pyelonephritis should ideally be hospitalised and treated with intravenous fluids and a combination of ampicillin and gentamicin.
- Non-responders must be investigated for underlying abnormalities in the urinary tract.
- UTI must be treated to reduce/avoid maternal and fetal complications.
- Antibiotic prophylaxis must be considered if preexisting urological complications are present.

QUESTIONS

Select the single most appropriate answer:

1. Dilatation of the renal calyces begins by
   a. 10 weeks c. 20 weeks
   b. 15 weeks d. 30 weeks
2. All of the following factors predispose to urinary tract infection *except*
   a. progesterone c. increased residual urine
   b. estrogen d. dilatation of renal calyces
3. In a clean void of urine, the criteria used to diagnose asymptomatic bacteriuria (ASB) is
   a. 1,000 bacteria/ml c. 100,000 bacteria/ml
   b. 10,000 bacteria/ml d. 1000,000 bacteria/ml
4. If asymptomatic bacteriuria is left untreated in a pregnant woman, the chances of developing pyelonephritis are
   a. 5% b. 15% c. 25% d. 35%
5. The antibiotic that must be used with caution to treat asymptomatic bacteriuria in pregnancy is
   a. amoxicillin
   b. nitrofurantoin
   c. cefotaxime
   d. cefuroxime

Select the appropriate answer using the following key:

a. if only responses 1, 2 and 3 are correct
b. if only 1 and 3 are correct
c. if only 2 and 4 are correct
d. if only 4 is correct
e. if all are correct

6. Acute pyelonephritis may be preceded by
   1. renal calculi
   2. urinary tract malformations
   3. sickle cell disease
   4. diabetes mellitus
7. In pregnancy complicated by acute pyelonephrits, the fetal complications include
   1. prematurity 3. intrauterine death
   2. neonatal anemia 4. respiratory infection

52

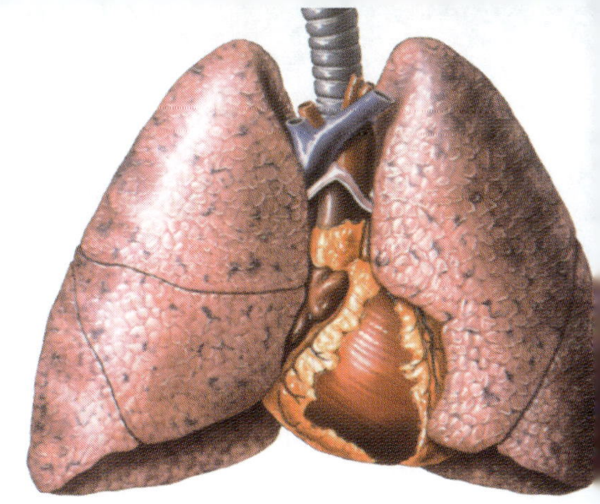

Sexually Transmitted Infections

Kapila Bharucha

LEARNING OBJECTIVES

At the end of this chapter, the reader should be able to:

- recognise that some sexually transmitted diseases (STDs) can affect the fetus adversely
- list the frequently encountered STDs
- enumerate the tests used for screening and confirmation
- describe the clinical features of the disease in the mother and the newborn
- describe the placental pathology
- outline the management for the mother and the newborn
- list the measures for the prevention of these infections

Introduction

Sexually transmitted infections (STI) are not infrequent during pregnancy; prevalence is on the rise, particularly among commercial sex workers and drug abusers (high-risk groups). The infection affects both the mother and the fetus adversely. Therefore, screening for some of these infections is part of routine antenatal care. In the women at risk, it is recommended that screening be extended to other STDs besides syphilis. If the test is positive, the woman can be treated with benefit to herself and the fetus.

Common STIs during pregnancy

The STIs seen in pregnancy are syphilis, gonorrhea, infection with chlamydia, hepatitis B virus, human immunodeficiency virus (HIV), bacterial vaginosis (BV), herpes simplex virus (HSV), human papilloma virus (HPV) and lymphogranuloma venereum (LGV).

Syphilis

Incidence

In the last few decades, there has been a decline in the incidence of syphilis in general. This may be attributed to the widespread use of antibiotics. Consequently, the incidence of congenital syphilis has also decreased. However, it has disastrous effects on pregnancy outcome.

Effect on the mother

A woman may become infected during pregnancy. The clinical course of the infection differs from that in the nonpregnant state: in pregnancy, the lesions on the genitalia are smaller and cervical chancre is more common.

Effect on the fetus and neonate

Syphilis during pregnancy is responsible for late abortion, stillbirth and neonatal infection.

A neonate affected by congenital syphilis has hepatosplenomegaly, ascites and jaundice. It can also suffer from 'snuffles' or rhinitis, nephrosis, lymphadenopathy and osteochondritis. Perinatal morbidity and mortality are high.

Infection of the fetus

The spirochetes cross the placenta easily, but not before 18 weeks. The fetus can be infected during any stage of syphilis, though it is usually infective in the primary, secondary or early latent stage. Practically every organ in the fetus is likely to be affected.

The spirochetes infect the placenta which becomes large and edematous; the villi lose their characteristic appearance of arborescence. Further, there is a decrease in the number of blood vessels and increased vascular resistance due to endoarteritis. Spirochetes are seen scattered throughout the placenta and the fetal organs.

Diagnosis

The serological test used for screening is the venereal disease research laboratory (VDRL) test. It is positive in the primary and secondary stages of syphilis. In India, screening for syphilis is recommended for every pregnant mother. Since this test lacks specificity, a *Treponema pallidum*-specific test is performed for confirmation of the diagnosis. In the fetus, diagnosis is made by demonstrating the presence of spirochetes in various organs and the placenta.

Treatment

Penicillin continues to be preferred. Benzathine penicillin G 2.4 million units is given as a single dose. If the woman is allergic to penicillin, either erythromycin or tetracyclines is given.

The neonate is treated with aqueous or procaine penicillin G administered intravenously for 10 days after testing the cerebrospinal fluid. If the mother was treated with erythromycin, the newborn must be considered to have congenital syphilis and treated.

Treating the neonate for syphilis will effectively prevent long-term sequelae.

Gonorrhea

Incidence

There is an overall decrease in the incidence of gonorrhea; its prevalence among pregnant women is variable and depends on the risk status of the population for STIs.

Effect on the mother

Gonococcal infection during pregnancy is limited to the lower urogenital tract; the urethra, periurethral and vestibular glands, and the endocervix are involved. Obliteration of the uterine cavity by pregnancy prevents the infection from spreading upwards; the fallopian tubes are therefore spared.

Effect on pregnancy outcome

Gonococcal infection can have deleterious effects on pregnancy in any trimester. Women infected with *Neisseria gonorrhea* are more prone to develop post-abortion sepsis, premature rupture of membranes, preterm delivery, chorioamnionitis and puerperal sepsis.

The newborn is at risk of developing gonococcal ophthalmia.

Diagnosis

This is essentially by smear examination and culture of discharge from infected sites. On Gram stain, Gram-negative intracellular diplococci are seen inside the polymorphonuclear leucocytes. Culture is the gold standard for detection and has 100% specificity. Gonococcal antigen is detected by an enzyme immunoassay. Polymerase chain reaction is a sensitive method to detect *N gonorrhea* from endocervical, urethral and urine samples.

Treatment

The woman is treated with one of the following antibiotics as a single dose:

- cefixime 400 mg orally

  or
- ceftriaxone 125 mg IM

  or
- ciprofloxacin 500 mg orally

All neonates are given prophylactic treatment to prevent ophthalmia neonatorum. Infants whose mothers test positive and are untreated, as well as infants who are infected should be investigated and treated with a single intravenous dose of ceftriaxone.

Chlamydial Infection

Incidence

The incidence of chlamydial infection is 2%–25%. It is caused by *Chlamydia trachomatis*, an obligate intracellular organism.

Effect on the mother

Symptoms of acute chlamydial infection in the woman are acute urethritis, mucopurulent cervicitis, salpingitis, Bartholinitis conjunctivitis and reactive arthritis. However, most pregnant women have a subclinical disease.

Effect on the neonate

There may be an increased risk of premature rupture of membranes and preterm delivery among women with chlamydial cervicitis. The risk of abortion is not increased. The newborn usually suffers from conjunctivitis and pneumonia.

Diagnosis

Diagnosis is confirmed by direct fluorescent antibody (DFA) test which has a sensitivity of 90%. There is no benefit in routine screening for *C trachomatis.*

Treatment

During pregnancy, the mother is prescribed erythromycin 500 mg four times a day orally for 7 days or amoxicillin 500 mg 3 times a day orally for 7 days. A single oral dose of azithromycin 500 mg is an accepted alternative treatment.

Herpes Simplex Infection

Herpes genitalis is caused by the herpes simplex virus, a DNA virus which is of two types, HSV 1 and HSV 2. The type 2 virus is transmitted sexually and is responsible for most genital infections.

Effect on the mother

The severity of the symptoms depends upon the type of the virus and the immune status of the woman. Patients complain of fever, headache, malaise and myalgia early in the course of the disease. The lesions start as bilateral, papular eruptions on the external genitalia; later, they ulcerate. The woman complains of itching, pain during urination, and vaginal or urethral discharge. The lesions become very painful and severe inguinal lymphadenopathy follows. Examination reveals mucopurulent bloody vaginal discharge and a friable ectocervix with ulcerative lesions.

Recurrent infection is common and occurs in spite of treatment of the primary infection with acyclovir.

Effect on the neonate

Infection in early pregnancy is not associated with an increased incidence of abortion, while in late pregnancy, it is likely to predispose to preterm labour.

The virus rarely crosses the placenta and the neonate becomes infected with the virus from the lower genital tract after rupture of membranes or during delivery. Three types of clinical manifestations are seen in the newborn: involvement of major organs, restricted involvement of the central nervous system, eyes and skin or the newborn could be completely asymptomatic.

To avoid neonatal infection, which can be severe, cesarean delivery has been advocated whenever genital herpetic lesions are suspected. The baby should be isolated and cultures taken for HSV. The mother can breastfeed but must be instructed about washing her hands and especially to avoid contact between her lesions, hands and the newborn.

Diagnosis

Infection with HSV is clinically apparent. However, recovery of the virus in tissue culture is the best test for confirmation; it has a sensitivity of 95%. Cytological examination of the cervical smear fixed in alcohol and with Papanicolaou stain is useful.

Polymerase chain reaction can be used to detect the genital herpes DNA.

Treatment

The administration of oral antiviral drugs is the mainstay of treatment; acyclovir is given 200 mg orally five times a day for 7–10 days. The addition of valacyclovir is useful in the latter part of pregnancy to obtain higher levels of acyclovir. Higher doses of acyclovir are recommended whenever there is associated HIV infection.

Severe pain and discomfort are controlled with analgesics and the application of local anesthetics.

Human Immunodeficiency Virus (HIV)

Human immunodeficiency virus (HIV) is a retrovirus that belongs to the subfamily of lentiviruses. The two main types are HIV 1 and HIV 2. HIV 1 is the more common of the two. The route of transmission is nearly always sexual; it could also be through sharing of needles among intravenous drug users and transfusion of blood and blood products. Perinatal transmission is one of the problems of HIV infection in pregnancy. In India, the the seroprevalence for HIV among pregnant women is less than 1%. Pregnancy has not been found to alter the course of the disease.

Effect on the mother

HIV infection does not increase the risk of abortion, prematurity or low birth weight. Pulmonary diseases like tuberculosis and fungal infections are common and are AIDS-defining illnesses. In developing countries, HIV may be associated with diseases like malaria.

Effect on the neonate

Parent-to-child transmission (PTCT) can occur antenatally, during labour and while breast-feeding. The risk of transmission ranges from 14% to 43%. In India, given a seropositivity of about 1% among pregnant women and with 25 million births annually, one may expect 75,000 HIV-infected newborns. Several factors like maternal viral load, maternal immune status, presence of genital tract infections and unprotected sexual intercourse influence the rate of PTCT. Obstetrical factors that enhance PTCT are premature rupture of membranes, preterm delivery, chorioamnionitis and vaginal delivery.

Diagnosis

Though HIV may be clinically suspected in high-risk groups, it is diagnosed only after the screening test is positive. The ELISA test is used for screening; it has a sensitivity of 99.5%. When ELISA is positive, the diagnosis is confirmed by a Western blot or immunofluorescence assay.

Other tests necessary are screening for other STDs, a pap smear and an X-ray chest. A complete blood count must be performed in women on antiretroviral therapy (ARV). If possible, a CD_4 count may be performed.

Measures to reduce parent-to-child transmission (PTCT)

Screening of all pregnant mothers: This is not ideal as it has far-reaching psychosocial consequences. However, when screened, the women should be counselled before and after the procedure. National AIDS Control Organisation (NACO) in India has taken up the task of screening all pregnant women after counselling and administration of ARV in an attempt to reduce PTCT under a programme called Prevention of Parent-to-Child Transmission (PPTCT).

Antiretroviral therapy: A number of drugs with effective antiretroviral activity are available. However, zidovudine (ZDV or AZT) is the mainstay of treatment. It is started after 14 weeks of pregnancy and is administered orally 100 mg five times a day during pregnancy and during labour; loading dose is 2 mg/kg body weight and maintenance is 1 mg/kg body weight.

If a woman presents late in pregnancy, nevirapine is given as a single oral dose of 200 mg; the newborn is administered an oral dose of 1 mg/kg within 72 hours of birth.

Antiretroviral therapy has an efficacy rate of 37%–51% in reducing PTCT.

Obstetric management: Since most infants acquire the infection in late pregnancy and labour, efforts must be made to reduce invasive interventions, avoid rupture of membranes early in labour and prolonged labour. The current recommendation is cesarean delivery.

Breastfeeding: The WHO guidelines recommend that the risks of breastfeeding must be explained to the mother and she should be advised to resort to breast-milk substitutes. In developing countries, breastfeeding may still be advantageous.

Hepatitis B Virus (HBV) Infection

Hepatitis B virus (HBV) is a hepatotropic virus and infection occurs through contact with infected body fluids like semen, cervical fluids, saliva and blood through the percutaneous, perinatal and sexual routes. The prevalence of the HBV antigen is high among those suffering from STDs and HIV infection, and about 3%–4% among the population. Because of its long-term adverse effects (chronic hepatitis and hepatocellular carcinoma), HBV infection is considered only second to tobacco as a killer. Usually the mother is a silent carrier. Those suffering from chronic hepatitis may not conceive.

Effect on the mother

The prevalence and the clinical course of HBV infection are unaltered by pregnancy.

Effect on the newborn

In acute hepatitis, transplacental viral transmission occurs in the first trimester. The percentage of fetuses affected increases with the duration of pregnancy. The extent of vertical transmission is directly related to the maternal HBsAg status. In chronic hepatitis, the neonate is infected when it ingests infected material during delivery or breastfeeding.

Diagnosis

Clinically, some women may present with features of hepatitis; others are asymptomatic. There are several immunological markers like surface antigen (HBsAg), core antigen (HBcAg) and HBeAg. After infection with HBV, the first marker is HBsAg in the serum; its persistence is characteristic of chronic infection.

Strategies for the prevention of neonatal infection

The following measures are recommended to prevent transmission to the newborn:

- All pregnant mothers should be screened for hepatitis B.
- If the woman tests negative and is at risk of infection, she should be vaccinated.
- When the mother is a chronic carrier of the virus, infection in the newborn can be prevented by administering hepatitis B immunoglobulins, followed by the administration of the hepatitis B vaccine.

Other Infections

Human papilloma virus (HPV)

Infection with this virus is not uncommon among women of the reproductive age. There are several types of HPV; types 16 and 18 are implicated in cervical and vaginal neoplasia. If pregnant women are infected with HPV 6 and 11, the infant may develop laryngeal papillomatosis. HPV infection may also be responsible for prematurity.

Several types of HPV affect mucocutaneous tissues and cause condyloma acuminata. The lesions grow rapidly during pregnancy and usually regress after delivery. Treatment consists of the topical application of trichloroacetic acid, followed by cryotherapy or laser ablation. Agents like podophyllin resin or 5-fluorouracil should not be used during pregnancy.

Lymphogranuloma venereum

Infection is caused by several types of *C trachomatis*. Inguinal lymphadenitis, suppurating infective lesions and lymphatic involvement of the genitalia and pararectal tissues occur with scarring and fibrosis leading to elephantiasis and rectal stricture. The drug of choice for treatment during pregnancy is erythromycin.

Trichomonal infection

This is common in pregnant women. Examination reveals a greenish yellow discharge and punctate vaginitis. Diagnosis can be easily confirmed by the demonstration of *T vaginalis* by microscopic examination of a wet smear of the vaginal discharge.

Trichomonal infection during pregnancy is associated with preterm premature rupture of membranes and preterm delivery. Metronidazole is an effective antitrichomonal drug. It is prescribed to the woman and her partner orally 200 mg 3 times a day for 7 days. The treatment of the partner is necessary to avoid reccurrence.

Bacterial vaginosis

This is the most common cause of vaginal symptoms among women in the reproductive age group. The normal vaginal flora is replaced with a mixed concentration of *Gardnerella vaginalis, Mycoplasma hominis*, anerobic Gram-negative rods and bacteroides. There is no inflammation of the vaginal epithelium; hence the term vaginosis is used.

The most common clinical manifestation is increased vaginal discharge. Some women are asymptomatic. On examination a there is thin, white, non-viscous, homogenous and vaginal discharge smelling of fish.

Diagnosis can be confirmed by one of the following tests:

- Microscopic examination of a wet smear reveals the presence of **clue cells** (epithelial cells with a granular appearance).
- **Whiff test** or **amine test**: A fishy odour emanates when a drop of 10% KOH is added to a drop of the discharge.
- Gram stain of vaginal smear is a simple and specific test: it shows the presence of three different bacterial morphotypes, including large Gram-positive rods (lactobacilli), small Gram-negative bacteroides and *Gardnerella vaginalis.*

Bacterial vaginosis during pregnancy has been associated with preterm labour, premature rupture of membranes and chorioamnionitis. If bacterial vaginosis is detected during pregnancy, it should be treated. The recommended regimen is oral metronidazole 500 mg twice a day for seven days.

KEY POINTS

- Sexually transmitted diseases are not uncommon during pregnancy. Their incidence is increasing due to an increase in HIV infections, drug abuse and failure to adopt safe sex measures.
- STDs affect the neonate during pregnancy if the organism crosses the placenta or during vaginal delivery when the organism is shed in the lower genital tract.
- Some STDs like bacterial vaginosis and trichomonal vaginitis are associated with preterm delivery.
- Pregnant women who are categorised as high-risk, should be screened for HIV after pretest counselling, followed by post-test counselling. Treatment with ARV, cesarean section and avoidance of breastfeeding are means of reducing perinatal transmission.

QUESTIONS

Select the single most appropriate answer:

1. In syphilitic infection during pregnancy, the spirochetes cross the placenta by
   a. 12 weeks b. 14 weeks c. 16 weeks d. 18 weeks
2. Syphilis during pregnancy is responsible for all of the following *except*
   a. first trimester abortion c. late abortion
   b. stillbirth d. neonatal infection
3. The antibiotic of choice in the treatment of gonorrhea is
   a. amoxicillin c. cefixime
   b. gentamicin d. penicillin
4. All of the following statements about HSV infection are true *except*

a. the virus rarely crosses the placenta.
b. newborn is infected after the rupture of membranes.
c. increases the risk of abortion.
d. cesarean section is advocated in the presence of herpetic lesions.

5. When a mother is a chronic carrier of HBV, the baby should be administered
   a. hepatitis B immunoglobulins
   b. hepatitis B vaccine
   c. hepatitis B vaccine followed by immunoglobulins
   d. hepatitis B immunoglobulins followed by vaccine
6. All of the following statements about bacterial vaginosis are true *except*
   a. preterm labour is uncommon.
   b. infection is with mixed flora.
   c. clue cells are characteristic.
   d. it should be treated with metronidazole.

In the following questions, there are two statements. Select the appropriate answer using the following key:

a. if both statements are true and causally related
b. if both statements are true but not causally related
c. if the first statement is true and the second is false
d. if the first statement is false and the second is true
e. if both statements are false

7. Screening for syphilis is recommended for every pregnant woman *because*

   If the woman tests positive, she and her offspring can be treated effectively.
8. A mother who is HIV-positive should not breastfeed her baby *because*

   Breastfeeding is associated with a very high transmission rate.

Select the appropriate answer using the following key:

a. if only responses 1, 2 and 3 are correct
b. if only 1 and 3 are correct
c. if only 2 and 4 are correct
d. if only 4 is correct
e. if all are correct

9. A woman with gonococcal infection is at risk of
   1. post-abortion sepsis
   2. chorioamnionitis
   3. puerperal sepsis
   4. premature rupture of membranes
10. In a woman who is HIV positive, the risk of mother-to-child transmission (PTCT) is enhanced by
    1. high viral load in the mother
    2. presence of genital tract infection
    3. low immune status of the mother
    4. abdominal delivery
11. Measures to reduce mother-to-child transmission include
    1. screening of all pregnant women for HIV
    2. antiretroviral therapy in the antenatal period
    3. abdominal delivery
    4. administration of antibiotics

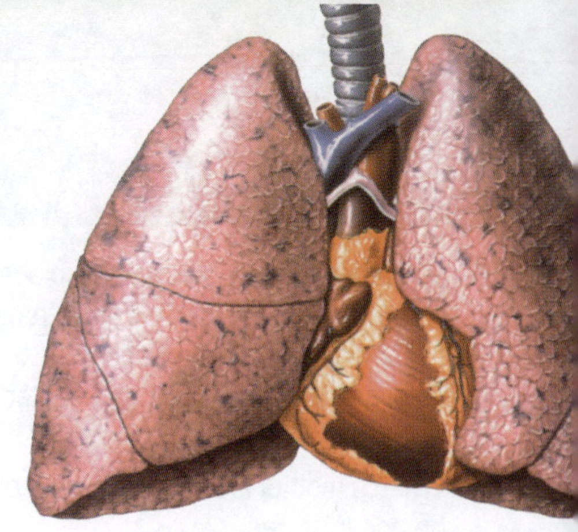

53

Tropical Infections

Asmita Rathore

LEARNING OBJECTIVES

At the end of this chapter, the readers should be able to:
- list the common tropical infections encountered in India
- describe the etiopathogenesis of these infections
- list their clinical features
- describe the adverse effects of these infections on pregnancy
- choose the laboratory investigations that help diagnose these infections
- outline the management of these infections
- list the principles of 'travel medicine' in pregnancy

Introduction

Most parasitic, bacterial and, viral infections occur in developing countries (located on the tropics) where environmental factors like hot and humid weather, overcrowding and poor hygiene combined with poor nutrition prevail. Pregnant women and children frequently experience a cycle of undernutrition and repeated infections.

This chapter deals with the clinical spectrum and management of common tropical diseases, their likely impact on pregnancy and existing intervention strategies for their control before or during pregnancy. Antiinfective drugs must be selected carefully keeping in mind the stage of pregnancy and the expected risks and benefits, with the ultimate goal of an optimal obstetric outcome.

Tropical infections may be grouped according to the main clinical manifestation.

Fever
Malaria
Typhoid/Enteric fever
Dengue fever
Visceral leishmaniasis (kala azar)
Filariasis

Intestinal disorders
Acute diarrhea
Amebiasis
Worm infestations: hookworm, roundworm

Other tropical diseases
Hydatid disease

MALARIA

Malaria is endemic in 91 countries and 40% of the world population is at risk. It is an important public health problem in India. In 2001, there were 0.98 million reported cases of malaria, of which 0.46 million were falciparum infections, and 431 deaths occurred. Malaria is an important cause of anemia in pregnancy, contributing to maternal mortality and morbidity.

Etiopathogenesis

Four species of the genus *Plasmodium* cause infections in humans: *P falciparum, P vivax, P ovale* and

P malaria. Most deaths are caused by *P falciparum.* It is a protozoan disease transmitted by the bite of an infected *Anopheles* mosquito and is communicable as long as the mature parasite is present in the circulating blood in sufficient density to infect the vector mosquitoes.

In malaria, there is hemolysis and infected red cells adhere to the capillaries; this results in profound hemolytic anemia during severe or prolonged attacks. In *P falciparum* malaria, red cells containing the parasite adhere to the capillary endothelium in the brain, liver, kidney, lungs and gut causing anoxia which is further aggravated by toxic and antigenic substances released by the rupture of the parasite, causing widespread organ damage.

Genetic disorders like sickle cell disease, thalassemia and G6PD deficiency confer protection against death by *P falciparum* malaria probably due to impaired parasite growth at low oxygen tension.

Clinical features

The severity of the disease depends upon the species of the parasite, patient's state of immunity, intensity of infection and associated conditions like malnutrition. A typical attack comprises:

- cold stage, which manifests with nonspecific initial symptoms like headache, fatigue, myalgia and abdominal discomfort
- hot stage, manifested by classical malarial paroxysms in which fever spikes, chills and rigors occur at regular intervals
- sweating phase, in which fever comes down, and is associated with tachycardia and sometimes delirium; nausea, vomiting and, orthostatic hypotension are common.

There are a few abnormal physical findings in uncomplicated malaria such as mild anemia and a palpable spleen. Splenic enlargement indicates repeated infections. Mild jaundice or petechial hemorrhages can sometimes occur.

Severe falciparum malaria is very dangerous and is associated with a high mortality rate. The main manifestations of falciparum malaria include cerebral involvement, hypoglycemia, renal failure, liver dysfunction, DIC and severe anemia.

Complications of chronic malaria are anemia, splenomegaly, nephropathy, Burkitt's lymphoma and Epstein–Barr virus infection.

Effect of pregnancy on disease

Pregnancy increases the risk of malaria 3–4-fold in women due to altered immunity. Pregnant women with little or no preexisting immunity are at high risk of severe disease. Severe hemolytic anemia and splenomegaly may develop in the second half of pregnancy. Infection with *P falciparum* is most hazardous particularly in primigravida. Women are at particular risk of cerebral malaria, hypoglycemia, pulmonary edema and severe hemolytic anemia.

Effect of disease on pregnancy

Malarial infection itself has a marked immunosuppressive effect. Asymptomatic infection is associated with placental parasitisation. It is a common cause of severe maternal anemia and low birth weight babies; abortion and preterm labour are common. Fetal and perinatal loss have been documented to be as high as 60%–70%.

Diagnosis

It is mainly by demonstration of the parasite in peripheral blood. Both thin and thick smears should be examined. Thick film facilitates the diagnosis of low level parasitemia while thin film is essential to confirm the diagnosis, to identify the species of the parasite and to quantify parasite load. If the smear is negative, it should be repeated after 12 and 48 hours when there is a high index of suspicion. The malarial fluorescent antibody test becomes positive about two weeks or later from primary infection and is therefore not useful in clinical practice but may be useful for epidemiological studies.

Treatment

Several drugs are available and the choice of drug depends on the likely sensitivity of the parasite. According to the drug treatment policy for malaria, under the National Anti-malaria Programme, any fever in endemic areas during transmission season without any other obvious cause may be presumed to be malaria and treated accordingly.

The principles of treatment of malaria during pregnancy are the same as in the nonpregnant state. Chloroquine is the mainstay of treatment; the dosage is as follows:

- day 1: tablet 600 mg
- day 2: tablet 600 mg
- day 3: tablet 300 mg

It is well absorbed when administered orally; the common side effects are nausea, vomiting, headache, dysphoria, pruritus and postural hypotension. It should not be given on an empty stomach. Major toxicity (with the parenteral route) includes cardiac arrhythmia, retinopathy and hypotensive shock. It is safe in pregnancy; there is no evidence of teratogenic effects.

The treatment options for chloroquine-resistant malaria are limited during pregnancy. **Primaquine** should not be given to pregnant women and those with G6PD deficiency. **Tetracycline** and **fansidar** are contraindicated in pregnancy. **Mefloquine** is advocated only in *P falciparum* malaria with proven resistance to chloroquine. **Pyrimethamine** is absorbed well when given orally and is tolerated well: major toxicity includes megaloblastic anemia and pancytopenia. Most authorities agree that it can be safely used in pregnancy. Infection with *P vivax* should be treated with chloroquine or amodiaquine which can be administered in a weekly dose of 300 mg until delivery and a full course of primaquine may be administered after delivery.

Acute falciparum malaria is hazardous both to the mother and to the fetus. Pregnant women with severe and complicated malaria should be hospitalised. Antimalarial therapy should be started immediately along with active treatment of complications like fluid–electrolyte and acid–base imbalance. The regimen is an infusion of quinine sulphate in a dose of 20 mg/kg body weight over four hours, followed eight hours later by 10 mg/kg infusion over four hours. It is desirable to switch to to from oral route at the earliest and the total duration of treatment should be seven days.

Quinine used in therapeutic doses has no abortifacient effect. Quinine and quinidine have been linked to stillbirth and congenital anomalies, but continue to have a place in the treatment of severe malaria.

Artemisinin derivatives, like artemether, which is used in severe, cerebral or chloroquine-resistant malaria, are embryotoxic in animals (no human studies have been conducted). The risks should be overlooked in life-threatening situations.

Prevention

The Government of India launched the National Malaria Control Programme (NMCP) in 1977 to reduce morbidity and mortality. Preventive strategies include regular personal protection (insecticide treated bed nets, insect repellents), vector control and chemoprophylaxis or intermittent preventive treatment with antimalarials.

Recommendations for chemoprophylaxis are as follows:

- Travellers from nonendemic areas should start taking the antimalarial drug at least one week before departure and should continue it for 4–6 weeks after leaving the endemic area.

For pregnant women living in areas where transmission is intense, chemoprophylaxis reduces the risk of severe antenatal anemia in the mother, improves birth weight and decreases perinatal mortality. The drugs used for prophylaxis are:

- **Chloroquine:** 300 mg of base orally once a week
- **Mefloquin:** 250 mg once a week. It is the antimalarial prophylactic agent of choice because it is very effective (90% protection), especially against multidrug-resistant falciparum malaria. It seems to be safe in pregnancy, but it is best to avoid its use during the first trimester.
- **Proguanil:** 200 mg daily combined with chloroquine provides 70% protection. It is safe in pregnancy but folate supplementation is recommended.

Other drugs like maloprim, fansidar, doxycycline and tetracyclines should not be used during pregnancy.

Typhoid Fever

Typhoid fever occurs in all parts of the world where water supply and sanitation are substandard; it is endemic in India.

Etiopathogenesis

The causative organisms are *Salmonella typhi* and paratyphi A and B which are transmitted by the feco-oral route. The average incubation period is 10–14 days. After a few days of bacteremia, the bacilli localise in the lymphatic tissue of the small intestine which swell, ulcerate and then heal and can sometimes perforate.

Clinical features

The patient presents with fever, headache, myalgia, relative bradycardia and constipation; a few days later she may develop diarrhea, cough, abdominal distension, rose spots on the trunk and splenomegaly. If untreated she can develop delirium, intestinal perforation, hemorrhage from the ulcer, pneumonia, cholecystitis, myocarditis, arthritis, meningitis, coma and even death. The course is shorter and milder in paratyphoid fever.

Effect of pregnancy on the disease

The course of the disease is not altered in pregnancy.

Effect of the disease on pregnancy

Salmonella typhi can cross the placenta, resulting in chorioamnionitis. Maternal–fetal infection with *S typhi* can lead to miscarriage, fetal death and neonatal infection. In order to avoid maternal complications and possible fetal transmission, treatment should be initiated at the earliest.

Diagnosis

The diagnosis may be difficult in the first week due to the absence of localising signs. Leucopenia and positive stool or blood culture will confirm the diagnosis. The organisms can be found in feces even after 2–3 weeks. The Widal test becomes positive after one week. However, it is not reliable and should be interpreted with caution, especially in vaccinated patients.

Treatment

Several antibiotics are effective in enteric fever. Third-generation cephalosporins like ceftriaxone and cefotaxime are the preferred first-line drugs; they are taken as 1–2 g, 12 hourly. Resistance to ampicillin and ciprofloxacin is common. Treatment should be continued for 14 days. Even with effective chemotherapy, there is a danger of complications, recrudescence of disease and development of chronic carrier stage.

Prevention

Improved sanitation and living conditions reduce the incidence of typhoid. Travellers to countries where the disease is endemic should be vaccinated. The antityphoid vaccine appears to have no untoward effect on pregnancy.

Dengue Fever

Dengue fever is an arthropod-borne viral disease associated with significant morbidity and mortality; serologic surveys confirm endemicity in India. Epidemics are on the rise due to the growing urban population, poor housing conditions, overcrowding and inadequate sanitation.

Etiopathogenesis

There are four serotypes of dengue viruses: all of these produce similar clinical syndromes. The principal vector is *Aedes aegypti*; it breeds in stagnant water.

Clinical features

The disease varies in severity from being asymptomatic to classical dengue hemorrhagic fever with or without shock. The prodromal phase lasts for about two days with vague symptoms like malaise and fever. This is followed by acute symptoms of fever, headache, arthralgia, generalised pains, anorexia, nausea, vomiting, depression, lymphadenopathy and scleral congestion. Fever, which may be continuous or of saddleback pattern with a break on fourth or fifth day, lasts for 7–8 days. The rash is transient; it is macular and then becomes maculopapular.

Dengue hemorrhagic fever is the severe form and hemorrhagic signs range from minor ones like petechiae, ecchymosis and, epistaxis to major ones like GIT bleeding, DIC and circulatory failure.

Effect of pregnancy on disease

Pregnancy does not alter the course of the disease.

Effect of disease on pregnancy

The incidence of dengue fever during pregnancy has increased due to frequent epidemics. Dengue fever during pregnancy seems to be associated with an increased frequency of low birth weight babies, prematurity and fetal distress.

Diagnosis

Clinical signs with hematological findings of leucopenia and thrombocytopenia are considered sufficient to establish clinical diagnosis. It can be confirmed by recovering the viral antigen from blood.

Management and prevention

The disease is self-limiting and the treatment is symptomatic and supportive. Paracetamol or opiates may be used for pain relief but aspirin should be avoided. Fluid and electrolyte replacement is the mainstay. Blood transfusion may be needed in case of shock.

There is no vaccine and prevention is mainly by abolishing breeding sites of mosquitoes and preventing mosquito bites.

Visceral Leishmaniasis (Kala Azar)

Visceral leishmaniasis (kala azar) is prevalent essentially in eastern India. Leishmaniasis may have visceral, cutaneous or mucocutaneous manifestations.

Etiopathogenesis

Leishmaniasis is caused by the protozoan *Leishmania donovani* and transmitted by the bite of the female phlebotomine sandfly. It is considered a nonzoonotic infection in India where the chief hosts are humans. The incubation period is about 1–2 months. Multiplication of leishmania takes place in macrophages, especially in the liver, spleen, bone marrow and lymphoid tissue. The disease is associated with malnutrition and immunosuppression.

Clinical features

Fever and hepatosplenomegaly are the main presenting symptoms. The onset is generally insidious with low grade fever but may sometimes be abrupt with high intermittent fever. Massive splenomegaly occurs with less marked hepatomegaly. If untreated, the patient becomes anemic and wasted. Cough, diarrhea, lymphadenopathy and dermal leishmaniasis may develop. Acute intercurrent pneumococcal or tuberculous infection is a common complication. Anemia is due to hemolysis, hypersplenism and ineffective erythropoiesis. Hepatocellular damage and bleeding are late complications.

Effect of pregnancy on the disease

The effect of pregnancy on the course of the disease is not known but reactivation of subclinical infection during pregnancy is possible.

Effect of disease on pregnancy

Little information is available regarding the effects of visceral leishmaniasis on pregnancy. Untreated visceral leishmaniasis may be associated with congenital transmission; it is imperative to treat pregnant women for kala azar.

Diagnosis

This can be established by demonstrating the parasite in stained smears of aspirates of the bone marrow, spleen or liver or by culture of these aspirates. The aldehyde test of Napier, caried out on venous blood, is a simple test and is widely used in India for the diagnosis of kala azar. Hematological tests show progressive leucopenia, thrombocytopenia, anemia, raised ESR and reversed albumin-globulin ratio. PCR is helpful in demonstrating the antigen. Antibody can be detected by ELISA, immunofluorescence or direct agglutination test in early disease. The leishmanin test based on the skin reaction to an intradermal injection distinguishes the immune from the nonimmune subject.

Treatment

Pregnancy is not a contraindication to treatment. Amphotericin B is effective in a dose of 2–3 mg/kg (a total of 21–24 mg/kg given in 7 days) but its toxicity and cost are limiting factors. Amphotericin B cures kala azar during pregnancy and is strongly recommended as the drug of choice. Specific treatment with pentavalent antimonials can also be started as soon as the diagnosis is established. Sodium antimony gluconate (pentosan) and, meglumine antimoniate are the drugs preferred in India due to lower cost, efficacy and familiarity. Usually a 10-day course is sufficient; sometimes a 30-day course may be required. The principal side effects of these drugs are myalgia, cardiac toxicity and pancreatitis. There is no report of adverse effects on the fetus by pentavalent antimonials and the risk of progressive deterioration of the mother and congenital transmission are avoided.

Measurement of spleen size, hemoglobin and serum albumin are useful parameters in monitoring.

Prevention

The kala azar control programme was launched in 1990 and the National Health Policy aims to eradicate kala azar by 2010. Early diagnosis and treatment of human infections reduce the reservoir and control epidemics. Serology is useful for case detection in the field. Sandfly control with DDT spray at regular intervals and personal protection play an important role in prevention. There is no vaccine.

Acute Diarrhea

Acute diarrhea is as important as respiratory infections as a cause of morbidity worldwide. It is a major public health problem in India and is common in pregnancy.

Etiopathogenesis

The organisms causing diarrhea are listed below: These are transmitted mainly by the feco-oral route.

- **Viruses:** Rotaviruses, astrovirus, adenovirus, calcivirus, coronavirus, Norwalk group virus, enterovirus
- **Bacteria:** *E coli*, Shigella, Salmonella, *Vibrio cholere*, *Campylobacter jejuni*, *Bacillus cereus*, Listeria.
- **Others:** *E histolytica*, *Giardia intestinalis*, trichuriasis, intestinal worms, Cryptosporidium spp.

Clinical features

Acute diarrhea is defined as the passage of loose, liquid or watery stools for 3–7 days; it is the predominant symptom of acute infective gastroenteritis. If blood is present in stools, the condition is called **dysentery**. Abdominal pain usually accompanies this condition. The patient may be febrile and signs of dehydration like tachycardia and dry tongue may be seen. Systemic examination is otherwise unremarkable. It is rarely fatal in adults but is associated with significant morbidity.

Effect of pregnancy on disease

Pregnancy does not alter the course of the disease.

Effect of disease on pregnancy

Frequent passage of stools with abdominal cramps may manifest as false labour. The risk of preterm labour may be increased. Dehydration and fever, if controlled promptly, should not have any adverse effect on pregnancy. Listeriosis is associated with bacteremia, focal placental infections and sometimes abortions.

Diagnosis

The diagnosis is based on symptoms. Stool microscopy shows the presence of leucocytes or the parasite. Stool culture should be performed to investigate bloody or persistent diarrhea.

Treatment

Maintaining proper fluid and electrolyte balance is the mainstay of treatment. Most cases are self-limiting and only require fluid and salt replacement. Oral rehydration solution (ORS) may be used in mild cases when vomiting is not present. In patients with severe gastroenteritis in pregnancy, hospital admission with intravenous fluid replacement is advised. Antibiotics should be used judiciously. Specific antibiotics should be given when the causative organisms are Shigella (norfloxacin 400 mg 12 hourly for three days), *Vibrio cholere* (ciprofloxacin 500 mg or norfloxacin 400 mg 12 hourly, erythromycin 500 mg 6–8 hourly) or listeria (amoxycillin 500 mg 8 hourly).

Prevention

Since transmission is by the feco-oral route, good personal hygiene and safe drinking water can significantly reduce the incidence.

AMEBIASIS

The term amebiasis has been defined by WHO as the condition of harbouring the protozoan parasite *Entameba histolytica* with or without clinical manifestations. Amebiasis affects about 15% of the Indian population.

Etiopathogenesis

It is caused by *E histolytica* and symptomatic disease occurs in less than 10% of infected individuals. The cysts of *E histolytica* are ingested through water or uncooked food. The incubation period ranges from two weeks to many years. Invasion of the colonic mucosa results in typical ulcers and the clinical syndrome of amebic dysentery. Extraintestinal amebiasis includes amebic liver abscess and cutaneous amebiasis.

Clinical features

Abdominal pain with two or more unformed stools is the common clinical presentation. Acute inflammatory diarrhea is seen in developing nations. There may be tenderness along the colon. In addition to acute and chronic colitis, ameboma can simulate a tumour of the large intestine and cause intussusception. Perforation of amebic ulcer may result in peritonitis.

Effect of pregnancy on disease

Amebic dysentery may take a fulminant course during pregnancy.

Effect of disease on pregnancy

Amebic colitis during pregnancy may present as false labour. Amebic liver abscess is rare, but when it does occur, it carries significant morbidity. It may be associated with preterm labour.

Diagnosis

It mainly depends on demonstration of motile trophozoites on stool microscopy. Sigmoidoscopy may reveal typical ulcers. Antibodies are detected by immunofluorescence in about 95% of cases of hepatic amebiasis and 60% of cases of intestinal amebiasis. Ultrasonography is helpful in the diagnosis of liver abscess.

Treatment

Metronidazole is the mainstay of treatment. It is known to cross the placenta and is teratogenic in animals, but should not be withheld in symptomatic pregnant women. Metronidazole 400 mg or 800 mg 8 hourly orally for five days or tinidazole 2 g daily for three days may be administered. Hepatic amebiasis requires hospitalisation; metronidazole 1.5 g is administered daily for three or more days. Large abscesses can be managed by ultrasound-guided aspiration or may need open drainage.

Prevention

Safe drinking water and thorough washing of vegetables will reduce the incidence.

HELMINTHIASIS

The prevalence of intestinal worm infestation in India varies from 5% to 76%, which is similar to that in other developing countries. These parasitic infestations are acquired by ingestion, inhalation or penetration of the skin by the infective forms.

Hookworm Infestation (Ancylostomiasis)

This is one of the main causes of anemia in tropical countries and is widely prevalent in India.

Etiopathogenesis: It is caused by *Ancylostoma duodenale* (commonly seen in north India) or *Necator americanus* (commonly seen in south India). The incubation period is about seven weeks for *Necator americanus* and five weeks for *Ancylostoma duodenale.* The infective material is feces containing the ova. The infective larva develops in soil and enters the body usually through the feet by penetrating the skin. It reaches the lungs, ascends the bronchi and is then swallowed; it settles in the small intestine. Allergic inflammation is caused at the site of entry (skin) of larva. Pulmonary eosinophilia can occur during passage through the lungs. In the small intestine, it attaches to the mucosa by its buccal capsule and sucks about 0.1 ml of blood daily. Severe or prolonged infection can cause varying degrees of anemia depending on the woman's nutrition.

Clinical features: Morbidity and mortality from hookworm infestation depend on the worm load and the individual's nutritional status. Symptoms are vague and variable like vomiting, epigastric pain and loose stools. Dermatitis may occur. Chronic blood loss and depletion of the body's iron stores lead to iron deficiency anemia; protein-losing enteropathy and hypoproteinemia may occur in malnourished women. High output cardiac failure may result from chronic iron deficiency anemia. Pulmonary eosinophilia may present as paroxysmal cough with blood-stained sputum and patchy pulmonary consolidation.

Pregnancy does not affect the course of the disease. In areas where hookworm infestation is endemic, 90% of pregnant mothers are anemic. Effects on pregnancy are due to anemia and will depend on the severity of anemia.

Diagnosis: Stool examination will show the presence of classical ova.

Management: The treatment of choice is mebendazole 100 mg 12 hourly for three days. It is not teratogenic in humans and routine use is recommended in anemic women. Single-dose treatment with albendazole 400 mg or levamisole 50–150 mg is also effective.

Roundworm Infestation (Ascaris lumbricoides)

It is the most common helminthic infestation. Its prevalence rates are 50%–75% in many Asian countries.

Etiopathogenesis: It is caused by *Ascaris lumbricoides*. It enters the human body as an ovum through contaminated food; the larvae migrate through the lungs and liver via bloodstream and ascend the bronchial tree and are swallowed to reach the intestine.

Clinical features: Intestinal ascariasis causes symptoms ranging from vague abdominal pain to malnutrition. The woman may give a history of passage of worms. The worms have a tendency to aggregate and due to their large size may occasionally cause intestinal obstruction. The tissue migration provokes local and general hypersensitivity reaction with cough and pneumonitis, eosiniphilic granuloma, bronchial asthma and urticaria.

Effect of pregnancy on disease: Pregnancy does not affect the course of the disease.

Effect of disease on pregnancy: There is no significant effect on pregnancy but associated malnutrition can cause problems if severe.

Diagnosis: History of passage of the worm or demonstration of ova in the stool confirms the diagnosis.

Treatment: Treatment is with mebendazole 100 mg 12 hourly for three days or single-dose treatment with albendazole 400 mg, levamisole 150 mg or pyrental palmoate 10 mg/kg body weight up to a maximum of 1 g as single dose.

Prevention of soil-transmitted helminthiasis: Preventing contact with fecally contaminated soil is very important. Adequate sewage disposal, clean drinking water and strict personal hygiene form the basis of control. Periodic deworming may be undertaken in high prevalence areas. Treatment during pregnancy should only be considered in the presence of symptoms.

Filariasis

The infection is widespread in India and lymphatic filariasis is a major public health problem; it is the most common cause of tropical pulmonary eosinophilia.

Etiopathogenesis

The species that cause disease are mainly *Wucheraria bancrofti* and *Brugia malayi*. The larval stage is inoculated by biting mosquitoes or flies, each specific to a particular filarial species. The larva develop into adult worms (2–50 cm long) which, after mating, produce millions of microfilaria (170–320 microns long) that migrate through blood and skin. The adult worm lives in lymphatics and microfilaria circulate in large numbers in blood. The clinical incubation period is 8–16 months but may be longer. An inflammatory response is evoked by the dead worm and microfilaria and secondary infection cause tissue destruction. Toxins released by the worm cause lymphangiectasia. Dilatation of the lymphatic vessels leads to lymphatic dysfunction and chronic clinical manifestations of lymphedema and elephantiasis.

Clinical manifestations

Lymphatic filariasis: The clinical outcome of infections with *Wucheraria bancrofti* and *B malayi* ranges from subclinical infection to hydrocele and elephantiasis. Acute filarial lymphangitis presents with fever, pain, tenderness and erythema along the inflamed lymphatic vessels. The episodes are recurrent and last for a few days. A chronic obstructive lesion develops 10–15 years later due to fibrosis and obstruction of the lymphatic vessels. Progressive enlargement, coarsening, corrugation and fissuring of the skin develops gradually into irreversible elephantiasis. Vulval elephantiasis is a rare manifestation of lymphatic filariasis in women.

Tropical pulmonary eosinophilia: This manifests mainly with paroxysmal cough, wheeze and fever. The chest radiograph shows miliary changes or mottled opacities. If untreated, this progresses to debilitating chronic interstitial lung disease.

Effect of pregnancy on the disease

Pregnancy does not change the course of the disease.

Effect of disease on pregnancy

Microfilariae cross the placenta in less than 10% of pregnancies. Though such transplacental transfer seems to be a rare phenomenon, prenatal exposure to maternal filarial parasite infection may result in cellular hyporesponsiveness in children.

Diagnosis

Clinical features, eosinophilia and positive filarial serology are the mainstay of diagnosis. Microfilaria can be demonstrated in peripheral blood film. Calcified microfilaria may be demonstrated by radiograph. Indirect fluorescence and ELISA detect antibodies in about 95% of active and 70% of chronic cases.

Management

Treatment is aimed at reversing and halting disease progression. Diethylcarbamazine (DEC) is given in a dose of 6 mg/kg body weight daily orally in three divided doses for 12 days. DEC is not associated with any teratogenic effect. Most adverse effects seen during treatment include fever, headache, nausea vomiting and, arthralgia and occur within 24–36 hours of the first dose of DEC. Ivermectin may also be used and a single oral dose of 200–400 µg/kg eliminates the microfilaria from blood. The safety of ivermectin in pregnancy is not established. Albendazole can also be used.

Prevention

As per revised filarial control strategy and WHO recommendations, treatment of the whole population in endemic areas with and annual single dose of DEC 100 mg for adults and 50 mg for children has reduced the disease. The use of DEC-medicated salt is a special form of mass treatment. Mosquito control programmes and personal protection measures are also crucial.

Hydatid Disease

It is an important zoonotic disease in humans and is recognised as a public health problem found in all sheep-raising countries. In India, foci are known to exist with high prevalence reported in Andhra Pradesh and Tamilnadu.

Etiopathogenesis

It is caused by infective larvae of the intestinal tapeworm *Echinococcus granulosus*. It follows a dog–sheep cycle; humans are accidental intermediate hosts. Humans may ingest eggs by handling a dog or drinking contaminated water. The embryo is released in the small intestine and enters the bloodstream to reach the liver. The resultant cyst grows slowly and gives rise to multiple cysts.

Clinical features

The symptoms of hydatid disease manifest several years after exposure. A large hydatid cyst typically causes pressure symptoms depending on the organ involved; the liver is involved in 75% of cases.

Effect of pregnancy on disease

Pregnancy seems to have no effect on the disease.

Effect of disease on pregnancy

A pelvic hydatid cyst can cause obstructed labour or be discovered incidentally during cesarean section.

Diagnosis

History of residence in an endemic area, close association with dogs, and the presence of a slowly growing cystic tumour suggest the diagnosis. Ultrasonography is the mainstay in diagnosis. Complement fixation and ELISA are positive in 70%–90% of cases.

Management

Symptomatic hydatid cyst should be excised surgically wherever possible. Great care should be taken to avoid spillage and cavities should be sterilised with silver nitrate or sodium chloride solution. Anaphylactic shock due to exposure to the fluid in the cyst can be fatal. Albendazole 400 mg 12 hourly for three months is used for inoperable disease and to reduce infectivity preoperatively. Praziquantel 20 mg/kg 12 hourly for 14 days kills protoscolices perioperatively; its teratogenicity is not established.

Prevention

The control of dogs, quality control over slaughter houses and meat inspection are the important steps in prevention.

Travel Medicine

Travel to tropical countries involves the risk of contracting diseases prevalent there.

The commonly recommended vaccinations are against cholera, hepatitis, typhoid, tetanus, tuberculosis and polio. No vaccine or immunoglobulin has established safety in pregnancy, particularly in the first trimester. There must be a clear indication for vaccination and chemoprophylaxis during pregnancy after risks and benefits have been considered. Acute illness, as a result of vaccination or infection, brings with it the risk of preterm labour or in utero infection, and consequent morbidity and mortality. No vaccine is completely effective and live vaccines should be avoided.

KEY POINTS

- Tropical infections have significant impact on the health of pregnant women and the fetus.
- In endemic areas, malaria is an important cause of anemia in pregnancy. The disease is associated with low birth weight babies.
- Severe falciparum malaria during pregnancy can result in maternal death, especially in nonimmune primigravida.
- It is safe to use chloroquine in pregnancy.
- Typhoid fever is a food-borne disease associated with significant maternal and fetal morbidity which can be reduced by early treatment.
- Dengue fever can affect pregnant women during epidemics.
- Prompt treatment of visceral leishmaniasis during pregnancy can prevent progressive maternal deterioration and congenital transmission.
- Diarrheal diseases are common during pregnancy, and associated dehydration and fever can cause problems to both the mother and the fetus.
- Amebic dysentery can take a fulminant course during pregnancy.
- Amebic liver abscess is a possible cause of abdominal pain during pregnancy.
- Hookworm infestation is a major cause of anemia in pregnancy in developing countries.
- Prenatal exposure to filarial infection may increase the risk of infection in childhood.
- Pelvic hydatid cyst is a rare cause of obstructed labour.
- Most drugs used in the treatment of tropical infections fall in categories B or C of pregnancy risk but treatment should not be withheld in severe illness; drugs with less risk should be chosen.
- While travelling to endemic areas, a pregnant woman should be advised to take chemoprophylaxis and vaccination. However, live vaccines should be avoided.

QUESTIONS

Mark true (T) or false (F) against each statement:

1. Pregnancy increases the risk of malaria.
2. Chloroquine is contraindicated in pregnancy.
3. Malaria during pregnancy can result in maternal death.
4. Malaria during pregnancy can cause low birth weight in the neonate.
5. Typhoid fever during pregnancy should be treated with ciprofloxacin.
6. Visceral leishmaniasis may result in vertical transmission to the fetus.
7. Acute diarrhea during pregnancy should always be treated with antibiotics.
8. Hookworm infestation can cause intestinal obstruction.
9. Metronidazole should not be used in the treatment of amebiasis in pregnancy.
10. Hookworm infestation is an important cause of anemia in pregnancy.
11. Hydatid disease does not cause any problems during pregnancy.

54

Epilepsy

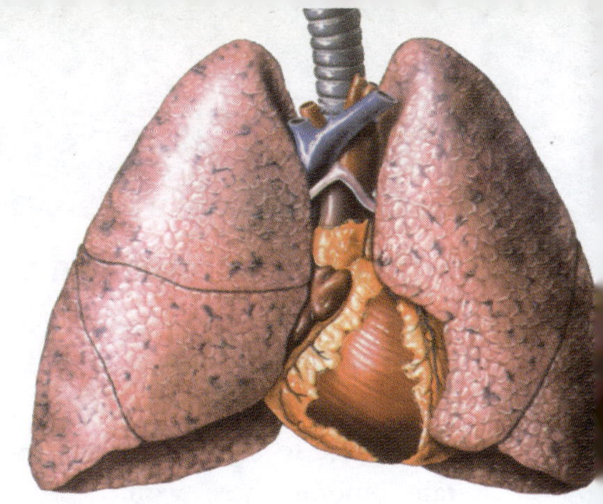

S Habeebullah

LEARNING OBJECTIVES

At the end of this chapter, the reader should be able to:

- recognise that epilepsy is the most common neurological disorder in pregnancy
- describe the reasons for an increased risk of seizures during pregnancy
- list the effects of epilepsy on pregnancy
- enumerate the adverse effects of epilepsy and antiepileptic drugs on the fetus and the baby
- counsel a woman with epilepsy who is planning a pregnancy
- outline the management of an epileptic pregnant woman
- enumerate the commonly used antiepileptic drugs in pregnancy
- advise the woman regarding the use of contraception

Introduction

In India, 2–3 million women suffer from epilepsy; of these, about two-thirds are in the reproductive age group. Considerable advances has been made in the care of epilepsy and more women now tend to bear children. Epilepsy is the most common neurological disorder complicating pregnancy and poses special problems for the mother, the fetus and the neonate. The incidence of epilepsy in pregnancy ranges 0.3%–0.6%. Since most of these pregnancies are unplanned, they pose a challenge to those caring for these women. Optimal maternal and perinatal outcome can be achieved through integrated care by the neurologist and the obstetrician.

Effect of pregnancy on epilepsy

In 50% of women with epilepsy, there is no change in seizure frequency during pregnancy; in about 30%, there is an increase. This is due to vomiting, decreased absorption of drugs, increased metabolic clearance and increased blood volume leading to decreased blood levels of antiepileptic drugs (AED), psychological stress and noncompliance. Prolonged duration of epilepsy (more than five years) is associated with increased seizure frequency during pregnancy. Status epilepticus may occur in 1%–2% and is associated with higher maternal and perinatal mortality.

Effect of epilepsy on pregnancy and delivery

Women with epilepsy are known to have reduced fertility. Polycystic ovarian syndrome (PCOS), premature menopause, hyperprolactinemia and anovulation are also more common in these women.

Epilepsy has minimal effects on the course of pregnancy. In women with epilepsy, there is an increased risk of abortions, preeclampsia and abruption. Though in the majority of women spontaneous labour and delivery occur, increased risk of preterm labour, PROM, APH, stillbirth and cesarean section has been noted.

Effect on the fetus and the neonate

The rates of major malformations are doubled in the infants of mothers with epilepsy. This may be due to epilepsy or AED. The number of drugs and their dosage play a role in causing anomalies. The malformation rate among these women is 4%–6%. These are markedly increased if more than two drugs are used. Valproic acid is associated with a tenfold increase in neural tube defects. A possible explanation for the increased anomalies is genetic predisposition, hypoxia due to repeated convulsions and folic acid deficiency. The most common anomalies are cleft lip and palate, neural tube defects, congenital heart defects like ASD and VSD and fetal antiepileptic syndrome. During convulsions, fetal asphyxia and death can occur. The drugs may cause hemorrhagic disease in the newborn due to vitamin K deficiency. Psychomotor retardation may be seen in infants. The children have an increased risk of epilepsy.

Management

Prepregnancy strategies: Women with epilepsy should be counselled before pregnancy, especially regarding the risk of major and minor anomalies: these are 2–3 times more common in this group. Seizures should be controlled for at least one year before pregnancy is planned. AED with higher risk of fetal malformations should be avoided. One should also consider stopping AED in those with a seizure-free period of 2–3 years. Monotherapy is preferred to multiple drugs and the lowest effective dose should be maintained to reduce the risk of anomalies. Periconceptional folic acid supplementation further reduces the risk of neural tube defects.

Antiepileptic drugs: The choice of AED depends on the type of epilepsy. Most AEDs belong to categories C and D of the FDA classification for the use of drugs during pregnancy. The most commonly used drugs and fetal effects are shown in **Table 54.1**. Valproic acid and newer drugs like lamotrigine, primidone and clonazepam should be avoided. The commonly used drugs are carbamazepine, phenobarbital and phenytoin.

Table 54.1 Commonly used antiepileptics during pregnancy and their potential toxic effects

Drug	Potential fetal/neonatal effects
Carbamazepine	Facial dysmorphism, neural tube defects, hypoplasia of distal phalanges
Phenobarbital	Neonatal withdrawal, neonatal coagulopathy
Phenytoin	Facial clefting, hypoplasia of distal phalanges, hypertelorism, neonatal coagulopathy
Primidone	Neonatal withdrawal, neonatal coagulopathy
Valproic acid	Facial dysmorphism, neural tube defects

The dosage of AED may have to be increased during pregnancy. The AED should be continued throughout pregnancy and labour. The dosage may be reduced to prepregnant levels one week after delivery. Folic acid supplementation with 4 mg/day should be continued and oral vitamin K 10 mg/day should be added in the last four weeks. Alternatively, it may be administered parenterally twice in the last month and during labour.

Labour: Spontaneous labour and vaginal delivery occur in the majority of women. Cesarean section is resorted to only for obstetric indications except in rare cases of uncontrolled convulsions which might jeopardise fetal wellbeing.

Care of the newbom: The newborn should receive a 1 mg injection of vitamin K soon after birth. Breastfeeding should be continued even though all AEDs find their way into breast milk. Lethargy, irritability and feeding difficulties may occur due to exposure to phenobarbital and phenytoin. The babies on artificial feeds may show signs of drug withdrawal.

Contraception: Antiepileptic drugs may reduce the effectiveness of low-dose oral contraceptive pills. Therefore, women with epilepsy are advised to use combined pills with 50 μg ethinyl estradiol instead of 20 μg or 30 μg. Barrier contraceptives and IUCDs may also be recommended.

KEY POINTS

- Epilepsy is the most common neurological disorder affecting pregnancy.
- Increased seizure frequency is seen in one-third of women during pregnancy.
- Increased pregnancy complications and fetal anomalies occur in women with epilepsy.
- Prepregnancy counselling, folic acid supplementation and changing to monotherapy and safer drugs will improve perinatal outcome.
- The newborn should be given vitamin K.
- If OCPs are considered for contraception, pills with 50 μg ethinyl estradiol should be recommended.

QUESTIONS

Select the single most appropriate answer:

1. Which of the following statements regarding pregnancy with epilepsy is *not* correct?
   a. seizure frequency increases in 90% of women
   b. there is increased frequency of fetal anomalies
   c. periconceptional folic acid should be given
   d. the newborn should get vitamin K injection
2. Which one of the following anticonvulsants is associated with an increased risk of fetal neural tube defects?
   a. phenobarbitone
   b. carbamazepine
   c. phenytoin
   d. sodium valproate
3. A pregnant woman with epilepsy is at an increased risk of
   a. abortion
   b. preeclampsia
   c. preterm delivery
   d. placental abruption

In the following questions, there are two statements. Select the appropriate answer using the following key:

a. if both statements are true and causally related
b. if both statements are true but not causally related
c. if the first statement is true and the second is false
d. if the first statement is false and the second is true
e. if both statements are false

4. Women on antiepileptic drugs should be advised not to take oral contraceptive pills *because*

   Antiepileptic drugs reduce the efficacy of oral contraceptive pills.
5. The rate of congenital malformation is doubled in women with epilepsy *because*

   In women with epilepsy, antiepileptic drugs and hypoxia during convulsions act as teratogens.

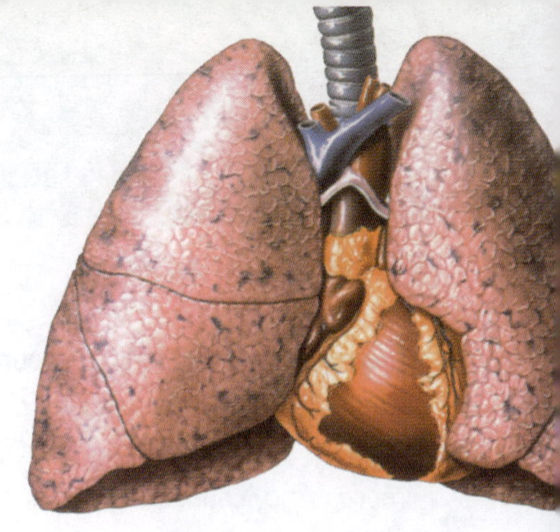

55

Psychiatric Disorders

R Raguram

LEARNING OBJECTIVES

At the end of this chapter, the reader should be able to:

- appreciate the behavioural and mental changes of the mother during pregnancy and puerperium
- identify psychiatric disorders associated with pregnancy and puerperium
- understand the issues involved in treating mentally ill women during pregnancy and lactation
- evaluate the role and safety of various psychotropic drugs in pregnant or lactating women
- establish an effective liaison with psychiatrists to initiate a comprehensive care plan for women with psychological problems during this period

Introduction

For many couples, the confirmation of pregnancy is accompanied by an overwhelming sense of excitement as they await the arrival of their baby. Even when the pregnancy has been carefully planned, there is a sense of wonder and surprise. However, mixed with these feelings, there are doubts and apprehensions about the major impending change in their lives. The unknown direction that a new life takes is both thrilling and scary for the new parents. It generates a cascade of emotional, psychological and social changes that affect a woman in many ways. Even though pregnancy is often considered to have a protective effect on the course of psychiatric illness, in reality it may exacerbate psychiatric disorders and adversely impact the emotional wellbeing of the individual. There is growing evidence that psychological problems during pregnancy and puerperium can cause significant morbidity for the mother, in addition to having an adverse impact on the development of the child.

PSYCHIATRIC DISORDERS DURING PREGNANCY

During pregnancy, a woman is likely to experience emotional changes. Some may also suffer from mood disorders.

Mood Disorders

Major depression

The most common mood disorder during pregnancy is major depression.

- 70% of pregnant women report experiencing at least one depressive symptom.
- Approximately 10% of them fulfill the criteria for the diagnosis of a major depressive episode.
- Two-thirds of women with a history of depression experience a depressive episode during pregnancy, especially when they discontinue treatment.
- Many women are likely to experience their first depressive episode during pregnancy.

Diagnostic features:

Major depression is characterised by:

- abnormal depressed mood
- loss of interest and pleasure
- appetite or weight disturbance: either weight loss or decrease in appetite; rarely weight gain or increase in appetite
- sleep disturbance, either insomnia or hypersomnia
- activity disturbance, either agitation or slowing
- excessive fatigue or loss of energy
- self-reproach or guilt
- poor concentration or indecisiveness
- morbid thoughts of death and suicidal ideas.

A diagnosis of major depression is made if at least **five** of these symptoms are continuously present for a two-week period. **Depression during pregnancy is frequently missed**. There are two main reasons for it. Firstly, the pregnant woman may manifest symptoms like low energy, fatigue and sleep disturbances, found in depression, but these are viewed as being 'normal problems' of pregnancy. Secondly, some medical disorders commonly seen during pregnancy like anemia and gestational diabetes may also have features suggestive of depression and lead to diagnostic confusion. However, the presence of features like anhedonia, guilt and suicidal ideation strongly indicate the presence of major depression.

Risk of untreated depression:

In the mother:

- risk of self-injurious or suicidal behaviour
- inadequate attention to nutrition
- poor compliance with antenatal care
- greater susceptibility to smoking or drinking alcohol

For the child:

- greater incidence of premature birth
- low birth weight
- smaller head circumference
- lower Apgar score
- children of depressed mothers are more prone to developing conduct problems and emotional instability later in life

The relationship between poor pregnancy outcome and depression becomes stronger when the mother is depressed during the late second to early third trimester. Depression during pregnancy also significantly increases the risk of postpartum depression.

Risk factors for antenatal depression

- history of affective illness
- marital discord or dissatisfaction
- inadequate psychosocial support
- recent adverse life events
- unwanted pregnancy

Bipolar Disorder

This condition is characterised by recurrent episodes of depression and mania. In the latter, there is a distinct period of abnormally and persistently elevated, expansive or irritable mood lasting for at least one week. In addition, at least three of the following symptoms should be present:

- inflated self-esteem or grandiosity
- decreased need for sleep
- more talkative than usual or pressure to keep talking
- flight of ideas or subjective experience that thoughts are racing
- distractibility (that is, attention too easily drawn to unimportant or irrelevant external stimuli)
- increase in non–goal-directed activity or agitation
- excessive involvement in pleasurable activities that have a high potential for painful consequences (such as unrestrained buying sprees, sexual indiscretions or foolish business investments).

The incidence of bipolar disorders in pregnancy is unknown. However, during pregnancy, there is a high risk of relapse in patients who have an established diagnosis of this disorder. Bipolar disorders cause a significant amount of distress and dysfunction and are often accompanied by substance abuse. There is also a significantly increased suicidal risk in these patients. Hence, accurate diagnosis and prompt treatment is very important in these disorders.

Schizophrenia

Schizophrenia is a severe and persistent mental illness characterised by the presence of two or more of the following symptoms for at least a month:

- delusions which are multiple, fragmented and bizarre
- hallucinations of commenting or commanding nature
- disorganised speech which is incoherent
- catatonic motor symptoms
- negative symptoms like apathy, avolition and amotivation.

The most common initial age of onset of schizophrenia is in the reproductive stage. There is little information about this disorder and its course during pregnancy. However, it is known that women who have schizophrenia experience more obstetric complications and are significantly more likely to deliver a low-birth-weight child. Maternal schizophrenia is also associated with high rates of perinatal death. The illness could impair a woman's ability to obtain appropriate and necessary prenatal care and may impede her ability to cooperate with caregivers during delivery.

Anxiety Disorders

Anxiety symptoms occur in at least one-third of women during pregnancy. The anxiety may be generalised or may occur in episodes as **panic attacks**. Predominant symptoms include nervousness, tremulousness, sweating, palpitations, nausea and dizziness together with an overwhelming sense of dread or apprehension. Occasionally, the woman may present with **phobias**: fears that are out of proportion to real risk, leading to avoidance of the feared object or situation. **Tokophobia** is the specific fear of labour and delivery.

Obsessive compulsive disorders are not uncommon during pregnancy. They are characterised by the presence of intrusive, unwelcome, anxiety-provoking thoughts which recur repeatedly in spite of resistance. Sometimes they are accompanied by compulsive motor acts often involving repeated cleaning or checking.

Despite their frequent occurrence, there is very limited information about the incidence and course of various anxiety disorders during pregnancy. However, it is known is that in women who report increased levels of anxiety during pregnancy, the symptoms continue during the postnatal period. It has also been suggested that the presence of anxiety disorders during late pregnancy is predictive of slow mental development in two-year-old children.

Adjustment Disorders

These are states of intense emotional distress often occurring in response to significant stressors. They may be associated with unwanted pregnancy or other major changes like separation from the partner. Often, there is an admixture of anxiety and depressive symptoms which are of mild intensity. These are usually transient and the symptoms abate with changes in the life situation of the woman.

Emotional Changes Associated with Pregnancy Loss

Early loss of pregnancy is common, occurring in about 12%–15% of pregnancies.

The grieving reaction of women to miscarriage will depend on the meaning of the loss to her. For most women, conception itself is a major event and loss of pregnancy is more than just loss of the product of conception. It can trigger off doubts about competence in procreation. The grieving process typically proceeds through several stages: initial shock followed by numbness, pining for the lost object, anger, acceptance and finally resolution. The psychological turmoil is intense in the first few weeks after the loss and resolves gradually in most women. However, it can persist in some women with superadded symptoms of depression and anxiety. One of the strongest predictors of prolonged or complicated grief is a previous episode of depression. Repeated miscarriages and lack of social support, especially from the partner, are added risks. Understandably, desirability of the pregnancy is an important determinant of the grieving process.

Substance Abuse

Substance abuse during pregnancy is often under-recognised. There has been a steady increase in substance abuse among women and it is not uncommon during pregnancy. Though a wide array of substances is often abused, alcohol deserves special attention.

Alcohol abuse during pregnancy

Women often drink alone, drink smaller quantities and binge less often. The progress from use to abuse is much faster in women. It has often been observed that women with multiple roles (for example, a mother who also works outside the house) are less likely to abuse alcohol. Approximately 14%–22% of women report drinking alcohol during pregnancy. There is no established safe level of alcohol consumption during pregnancy. Even low levels of prenatal exposure can affect the fetus.

Effect on the fetus: Drinking during pregnancy is associated with major neuro-developmental and other birth defects. **Fetal alcohol syndrome** (FAS) has been reported in the offspring of alcoholic mothers and includes features of gross physical retardation with onset prenatally and continuing after birth. At least one characteristic from each of the following three categories has to be present for a valid diagnosis of the syndrome:

- growth retardation before and/or after birth
- facial anomalies, including small palpebral fissures, indistinct or absent philtrum, epicanthic folds, flattened nasal bridge, short nose, thin upper lip, low-set, unparallel ears and retarded midfacial development
- central nervous system dysfunction including microcephaly, varying degrees of mental retardation or other evidence of abnormal neurobehavioural development, such as attention deficit disorder with hyperactivity.

None of these features is individually pathognomonic for fetal alcohol exposure. Confirmatory evidence for this diagnosis is a history of heavy maternal drinking during pregnancy.

Alcohol-related neurodevelopmental disorder (ARND) refers to the appearance of several signs of brain damage in the absence of other indications of fetal alcohol syndrome. These include malformations and dysplasias of the heart, bone, kidneys and vision or hearing systems.

Detection of alcohol abuse during pregnancy: In light of the significant adverse effects of alcohol on the growing fetus, it is mandatory to recognise alcohol abuse in pregnancy early. Pregnant and postpartum women who abuse alcohol or other drugs experience considerable degree of stigma and therefore may deny their habit. A skillful and empathic enquiry is essential for detecting and resolving these problems.

PSYCHIATRIC DISORDERS DURING PUERPERIUM

The puerperal period is clearly a time of increased vulnerability to psychiatric illnesses in women. Although postpartum psychiatric disorders were initially conceptualised as being distinctly different from other types of psychiatric illnesses, the two groups are clinically indistinguishable.

Postpartum Blues

In the initial week after delivery, many women experience a brief period of affective instability, commonly referred to as **postpartum blues or maternity blues**. As many as 50%–85% of mothers experience postpartum blues. It begins 3–5 days after delivery, peaks between days 5 and 7 and usually subsides by the end of the second week. Some women with severe blues may go on to develop postpartum depression. The prominent symptoms are dysphoric mood, lability of emotions, tearfulness, irritability and exaggeration of dependency needs. It may be appropriate to consider this as a normal experience associated with childbirth rather than as a psychiatric disorder.

Postpartum Depression

In contrast to postpartum blues, postpartum depression is more pervasive and significantly interferes with a mother's ability to function and take care of the child.

It occurs in 10%–15% of women. Onset is usually within four weeks of delivery. Clinical features of this disorder are indistinguishable from that of major depression. Women often express ambivalent or negative feelings towards the infant and are doubtful about their ability to care for them. Anxiety symptoms may be prominent. Often, there are intrusive, obsessive ruminations of a violent nature involving the child, like thoughts of smothering the child or throwing the child down.

Table 55.1 outlines the main differences between postpartum blues and postpartum depression.

Screening for postpartum depression

Despite multiple contacts with medical professionals during the postpartum period, patients and caregivers often overlook postpartum affective illness. Often, postpartum depression is dismissed as a normal or natural consequence of childbirth. Women commonly report the persistence of depressive symptoms for many months before the initiation of treatment. Although symptoms of depression may remit spontaneously, many women are even depressed a year after childbirth.

It is difficult to predict who is at risk of postpartum psychiatric illness. Risk factors for the development of postpartum depression include:

- history of major depression
- previous occurrence of postpartum depression
- depressive symptoms during pregnancy
- family history of depression
- marital difficulties
- ambivalence about the pregnancy
- limited social support
- stressful life events.

Postpartum Psychosis

Puerperal psychosis is a rare event, occurring in 1–2 per 1000 women after childbirth. Its presentation is often dramatic; symptoms set in within the first few days of delivery. Most commonly, it is an affective illness, usually a bipolar disorder. The symptoms closely resemble those of a rapidly evolving manic or mixed episode. The earliest signs are restlessness, agitation, irritability and sleep disturbances. Often there is rapid shifting of mood, disorientation, confusion and disorganised behaviour. Delusional beliefs are common and focus on the baby. Auditory hallucinations instructing the mother to harm herself or the child are sometimes present. Risk of infanticide as well as suicide is high.

Problems in the Mother–Infant Relationship

The most important aspect of childbirth is the development of a close relationship between the mother and the child. Sometimes there may be disruptions in this process. Disturbances in the

Table 55.1 Differences between postpartum blues and postpartum depression

Characteristic	Postpartum blues	Postpartum depression
Incidence	50%–80%	10%–15%
Onset	3–5 days after delivery	Within 3–6 months
Duration	Days to weeks	Months to years (if untreated)
Associated stressors	No	Yes (especially lack of support)
Sociocultural influence	No	Yes
History of mood disorder	No association	Strong association
Tearfulness	Yes	Yes
Sleep disturbance	Sometimes	Almost always
Suicidal thoughts	No	Almost always
Thoughts of harming the baby	Rarely	Often

mother–infant relationship occur in 10%–25% of women. In extreme cases, there might even be total rejection of the child. Often there is a wish that the child could disappear, accompanied by neglect in caring for the child. It could lead to child abuse and long-term psychiatric sequelae in children. Impairments in bonding may not be the result of depression alone. Frequently, there is marital disharmony and significant psychopathology in the mother.

Anxiety Disorders

Sometimes, mothers can feel extremely anxious about the care and welfare of the infant. Many become excessively preoccupied with the health and safety of the newborn. The main manifestation is one of nocturnal vigilance. The mother lies awake listening to the infant's breathing and often keeps checking as to what is happening to the child. This can last for months, leading to sleep deprivation, irritability and labile mood. This could be a major problem in women who are psychologically unprepared for the arrival of the child and who themselves are unduly health conscious. It may be accentuated in isolated, nuclear families. Support from close family members or nursing staff is required to address the problem.

Management of Psychiatric Disorders During Pregnancy and Puerperium

The importance of involving a psychiatrist in the management of these disorders cannot be overemphasised.

Planning and initiation of management

In order to plan and initiate an effective treatment for patients, the clinician has to address several questions:

- Does the patient have a diagnosable psychiatric disorder or a transient psychological reaction?
- If she has a psychiatric problem, what kind of disorder is it? Is it a depressive or anxiety disorder or a psychotic illness?
- Does she require treatment for the problem? This may require active consideration, especially in managing psychiatric illnesses during the first trimester.
- If she requires treatment, can it be handled through non-pharmacological intervention strategies? Non-pharmacological therapies may eliminate or minimise the need for medications in handling anxiety or depressive disorders.
- Is pharmacotherapy indicated?

Non-pharmacologic treatment methods

Until recently there was a paucity of data on the role of non-pharmacological treatment in the management of psychiatric disorders during pregnancy and puerperium. Since pharmacological treatment during this period is associated with some risk, it is important to consider the role of these options before initiating drug treatment. They not only provide symptom relief but also enhance the individual's coping mechanism and facilitate better adaptation.

- **Supportive psychotherapy:** This is particularly useful in handling adjustment disorders and grief and can also complement other intervention strategies to address common psychological problems during pregnancy and puerperium.
- **Cognitive behaviour therapy:** This is a very useful treatment method to handle mild to moderate degrees of depression and anxiety states. It is based on the concept that changing negative thinking patterns can have a powerful effect on influencing the emotional state of the person. The dysfunctional thinking patterns are identified and, the therapist guides the patient to restructure them in a rational, reality-oriented fashion.
- **Interpersonal therapy:** This is a short-term intervention and is being increasingly used in the management of depression during pregnancy and puerperium. The interpersonal therapy approach focuses on the mother's past and present relationships, including the relationship with her own mother, and helps her to relate problematic aspects of these relationships to her current depression.

General principles of pharmacotherapy during pregnancy and puerperium

1. A drug is chosen based on evidence.
2. The guidelines for the use of the drug are considered. Most psychotropic medications are included in category C. No psychotropic drug is classified as being absolutely safe during pregnancy (group A).
3. The woman and the relatives are counselled about the known benefits and risks.
4. A drug that the woman has already been exposed to and to which there has been a good response in the past is chosen.
5. The lowest effective dose is used. It must be remembered though, that to maintain serum levels within the therapeutic range, particularly in the third trimester, the dose of some drugs like antidepressants should be increased 1.5 times the mean doses required when the patient is not pregnant.
6. The treatment decisions are individualised to the needs of the particular patient.

Evaluating the risks and benefits for the use of medication during pregnancy

Risks: All currently available psychopharmacologic agents and their metabolites cross the placenta. They can potentially affect the fetus in three different ways:

- **Structural teratogenesis** causes organ malformations.
- **Perinatal syndromes** refer to a spectrum of physical and behavioural symptoms observed in the infant immediately after delivery which are attributed to drug exposure during pregnancy. Usually they take the form of withdrawal symptoms from a particular drug.
- **Behavioural teratogenicity** refers to the potential of psychotropic drugs to cause long-term neurobehavioural sequelae.

Benefits: Though the benefits are difficult to discern, they are increasingly becoming a focus of interest.

Psychotropic drugs and breastfeeding

All psychotropic medications are excreted in breast milk in varying amounts and are passed on to the nursing infant. Thus, when pharmacotherapy is indicated for a lactating woman, the potential risks of medication exposure has to be weighed against the risk of untreated mental illness in the mother and its impact on infant attachment and development. The aim is to safeguard the mental health of the mother while ensuring the wellbeing of the infant.

PLANNING MENTAL HEALTH CARE DURING PREGNANCY AND PUERPERIUM: IMPLICATIONS FOR PRACTICE

Concepts of motherhood and the expectations associated with it vary according to the cultural context. For instance in many parts of India, the postpartum period is considered as a phase of extreme vulnerability and women and the neonates are largely confined to the home. In addition, various dietary and lifestyle modifications take place during these periods, which are largely influenced by cultural beliefs concerning pregnancy and motherhood. The descriptions and labels used to describe psychological changes during this period, as well as the help-seeking behaviour, are all linked to sociocultural attitudes towards these problems. When mental illness itself is enmeshed in a considerable degree of stigma, emotionally disturbed mothers would find it exceedingly difficult to voice their distress or seek appropriate help. Hence, in planning appropriate mental health care for women during pregnancy and puerperium, it is essential to move beyond the traditional and restrictive focus on clinically diagnosable disorders and address the larger sociocultural dimensions of the problem as well. One way to do this is to pay attention to these issues during prenatal and postpartum appointments.

Unfortunately during these visits, hardly any attention is paid to the psychological dimension. There could be many reasons for such an omission: lack of time, pressure of work and poor exposure to psychological aspects during training. Raising levels of awareness and enhancing the skills within the profession are of vital importance. It must be remembered that one will not make women depressed by asking them how they feel! But whoever asks this question needs to feel comfortable and confident that they can handle the response! An effective liaison with mental health professionals is crucial for early identification and initiation of appropriate care for women during this critical period in their lives.

Appropriate management of psychiatric disorders during pregnancy and puerperium:

- minimises the morbidity associated with the illness
- enhances the quality of life of women during these critical periods
- facilitates adherence to prenatal care programmes
- improves positive pregnancy outcome
- reduces the occurrence of neonatal complications
- sets the stage for the development of an effective mother–child relationship
- promotes a closer empathic bonding between the mother and the child
- increases the capacity for effective parenting
- minimises negative mental health outcome and facilitates optimal infant development.

KEY POINTS

- Pregnancy is a state of significant psychological changes.
- These may range from simple mood changes to severe psychosis.
- The disorders may be missed or diagnosed late.
- Psychiatric disorders have a significant effect on the mother and the fetus.
- Early intervention can minimise adverse effects.
- Non-pharmacological treatment has an important role.
- The caregivers should be conscious of possible psychological problems and seek psychiatric consultation early.

QUESTIONS

Select the single most appropriate answer:

1. In postpartum blues, the treatment of choice is
   a. reassurance and family support
   b. antidepressants
   c. electroconvulsive therapy
   d. lithium
2. The organic cause of postpartum psychosis is
   a. past history of affective disorders
   b. drug reactions, for example, scopolamine or barbiturates
   c. exhaustion
   d. Sheehan syndrome
3. Which of the following statements is *not* true?
   a. pregnancy may have a protective effect on the course of a psychiatric illness
   b. psychiatric illnesses have no effect on the health of the fetus
   c. some psychiatric illnesses may worsen in pregnancy
   d. there are several emotional changes during pregnancy
4. The most common psychiatric mood disorder in pregnancy is
   a. schizophrenia c. mania
   b. bipolar disorder d. depression
5. Diagnostic features of depression include the following except
   a. mania c. excessive sleep
   b. loss of interest d. guilt
6. Inflated self-esteem or grandiosity is usually indicative of
   a. depression c. mania
   b. anxiety d. bipolar disorder
7. Schizophrenia *may not be* associated with
   a. negative symptoms like apathy
   b. hallucinations and delusions
   c. excessive sleep
   d. disorganised speech
8. Panic attacks are characteristic of
   a. depression c. mania
   b. anxiety disorders d. schizophrenia
9. Recurrent, intrusive, unwelcome and anxiety-provoking thoughts occur in
   a. obsessive compulsive disorder
   b. depression

c. schizophrenia
d. bipolar disorder

10. Adjustment disorders include all of the following *except*
    a. alcoholism
    b. grief
    c. drug dependence
    d. delusions

11. Which of the following statements about postpartum blues is not true?
    a. it is very common
    b. labile emotions may be a feature
    c. it may persist even months after delivery
    d. dependency or attention seeking may be exaggerated

12. Postpartum depression
    a. may not have stressors
    b. can persist for months or years
    c. may not be associated with a mood disorder
    d. may not produce suicidal thoughts

56

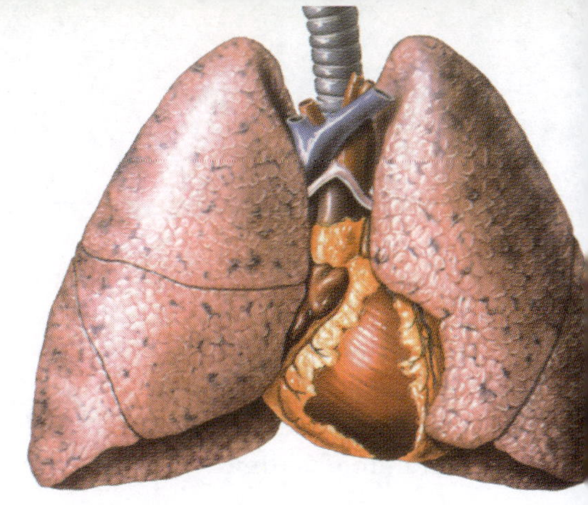

Diseases of the Liver

Asmita Rathore

LEARNING OBJECTIVES

At the end of this chapter, the reader should be able to:

- describe the important changes in the hepatobiliary system during pregnancy
- interpret the liver function tests during pregnancy
- list the diagnostic features of common liver diseases specific to pregnancy
- outline the management of these diseases
- detect and outline the management of liver diseases like acute viral hepatitis and fulminant hepatic failure during pregnancy
- manage pregnancy in women with chronic liver disease
- list the salient clinical features of acute cholecystitis and biliary tract calculous disease and outline the principles of management

Introduction

Liver dysfunction during pregnancy may be due to conditions that are specific to pregnancy or to liver diseases that occur coincidentally during pregnancy. The interaction between the physiologic changes induced by pregnancy and the pathophysiologic changes of liver disease is complex. Liver disease in pregnancy poses a challenge to the treating physician because of several diagnostic possibilities and the substantial maternal and fetal risk. A multidisciplinary approach can help optimise the outcome.

The liver in normal pregnancy

The hepatobiliary system undergoes physiological changes during pregnancy but there is no gross change in the morphology of the liver. Spider nevi and palmar erythema may occasionally be seen during pregnancy; they disappear after delivery.

Liver function tests in pregnancy

It is important to understand the changes in biochemical liver function tests (LFT) during pregnancy to interpret the results correctly. The alterations in the functions are depicted in **Table 56.1**.

LIVER DISORDERS SPECIFIC TO PREGNANCY

These disorders occur for the first time during pregnancy and often recur in subsequent pregnancies. They include intrahepatic cholestasis of pregnancy (IHCP), acute fatty liver of pregnancy (AFLP), PIH, HELLP syndrome and hyperemesis gravidarum.

Intrahepatic Cholestasis of Pregnancy

Intrahepatic cholestasis of pregnancy (IHCP) or recurrent jaundice of pregnancy is a condition peculiar to pregnancy.

Table 56.1 Changes in liver function tests in pregnancy

Unchanged
Serum bile acids Prothrombin time Coagulation tests
Increased
Alkaline phosphatase Globulins Lipids: Cholesterol, triglycerides, VLDL Ceruloplasmin
Decreased
Serum bilirubin Aminotransferases (AST/ALT) Albumin

Etiopathogenesis

The exact etiopathogenesis is not known. Genetic factors play an important role with a suggestion of a Mendelian dominant pattern and probably involve mutations in genes that code for the bile acid transporter protein. Estrogen appears to be the main provoking factor in genetically susceptible women. Incomplete clearance of bile acids by the liver and inefficient canalicular transport result in raised level of bile acids. The fetus too is affected because of disturbed fetal-to-maternal transfer of bile acid across the placenta resulting in accumulation of bile acids which are toxic to the fetus.

The histological features of IHCP are mild cholestasis with bile plugs in centrilobular hepatocytes and canaliculi without inflammation or necrosis.

Clinical features

The most common presenting symptom is pruritus without rash. Usually the patients present in the third trimester of pregnancy. Women may complain of dark urine but very few develop jaundice. Anorexia, malaise, epigastric discomfort, steatorrhea and insomnia are other symptoms. The illness resolves very soon after delivery. Family history is present in 50% of cases. Multiple pregnancies increase the severity of disease. It is not associated with permanent liver damage.

Effect on the mother and fetus

This condition has no deleterious effects on the mother but fetal prognosis is poor as the fetus is unable to eliminate the bile acids transferred across the placenta. The fetus is at risk of prematurity, sudden intrauterine death, peripartum hemorrhage, and fetal distress during labour. The mother may be at increased risk of postpartum hemorrhage, probably due to prolongation of prothrombin time.

Diagnosis

Diagnosis is based on the presence of pruritus and elevated levels of serum bile acids in an otherwise healthy pregnant woman. The serum bile acid concentration increases 10- to 100-fold and is the most specific test. Alkaline phosphatase is raised and the transaminases are normal or moderately raised. Prolongation of prothrombin time is due to vitamin K deficiency and is easily corrected by replacement.

Differential diagnosis

Pruritic skin diseases, viral hepatitis and other causes of jaundice should be considered.

Management

In the presence of IHCP, the pregnancy should be managed as a high-risk one. The goals of management are relief of pruritus, correction of coagulopathy, fetal surveillance and delivery at 37–38 weeks to prevent sudden intrauterine death.

Ursodeoxycholic acid (UDCA) is currently the first choice of therapy. It is effective in improving symptoms, liver function and probably fetal prognosis. UDCA reduces bile acid content in both maternal and fetal compartments. The dose is 1,000 mg/day for 7–10 weeks or till delivery.

Cholestyramine also effectively relieves itching. It is a nonabsorbable anion exchange resin that binds bile acids and fat-soluble vitamins. The maximum dose is 20 g/day. Both drugs are considered safe in pregnancy, but have not been approved for use in pregnancy. The most serious side effect is prolongation of prothrombin time; hence women taking this drug should be given vitamin K 10 mg orally daily from week 36 till delivery. The mother should be monitored weekly for liver function and clotting tests.

Fetal surveillance should be started once diagnosis of IHCP is made; pregnancy should be terminated by 37–38 weeks of gestation to avoid sudden intrauterine death. The incidence of fetal distress is higher in labour, and in 40% of cases meconium is passed. The neonate should be administered injection 1 mg vitamin K to prevent intracranial hemorrhage.

Women with IHCP are prone to postpartum hemorrhage and one should take measures to prevent PPH. They should be warned that the chances of recurrence are high in a subsequent pregnancy.

Acute Fatty Liver of Pregnancy

Acute fatty liver of pregnancy (AFLP) is considered a rare disease with high mortality. However, early diagnosis and management have improved the outcome.

Pathogenesis

Current evidence suggests that most patients with AFLP have partial defects in fatty acid oxidation. These mothers have point mutations in the gene that controls the enzyme, long chain 3 hydroxyacyl-CoA dehydrogenase (LCHAD), involved in the beta oxidation of fatty acids. Stressful situations such as pregnancy can reveal latent deficiencies of fatty acid metabolism in a heterozygous mother. When such women become pregnant with a fetus who is homozygous for LCHAD deficiency, fatty acids from the fetal liver traverse the placenta to reach the mother and overburden her capacity for fatty acid oxidation, resulting in marked fatty infiltration of the liver in the third trimester. Estrogens further suppress fatty acid oxidation and increase VLDL secretion by the liver.

The liver is small and yellow on gross presentation. Histological changes in AFLP are characterised by microvesicular fatty infiltration (more marked in centrilobular areas; the hepatocyte nuclei remain central). It is commonly accompanied by intrahepatic cholestasis.

Clinical features

The women are obese and in the third trimester of pregnancy. The initial symptoms are anorexia, nausea, headache and fatigue followed by jaundice, abdominal pain localised to the right upper quadrant and vomiting. As the disease worsens, mental confusion, disseminated intravascular coagulation (DIC), renal failure with azotemia, hypoglycemia, coma and death may occur. The risk of perinatal mortality rises with the quantity of fat, elevation in serum uric acid and reduction in platelet count. The disease may recur in subsequent pregnancies.

Effect on the mother and fetus

The maternal and fetal effects on pregnancy are due to hepatic dysfunction. Maternal mortality may occur in up to 25% cases and perinatal mortality is even higher. There is an increased incidence of preterm labour, both spontaneous and induced.

Diagnosis

Clinical features and liver function tests help in the diagnosis. There is moderate elevation in serum bilirubin (generally up to 10 mg/dl) and aminotransferases, and a marked rise in serum alkaline phosphatase. Serum ammonia is elevated even in early disease and may be up to ten times higher in comatose patients; this is considered characteristic of AFLP. Increased serum uric acid levels in the absence of hypertension is strongly suggestive of AFLP. Coagulation tests are abnormal with prolonged prothrombin time (PT) and partial thromboplastin time (PTT). Thrombocytopenia and reduced antithrombin activity precede the onset of disease and may be useful for identifying women at risk of AFLP. Total leucocyte count may be increased to 30,000/mm^3. Blood smear may show evidence of intravascular hemolysis with presence of schistocytes, burr cells and normoblasts. Levels of fibrinogen and antithrombin III are reduced with an increase in fibrin degradation products.

Differential diagnosis

It can be differentiated from HELLP syndrome by the markedly raised serum ammonia levels, which is rare in HELLP.

Fulminant hepatic failure (FHF) may be confused with AFLP in some cases, but in FHF, abdominal pain is absent and transaminases are markedly elevated without a significant increase in alkaline phosphatase and uric acid.

Management

Once diagnosis is established, aggressive therapy should be started. Maternal hypoglycemia and acidosis should be corrected. Fresh frozen plasma, platelets and red blood cells are administered to correct coagulopathy, and PT and PTT are monitored. Lactulose can be given to patients with hepatic encephalopathy. Intensive care facilities should be available.

Once the patient is stabilised, delivery should be accomplished promptly. Cesarean section can be performed if vaginal delivery is not accomplished in a reasonable time, and if the maternal condition deteriorates or for an obstetric indication. Despite treatment, liver disease may progress and liver transplantation may be considered if appropriate.

Infants born to mothers with AFLP may have LCHAD deficiency and may be screened for it. Recurrence in subsequent pregnancies depends on the LCHAD status of the fetus.

Pregnancy-induced Hypertension

Pregnancy-induced hypertension (PIH) is the most common cause of hepatic dysfunction during pregnancy. Hepatic dysfunction is considerable in HELLP syndrome. The clinical features, effects on pregnancy and management are mainly those of PIH rather than liver disease and details are dealt with in the chapter on PIH (see Chapter 52).

Hyperemesis Gravidarum

Hyperemesis gravidarum is a severe and intractable form of vomiting in pregnancy, in which the liver and brain may be affected when the condition is very severe. The liver function tests show serum bilirubin rarely exceeding 5 mg/dl and a less than fivefold elevation of transaminases. Alkaline phosphatase and prothrombin time are usually normal (see Chapter 38).

LIVER DISEASES COINCIDENTAL TO PREGNANCY

Acute Viral Hepatitis

Viral hepatitis is the most common cause of jaundice in pregnancy.

Pathogenesis

Several viruses are known to cause acute hepatitis; the main ones are hepatitis viruses A, B, C, D and E. The mode of transmission, incubation period and the course of the disease is presented in **Table 56.2**.

Histopathological findings in patients with uncomplicated hepatitis show spotty necrosis throughout the liver lobule. The inflammatory cell infiltrate is mainly composed of lymphocytes.

Clinical features

The clinical features are similar, regardless of the type of the infecting virus. A prodromal phase is characterised by symptoms like low-grade fever, arthralgia and rash. Onset is abrupt with hepatitis A and E and more insidious with hepatitis B and C. Most patients seek medical attention when jaundice appears. However, anicteric disease occurs in about half the cases. Anorexia, nausea and altered bowel habits are common symptoms. Improvement begins after 1–2 weeks and the disease resolves within a few weeks in over 90% of cases. All of them can result in fulminant hepatic failure.

Course of the disease

The course of the disease varies with the type of hepatitis (**Table 56.2**).

Hepatitis A and B: Most patients recover within 3–4 months of onset; the illness may be prolonged in some upto 6–12 months

Hepatitis C: It is the main cause of non-A non-B hepatitis. It is a slowly progressive disease with significant long-term sequelae including cirrhosis, liver failure and hepatocellular carcinoma. More than half the patients with acute hepatitis C develop chronic hepatitis and up to 25% of them develop cirrhosis.

Table 56.2 Features of viral hepatitis

	Hepatitis A	Hepatitis B	Hepatitis C	Hepatitis D	Hepatitis E
Virus type	RNA	DNA	RNA	RNA	RNA
Route of transmission	Feco-oral	Parenteral	Parenteral	Parenteral	Feco-oral
Incubation period (days)	14–50	14–180	14–180	14–180	14–63
Fulminant hepatic failure	Yes	Yes	Yes	Yes	Yes
Chronic hepatitis, Cirrhosis	No	Yes	Yes	Yes	No
Carrier state	No	Yes	Yes	Yes	No
Maternal–fetal transmission	Rare	Frequent	Uncommon	Rare	Frequent

Hepatitis D (delta hepatitis): The virus peculiarly infects only those who have already had hepatitis B.

Hepatitis E: It is encountered most commonly in tropical and subtropical countries and is responsible for epidemics and sporadic cases of acute hepatitis. The disease is more severe in pregnant women, especially those infected in the third trimester. Case fatality could be a high as 20% and hepatitis E is an important cause of maternal death in India.

Effect on the mother and fetus

Acute hepatitis is associated with an increased risk of fulminant hepatic failure during pregnancy which may occur in up to 20% of cases; fetal mortality may be as high as 50%. A mother with acute hepatitis is prone to preterm labour and postpartum hemorrhage due to coagulopathy.

Maternal–fetal transmission is a major risk with hepatitis B. More than 50% of infants born to such mothers test positive for HBsAg and HBeAg and develop hepatitis. The risk of these babies developing cirrhosis and hepatocellular carcinoma in adolescence and adulthood is as high as 25%. Although the risk of infection is low when HBeAg is negative, it may still be about 25%. With hepatitis C, vertical transmission has been reported to be approximately 5%; the risk increases to about 15% when the mother is infected with HIV. In hepatitis E, vertical transmission is reported in up to 50% of pregnancies; the newborn may have icteric or nonicteric hepatitis.

Diagnosis

The clinical features and liver function tests help in arriving at the diagnosis.

Liver function tests: Regardless of the type of infection, the levels of transaminases usually exceed 500 U/l. Serum bilirubin may be raised. Serum proteins and prothrombin time usually remain normal.

Serologic diagnosis of types of hepatitis: Serologic tests help in identifying the virus and is useful in predicting long-term prognosis; they also help in deciding neonatal prophylaxis.

Hepatitis A: In the acute stage, IgM antibodies develop shortly after onset of the illness and persist for a few months. IgG antibodies develop gradually but persist throughout life, serving as markers of previous infection.

Hepatitis B: About 95% of patients with acute hepatitis B will have the hepatitis B surface antigen (HBsAg) in the prodromal phase. HBeAg, which indicates viral replication, becomes positive at the same time but persists only for a few days. Hepatitis B DNA appears briefly and provides quantitative measurement of viral replication. Antibodies to the hepatitis B core antigen (anti-HBcAg) develop after the onset of jaundice.

Hepatitis C: Hepatitis C RNA tests measure the components of the C virus and provide evidence of circulating virus in the patient's serum. Antibodies to hepatitis C can be detected by second-generation EIA tests 3–4 weeks after the onset of disease.

Hepatitis D: Antibodies to hepatitis D are detected in patients with hepatitis B who are infected with hepatitis D.

Hepatitis E: Currently no tests are available to detect these viral antibodies, though many tests are under development.

Management

Management of acute hepatitis in pregnancy is similar to that in the nonpregnant state except with greater surveillance for fulminant hepatic failure. The patient is preferably hospitalised for rest and monitoring for fluid and dietary intake. Universal precautions should be taken to protect health care providers.

Since mother-to-fetus transmission is low in hepatitis A, administration of immune serum globulin to the neonate at birth is optional. For mothers with hepatitis B, the risk of transmission to the fetus is significant and prophylactic measures can prevent neonatal transmission in up to 90% of cases. Universal screening of pregnant women for HBsAg and administration of the hepatitis B immunoglobulin (HBIg) and hepatitis B vaccine to infants born to hepatitis B-positive mothers is advocated. Guidelines for prophylaxis for hepatitis C and D are not clearly established and administration of immune serum globulin is optional.

Prevention

Viral hepatitis is a public health problem and epidemics of hepatitis A occur in various parts of India. Safe drinking water and personal hygiene are important in reducing epidemics due to hepatitis A and E. Vaccines for hepatitis A and B are available. India has a high carrier rate for hepatitis B, 5%–7% in the general population and about 10% in hospital staff. Other preventive measures include screening of blood donors, use of disposable needles and vaccination of children.

Fulminant Hepatic Failure

Fulminant hepatic failure (FHF) is a rare but life-threatening complication of several types of liver diseases.

Clinical features

These include progressive jaundice leading to the rapid development of hepatic encephalopathy. Ascites, peripheral edema and sepsis in the form of urinary tract infection (UTI) or pneumonia develop. Progressive liver failure results in hepatic coma, gastrointestinal hemorrhage, renal failure, cerebral edema and death.

Effect on the mother and fetus

Case fatality could be as high as 80%–90%. The risk of preterm labour and stillbirth is markedly increased.

Diagnosis

There is gross increase in transaminases and prolongation of prothrombin time. Serum bilirubin may increase to 20–30 mg/dl. Aminotransferases may decrease when the disease enters the pre-terminal stage. Serum ammonia levels may be high.

Differential diagnosis

Fulminant hepatic failure may be confused with AFLP and PIH, especially when it occurs in late pregnancy. In FHF, aminotransferases are very high but the rise in alkaline phosphatase is less.

Management

Treatment is essentially supportive. The patient should be managed in an intensive care unit and treatment may include administration of corticosteroids, plasma exchange and hemoperfusion. These measures are generally ineffective and liver transplantation has been proposed by some groups. Patients with AFLP- and PIH-related liver injury may benefit from termination of pregnancy.

Chronic Liver Disease in Pregnancy

Pregnancy is rare in advanced liver disease; in milder disease, the outcome will depend on the extent of liver damage and the causative factors.

Chronic Hepatitis

It includes a group of necroinflammatory diseases, usually persisting for more than six months and varying in severity. Hepatitis B and C infections, autoimmune hepatitis, alcoholic hepatitis and idiopathic chronic hepatitis may result in chronic hepatitis. The diagnosis and classification into mild, moderate and severe is histopathological regardless of the cause.

Clinical features

The clinical features will vary according to the severity of the disease, ranging from asymptomatic or mild fatigue to severe illness with jaundice, ascites and hepatic encephalopathy. Liver chemistry also varies widely and may reveal elevated of serum bilirubin, prolonged of prothrombin time and reducted serum albumin.

Patients with mild autoimmune hepatitis have good prognosis but prognosis for hepatitis B is unclear.

Effect on the mother and fetus

There is no increase in the risk to mother or the child in mild chronic hepatitis, except for hepatitis B where fetal transmission can occur. In severe chronic hepatitis, the risk of maternal and fetal death is increased.

Diagnosis

Since histological severity is the key prognostic indicator, a liver biopsy should be performed. Liver function tests can help monitor the course of the disease.

Management

Women with autoimmune and idiopathic chronic hepatitis show marked clinical improvement with corticosteroids, which should be started for those who are serologically negative for viral markers. Interferon therapy may delay disease progression and the development of cirrhosis but is not indicated in pregnant women.

Cirrhosis and Portal Hypertension

Cirrhosis is the terminal stage for a variety of hepatic diseases and is the main cause of intrahepatic portal hypertension. Non-cirrhotic portal hypertension may be caused by sarcoidosis, tuberculosis, schistosomiasis, metastatic malignancy, polycystic liver disease and Gaucher's disease.

Clinical features

Clinical features include varying degrees of jaundice, edema, ascites, coagulopathy and metabolic abnormalities. Portal hypertension manifests as hematemesis due to esophageal varices and splenomegaly.

Effect on the mother and fetus

Maternal prognosis depends on the degree of hepatic dysfunction and the cause of liver damage. Well-compensated biliary and postnecrotic cirrhosis carry the best prognosis. About half the women with documented cirrhosis who become pregnant deliver successfully.

In early pregnancy, the risk of spontaneous abortions is increased. Bleeding from esophageal varices is the most significant complication in pregnancy. Hepatic dysfunction can result in complications like uterine hemorrhage, hepatic coma, ascites and bacterial peritonitis. The maternal mortality rate is 10%–20% and is mainly due to gastrointestinal bleeding. Fetal loss is high in advanced cirrhosis. The incidence of IUGR, stillbirths and neonatal death is increased.

Diagnosis

The diagnosis is easily made based on history, liver function tests, ultrasound of the liver and biopsy.

Management

This includes rest, vitamin supplementation and high a carbohydrate, high-fibre, low-protein diet. Hypoglycemia, constipation and hypotension can precipitate encephalopathy. Severe bleeding from the varices can be managed by balloon tamponade or endoscopic procedures like banding and injecting sclerosing agents.

Additional medical therapy like corticosteroids for autoimmune chronic hepatitis, D penicillamine for Wilson's disease and abstinence from alcohol in alcoholic cirrhosis may induce remission even in the presence of large varices. Ascites can be managed by restricting dietary sodium and diuretics like aldactone or spironolactone and tapping.

Obstetric management: Pregnancy with well-compensated cirrhosis without jaundice and impaired liver function should be allowed to continue till term. Delivery should take place in a centre which can manage bleeding esophageal varices, and vitamin K, fresh frozen plasma and coagulation factors should be readily available. During labour, the second stage should be cut short to avoid and increase in portal pressure. Postpartum hemorrhage should be anticipated and managed promptly. Sedatives and anesthetic agents should be used with caution as they can precipitate encephalopathy. Cesarean section should be reserved for obstetric indications. Medical termination of pregnancy should be considered only for decompensated cirrhosis in the first trimester.

Drug-induced Hepatitis

Drug-induced hepatitis (DIH) is uncommon during pregnancy and may be caused by isoniazide antiemetics, antibiotics, sedatives and analgesics. The features are similar to mild hepatitis and most patients improve once the drug is discontinued. Cimetidine or ranitidine prescribed for heartburn can produce mild hepatocellular injury or cholestasis which promptly remits on withdrawal of the drug. Alpha methyl dopa, used in the treatment of hypertension in pregnancy, is hepatotoxic and LFT should be carried out when these drugs are prescribed.

Acetaminophen is a commonly used drug which causes acute liver failure when ingested in very high doses; treatment includes administration of the antidote N acetylcysteine (NAC) along with supportive therapy.

KEY POINTS

- Liver function tests are altered during pregnancy: these values should be interpreted with caution.
- Intrahepatic obstetric cholestasis is a mild disease associated with pregnancy that affects the fetus.
- Acute fatty liver of pregnancy is a rare but severe disease specific to pregnancy and is associated with significant maternal and fetal mortality.
- The liver is commonly involved in pregnancy-induced hypertension, with severe derangement in hepatic function in the help syndrome.
- Acute viral hepatitis in pregnancy is an important indirect cause of maternal death in India.
- Fulminant hepatic failure occurs more frequently in pregnant women.
- In women with hepatitis B in pregnancy, neonatal prophylaxis is recommended to reduce mother-to-child transmission.
- Pregnancy is uncommon in severe chronic liver disease; in less severe disease, the outcome depends on the liver function and the cause of liver injury.
- The main risk in cirrhosis and portal hypertension during pregnancy is variceal bleeding.
- Acute cholecystitis is not uncommon during pregnancy and responds well to conservative management.
- A multispecialty team should manage disorders of the liver and gall bladder in pregnancy.

QUESTIONS

Mark true (T) or false (F) against each statement:

1. Intrahepatic cholestasis of pregnancy is associated with high maternal mortality.
2. The diagnostic test for IHCP is raised serum bile acids.
3. Acute fatty liver of pregnancy is associated with high perinatal mortality.
4. The differential features which distinguish AFLP from other liver diseases are abdominal pain and hypoglycemia.
5. Hepatic involvement in pregnancy-induced hypertension is the common cause of liver dysfunction in pregnancy.
6. The course of acute viral hepatitis in pregnancy is more severe in developed countries than in developing countries.
7. Hepatic encephalopathy is associated with high maternal mortality.
8. Mother-to-fetus transmission of hepatitis A is rare.

9. Neonatal prophylaxis significantly reduces the risk of vertical transmission of hepatitis B.
10. The main risk of cirrhosis and portal hypertension in pregnancy is of hepatic failure.
11. In a case of IHCP, it is wise to wait till 40 weeks of pregnancy for spontaneous vaginal delivery.
12. Drug-induced hepatitis is common during pregnancy.
13. In mild chronic hepatitis B, fetal transmission is possible.
14. In acute viral hepatitis during pregnancy, case fatality is very high.
15. In normal pregnancy the transaminases are elevated.
16. IHCP is likely to recur in subsequent pregnancies.

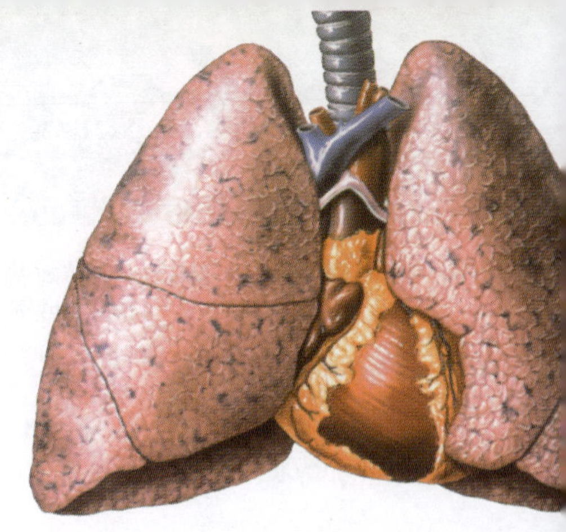

57

Common Surgical Causes of Acute Abdomen in Pregnancy

N Ananthakrishnan

LEARNING OBJECTIVES

At the end of this chapter, the reader should be able to:

- define acute abdomen
- enumerate the common causes of acute abdomen in pregnancy
- appreciate the difficulties in the diagnosis of surgical conditions in pregnancy
- diagnose, investigate and understand the management of common surgical causes of acute abdomen
- appreciate that abdominal surgery during pregnancy carries a definite but acceptable risk
- recognise that any delay in surgical intervention where necessary can be detrimental to the mother and the fetus
- know the dose of radiation exposure to the fetus for common radiological procedures
- appreciate the role of laparoscopic surgery in the management of acute abdomen

Introduction

Acute abdomen is characterised by abdominal pain of moderate to severe intensity, associated with tenderness and, occasionally, guarding or rigidity of the abdominal musculature and may or may not need surgical intervention. Among the many surgical causes of acute abdomen, some are particularly common in pregnancy; these are in addition to obstetric and gynecological conditions which can also present with an acute abdomen in pregnancy. The primary importance of these conditions is that the normal diagnostic signs and symptoms of these surgical conditions may be mistaken for features of normal pregnancy like vomiting and nausea and the classical signs may not be present due to displacement of abdominal organs by the gravid uterus. In this chapter, the common surgical causes of acute abdomen in pregnancy and the variations in presentation and management of these conditions as compared to nonpregnant patients are discussed.

Causes of acute abdomen

The common causes of acute abdomen in pregnancy include surgical and gynecological/obstetrical disorders.

Surgical causes:

- acute appendicitis
- acute cholecystitis
- intestinal obstruction
- acute pancreatitis
- urolithiasis

Obstetric and gynecological causes:

- ectopic pregnancy
- abruptio placentae
- acute polyhydramnios
- twisted ovarian cyst

Acute abdomen in pregnancy: Difficulties in diagnosis

Delay in diagnosis and definitive treatment of the surgical acute abdomen is the root cause of increased morbidity and mortality in the fetus and the mother. The causes for this delay are:

- Symptoms and signs of acute abdomen due to surgical disorder is often attributed to symptoms and signs unique to pregnancy.
- Presence of a gravid uterus makes evaluation of signs difficult because of displacement of organs.
- There is a natural tendency to be overcautious in the treatment of these patients and a conservative line of therapy is often preferred to surgical intervention, even when surgery is indicated, due to the risk of preterm labour.

Intraabdominal surgery during pregnancy as such carries an acceptable risk to the mother and the fetus. However, complications consequent to delay in diagnosis and treatment of the condition enhances the risk to the mother and the fetus. The overall risk of preterm labour with pelvic or abdominal surgery is 4%–6% and may be as high as 20%.

Acute Appendicitis

Incidence and clinical features

Acute appendicitis is the most common surgical cause of acute abdomen in pregnancy: the estimated case-to-delivery ratio is 1 in 1,500 to 1 in 2,000 deliveries. Acute appendicitis is most common in the first and second trimesters. Delay in diagnosis during pregnancy can lead to an increase in the incidence of perforation and abscess formation and a consequent increase in morbidity.

The clinical features of acute appendicitis in pregnancy are not typical. Many of the symptoms of appendicitis like anorexia, nausea, vomiting and abdominal pain may be due to pregnancy itself, thus delaying diagnosis. The pain of appendicitis lies in the right lower quadrant in the first trimester and shifts up in the second trimester due to displacement by the gravid uterus. In the third trimester, the pain is felt in the right upper quadrant of the abdomen and can simulate pain due to cholecystitis. In patients with a retrocecal appendix, this upward shift of pain is felt in the loin and mimics ureteric colic or pyelonephritis.

The classic signs of appendicitis include tenderness at McBurney's point, rebound tenderness and localised guarding in the right iliac fossa. These signs are due to inflammation of the parietal peritoneum due to contact with the inflamed appendix and is more severe in intensity than the visceral pain at onset (which is of low intensity and felt in the central abdomen). As the gravid uterus lifts the abdominal wall away from the abdominal viscera, the appendix may not come in contact with the parietal peritoneum and the classic signs of appendicitis may not be present in half the patients. Appendicular tenderness should be differentiated from uterine tenderness. The latter tends to shift with posture whereas appendicular tenderness in pregnant women remains fixed when the position of the patient is changed during examination. Psoas muscle spasm or rectal tenderness may be present in pelvic appendicitis.

Investigations

As leucocytosis is a feature of pregnancy, its value in diagnosing appendicitis is limited. Ultrasonography is useful: the criteria for the diagnosis of acute appendicitis are the presence of a fecolith and loss of continuity of the echogenic submucosa. When there is localised perforation, a periappendiceal collection or mass formation can be seen. In the presence of appendicular perforation with generalised peritonitis, free fluid in the abdomen with interloop collection may be detected on ultrasound.

An erect skiagram of the abdomen with both domes of the diaphragm might show pneumoperitoneum in patients with appendicular perforation. However, this finding is very rare. In equivocal cases when a perforated appendix is suspected, a diagnostic peritoneal lavage (DPL) may help avoid a non-therapeutic laparotomy. CT scan can also be used for the diagnosis of appendicitis. An abnormally turgid appendix with periappendiceal inflammation is suggestive of appendicitis. Radiological investigations must be used with care in view of the risk to the fetus.

Treatment

Due to difficulties in the diagnosis of appendicitis in pregnant patients, the chance of finding a normal appendix at laparotomy for acute appendicitis in pregnant patients is higher (25%–30% compared to about 15% in the nonpregnant). This higher negative laparotomy rate is acceptable when balanced against the consequences of a delay in treatment leading to perforation or abscess formation. When surgery is delayed, the fetal mortality rate rises significantly from 3% to 5% in non-perforated appendicitis to more than 20% in patients with perforated appendix. Maternal mortality is also higher in fecal peritonitis. Hence, surgery should be considered at the earliest when the diagnosis of appendicitis is made, as the incidence of perforation is directly related to the delay in surgery.

If an appendicular mass is found, the conservative regimen of Ochsner Sherren is used. This comprises antibiotics and close observation for resolution of the mass. If there is no resolution of the mass or it progresses to an abscess, percutaneous or open drainage may be done.

Conventionally, appendectomy is done by a transverse incision over the area of maximum tenderness. A midline incision is used when perforation is suspected or the diagnosis is not clear. Alternatively, a laparoscopic appendectomy may be done. Surgery carries a risk of preterm labour of 10%–15% both during surgery and up to one week after surgery. Hence, careful postoperative monitoring is mandatory.

Acute Cholecystitis

Incidence

Acute cholecystitis is the second most common surgical disorder seen in pregnant patients, with a case-to-delivery ratio of 1 in 2,000 to 1 in 5,000 deliveries. Although the hormonal changes during pregnancy may predispose to gall stone formation by promoting stasis and hypersaturation of bile, there is no significant increase in the incidence of cholecystitis in pregnancy.

Clinical features

The pain of biliary colic is felt in the right upper quadrant usually following a fatty meal and may or may not radiate to the upper back or right scapula. The pain lasts for a few hours but rarely extends beyond 24 hours. It might be associated with nausea, vomiting and intolerance to fatty foods. When acute cholecystitis sets in, the pain is often localised to the right hypochondrium and may be associated with fever. The Murphy sign can be elicited in these patients. If continuous gentle pressure is applied over the right hypochondrium and the patient is asked to take a deep breath, there is a sudden catch in the breath on deep inspiration due to the inflamed gall bladder touching the palpating hand. As stated earlier, the presentation can simulate appendicitis in the third trimester. When localised peritonitis occurs, patients have rebound tenderness and guarding in the right upper quadrant. Sometimes, there may be a palpable mass due to a pericholecystic phlegmon similar to an appendicular mass.

Investigations

Since leucocytosis may be a feature of pregnancy, it is not very useful in diagnosis (as for acute appendicitis). Ultrasound is the investigation of choice to diagnose acute cholecystitis. The sonographic findings of cholelithiasis include findings of an acoustic shadow due to the presence of gall stones in the gall bladder and gravity-dependent movement of the stones in the gall bladder. Apart from these findings, in the acute phase, thickened and edematous gall bladder wall and, perigall bladder edema or collection is suggestive of acute cholecystitis. The Murphy sign is observed by eliciting tenderness when the sonographic probe is placed in the right hypochondrium, just beneath the costal margin. Dilatation of the common bile duct with presence of stones is suggestive of choledocholithiasis. CT scan or MRI is generally not required.

Treatment

Once the diagnosis of acute cholecystitis is made, initial therapy in pregnancy is usually conservative. This includes withholding oral feeds, intravenous fluids, nasogastric suction, appropriate antibiotics and analgesics: most patients respond to this conservative line of therapy. Once the patient has recovered from the acute attack, an elective cholecystectomy is recommended after 6–8 weeks. Currently, early cholecystectomy during acute cholecystitis is being recommended. This aggressive approach has been advocated since the traditional conservative therapy is associated with an extended hospital stay and repeated admissions due to recurrent attacks of cholecystitis before an elective cholecystectomy is done. Recurrent attacks of cholecystitis or associated gall stone pancreatitis can also induce premature labour. In pregnant patients, morbidity is due to the disease and not due to surgery; hence, early cholecystectomy is preferred, especially in the second trimester. However, recent evidence supports surgical intervention as the first modality of therapy for acute cholecystitis in the first and third trimesters also.

At present laparoscopic cholecystectomy is the preferred procedure for acute cholecystitis. Other complications of gall stone disease could be empyema of the gall bladder or gall bladder perforation with generalised peritonitis which needs immediate surgical intervention.

Occasionally, acute acalculous cholecystitis may occur. The exact cause is not known: gall bladder stasis and ischemia have been suggested as causative factors. The presentation is similar to calculous cholecystitis. Cholecystectomy is the treatment once the condition is diagnosed but the chances of complications in the form of empyema, gangrene and perforation are higher with acalculous cholecystitis, resulting in increased mortality and morbidity.

Pancreatitis

Incidence

The case-to-delivery ratio of acute pancreatitis ranges from 1 in 2,000 to 1 in 3,000 deliveries.

Clinical features

Acute pancreatitis presents with sudden onset upper abdominal pain, nausea, vomiting and occasionally low-grade fever. Pain might persist for several hours and may radiate to the back. In alcohol-associated pancreatitis, the pain may begin a few hours after the intake of alcohol. This may be associated with jaundice. Gall stone pancreatitis is more likely to be associated with jaundice.

On physical examination, the patient has tenderness in the upper abdomen and umbilical region. Guarding may be present depending on the severity of pancreatitis. In a mild attack, bowel sounds and the patient's general condition may be stable. However, during a severe attack of pancreatitis, the patient is very sick, with abdominal distension due to free fluid and paralytic ileus and unstable vital signs, besides multiple metabolic derangements. The circulatory instability is due to reduced peripheral resistance, hypovolemia and decreased venous return to the heart. Sometimes, patients may have pleural effusion and acute pulmonary failure.

Investigations

Diagnosis is based on the estimation of serum amylase in the early phase of the disease. Although pregnancy too can lead to elevation of serum amylase, a gross increase is suggestive of pancreatitis. Imaging modalities that could be used are ultrasound examination of the abdomen, CT scan and MRI. Although sonography may show free fluid and identify gall stone disease, imaging of the pancreas could be hampered by the presence of the overlying air-filled bowel and stomach and consequent lack of a sonographic window. Currently, contrast-enhanced CT scan is the investigation of choice. Pancreatic edema, peripancreatic collection and pancreatic necrosis can be documented well with CT scan. MRI also can be used for demonstrating peripancreatic collections and for follow-up in pregnant patients, as MRI does not expose the patient to ionising radiation unlike CT.

Treatment

The initial therapy is always conservative. The patient is kept on nil oral, intravenous fluids and nasogastric suction. Correction of fluid–electrolyte balance and non-narcotic analgesics is important. Nasogastric suction reduces the acid load into the duodenum, thus reducing the stimulus to secretin release which stimulates exocrine secretion of the pancreas and exacerbation of symptoms. The role of proton pump inhibitors is yet to be proven. Antibiotics are usually given in moderate to severe attacks. Hyperglycemia and hypercalcemia may require treatment. Oral intake is started when abdominal pain and tenderness improve, vomiting (if present) stops, guarding resolves and bowel sounds become normal. In biliary pancreatitis, cholecystectomy is postponed and performed as an elective procedure. Surgical intervention in acute pancreatitis is indicated when the diagnosis is in doubt or when hollow viscus perforation or mesenteric ischemia cannot be ruled out. It is also indicated for complications like infected necrosis and pancreatic abscess.

Overall, a mild attack of pancreatitis resolves with conservative treatment in most patients in about a week, and has good prognosis. However, as the severity of the disease increases, the maternal mortality may be as high as 35%. Complications of pancreatitis are also associated with high maternal and fetal morbidity and mortality.

Intestinal Obstruction

Incidence

Intestinal obstruction can occur with a case-to-delivery ratio of 1 in 1,500 to 1 in 5,000 deliveries. Adhesive intestinal obstruction and volvulus are the common causes of intestinal obstruction in pregnancy. Other rare causes are intussusception, obstructed inguinal or femoral hernia and cancer.

In more than half the patients with intestinal obstruction in pregnancy, the cause is adhesions due to previous surgery such as appendectomy or gynecologic surgery or due to pelvic inflammatory disease. Volvulus, sigmoid or less commonly cecal volvulus, is the next most common cause of intestinal obstruction in pregnancy and is seen in one-fourth of patients. The cause of volvulus is mechanical displacement due to the gravid uterus; incidence increases with the length of gestation. During puerperium, a rapid reduction in the size of the uterus can lead to a change in the position of the gut, predisposing to volvulus.

Clinical features

Intestinal obstruction is characterised by the four cardinal features:

- colicky abdominal pain
- vomiting
- abdominal distension
- absolute constipation (obstipation).

If a patient has vomiting late in pregnancy, the possibility of intestinal obstruction should be suspected especially if she has had previous surgery. The nature of the vomitus is important as feculent and foul-smelling vomitus is suggestive of complete obstruction for 2–3 days. Rapid onset abdominal distension with a tympanitic note on percussion indicate possible sigmoid or cecal volvulus. When the obstruction is complete, the patient will have obstipation, that is, not passing flatus and feces. Colicky abdominal pain becoming continuous with diminishing or absent bowel sounds associated with guarding or rebound tenderness of the abdomen is an indicator of bowel strangulation. Intussusception presents with colicky abdominal pain and a mass in the abdomen which changes its position without gross abdominal distension. Hernial sites should be carefully examined to rule out an obstructed or strangulated groin hernia.

Investigations

Once intestinal obstruction is suspected, a plain skiagram of the abdomen in the erect and supine positions should be done to confirm the diagnosis. Multiple air-fluid levels are diagnostic of intestinal obstruction. In sigmoid volvulus, the classical 'bent inner tube sign' or the 'coffee bean sign' due to the distended loop of the sigmoid colon arising from the pelvis would be seen. In cecal volvulus, a hugely distended and displaced cecum would be seen, especially to the left of the abdomen, with a bird's beak image at the point of the torsion. Ultrasound examination may be useful for the diagnosis of intussusception.

Treatment

If the intestinal obstruction is due to adhesions, a short duration of conservative line of therapy can be tried, provided the patient does not have evidence of strangulation. Conservative treatment comprises withholding oral feeds, intravenous fluids, nasogastric suction, monitoring of abdominal girth and a close watch for signs of strangulation. If the patient responds to these measures within 24–48 hours, then surgical intervention can be avoided. If the patient shows no signs of improvement, a laparotomy and adhesiolysis should be done. This procedure may also be performed laparoscopically. In pregnancy, a trial of conservative therapy should be of shorter duration compared to nonpregnant patients due to an increase in maternal and fetal mortality associated with complications of intestinal obstruction such as perforation and strangulation. Sigmoid volvulus needs surgical intervention if the bowel cannot be decompressed by insertion of a rectal tube or by colonoscopy. Strangulation should be ruled out before attempting decompression of the volvulus. After reduction, an elective procedure is necessary as the possibility of recurrence is very high. Cecal volvulus usually needs immediate surgical intervention. Resection is the preferred choice although cecopexy has also been tried. When the bowel is gangrenous, resection is the only alternative.

Intussusception is managed by resection if the involved segment is ischemic or if the intussusception is secondary to a primary pathology such as a tumour. Hernias are managed by mesh repair and bowel resection when the bowel is strangulated. Appropriate antibiotics are required after resection for gangrene of the gut. If obstruction occurs after 24 weeks of gestation, close fetal monitoring is required in the postoperative phase. The maternal mortality rate for intestinal obstruction in pregnant patients is significantly higher than for nonpregnant patients and ranges around 12%. The fetal mortality rates are higher, ranging from 30% to 50% and could go up to 60% in the third trimester.

UROLITHIASIS

Incidence

Urolithiasis may occasionally present as acute abdomen in pregnant patients. The case-to-delivery ratio is in the range of 1 in 1,500 to 1 in 2,000 deliveries.

Clinical features

Renal colic is the presenting symptom. This consists of moderate to high intensity, localised pain in the flank which radiates from the loin to the groin and is sometimes associated with nausea and vomiting. There may be associated dysuria, urgency, microscopic or gross hematuria and tenderness in the renal angle. If urinary tract infection is present, the patient may have fever.

Investigations

Urine examination for microscopic hematuria, presence of pus cells and detection of microcalculi in the urine helps in the diagnosis of the condition. A kidney-ureter-bladder film may show the presence of a stone as almost 90% of urinary calculi are radiopaque. Ultrasound examination of the urinary tract can show hydronephrosis and calculi in the urinary tract. Physiologic dilatation of the urinary tract, particularly on the right side, during the second half of pregnancy should not be mistaken for a pathological obstruction.

Treatment

Treatment of urolithiasis depends on the size, location and composition of the urinary calculi, degree of obstruction, severity of symptoms and concomitant infection. Pain from renal colic may be relieved by anti-spasmodic drugs in combination with NSAIDs. In most patients, the calculi will pass with hydration therapy especially when they are less than 5 mm in size and located in the distal ureter. Intervention may be necessary if intractable pain, high-grade obstruction the recurrent urinary tract infection are present. More than 95% of the patients with urolithiasis can be managed by minimally invasive techniques. These include rigid or flexible ureteroscopy with basket extraction of stones or the use of electrohydraulic or laser lithotripsy. Percutaneous nephrostolithotomy (PCNL) with nephrostomy can be used for stones larger than 3 cm in the kidneys. The safety of extracorporeal shock wave lithotripsy (ESWL) in pregnancy has not been established. Open surgery for urolithiasis is only necessary in a select group of patients when the minimally invasive techniques have failed or in the presence of large stones in the renal pelvis which might be difficult to remove by other methods.

Risk of abdominal surgery during pregnancy

Abdominal surgery during pregnancy may be complicated by abortion, preterm labour, fetal death, sepsis and, paralytic ileus depending on the period of gestation and the condition warranting laparotomy. The drugs used, anesthetic agents and surgical manipulations all contribute to the adverse effects on pregnancy. The outcome is best during the second trimester, especially if the procedure is electively planned and performed. However, the acute nature of the condition may not permit ideal conditions for surgery.

Danger of delayed treatment

While surgical treatment in pregnancy carries a risk, delay in treatment where it is indicated will increase the risk. Physicians are reluctant to resort to surgery during pregnancy, and may wish to postpone it. Most of the causes of acute abdomen will lead to dangerous complications like rupture or gangrene of organs, peritonitis, septicemia and shock: these will increase the risk to higher livels than that of surgery done early.

Fetal exposure due to radiological procedures for diagnosis

While ionising radiation in the evaluation of patients who are pregnant is often a source of anxiety for the practising clinician, radiograph exposure from a single diagnostic procedure will not result in harmful fetal effects. As ionising radiation with multiple exposures can lead to an increase in fetal anomalies or fetal loss, it should only be used when absolutely necessary for the diagnosis of the cause of the acute abdomen. Other imaging procedures such as ultrasound should be preferred over radiographic procedures. An exposure of less than 0.05 Gy has not been associated with any known detrimental effect to the fetus.

The estimated fetal exposure for some common radiographic procedures is given below:

Abdominal film (single view)	0.1 cGy
Intravenous urography	less than 1 cGy
Barium enema	less than 4 cGy
CT head/chest	less than 1 cGy
CT abdomen	about 4 cGy

Magnetic resonance imaging (MRI) can be used (more frequently compared to CT) as no ionising radiation is used in this modality. However, in the first trimester, even MRI is not commonly recommended.

Safety of therapeutic laparoscopy in pregnancy

Laparoscopic cholecystectomy is the most common procedure performed in pregnancy and accounts for half of the therapeutic laparoscopic procedures carried out in pregnancy. One-fourth of laparoscopic procedures in pregnancy are for adnexal masses and another 25% for appendectomy and other miscellaneous conditions. Most of these procedures are performed in the second trimester. The maternal and fetal complications following laparoscopic surgery in pregnancy are comparable to the general nonpregnant population, suggesting that laparoscopic surgery does not increase the possibility of premature labour.

The initial reservation about laparoscopic surgery in pregnancy was about:

- whether there can be safe access to the celomic cavity in the presence of a gravid uterus
- whether a gravid uterus would interfere with the procedure through the conventional port sites
- the adverse effects of CO_2 pneumoperitoneum on fetal physiology and blood flow.

The Hasson technique of access to the celomic cavity using a special trocar is now standard practice in pregnancy. Alternatively, a conventional trocar with a vaseline gauze pad sutured around the port can be used. The port sites can be adjusted according to the requirements of the procedure in the presence of a gravid uterus so that access to the target organ is not compromised.

In pregnancy, pneumoperitoneum affects the fetus by increasing the pressure on the uterus and altering maternal hemodynamics and acid–base balance. Studies have shown that there can be fetal hypercarbia, acidosis, tachycardia and increase in fetal arterial pressure with the use of CO_2 pneumoperitoneum. However, the long-term effects of these physiological alterations are currently not known. During laparoscopic surgery, it is imperative that the fetal condition should be closely monitored and corrected to avoid adverse effects.

KEY POINTS

- Acute appendicitis, acute cholecystitis, pancreatitis, intestinal obstruction and urolithiasis are the common causes of surgical acute abdomen in pregnancy.
- In patients with acute abdomen in pregnancy, the clinical features might not be as characteristic as in nonpregnant patients. Many of the symptoms of acute abdomen like anorexia, nausea, vomiting and abdominal pain could be due to pregnancy itself. Signs can also be masked or altered due to the gravid uterus.
- Intraabdominal surgery during pregnancy carries an acceptable risk to the mother and the fetus. However, the complications associated with delay in diagnosis and therapy of the condition leads to a significant increase in disease severity and enhances the risk to the mother and the fetus.
- An open approach with timely surgical interventions when necessary should be carried out to prevent complications due to delay in diagnosis and therapy.
- Limited use of radiologic procedures when necessary is not contraindicated. An exposure of less than 0.05 Gy has not been associated with any effects detrimental to the fetus.
- Advances in laparoscopic surgery have made therapeutic laparoscopic procedures like cholecystectomy, excision of adnexal masses and appendectomy safe in pregnancy.

QUESTIONS

Select the single most appropriate answer:

1. All of the following are common causes of acute abdomen in pregnancy *except*
   a. acute appendicitis
   b. gastric volvulus
   c. acute cholecystitis
   d. acute pancreatitis
2. The incidence of acute appendicitis in pregnancy is approximately
   a. 1 in 250 to 1 in 500 deliveries
   b. 1 in 500 to 1 in 1,000 deliveries
   c. 1 in 1,500 to 1 in 2,000 deliveries
   d. 1 in 2,000 to 1 in 5,000 deliveries
3. In acute appendicitis in pregnancy, a positive Adler sign is
   a. Tenderness persisting in McBurney's point
   b. Tenderness shifting to the left with change in posture
   c. Pain at the McBurney's point on pressure over the left iliac fossa
   d. Pain on internal rotation of the thigh
4. Estimated fetal exposure due to a single abdominal skiagram during pregnancy is
   a. 0.1 cGy
   b. 0.2–1.0 cGy
   c. 1–4 cGy
   d. more than 4 cGy
5. The investigation of choice for the diagnosis of acute cholecystitis in pregnancy is
   a. demonstration of leucocytosis
   b. LFT
   c. abdominal sonography
   d. HIDA scan
6. Intestinal obstruction in pregnancy is best diagnosed by
   a. diagnostic laparoscopy
   b. CT scan
   c. abdominal sonography
   d. plain skiagram of the abdomen

7. Delayed surgery for perforated acute appendicitis in pregnancy may result in fetal mortality rates in excess of
   a. 1%–5%
   b. 5%–10%
   c. 10%–15%
   d. More than 20%

In the following questions, there are two statements. Select the appropriate answer using the following key:

a. if both statements are true and causally related
b. if both statements are true but not causally related
c. if the first statement is true and the second is false
d. if the first statement is false and the second is true
e. if both statements are false

8. Symptoms and signs of acute abdomen in a pregnant woman are often atypical *because*

   Presence of a gravid uterus results in displacement of abdominal organs.

9. In pregnancy, early cholecystectomy is the treatment of choice for acute cholecystitis *because*

   Conservative therapy is associated with an extended hospital stay and repeated admissions due to acute cholecystitis.

10. Sonography is the best method for the diagnosis of pancreatitis in pregnancy *because*

    It is always possible to find a clear acoustic window for imaging due to the enlarged uterus.

58

Gynecological Disorders Complicating Pregnancy

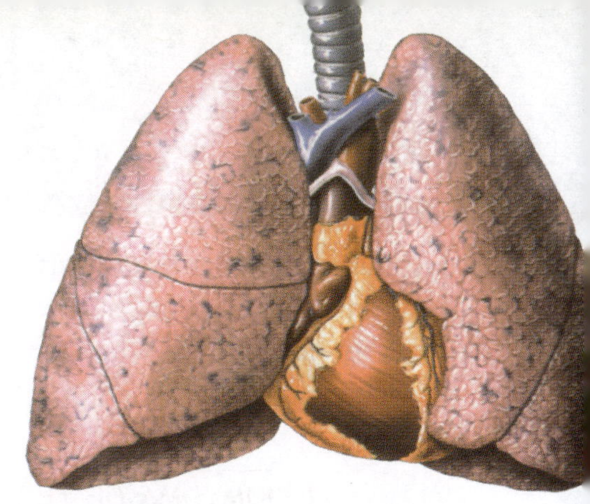

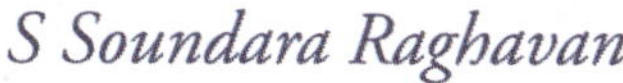

S Soundara Raghavan

LEARNING OBJECTIVES

At the end of this chapter, the reader should be able to:

- list the common gynecological conditions in pregnancy
- understand the effects of Mullerian anomalies on pregnancy and suggest appropriate measures when they are encountered
- appreciate the difficulty in diagnosing uterine leiomyoma complicating pregnancy
- list the complications of leiomyoma in pregnancy and the effects of pregnancy on leiomyoma
- explain the basic principles in the diagnosis and treatment of ovarian tumours in pregnancy
- list the changes pregnancy can cause on uterine prolapse and suggest treatment options for the condition
- be aware that the antenatal period provides an opportunity for the early screening and diagnosis of cancer of the uterine cervix
- list the effects of treatment and refer the patient appropriately

Introduction

Diseases of the reproductive tract can complicate pregnancy, just as diseases of other systems can. The reproductive system undergoes the most significant changes during pregnancy and these conditions can have adverse effects on the pregnancy, or sometimes may be affected by it too. This chapter deals with some common gynecological conditions that may be seen during pregnancy.

Mullerian Defects

Mullerian duct development defects are uncommon. There is also a wide range of defects, ranging from total agenesis (such as Rokitanski–Kustner–Hauser syndrome) to very minor forms like arcuate uterus. The effect of these defects will vary from amenorrhea and infertility in severe conditions like agenesis to almost no effect as in arcuate uterus. Some of the minor defects may only be diagnosed incidentally at cesarean section or may come to light if it was already known to be present in the prepregnant state. Some rare conditions like pregnancy in a rudimentary horn may result in life-threatening conditions like rupture. About 20% of Mullerian defects may be associated with cervical insufficiency and may cause recurrent abortion. Apart from these, Mullerian duct defects may cause preterm labour, malpresentations, dysfunctional labour, antepartum hemorrhage and postpartum hemorrhage. The need for operative intervention increases when these defects complicate pregnancy.

Leiomyoma of the Uterus

Leiomyomas are extremely common, and are found in almost one-third of all women. They usually do not produce any symptom; mere detection of their presence does not warrant treatment. With increasing use of ultrasound, more leiomyomas are diagnosed. A woman who knows she has a leiomyoma is often anxious about it and is made to believe it needs to be removed. The situation is even worse when pregnancy occurs along with a leiomyoma. Small leiomyomas may be detected for the first time during pregnancy, because ultrasound examination is increasingly performed for pregnant women. Some leiomyomas may increase in size during pregnancy because of increased vascularity and edema. Others, which were known to be present before pregnancy, may not be identified during pregnancy, because they may not be differentiated from the surrounding myometrium or they may get slightly displaced as the uterus enlarges during pregnancy.

Apart from the increase in size, a leiomyoma may undergo red degeneration, a condition peculiar to pregnancy and puerperium. The woman may report pain and fever, and may have leucocytosis. Treatment of this condition is essentially conservative: rest and pain relief are advised. Occasionally, in a woman with submucous fibroid with evidence of sepsis in the postnatal period, an antibiotic may be indicated.

The effect of leiomyoma on pregnancy will depend on the size, number, proximity to the placenta and location of the uterine fibroid. Though rare, abortion, preterm labour, dystocia, antepartum hemorrhage, postpartum hemorrhage, subinvolution and puerperal sepsis may occur in women with fibroid complicating pregnancy. Cesarean section may be necessary if the fibroid obstructs labour. Traditionally, a fibroid (except a pedunculated subserous one) is not surgically treated if encountered during a cesarean section for fear of massive bleeding. However, currently, there is an increasing trend to remove leiomyomas during cesarean section.

Ovarian Tumours

The ovaries may enlarge and become cystic during pregnancy due to the placental hCG-producing theca lutein cysts. These are more common with trophoblastic disease and multiple pregnancy and may be mistaken for pathological (neoplastic) ovarian cysts. Enlargement of the ovary up to 6 cm is considered physiological. Ovarian cysts measuring 10 cm or more are definitely considered abnormal and surgery is advised. Those which measure 6–10 cm may be followed up.

The most common tumours of the ovary seen during pregnancy are serous cysts, which are of average size, uniloculated and do not contain internal echoes or septa. Benign cystic teratomas or dermoid cysts are also not uncommon.

Unless their presence was already documented or the tumours are ovarian cysts, they may be missed during clinical examination. Some of them may be detected during routine early obstetric ultrasound. USG may help not only in the diagnosis, but also to identify the benign or malignant nature of the tumour.

Unless large, the cyst may not produce any effect on pregnancy. The combined effect of the size of the uterus and cyst may cause pressure symptoms. Rarely, they may become impacted in the pelvis and cause dystocia.

The cyst may undergo torsion, which is the most common complication during pregnancy and puerperium, apart from rupture. These are acute complications which will affect both maternal and fetal outcome adversely.

The duration of pregnancy, size of the tumour, presence of any complication or suspicion of malignancy will determine the mode of treatment. Generally, second trimester and early third trimester are considered safe for elective surgery during pregnancy. In malignancy, pregnancy may be disregarded and the tumour treated at a specialised centre. If a tumour is encountered during cesarean section, it can easily be excised (cystectomy or ovariotomy).

Laparoscopy is being increasingly used during pregnancy to deal with ovarian cysts of medium size.

Uterovaginal Prolapse

Uterovaginal prolapse is a fairly common gynecological condition in India and complicates about 4–5 per 1,000 pregnancies. Usually, only minor degrees of prolapse are seen, and pregnancy is not significantly affected. Procidentia is rarely seen during pregnancy as pregnancy is unlikely to occur. As pregnancy advances, the growing uterus may drag the cervix upwards and prolapse may reduce. Occasionally, the increasing edema and vascularity may enhance anatomical changes like hypertrophy and the prolapse may become irreducible. Vaginal discharge may become copious, decubitus ulcer may appear for the first time or worsen. It is not clear if there is an increased risk of abortion. There may be a greater risk of chorioamnionitis, preterm rupture of membranes, preterm labour, dystocia due to non-dilatation of the cervix in labour, cervical injury, need for surgical intervention and sepsis.

If the cervix is outside the introitus and the woman experiences discomfort by its physical presence, it may be kept reduced with a pessary. However, it is important to keep in mind that pessary treatment during pregnancy may cause ulceration of the vagina. Antiedema measures may help reduce the size and keep the cervix inside the vagina. Surgical treatment for prolapse should not be considered in pregnancy or puerperium.

Pre-invasive and Invasive Cancer of the Cervix

Pregnancy affords a very good opportunity for health care professionals to perform a speculum examination or to take a pap smear; unfortunately, this is not often done. Invasive cancer cervix is seen in about 1 in 2,000 pregnancies. Pregnancy does not seem to have any effect on the course of the disease. Invasive disease may increase the risk of abortion, preterm labour, hemorrhage and sepsis during pregnancy.

In low-grade squamous intraepithelial lesions (LGSIL) and atypical squamous cells of unknown significance (ASCUS), colposcopy may be postponed for six weeks after delivery. High-grade squamous intraepithelial lesions (HGSIL) warrant immediate colposcopy. Biopsy of the cervix during pregnancy may result in profuse bleeding.

Invasive cancer needs to be treated promptly. In the first half of pregnancy, it should be terminated and the disease treated according to the protocol followed in the nonpregnant woman. Treatment of the disease diagnosed later in pregnancy needs to be individualised. Radical hysterectomy with pregnancy in situ can be done in early pregnancy for the early stages of the disease.

Invasive cancer may cause severe bleeding and the disease may spread during vaginal delivery or lower segment cesarean section; hence, classical cesarean section has been advocated in the presence of invasive cervical cancer complicating advanced pregnancy. Prognosis of the disease is similar to that in the non-pregnant state except possibly for an increased risk of hemorrhage. Radiotherapy, where indicated, may be administered four to six weeks after termination of pregnancy.

KEY POINTS

- Abnormalities of the reproductive tract complicating pregnancy may include developmental defects like Mullerian duct defects.
- The effect of Mullerian defects may range from no effect to rupture of the rudimentary horn.
- Leiomyomas are quite common in women and may complicate pregnancy.
- Most leiomyomas do not need to be treated during pregnancy.
- Red degeneration of the fibroid is a complication peculiar to pregnancy and puerperium.
- Ovarian tumours may occasionally be seen during pregnancy.
- Benign tumours like serous cyst or cystic teratomas are common.
- If ovarian cysts present with torsion or if they are suspected to be malignant, they should be operated.
- Uterine prolapse can on reduced or may become edematous and irreducible during pregnancy.
- It can cause cervical dystocia or result in cervical injury during labour.
- Screening for cancer cervix should be routinely done during antenatal care.
- LGSIL and ASCUS seen during pregnancy can be treated six weeks after delivery.
- HGSIL and invasive cancer should be promptly treated.

QUESTIONS

Select the single most appropriate answer:

1. Mullerian defects complicating pregnancy can result in all of the following *except*
   a. abortion
   b. preterm labour
   c. malpresentations
   d. hydatidiform mole
2. The complication peculiar to pregnancy or puerperium in a fibroid is
   a. hyaline degeneration
   b. red degeneration
   c. cystic degeneration
   d. malignant change
3. Red degeneration is best treated by
   a. immediate myomectomy
   b. antibiotics
   c. rest and analgesics
   d. GnRH analogue
4. The safest period for any elective surgery during pregnancy is
   a. first three months
   b. second trimester
   c. at 32 weeks
   d. along with cesarean section
5. The most common complication of ovarian cyst in pregnancy is
   a. torsion
   b. rupture
   c. infection
   d. malignant change
6. The most common ovarian tumour in pregnancy is
   a. dysgerminoma
   b. mucinous cystadenoma
   c. endometrioma
   d. serous cystadenoma
7. Prolapse of the uterus complicating pregnancy may be associated with all of the following *except*
   a. cervical dystocia
   b. chorioamnionitis
   c. premature rupture of membranes
   d. malpresentation
8. Which of the following conditions diagnosed during pregnancy warrants immediate treatment?
   a. low-grade squamous intraepithelial lesion
   b. atypical squamous cells of unknown significance
   c. human papilloma virus associated changes
   d. invasive cervical cancer

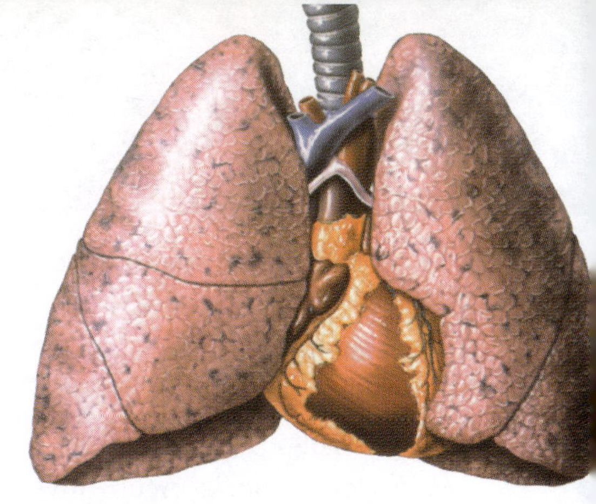

59

Shock in Obstetrics

Asha Oumachigui

LEARNING OBJECTIVES

At the end of this chapter, the reader should be able to:

- define shock
- explain how maternal changes in pregnancy protect the woman from succumbing to shock
- list the causes of shock
- describe the pathophysiology of shock
- list the clinical features and complications of shock
- describe the management of hypovolemic shock
- explain the management of septic shock
- outline the management of shock due to other causes

Introduction

Shock is an acute, life-threatening condition in which there is a sudden drop in blood flow through the body which results in a generalised decrease in tissue perfusion; blood flow is lower than the level needed to deliver oxygen and nutrients for normal cell function. It is defined as a syndrome initiated by acute tissue hypoperfusion leading to tissue hypoxia and dysfunction of vital organs.

Reduced tissue perfusion occurs either due to an overall decrease in circulatory volume as in hemorrhage or due to poor distribution as in septic shock. While managing shock in a pregnant woman, it is important to keep two factors in mind: the physiological changes in pregnancy and that there are two patients to be dealt with, the mother and her child. The aim is to protect both.

Cardiovascular Changes in Pregnancy

Some of the cardiovascular changes that take place during pregnancy protect a woman from shock to some extent. Blood volume increases by almost 50%, plasma volume by 45% and red blood cell volume by 20%. Total increase in circulatory volume is 1–1.5 l.

- Significant sodium retention (1000 mEq) is caused by an increase in steroidal hormones. Subsequently, total body water increases by 6–8 l.
- Blood pressure decreases midtrimester. A fall in systemic vascular resistance occurs and reaches a nadir around 24 weeks.

Causes of shock

There are several causes of shock. The presence of a placenta and increased vascularity make the pregnant woman prone to hemorrhage and the raw placental site in the uterus to infection. However, a pregnant woman may suffer from shock due to other causes as in the nonpregnant state.

The types and causes of shock are classified as follows:

Hypovolemic shock: Hemorrhage, hyperemesis gravidarum, gastroenteritis

Septic shock: Intrapartum/postpartum sepsis, septic abortion, pyelonephritis

Cardiogenic shock: Cardiomyopathies, obstructive or regurgitative valvular lesions, myocarditis and dysrhythmias

Neurogenic shock: Acute inversion of the uterus, intrauterine manipulations without anesthesia, anaphylaxis, regional anesthesia

Pathophysiology

The human body responds to acute hemorrhage by activating the hematologic, cardiovascular, renal and neuroendocrine systems. The coagulation cascade is activated and there is vasoconstriction. There is an increase in heart rate and myocardial contractility. Blood is redistributed to the brain, heart and kidneys and away from the skin, muscles and alimentary tract. An increase in renin secretion converts angiotensinogen to angiotensin I (which is later converted to angiotensin II) which has two main effects: vasoconstriction of arteriolar smooth muscle and stimulation of aldosterone secretion by the adrenal cortex. Aldosterone is responsible for active sodium reabsorption and subsequent water conservation. Fall in blood pressure and loss of sodium also increase the secretion of the antidiuretic hormone (ADH), which results in increased reabsorption of water and sodium.

Septic shock may occur if abortions and deliveries are conducted by unskilled birth attendants. Shock in sepsis is essentially due to widespread inflammatory response which results in extensive vasodilatation, decreased systemic vascular resistance, increased capillary permeability, cardiac depression and hypotension culminating in decreased tissue perfusion. In addition, poor oxygen utilisation by the tissues leads to tissue hypoxia, which in turn leads to multiple organ failure and death.

The cell walls of the infecting Gram-negative and Gram-positive bacteria induce the release of **cytokines** in the host cells like macrophages, monocytes and neutrophils. The cytokines play an important role in the occurrence of shock.

The cytokines initiate coagulation by activating the tissue factor through the extrinsic coagulation pathway. This is followed by thrombin production, cleavage of fibrinogen to produce fibrin and the formation of microvascular thrombi. The condition further worsens as the cytokines disrupt the body's modulators of coagulation, leading to suppression of fibrinolysis.

The performance of the heart is reduced by the depressant substances, pulmonary hypertension, cytokines, nitric oxide and β receptor downregulation.

Abnormalities in peripheral blood flow are the result of an imbalance between the local regulation of arterial vascular tone and the activity of central mechanisms. Arteriovenous oxygen difference is reduced and the blood lactic levels increase. The end result in septicemia is disturbance in microcirculation, poor oxygenation and lactic acidemia.

Clinical features

Symptoms include weakness, lightheadedness, lethargy, confusion and palpitations. There may be air hunger and cold clamminess.

On examination, the patient may be found to have tachycardia, low volume pulse and hypotension. There may also be tachypnea. In hemorrhagic shock, pallor will be a notable feature; if it is due to fluid loss, dehydration (dry tongue and sunken eyes) may be noted.

Complications

Tissue hypoperfusion leads to renal failure which is reversible in the initial stages, but may become irreversible if cortical necrosis develops.

In massive hemorrhage, DIC may cause complications. If corrective measures are not taken in time, multiorgan failure results and the outcome is grave. In septicemic shock, vascular endothelial injury may lead to ARDS.

Immediate management

Sound initial management is absolutely essential for ensuring the health of the mother and her unborn child. The outcome also depends on the stage in which the patient presents. Management of shock requires a team approach; if necessary, the obstetrician must seek the help of other colleagues like physicians and anesthetists. Any intervention should be directed towards optimal stabilisation of the mother's condition.

Resuscitation follows the ABC pattern adopted in any medical emergency:

The first step is to ensure a patent **Airway**. Endotracheal intubation is required in potentially compromised patients.

Breathing should be monitored closely and supported if necessary.

Circulation: The following measures are instituted to maintain adequate circulation:

- access to a large vein
- collection of blood for crossmatching and for other laboratory investigations like serum electrolytes and coagulation profile
- administration of crystalloids, preferably Ringer lactate
- blood be transfused as soon as available; response to therapy monitored closely using clinical parameters: pulse, respiration and blood pressure, urine output and oxygen saturation
- patient positioned in the left lateral position to avoid aortocaval compression which can worsen hypotension.

Once resuscitation is initiated, efforts must be made to ascertain the underlying cause of shock.

Specific management

Hemorrhage and hypovolemia: In obstetrics, the most common cause of hypovolemia is hemorrhage. It could be during pregnancy or after delivery.

The conditions responsible for hemorrhage are summarised below:

The mainstay of treatment of hemorrhagic shock is blood transfusion and arrest of bleeding at the earliest. In other words, the treatment of the specific cause of hemorrhage should be instituted. The management of each cause has been discussed in the relevant chapter.

Nonhemorrhagic causes of hypovolemia

Nonhemorrhagic hypovolemia is seen in severe hyperemesis and gastroenteritis. The principles of management consist of controlling vomiting and diarrhea and restoring the fluid–electrolyte balance.

Septic shock

Laboratory tests reveal abnormal white cell count, low platelet count, coagulopathy, abnormal liver and kidney function and metabolic acidosis.

The general management is the same as for hypovolemic shock. The aim is to correct hypovolemia and maintain tissue perfusion. Broad spectrum antibiotics are administered parenterally after taking blood and swabs from sites of infection for isolation of organisms. Inotropic drugs like dopamine are given to restore or maintain tissue perfusion. Corticosteroids are of no benefit in septic shock.

Cardiogenic Shock

In cardiogenic shock, the cardiac output is inadequate and results in underperfusion of tissues. This phenomenon most commonly occurs at 28–32 weeks of pregnancy when the blood volume is highest. Cardiac disease prior to pregnancy and peripartum cardiomyopathy increase the risk of cardiogenic shock.

Neurogenic Shock

Acute inversion of the uterus and intrauterine manipulations without proper anesthesia can lead to neurogenic shock. Therefore, adherence to the correct practice of obstetrical procedures and the use of anesthesia where appropriate can prevent this condition.

Anaphylaxis is defined as a serious allergic reaction that is of rapid onset and may cause death. There is an exaggerated immunological response to an antigen which could be a drug or food material to which an individual has been exposed earlier. The reaction is responsible for the breakdown of mast cells and basophils, which release mediators like histamine, serotonin, bradykinin, thromboxane, tryptase and leukotrienes into the plasma. These substances are responsible for increased secretions from mucous membranes, increased capillary permeability and leakage, marked vasodilatation and bronchospasm.

Clinically, besides the features of shock, there are cutaneous manifestations and signs like wheezing and stridor.

The steps in the management are:

- withdrawal of the offending substance/drug
- secure the airway
- Trendelenburg position to promote venous return
- injection of adrenaline intramuscularly, and intravenously if needed
- infusion of crystalloids to expand to intravascular volume
- antihistaminics, β blockers and corticosteroids

Amniotic fluid embolism is a rare, but near-fatal complication in obstetrics. The exact pathophysiology is unknown. The entry of amniotic fluid in to pulmonary circulation causes pulmonary vasospasm and hypertension, and results in hypoxia. The clinical picture is characterised by:

- hypotension
- sudden and severe dyspnea
- cyanosis
- DIC
- maternal death

Management consists of:

- basic measures to manage shock
- intensive management for cardiac failure and DIC

Shock Following Administration of Anesthesia

The main defect here is massive vasodilatation resulting in relative hypovolemia, reduced tissue perfusion and consequent tissue hypoxia. The underlying cause is sympathetic dysfunction leading to vasodilatation in regional anesthesia. In general anesthesia, the shock is a result of an anaphylactic reaction to administered anesthetic agents.

- High spinal is due to the use of overdose of local anesthetics and excessive spread of intrathecal administration. Hypotension can also result from incorrect positioning, like not providing a lateral tilt; this leads to aortocaval compression and hypotension.
- Local anesthetic toxicity is the result of inadvertent/accidental intravenous injection of local anesthetic. It may also be due to excessive and rapid absorption.
- Management is essentially as in the basic management of shock. In addition, it is important to institute life support measures like the use of vasopressor drugs; anticonvulsants should be used if the patient has convulsions.

KEY POINTS

- Shock is an acute life-threatening condition where tissue perfusion is reduced due to hypovolemia or abnormal distribution.
- Hemorrhage and sepsis are leading causes of shock.
- Pallor, tachycardia, hypotension and dehydration are the prominent features.
- Renal dysfunction may lead to oliguria and anuria.
- ARDS may be a feature of septic shock.
- Early resuscitative measures will help reduce mortality and morbidity.
- Replacement of blood is the mainstay of treatment in hemorrhagic shock.
- Crystalloid replacement, inotropic support, appropriate antibiotic therapy and correction of fluid–electrolyte, acid–base imbalance are important aspects of management of septic shock.
- The cause of shock should be simultaneously treated.
- Anaphylaxis, amniotic fluid embolism and anesthetic accidents are uncommon causes of shock.

QUESTIONS

Select the single most appropriate answer:

1. The most common cause of shock in obstetrics is
   a. infection c. cardiac disease
   b. hemorrhage d. eclampsia
2. All of the following are end results of septicemia except
   a. lactic acidemia
   b. disturbance in microvascular circulation
   c. respiratory alkalosis
   d. poor oxygenation
3. In a patient who is in shock the most recommended IV fluid is
   a. 5% dextrose
   b. normal saline
   c. 10% dextrose
   d. ringer lactate
4. Cardiogenic shock in a pregnant woman occurs most frequently at
   a. 14 to 18 weeks
   b. 20 to 24 weeks
   c. 28 to 32 weeks
   d. 34 to 38 weeks
5. Amniotic fluid embolism is associated with all the following *except*
   a. sudden dyspnea
   b. hypertension
   c. cyanosis
   d. disseminated intravascular coagulation

In the following questions there are two statements. Select the appropriate answer using the following key:

a. if both statements are true and causally related
b. if both statements are true but not causally related
c. if the first statement is true and the second is false
d. if the first statement is false and the second is true
e. if both statements are false

6. In shock delivery of oxygen and nutrients to tissues is reduced *because*

   There is drop in blood flow leading to acute hypoperfusion
7. In septic shock there is decrease in tissue perfusion *because*

   In septic shock there is an overall decrease in circulatory volume

60

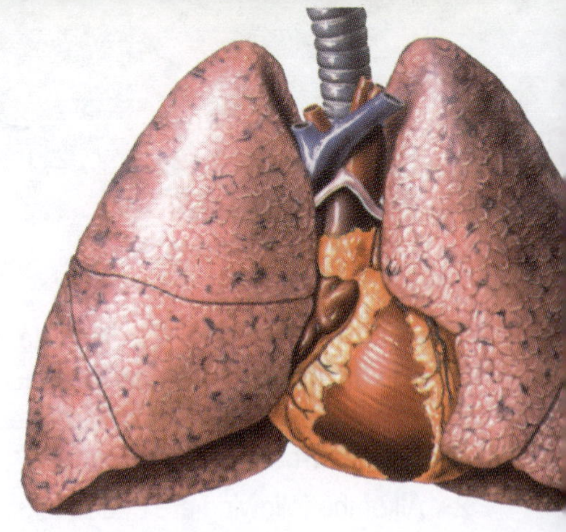

Disseminated Intravascular Coagulation

S Habeebullah

LEARNING OBJECTIVES

At the end of this chapter, the reader should be able to:
- recapitulate the normal coagulation mechanism
- list the obstetric conditions that predispose to DIC
- appreciate the adverse effects of DIC
- describe the pathophysiology of DIC
- list the investigations useful in the management
- enumerate the principles of the management of DIC

Introduction

During pregnancy and childbirth, a woman is at high risk of hemorrhage. As a protective mechanism, apart from an increase in blood volume, major changes occur in the coagulation system. There is a rise in the level of plasma fibrinogen, from 300 mg/dl in the nonpregnant state to 450–600 mg/dl. The circulating levels of factors VII, VIII, IX and X also rise remarkably. There are no significant changes in the levels of other circulating factors and platelets. The levels of factor XI and XII decrease. Another important change is a reduction in fibrinolytic activity which returns to normal within an hour of delivery of the placenta. The increased coagulation factors and reduced fibrinolytic activity make pregnancy a 'hypercoagulable' state. Normally, a fine dynamic balance exists between procoagulants (fibrinogen) and anticoagulants (fibrinolysins) in vivo. However, in certain complications of pregnancy, this balance is disturbed leading to widespread coagulation in blood vessels, called disseminated intravascular coagulation (DIC), paradoxically resulting in hemorrhage. More than half the cases of DIC are of obstetric origin.

Physiology of Coagulation

The normal hemostatic mechanism is complex. It includes intact vasculature, normal platelets, procoagulants and anticoagulants. Intact endothelium (vasculature) plays an important role in preventing coagulation inside the vasculature.

The four important steps in the coagulation pathway are:
1. Activation of factor X
2. Conversion of prothrombin to thrombin
3. Formation of fibrin and its stabilisation
4. Resolution of fibrin by fibrinolysins once the purpose is achieved.

The physiology of coagulation is shown in **Fig. 60.1**.

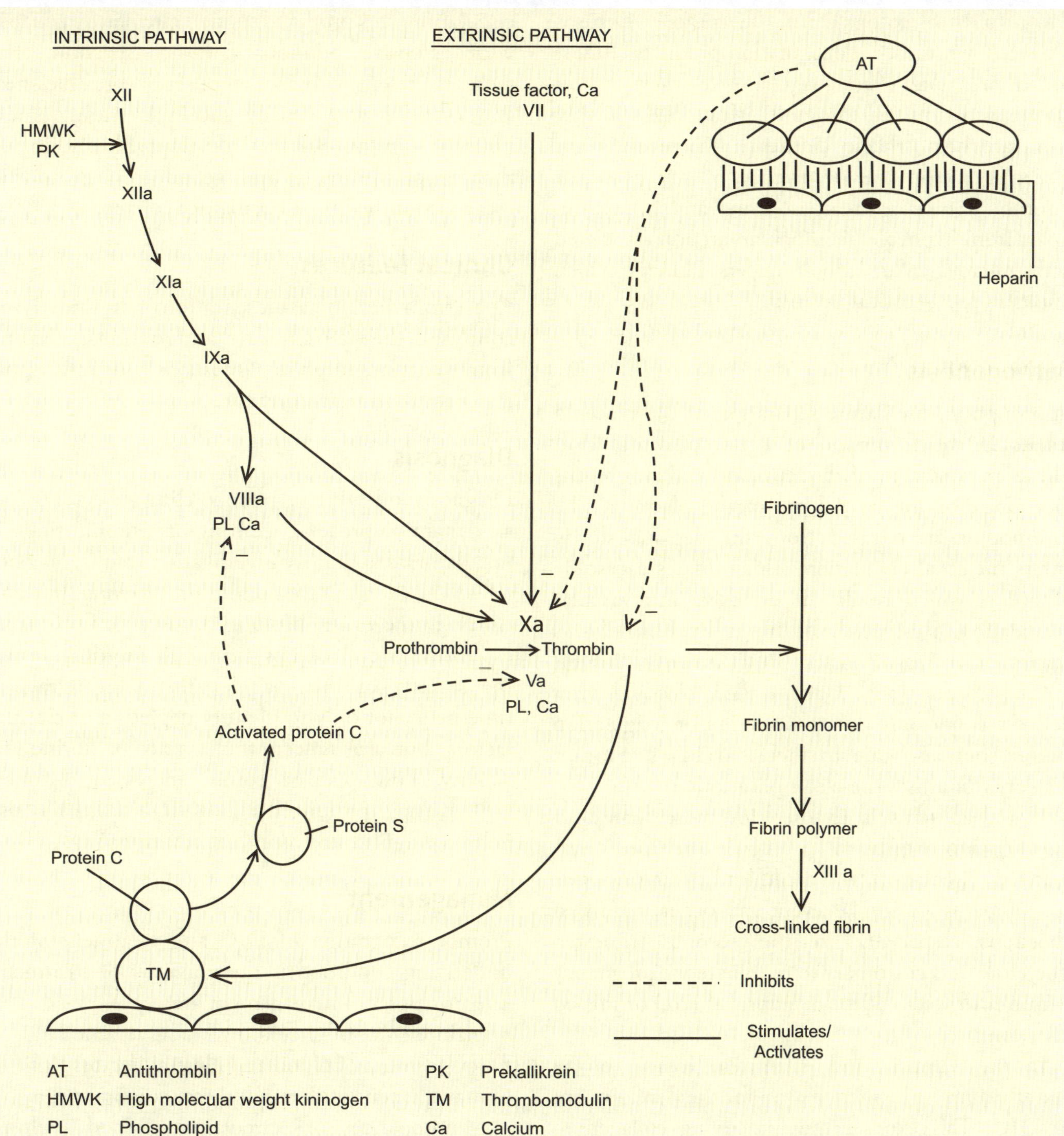

Fig. 60.1 Normal coagulation cascade.

Causes of DIC

Disseminated intravascular coagulation, also known as **consumptive coagulopathy** in obstetrics, is always secondary to an underlying problem. The common causes are abruptio placentae, amniotic fluid embolism, prolonged retention of a dead fetus, septic abortion, preeclampsia/eclampsia, missed abortion and chorioamnionitis.

In 1901, Dee Lee described DIC following abruption as 'temporary hemophilia'. In DIC there is extensive coagulation which results in the consumption of all coagulation factors, leading to uncontrolled bleeding. During the process, fibrin is broken down to fibrin degradation products (FDPs) which are potent anticoagulants as they inhibit platelet function and thrombin. Thus, FDPs further aggravate hemorrhagic diathesis. Whatever is the initiating factor, the occurrence of microvascular thrombi results in organ ischemia and infarction. Apart from hypovolemic shock, infarction associated with microvascular emboli targets kidneys which results in renal cortical necrosis.

Pathogenesis

In abruption, premature separation of the placenta results in the formation of a retroplacental clot. The slow expansion of the retroplacental clot results in rupture of the basal plate of the placenta. The thromboplastin released from the decidua slowly enters maternal circulation. This initiates a cascade of events which results in extensive intravascular coagulation. Resolution of fibrin by fibrinolysins results in increased FDPs. FDPs strongly inhibit uterine contractions. Uncontrolled bleeding after delivery is not only due to depletion of coagulation factors, but also due to increased FDPs. Prompt delivery minimises these complications.

If a dead fetus is retained for more than four weeks, thromboplastin is slowly released into maternal circulation, and could lead to consumptive coagulopathy. A similar event can occur in missed abortions, especially in the second trimester. Therefore, it is customary to terminate the pregnancy within **four** weeks of the diagnosis of IUD or missed abortion.

In preeclampsia and eclampsia, injury to the endothelium is the main reason for the development of DIC. This exposes the underlying collagen to procoagulant factors.

In septicemia, multiple factors contribute to DIC. Most important are endothelial damage due to endotoxins and activation of the extrinsic pathway due to the expression of tissue factors.

Amniotic fluid embolism is very rare but is almost fatal in about 50% of cases. It is usually associated with strong uterine contractions. This forces the amniotic fluid and its components into maternal circulation; this produces sudden circulatory collapse with extensive pulmonary vasoconstriction. The patients present with sudden onset of breathlessness and cyanosis and usually succumb within a few hours. Coagulation failure develops rapidly due to thromboplastin release and manifests in those who escape from the initial circulatory collapse.

Clinical features

Apart from the clinical presentation of the underlying condition, the main clinical manifestation is bleeding from venepuncture sites, epistaxis, purpuric spots and postpartum hemorrhage.

Diagnosis

Diagnosis of DIC is mainly clinical. As DIC is a dynamic process, continuous monitoring is mandatory. Laboratory investigation results may not reflect the extent of the condition. Bleeding time and clotting time will be prolonged. Reduced fibrinogen, especially a level of less than 100 mg/dl indicates the severity of the coagulopathy. Clot retraction time helps not only to identify depletion of clotting factors, but also reflects the severity of fibrinolytic activity. Low platelet count, increased d-dimers (>80 μg/ml), prolonged PT (INR) and aPTT also help to diagnose and assess the severity of DIC.

Management

Prompt recognition of DIC and treatment of the underlying condition is the mainstay of treatment. The principles of management are:

- maintenance of circulating blood volume
- replacement of blood and clotting factors
- management of the underlying condition.

Maintenance of circulating blood volume by crystalloid, colloid and blood is of prime importance because it not only maintains perfusion to vital organs but also helps to clear the FDPs from the circulation. Dextran should not be used as it interferes with platelet function and can aggravate DIC and bleeding. Prompt fluid replacement also prevents renal failure.

Packed cell transfusion alone is not sufficient as it lacks clotting factors. Fresh frozen plasma (FFP)

200–250 ml contains all clotting factors except platelets and one unit of FFP increases the fibrinogen by 100 mg. Cryoprecipitate 20–40 ml contains mainly fibrinogen apart from factors VIII and XIII, and one unit increases the fibrinogen by 10 mg.

Platelet transfusion is necessary if platelet count is less than 50,000/mm^3. Each unit (50 ml) provides 5,000–10,000 cells/mm^3.

In general, heparin and antifibrinolytics have no role in the management of DIC.

Management of the underlying condition is the most essential part in the management of DIC. In abruption, prompt delivery should be achieved by amniotomy and oxytocin. Most of the IUDs will be expelled spontaneously within two weeks. Nowadays it is rare to encounter DIC in cases of IUD as labour is induced in all cases soon after diagnosis. It is customary to perform basic investigations along with plasma fibrinogen before induction.

As amniotic fluid embolism is difficult to predict and diagnose, it is very difficult to manage. Cardiopulmonary support and replacement of clotting factors are vital. In septic abortion and chorioamnionitis, treatment with broad-spectrum antibiotics along with removal of septic foci are essential to prevent the development of DIC.

KEY POINTS

- Pregnancy is a hypercoagulable state.
- Obstetrical complications contribute significantly to the occurrence of DIC.
- Release of thromboplastin and/or endothelial injury are responsible for initiating intravascular coagulation.
- Fibrinogen level of <100 mg/dl, presence of FDPs, platelet counts <50,000/mm^3 and D-dimer >80 µg/ml help in diagnosing DIC.
- Treatment consists of circulatory support, replacement of coagulation factors and management of the underlying obstetric condition.

QUESTIONS

Select the single most appropriate answer:

1. In pregnancy, levels of all the following are increased *except*
   a. fibrinogen
   b. platelet count
   c. factor IX
   d. factor X
2. All of the following may be associated with disseminated intravascular coagulation *except*
   a. threatened abortion
   b. amniotic fluid embolism
   c. abruptio placentae
   d. prolonged retention of dead fetus
3. During pregnancy fibrinolytic activity is reduced, but it returns to normal how many hours after delivery?
   a. 1 hour b. 2 hours c. 3 hours d. 4 hours
4. Which of the following statement is *false* about pathogenesis of DIC?
   a. in placental abruption thromboplastin is released from the decidua
   b. level of fibrin degradation products (FDPs) is increased
   c. FDPs do not inhibit uterine contractions
   d. there is uncontrolled bleeding from the uterus
5. In a case of DIC it is best to transfuse
   a. whole blood
   b. packed cells
   c. fresh frozen plasma
   d. platelets

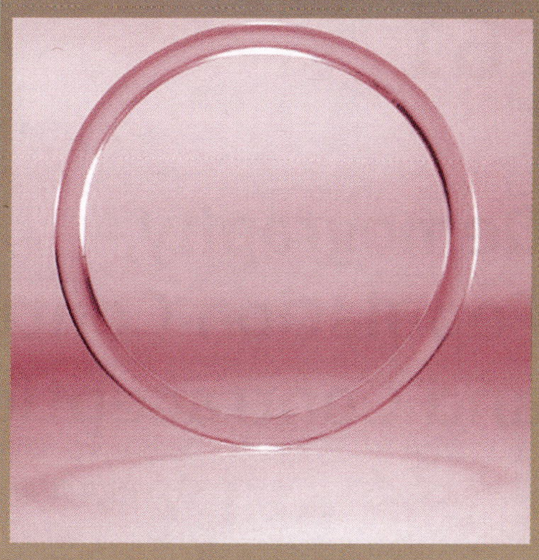

Part VII Contraception

61

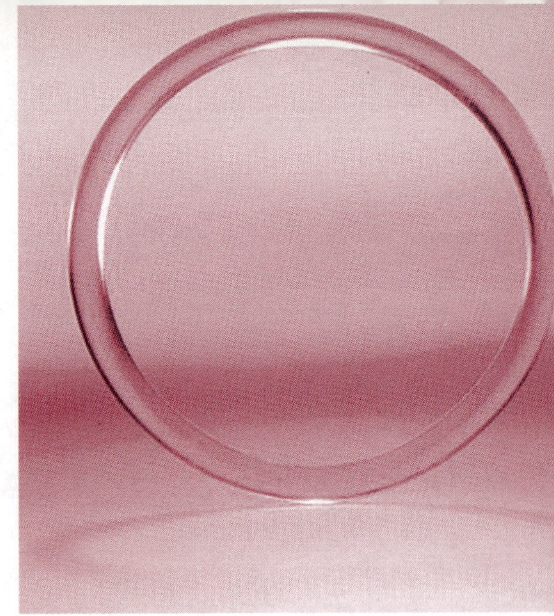

Demography, Population Control and Contraception

S Soundara Raghavan

LEARNING OBJECTIVES

At the end of this chapter, the reader should be able to:

- understand population dynamics and its effect on development
- define demography and the common terminology used in relation to demography
- list the initiatives taken by the Government of India (GOI) for population control
- appreciate the role of contraception in population control
- list the indices for measuring contraceptive effectiveness

Introduction

The world's population has been growing rapidly and it is about 7 billion at present. The population of India is about 1.2 billion, which is approximately 16% of the world's population, but India has only 2.5% the land area of the world (**Fig. 61.1**).

The population of India has been growing at a rate of 1.9% every year. It is widely recognised that population growth is inversely related to development. Population control is one of the measures to aid in the development of a nation. Women and children directly and family and community indirectly will benefit from fertility control measures. Apart from improving the standard of living, it will bring down maternal and infant mortality which will further improve contraceptive acceptance, resulting in a healthy cycle.

Unfortunately poor nations are the ones most affected by illiteracy and consequent lack of awareness, inadequate services, difficulty in accessing even the available services, high parity and poor health of the mothers and children. This forms a vicious cycle difficult to break. Awareness about these factors will help in better understanding of the need for population control measures.

Demography

Demography is the study of population, its size, distribution, determinants and changes.

Population is not constant or static, but is constantly changing. Births, deaths, migration or social mobility, marriage and fertility are responsible for the dynamics of population. Knowledge about these aspects of population will help to plan measures for population control.

Common demographic terms

- **Birth rate** is the number of births per 1,000 mid-year population.

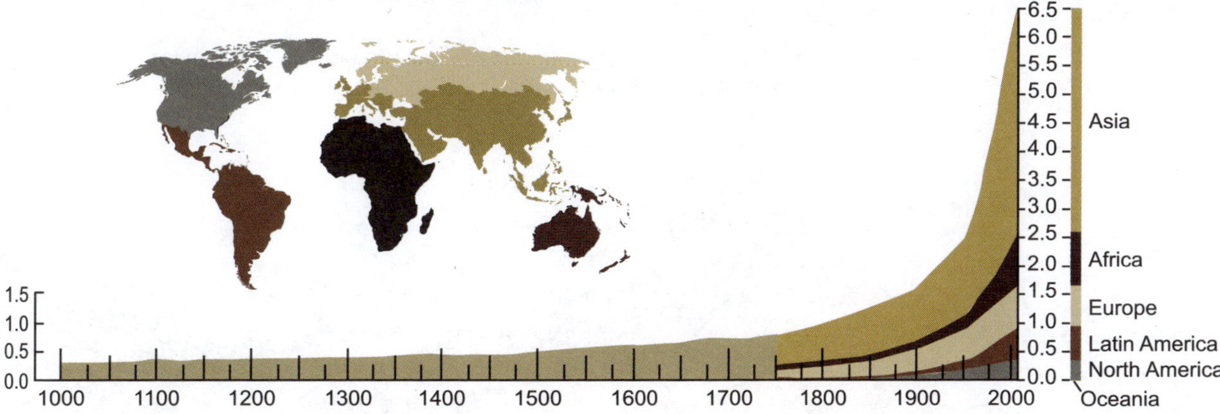

Fig. 61.1 Population, its growth and density (*From the United Nations Secretariat, Population Trends, 2004*). *Source:* 1. The world at six billion: Population division of the Department of Economic and Social Affairs of the United Nations Secretariat; World Population Prospects: The 2004 Revision and World Urbanisation Prospects: The 2003 Revision <http://ea.un.org/unpp> 2. United Nations, 1973. *The Determinants and Consequences of Population Trends,* Vol. 1 (United Nations, New York) (forthcoming); World population prospects: The 1998 Revision (United Nations, New York). <http://www.geohive.com/global>

- **Death rate** is the total number of deaths per 1,000 mid-year population.
- **Growth rate** is birth rate minus death rate.
- **Total fertility rate** is the average number of children that would be born to a married woman through the reproductive years (15–44 years).
- **Net reproduction rate** is the number of daughters a girl will bear in her lifetime.
- **Couple protection rate** is the number of couples effectively protected against pregnancy per 100 couples.

There are several other terms used in demography which help one to study and compare population and its subdivisions. One of the main reasons for the growth in world population is declining death rates without a concomitant reduction in birth rates.

India and population

Like any other developing country, India has its share of problems caused by the rapid rise in its population. The death rate in India has declined significantly from 24 to about 8. While there has been a decline in birth rate from 48 to 23 in the last few decades, India still adds one Australia to its population every year, resulting in a high growth rate, thus slowing down economic development and modernisation. In addition, being a very large country with a wide distribution of people from differing geographical and cultural backgrounds, some areas are less developed than the others (**Fig. 61.2**). The literacy rates and health indicators vary widely between different states.

Government initiatives for population control

India became the first country in the world to formulate a government sponsored programme for population control, called the National Family Planning Programme, in 1952. The programme was made time-bound and target-oriented to make it more focused. In 1969, the All-India Hospital Postpartum Programme was launched, as a hospital-based, maternity-oriented programme to give more attention to pregnant and postpartum women with the hope that this section of people will accept contraception better. In the late 1970s, the term 'Family Planning' was changed to 'Family Welfare Programme' to include other aspects of the care of women and children, like care during pregnancy and delivery. The observation that reduction in maternal and infant mortality resulted in reduction in fertility led to the Maternal and Child Health Programme, further strengthened as the Child Survival Safe Motherhood Programme which also included

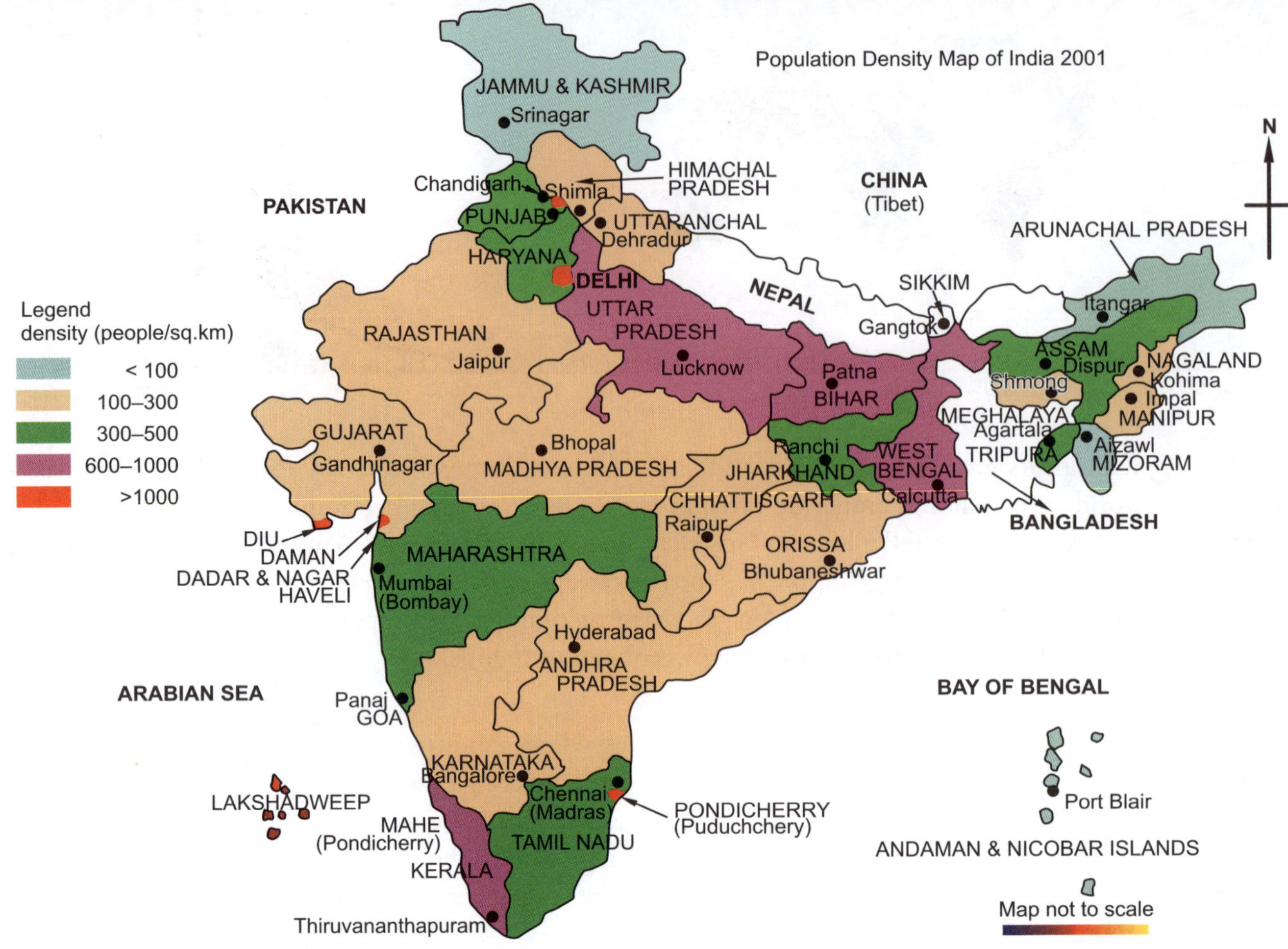

Fig. 61.2 Population distribution in India.

postnatal care, immunisation services for the mother and child, control of diarrheal diseases and respiratory infections and birth control methods focusing on spacing between pregnancies. In the last 15 years or so, the focus has been on Community Need Assessment Approach (CNA) to ensure better community participation in the Reproductive and Child Health (RCH) programme.

The revised National Health Policy of 2000 has set the following goals for 2010:

- fulfilling the unmet need for RCH
- free and compulsory education for children under 14
- reducing the school dropout rate to 20%
- reducing IMR to less than 30
- reducing MMR to less than 100
- increasing immunisation to 100%
- increase in average age at marriage of girls to more than 18 years
- increasing institutional deliveries to 80%
- ensuring a skilled birth attendant for all deliveries
- making the contraceptive of choice available to all

The National Rural Health Mission was launched in 2005 and will end in 2012. It is an omnibus broadband programme integrating all vertical health programmes for effective implementation.

Contraception and Population Control

Fertility control at the individual level will translate to population control at community and, consequently, at national and international levels. Fertility control includes contraception as well as termination of pregnancy. While contraception prevents unwanted pregnancy, termination of unwanted pregnancy is associated with more morbidity and possibly mortality. Hence, contraception should be the first option for population control. While contraception may be adopted for a variety of reasons like limiting family size, spacing between pregnancies or other eugenic reasons, at the macro level, it will bridge the gap between developing and developed countries.

Methods of contraception

There are several temporary and permanent contraceptive methods available for men and women. But in practice, it is the women who adopt these methods more readily than men.

These are:

- **Reversible**
  - Natural methods
  - Barrier methods
  - Intrauterine devices
  - Hormonal methods
    - Oral
    - Injectables
    - Implants
  - Vaginal rings
  - Transdermal patches
  - Intrauterine releasing systems
- **Permanent**
  - Female sterilisation
  - Male sterilisation

Effectiveness of contraception

Contraceptive efficacy can be measured by any of the following methods.

- **Pearl index:**
  - Failure rate per HWY

$$= \frac{\text{Total accidental pregnancies}}{\text{Total months of exposure}} \times 1200$$

- **Life table technique:**
  - Expressed as per 100 women per year
  - Eliminates bias in Pearl index

The most commonly used measureS at present are:

Total fertility rate: Average number of children a woman would have assuming current birth rates exist throughout reproductive years.

Net pregnancy rate: Multiple-decrement probability involving method failure and compliance

While a lot has been achieved, much remains to be done. Health, particularly reproductive health, cannot be looked at in isolation, and a number of social, cultural and economic factors are closely interlinked. Improvement in literacy, economic status, curbing unemployment, raising the age of marriage and eliminating gender bias will all contribute towards this goal. Family Planning has to become a way of life at the family level to meaningfully translate to developmental changes at community, national and international levels.

KEY POINTS

- Demography is the study of population and its characteristics.
- Population is affected by birth, death and migration.
- Rising population affects development adversely.
- Population control has been recognised to be essential for the improvement of health status.
- Contraception forms an important component of population control.
- Several contraceptive choices are available for men and women.
- Contraceptive efficacy is measured by the Pearl index and by life table analysis.

QUESTIONS

Select the single most appropriate answer:

1. Of world population, India's population accounts for
   a. 5% b. 10% c. 16% d. 25%
2. The National Family Planning programme was launched by Government of India in the year
   a. 1947 b. 1952 c. 1971 d. 1983
3. The National Rural Health Mission was launched in the year
   a. 1983 b. 1987 c. 2000 d. 2005
4. Contraception should be preferred over medical termination of pregnancy for population control *because*
   a. MTP has higher morbidity and possibly mortality
   b. medical method of abortion needs expertise
   c. contraception is difficult to adopt
   d. MTP is not widely available
5. Surgical contraception includes all of the following *except*
   a. laparoscopic sterilisation
   b. no-scalpel vasectomy
   c. hormonal implant
   d. minilap sterilisation

62

Natural and Conventional Methods of Contraception

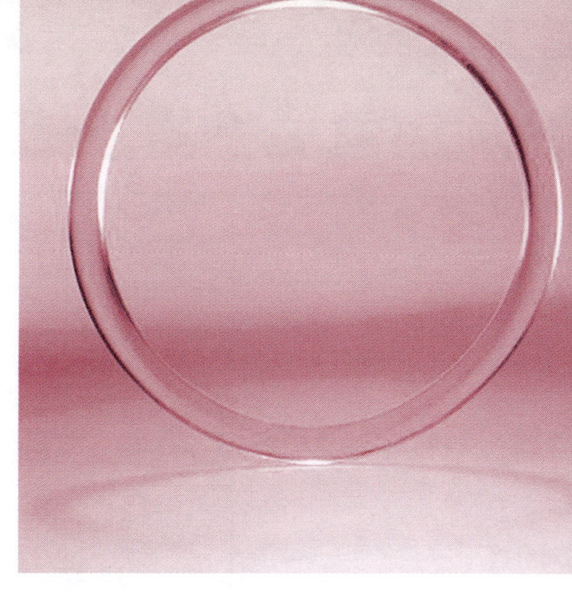

N Sundari

LEARNING OBJECTIVES

At the end of this chapter, the reader should be able to:

- describe the principles that govern the methods of NFP
- enumerate the different methods of NFP
- enumerate the advantages and disadvantages of NFP methods
- describe the principles underlying the use of conventional contraceptives
- list the commonly used conventional contraceptives
- enumerate the advantages and disadvantages of these methods

Introduction

Natural family planning (NFP) methods and conventional contraceptives (CC) have been used by couples over the last few centuries. Natural family planning methods are those which do not use any appliance or medicine. Some of these methods have been practised since prehistoric times. They are specifically adopted by those who have a religious objection to contraceptives that interfere with fertilisation and require implantation. Conventional contraceptive methods are those that are used at the time of intercourse. As compared to contraceptive methods based on medication or surgery, they have a higher failure rate, but the side effects are negligible. These methods are used even today by millions of couples throughout the world.

Natural Methods of Family Planning

Principle

The NFP methods are based on the timing of ovulation, which determines the fertile and infertile periods in a woman's menstrual cycle. The relationship between the cyclical changes in the genital tract and the clinical, hormonal and ultrasound events are described in **Fig. 62.1**.

- Ovulation takes place 14 days before the first day of the next menstrual cycle. The ovum survives on an average for 24 hours. During exclusive breastfeeding, there is absence of ovulation for the first six months.
- Cervical mucus, under the unopposed action of estrogen, becomes increasingly thin and receptive

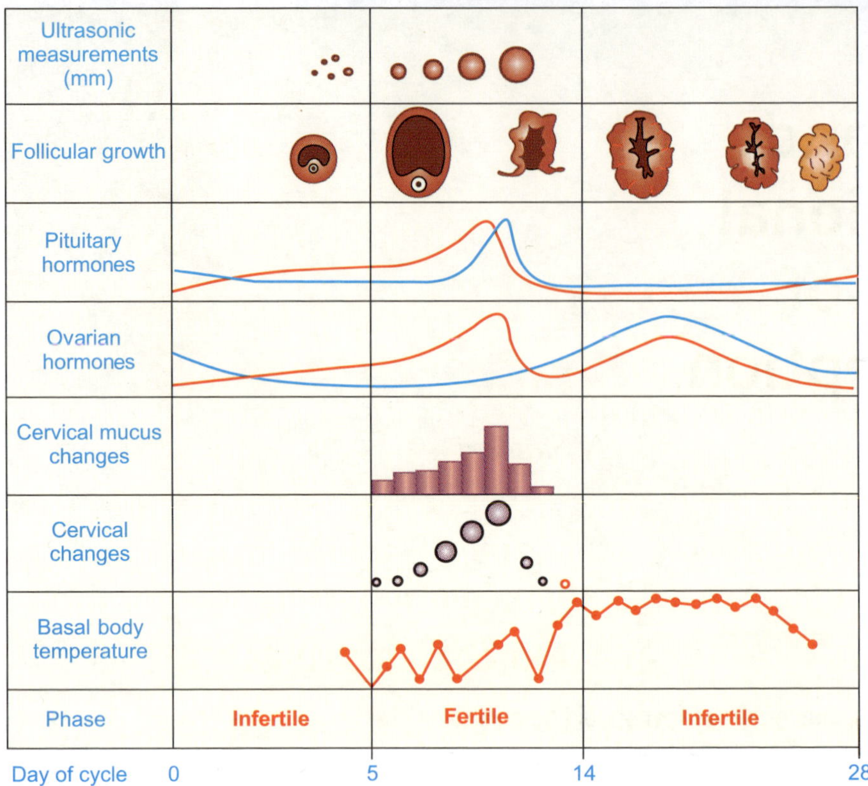

Fig. 62.1 Relationship during the cycle of serial ultrasound measurements, hormonal control and clinical indicators of fertility.

to sperms. It is slippery and can be stretched to a few centimetres.

- Sperms survive on an average for 48–72 hours in the woman's body.

Methods of NFP

Sexual behaviour is modified to avoid intercourse at the time of ovulation. Based on these physiological facts, the following methods of NFP are practised.

Rhythm method: It is also known as the calendar method. In this method, the woman needs to calculate the day of ovulation and determine the fertile period. Few women have regular cycles and therefore the following steps should be adopted to determine the fertile period:

- The woman should define the shortest and longest cycle over the previous 12 cycles
- She should subtract 20 days from the length of the shortest cycle to derive the first day of the fertile period.
- She should subtract 11 days from the longest cycle to derive the last day of the fertile period.

For example if her recorded cycles vary from 26 to 32 days, the fertile period will be from 26–20 = 6 to 32–11 = 21 days. The couple should avoid unprotected intercourse from day 6 to day 21.

Even with good compliance, this method has a high failure rate. Moreover, since many women tend to have irregular periods, the long and continuous period of abstinence is unacceptable to many couples.

The next two methods make use of the clinical indicators of ovulation. Compliance is influenced by the woman's ability to accurately detect and note the indicator.

Cervical mucus method: This is popularly known as **Billing's method.** It is based on recognising when the scanty and thick cervical mucus in the preovulatory phase becomes profuse, transparent and watery. The discharge can be drawn out into a thread between the fingers (spinnbarkeit test). The woman also experiences a 'wetness' at the vulva. The discharge becomes scanty and thick once again in the postovulatory phase. Women are trained to recognise the type of discharge and record the changes on paper or preferably on a chart. The 'dry' days refer to the infertile period when intercourse can be practised: the couple is advised to abstain once the 'wet' days begin.

Basal body temperature (BBT) method: This is based on the clinical indicator of the biphasic nature of the temperature caused by metabolites of progesterone. The woman records her body temperature under basal conditions as she wakes up from sleep, without getting out of bed or having a drink. There is a preovulatory drop of 0.5 °C and a postovulatory rise of 0.2–0.6 °C; hence it is advisable to use a special expanded-scale mercury thermometer or a modern electronic version. The results are recorded daily to measure the rise. It is generally accepted that ovulation occurs just before the temperature rise.

The disadvantages of this method are as follows:

- The temperature has to be recorded meticulously.
- If the woman has fever, the method is invalid.
- The end of the preovulatory safe period cannot be determined.

Symptothermal method: As the name suggests, it uses all the clinical indicators discussed above, apart from other symptoms like midcycle pain, and bleeding to predict the time of ovulation. The woman is advised to maintain a chart where all the changes are noted. Therefore, it is more reliable in determining the safe period. The drawback is that the woman has to be highly motivated to note the changes and record them on a chart.

Effectiveness of NFP methods

The typical failure rates are estimated to be 20 per 100 woman years (20/HWY) in the first year of use. Later, the failure rates are reduced to 1–9/HWY.

Advantages

The greatest advantage is that no medication, device or surgery is used, and therefore the risk of side effects is nonexistent. Control of fertility is entirely in the hands of the couple.

Disadvantages

The partners need to be highly motivated and cooperative. The couple requires training and help. In some cases, the period of abstinence could be long and hence unacceptable. Should a pregnancy occur, there might be an increased risk of fetal malformation, spontaneous abortion or ectopic pregnancy, but this risk has not been proven.

Contraindications

The NFP method cannot be adopted by women who have very irregular periods, have undergone surgical procedures on the cervix, are suffering from pelvic inflammatory disease and whose partners are not cooperative.

Lactational amenorrhea method (LAM)

Mechanism of action: This method of contraception is based on the fact that there is no ovulation when a woman is breasteeding and has amenorrhea. She is unlikely to become pregnant if she is **exclusively** breastfeeding her baby. It is noted that during lactation there is excessive secretion of prolactin. The high levels of prolactin in the blood inhibit the secretion of LH from the pituitary, but have no effect on the secretion of FSH. The ovaries are refractory to LH and FSH with the result that ovulation and menstruation do not occur. The more the woman suckles her baby, the higher the secretion of prolactin and the fewer the chances of ovulation.

Counselling: Women who are breastfeeding should be counselled that the contraceptive effect of lactation is closely linked to exclusive breastfeeding, on demand through 24 hours. It is difficult to estimate the exact duration of protection against pregnancy, but amenorrhea provides a high degree of protection. The contraceptive effect of lactation declines with the onset of menstruation. In brief, LAM is most effective for six months if the woman is exclusively breastfeeding. After six months or with the first menstruation, the woman should be advised to adopt other methods of contraception.

Effectiveness: The failure rates for six months are 2/HWY, but may be higher.

Advantages: LAM has all the advantages of NFP. In addition, the woman who exclusively breastfeeds her child is less likely to develop breast cancer. In addition, the use of other contraceptives can be postponed during this period.

Disadvantages: Contraceptive efficacy is uncertain.

Contraindications: These are the same as for breastfeeding like when the woman is HIV positive, is on drugs that are secreted in breast milk or is seriously ill.

Conventional Methods of Contraception

Conventional methods of contraception are those that require action just before or at the time of sexual intercourse. There are various physical and chemical methods that can be used singly or in combination. These are effective only when they are used consistently and carefully.

Types of contraceptives

A variety of methods are available for both men and women. They can be classified as follows:

- **Barrier or physical methods:** Condoms, diaphragms and vaginal sponges
- **Chemical methods:** Foams, tablets, creams, jellies and suppositories
- Combined methods

Male condom

A condom is a close-ended stretchable tubular device designed to cover the erect penis and physically prevent the deposition of sperms in the vagina. It is made of vulcanised latex rubber or silicon which is as thin as possible while maintaining adequate strength; it is often lubricated to minimise loss of 'sensitivity'. They are 15–20 cm long, 3–3.5 cm in diameter and 0.003–0.007 cm in thickness. They are available in dry, semi-dry and, pre-lubricated forms or as spermicidal condoms (coated with nonoxynol 9). Condoms are packed rolled on to the rim and usually sealed in aluminium or plastic foil.

In India, condoms are manufactured and supplied free of cost by the Ministry of Health and Family Welfare, Government of India, under the brand name 'Nirodh'. In the market, lubricated condoms are available under names like Nirodh Lubricated, Kamasutra and Kohinoor; brands lubricated with spermicides are Rakshak or Share. The average shelf-life of condoms is five years from the time of manufacture. They should be stored in a cool dry place.

Effectiveness: The failure rates are variable and pregnancies occur more due to user failure than method failure. When used correctly every time, failure rates are 1–3 per HWY; otherwise, the rates are 8–14/HWY.

Advantages: These are listed below.

- free of medical risks
- easily available and relatively inexpensive
- effective if used consistently and correctly
- suitable for couples who have infrequent coitus, during lactation or who cannot tolerate oral contraceptive pills or intrauterine devices
- involves the male partner in contraceptive responsibility
- protects against STDs
- may reduce the risk of cervical dysplasia and cervical cancer.

Disadvantages: There are almost no disadvantages. However, some men may experience the following:

- allergy to latex/lubricant
- interruption of the sexual act and decreased sensitivity during coitus
- reduced sexual pleasure
- higher failure rates
- storage and disposal, a problem particularly in rural areas.

Directions for use

- Damaged condoms should be avoided. Lubricants like baby oil or vaseline should not be used. KY jelly or a spermicidal product may be used.
- The condom is put on the erect penis before any genital contact. If there is no teat, the end of the sheath is pinched to make room for the semen.

- After intercourse, the penis is withdrawn before it becomes too soft, holding the base of the penis and taking care not to spill any semen.
- Each condom is used only once.
- For maximum effectiveness the female partner should use a spermicide.
- In case the condom breaks or slips off around the fertile period, the female partner should take emergency contraception within 72 hours.

Female condom

The female condom is a disposable barrier contraceptive for women. It is made of polyurethane, and is a thin, loose sac 15–17 cm long with an outer ring to prevent it from advancing beyond the vulva, and an inner ring that helps to retain the device in the vagina (**Fig. 62.2**).

The main advantage is that it is woman-controlled, secondly it is inserted before intercourse and and most importantly it protects the woman against sexually transmitted diseases.

Occlusive caps

These are contraceptives that a woman places in the vagina shortly before intercourse. They are not as effective as sperm-proof mechanical barriers like condoms, but are used as a means to retain spermicides in contact with the cervical os. They are usually made of rubber.

There are four types of caps (**Fig. 62.3**). The last three are not commonly used.

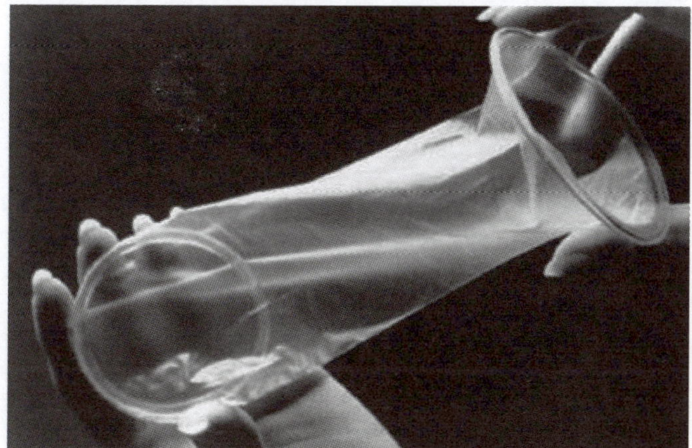

Fig. 62.2 Female condom.

- vaginal diaphragm (most common)
- vault cap: no metal spring at the rim
- cervical cap
- vimule cap

The vaginal diaphragm is a thin, nearly hemispherical dome made of rubber or latex with a circular, covered metal spring at the periphery. When properly placed, they block sperms. They should not be used in the following conditions where the appliance does not fit:

- genital prolapse
- cystocele
- cervix too short or too long or badly lacerated
- gross retroversion of the uterus.

Effectiveness varies depending on correct and consistent use. A failure rate of 5–25/100 per HWY has been reported in the first year of use. Failures are due to improper fitting, non-use of spermicides, defective occlusive caps and displacement of cervical cap during coitus.

The following instructions are essential to improve the effectiveness of these barrier methods:

- The health care provider prescribes the correct size after a pelvic examination.
- The client should be taught the right method of insertion, removal and storage of the device.
- The woman should smear 5 cm of cream or jelly (spermicide) on the inner and outer surfaces before introduction.
- To be introduced only two hours before the sexual act. If delayed beyond two hours, spermicidal jelly should be reintroduced.
- The device should not be removed before six hours after the act and should not be kept for more than 24 hours.

After removal, the device should be cleaned with soap water, dried, powdered and kept in a proper container.

There are some **disadvantages** associated with these devices:

- requires pelvic examination and prescription for proper of fitting device by a health care provider
- allergy to rubber or the spermicidal agent
- suitable only for highly motivated women
- may need a different size of diaphragm after childbirth

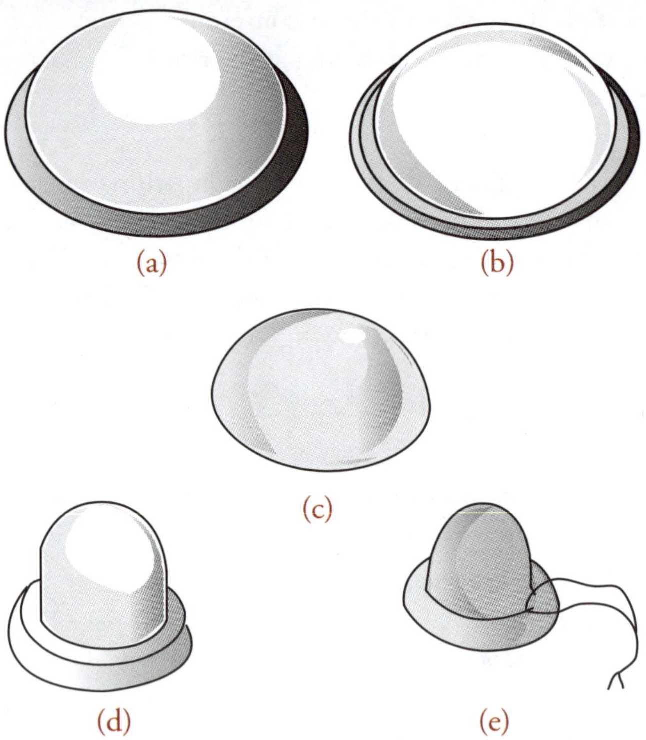

Fig. 62.3 a: and b: Vaginal diaphragm c: Vault cap d: Cervical cap e: Vimule cap.

- need careful storage to avoid damage
- may not prevent STDs.

Spermicides or chemical contraceptives

These contraceptives are chemical agents capable of destroying sperms. The commonly used agents contain nonionic surfactants which alter permeability of the sperm surface and kill them. Most contain nonoxynol 9, the best known spermicide. The spermicides are **not** very effective in preventing pregnancies when used alone; the failure rate is 6–36/HWY in the first year of use. Their main role is to improve the contraceptive effect of barrier methods. Spermicides are available as suppositories, creams, jellies and foam tablets. The foam tablets incorporate an active spermicide with foaming ingredients which effervesce when they come in contact with vaginal moisture.

Directions should be given clearly and the client warned of the failure rates. The client should be instructed to use the spermicide along with a barrier method, the tablet should be inserted at least 10 minutes before sexual intercourse and she should not wash herself for six hours.

Spermicides are available over the counter and there is no need to consult a health care provider. They do not have any side effects except an occasional allergic reaction. They protect against sexually transmitted diseases to some extent.

KEY POINTS

- Natural family planning (NFP) methods are those that do not use any medication or appliance.
- NFP is based on the timing of ovulation and on the duration of survival of sperms.
- The time of ovulation can be determined by any of three methods: rhythm/calendar, cervical mucus and basal body temperature (BBT).
- NFP has the great advantage of not having any side effects. The disadvantage is that the couple needs to be highly motivated and well trained in the use of NFP.
- Lactational amenorrhea is effective as a contraceptive for six months postpartum if the woman is exclusively feeding the baby.
- Conventional methods are those when the contraceptive device is used by one or both partners just before or at the time of sexual intercourse.
- The most common contraceptives are male condoms. If used correctly and consistently, the method is effective.
- There are no side effects, but the disadvantage is interruption during sexual intercourse.
- The effectiveness of barrier methods for women is variable. The woman needs to consult a health care provider to ascertain the correct size of the device.
- Nonxynol 9 is the best spermicide.
- Both male and female condoms protect the partners against sexually transmitted diseases.

QUESTIONS

Select the single most appropriate answer:

1. The term conventional contraceptives refers to
   a. those used traditionally
   b. calendar method
   c. coitus interruptus
   d. those used at the time of sexual intercourse
2. Which one of the following statements is true about natural contraceptive methods?
   a. they are based on religious teaching
   b. natural products are used
   c. they do not involve use of a drug or an appliance
   d. they are highly effective
3. Natural family planning methods are based on
   a. timing of ovulation
   b. use of natural products
   c. douching after intercourse
   d. use of condoms
4. An example of a conventional contraceptive is
   a. basal body temperature method
   b. condom
   c. cervical mucus method
   d. coitus interruptus
5. Natural method of contraception is most suitable for women
   a. with irregular periods
   b. with lactational amenorrhea
   c. with uncooperative partners
   d. with regular menstruation
6. Lactational amenorrhea has a contraceptive effect because it
   a. causes thickening of cervical mucus
   b. has spermicidal action
   c. inhibits ovulation
   d. decreases libido
7. Lactational amenorrhea method of contraception is most effective for
   a. 6 weeks
   b. 3 months
   c. 6 months
   d. 12 months
8. Conventional methods of contraception include all of the following *except*
   a. intrauterine device
   b. condom
   c. chemical methods
   d. female condom
9. The additional advantage of condom is that it
   a. is highly effective
   b. increases sexual pleasure
   c. is reusable
   d. prevents sexually transmitted infections
10. The efficacy of condom is improved by
    a. increasing the cost
    b. making it dotted
    c. adding a chemical coating of spermicide
    d. making it thinner

63

Hormonal Contraceptives

Raksha Arora

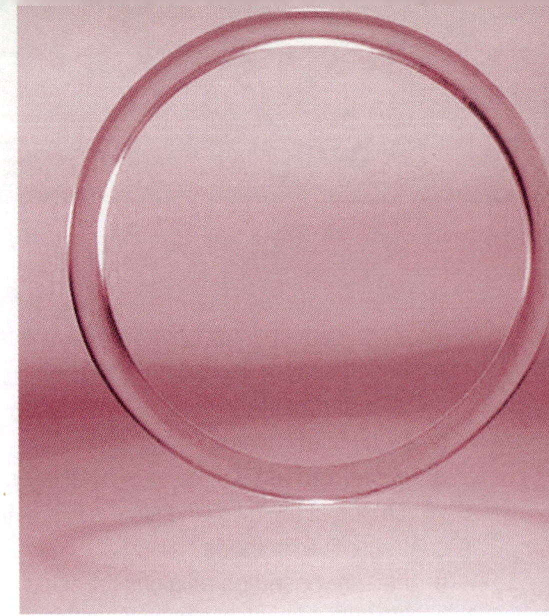

LEARNING OBJECTIVES

At the end of this chapter, the reader should be able to:

- explain the mechanism of action of hormonal contraceptives
- list the available preparations
- describe the effectiveness of various methods.
- list the advantages and disadvantages of combined oral contraceptives (COCs)
- explain the beneficial and adverse effects and contraindications of COCs
- describe the drug interactions
- list the progestogen-only contraceptives and their advantages and disadvantages
- describe the non-oral delivery systems of hormonal contraceptives

Introduction

Hormonal contraceptives were introduced in 1960. They essentially consist of a combination of synthetic estrogen and progesterone, or progesterone alone. They are available as oral pills, injectables and implants. In addition to being effective and reversible, hormonal contraceptives have several noncontraceptive benefits when compared to other methods.

Hormone Preparations used for Contraception

The estrogen found in all contraceptives is **ethinyl estradiol** (EE). The most commonly used progestogen is **levonorgestrel** (LNG). In an effort to reduce the estrogenic, antiestrogenic and androgenic effects of progestogens, desogestrel is used instead of LNG. There are two types of hormonal contraceptives:

- Combined estrogen and progestogen contraceptives: oral pills, injectables and transdermal patches.
- Progestogen-only contraceptives: pills, injectables, implants, intrauterine devices and vaginal rings

Combined Oral Contraceptive (COC) Pills

The COC pills are of two types: one preparation has a fixed dose of EE and progestogen. A second variety contains varying doses of the hormones to reduce the total dose of hormones ingested in a cycle. Previously, the dose of EE was 50 µg. Since most side effects of COC are estrogen dose–related, the estrogen content has been reduced to 30 µg or even 20 µg.The dose of LNG is 150 µg/300 µg. Another advance is the use of progestogens like desogestrel which are more selective and thus unwanted side effects like acne are minimised. More recently, drosperinone is being used.

Most modern pills are 'low-dose' varieties; that is, the dose of each hormone is the lowest possible to achieve reliability, cycle control and safety. The different preparations of low-dose combined pills available in India are listed in **Table 63.1**.

Mechanism of action: The COCs act mainly by suppressing ovulation by inhibiting GnRH and gonadotropin release. They also make the endometrium unfavourable for implantation by premature decidualisation. The progestogen component thickens the cervical mucus, thus inhibiting sperm penetration.

Effectiveness: Combined pills are the most effective method of all temporary methods of contraception. The failure rate, when used appropriately and consistently, is only 0.1% or 1 in 1,000 in the first year of use. However, the typical failure rate is 1.8%. Failure is often due to missed pills, delay in starting the next course and stoppage of the drug due to side effects.

Metabolic effects: The hormones in the COCs affect the metabolism and cause some adverse effects. However, with reduced doses of both EE and progestogen, proper selection of clients and follow-up, these effects can be minimised.

The metabolic effects influance almost all systems.

- COCs increase the levels of triglycerides and total cholesterol. The extent of increase depends on the dose and duration of use.
- COCs increase glucose intolerance and may increase the severity of existing diabetes or induce diabetes in susceptible women. For example, women with a history of gestational diabetes are likely to develop diabetes if they use COCs.
- Estrogen in the COCs is responsible for the increased production of globulins by the liver. There is also an increase in the production of angiotensinogen, leading ultimately to hypertension (pill-induced).
- Fibrinogen and other coagulation factors are increased and the rise is directly proportional to the dose of estrogen.
- Cholestasis and cholestatic jaundice are increased among COC pill users.

Other effects: These are as follows.

- There is documentation that, in rare cases, hepatic focal nodular hyperplasia and tumour formation may occur.The relationship between the use of COCs and breast cancer is unclear.
- COCs produce cervical mucorrhea due to cervical ectopy. The users are likely to suffer from vaginal candidiasis.

Beneficial effects

Contraceptive benefits

- very effective and consistently protects against both intrauterine and ectopic pregnancy
- safe and easy to use at any age from adolescence to menopause
- reversible and use can be discontinued at any time
- use is unrelated to sexual activity.

Noncontraceptive benefits

- ensures a regular 28-day menstrual cycle
- decreases menstrual blood loss and duration and thus prevents anemia
- reduces symptoms like premenstrual tension, spasmodic dysmenorrhea and midcycle ovulation pain

Table 63.1 Different preparations of low-dose combined pills

Combined pills	Estrogen (ethinyl estradiol)	Progestogen
Mala D (or Ovral-L)	30 μg	0.15 mg levonorgestrel
Novelon	30 μg	0.15 mg desogestrel
Femilon or Elogen	20 μg	0.15 mg desogestrel
Mala N	30 μg	0.30 mg levonorgestrel
Triquilar (triphasic pill)	30 μg for 6 days	0.05 mg levonorgestrel
	40 μg for 5 days	0.075 mg levonorgestrel
	30 μg for 10 days	0.125 mg levonorgestrel

- reduces the risk of pelvic inflammatory disease
- decreases the incidence of rheumatoid arthritis
- protects from ovarian and endometrial cancers
- protects from functional ovarian cysts
- protects from benign breast conditions such as fibroadenoma and fibrocystic disease.

Advantages

- ease of administration
- client controlled
- high efficacy
- several noncontraceptive benefits
- ideal for long-term use

Disadvantages

- the pill has to be taken every day: it may be difficult to remember to take it.
- it does not protect against sexually transmitted diseases like HIV.
- it is not appropriate for mothers who are breastfeeding.

Side effects: Minor side effects are common in the first three months of use; they usually disappear with continued use.

- nausea
- headache
- weight gain
- breast tenderness
- amenorrhea (postpill amenorrhea)
- intermenstrual bleeding or spotting (breakthrough bleeding)

Serious side effects such as venous thrombosis, liver problems like cholestasis, heart attack and stroke are rare with current COCs that have very low doses of estrogens and progestogens. However, the risk is high among women who smoke, particularly those over 35 years. However, women, who smoke, irrespective of the use of COCs, are at increased risk for the above complications.

Management of side effects

Amenorrhea: Whenever a client presents with amenorrhea, the following should be considered:

- check that no pill has been missed
- check if the client is suffering from diarrhea/ vomiting or is on antitubercular, antiepileptic drugs or antibiotics
- rule out pregnancy and reassure the client.

Spotting or intermenstrual bleeding: Reconfirm that the client has been taking the pills regularly and instruct her to continue the second packet. Lesions in the lower genital tract should be excluded.

Nausea: This is a common side effect, but is usually mild. The pill may be taken in the night to overcome this effect.

Headache: Organic causes of headache like migraine, ocular causes and hypertension should be ruled out. Mild analgesics may be prescribed.

Weight gain: Slight weight gain can be expected in the first few months. However, it may be ensured that the weight gain is not due to dietary indiscretion.

Breast tenderness: Some women experience breast discomfort or heaviness. A breast examination is performed to exclude a lesion, and the client is advised breast support and mild analgesics; she should also be reassured.

Indications: Combination contraceptive pills may be used not only for contraceptive benefits, but in particular may be selected for women suffering from certain gynecological problems. They are used by the following:

- those in the reproductive age group, who desire a highly effective contraceptive
- immediately after abortion
- those with menstrual cramps, menorrhagia or irregular cycles
- those with anemia
- those with a history of functional ovarian cysts.

Contraindications: The contraindications for the use of COC pills are discussed below.

Absolute contraindications

- thromboembolic disorders in the present or past
- cardiac disorders like ischemic heart disease, cardiac failure, valvular heart disease
- severe hypertension
- severe headache or migraine with focal neurological symptoms
- diabetes with vascular disorders such as retinopathy, nephropathy or neuropathy
- age above 35 years and heavy smoking
- active liver or gall bladder disease or a history of jaundice in the previous six months or recurrent jaundice in pregnancy

- breastfeeding
- unexplained vaginal bleeding
- history or suspicion of carcinoma of the breast.

Relative contraindications

- age over 40 years
- mild hypertension
- hyperlipidemia
- on antituberculous, antiepileptic or antibiotic therapy
- discontinued at least four weeks before planned surgery
- adolescents who have not reached menarche.

Drug interactions: Combination contraceptive pills interfere with the action of some drugs. For example, the efficacy of aspirin, methyl dopa, oral hypoglycemics and oral anticoagulants is decreased; that of benzodiazepines may be increased or decreased. Conversely, COCs increase the efficacy of drugs like aminophylline, theophylline, corticosteroids and caffeine.

Some drugs interfere with the efficacy of COCs, for example, phenytoin, barbiturates, carbemazepine, rifampicin, ketaconazole and primidone. Since the efficacy of COCs is decreased, women on any of the above drugs must be advised to use a back-up method.

Counselling for COC: Counselling is extremely important and must be done not only on the first visit, but also whenever the client comes for fresh supplies. Counselling is invaluable as it increases client satisfaction and ensures continuation.

Clinical assessment before prescribing oral contraceptive pills: Oral pills should only be provided after thorough clinical evaluation. History must be taken keeping in mind the metabolic and other effects of COCs. This is followed by a physical examination and a pap smear. Blood biochemistry and other investigations are requested whenever indicated.

Instructions for COC use: The client must be briefed about the method of taking the pill properly (**Fig. 63.1**). The combined pill can be started on the first or any of the first five days of the cycle, or the day of MTP or abortion.

- If the packet contains 28 tablets, the next packet is to be started without any break. In case of packets with 21 tablets, the next packet may be started after a gap of seven days or on the first day of withdrawal bleeding.
- The pill must be taken at a fixed time of the day. If one pill is missed, it must be taken as soon as possible and next pill should be taken as per the original schedule. If more than one pill is missed, an additional method should be adopted.
- The recommended schedule for follow-up is: first visit at three months; subsequent visits yearly. The client may be advised to report any untoward symptom or other concerns.

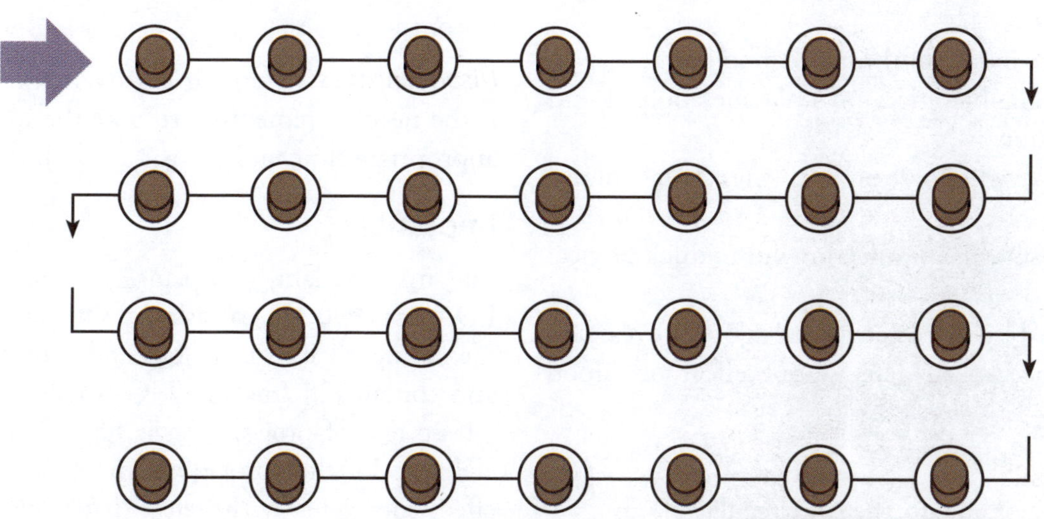

Fig. 63.1 The order in which the pills have to be taken is indicated on the pack.

Progestogen-only contraceptives (POPs)

These contraceptives were introduced mainly to avoid the adverse effects seen in COCs (due to estrogen). They are available as tablets, injectables, implants, intrauterine devices and vaginal rings.

Mechanism of action: The progestogen-only contraceptives act by:

- thickening of cervical mucus and thus making it impermeable to sperms
- thinning and atrophy of endometrium, thus making it unfavourable for implantation
- suppressing ovulation in some cycles.

Effectiveness: These contraceptives, when consistently used, have a failure rate of about 0.5%.

Progestogen-only pills are also referred to as 'mini pills'. Each pill contains progestogen in a small dose, nearly half of that in COCs. In India, these are available as Zerogen or Cerazette (28 tablets) and contain desogestrel 75 μg.

Administration: The mini pill must be taken daily at the same time every day, continuously from the first day of menstruation. A back-up method (condoms) must be used for the first seven days. In women who are breastfeeding, mini pills can be started six weeks after delivery and no back-up method is necessary.

Advantages:

- do not affect lactation; rather, they may increase milk production
- no increase in risk of thromboembolism
- have a negligible effect on lipid metabolism and liver function
- decrease dysmenorrhea and menstrual blood loss
- protect against pelvic infection due to thick cervical mucus
- can be used by women over the age of 40 years
- no evidence to suggest adverse effect on blood pressure.

Disadvantages:

- occurrence of amenorrhea or irregular bleeding
- higher failure rate than the COCs
- higher risk of ectopic pregnancy.

Injectable contraceptives

Injectable contraceptives are synthetic hormones administered intramuscularly at intervals of 1–3 months. The 2- and 3-monthly injections contain only progestogens and the monthly injection contains both progestogen and estrogen.

The following injectable contraceptives are available:

- Depot medroxy progesterone acetate (DMPA) is available as Depo Provera, 150 mg. The advantage of DMPA is that it can be used every three months, and provides immediate protection against pregnancy.
- The new lower dose formulation of Depo Provera (104 mg/0.65 ml) is administered subcutaneously rather than intramuscularly, and is expected to have the same therapeutic efficacy and tolerability.
- NET-EN (norethisterone enanthate) is available as Noristerat, 200 mg and is to be administered every two months.
- Cycloprovera (Cyclofem) is a combination of 25 mg of DMPA and 5 mg of estradiol cypionate. It is administered once a month.
- Mesigna is a combination of 50 mg norethisterone enanthate (NET-EN) and 5 mg estradiol valerate.

Advantages:

- The main advantage of injectable contraceptives is that the client need not take a pill every day.
- With combination injectables, menstrual abnormalities like amenorrhea and irregular bleeding are much less than with progestogen-only contraceptives.

Disadvantages: The main disadvantages of injectables is the need to remember to take the injection at the appropriate time and to visit a health facility.

Implants

The first implant, Norplant, was approved by the FDA in 1990. It consists of six silastic rods, each measuring 34 mm in length and 2 mm in diameter, and contains 36 mg of LNG (totally 216 mg). The release rate of progestogen is 85 μg/day for the first eight weeks, thus providing immediate contraceptive effect; subsequently, the release is 50 μg/day, decreasing gradually to 25–30 μg/day by the end of five years. The rods are inserted under the skin on the inside of the upper arm and have to be surgically removed after five years or whenever the woman wants to discontinue its use. The new system of norplant contains two rods and is called Jadelle or the LNG rod.

Implanon is a single rod containing 67 mg of 3-keto-desogestrel. It is placed subcutaneously in the inner side of the upper arm. It releases 30 µg of the drug daily and is effective for three years (**Fig. 63.2**).

Intrauterine devices

Incorporation of progestogen has added a new dimension to the intrauterine device (IUD). Progestasert and LNG-IUD release progestogen into the uterine cavity. They reduce the risk of pelvic infection (see Chapter 64).

Vaginal rings

Vaginal rings, recently approved by the FDA, offer a new way to deliver hormones into the bloodstream to prevent pregnancy. Combined estrogen and progestin rings offer better cycle control and deliver hormones more steadily than COCs (**Fig. 63.3**).

The ring is inserted by the woman into the upper part of the vagina. The ring remains in place and requires no further attention. If necessary, the ring can be removed for up to three hours for comfort during sexual intercourse or for cleaning.

Vaginal rings have a failure rate of 1.2–1.5 pregnancies per HWY.

Transdermal contraception

This is a newer delivery system approved by the FDA and is not yet available in India. The skin patch contains a combination of progestin and estrogen. This can be controlled by the woman and needs to be changed just once a week (**Fig. 63.4**).

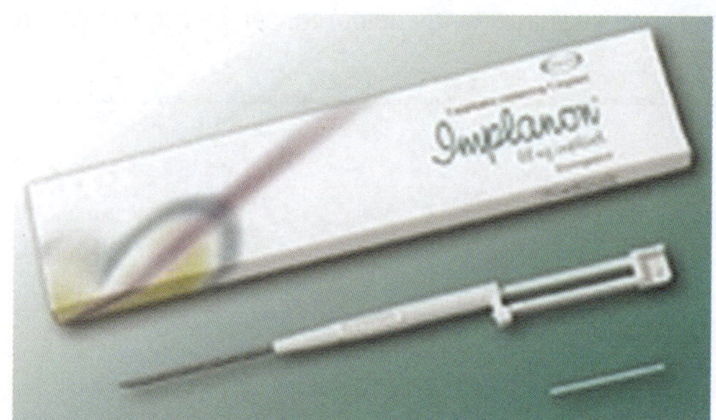

Fig. 63.2 Implanon.

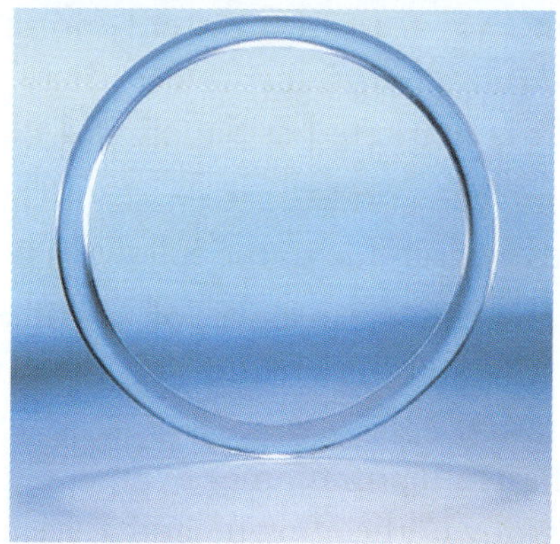

Fig. 63.3 Vaginal ring.

The combined hormonal patch delivers 150 µg of the progestin norelgestromin and 20 µg of the estrogen ethinyl estradiol per day. The woman wears a patch for one week after which she must replace it with a new one. The schedule is three weeks of patch use followed by one patch-free week. The hormones in the patch protect against pregnancy by preventing ovulation and by thickening the cervical mucus.

Centchroman

Centchroman is ormeloxifene developed by the Central Drug Research Institute, Lucknow. It is a Selective Estrogen Receptor Modulator (SERM) with antiestrogenic action on breasts, uterus and ovaries but estrogenic action on the bones.

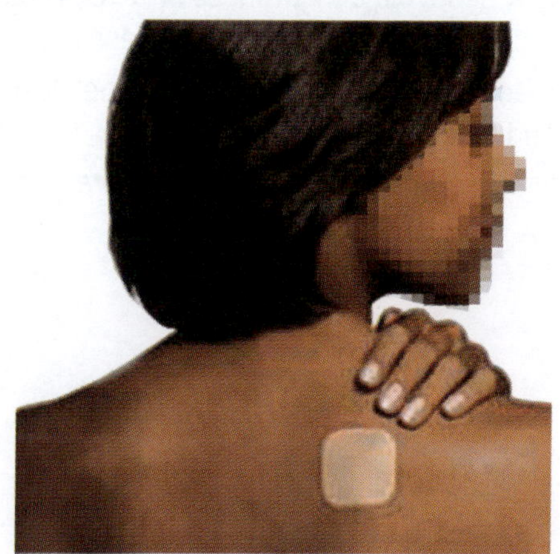

Fig. 63.4 Transdermal patch.

It has been shown to be a potent, nonhormonal, nonsteroidal oral contraceptive with a failure rate of 1.6%. It is marketed as Saheli and Novex-DS.

Mechanism of action: Centchroman has the contraceptive effect due to the following actions.

- It hastens the transport of fertilised ovum before the endometrium is favourable for implantation.
- It may hasten maturation of ovum.
- It slows down the growth and development of the endometrium making it unfavourable for implantation.

Dosage: For the first three months, the woman is advised to take centchroman, one tablet of 30 mg twice a week (for example, on a Sunday and Wednesday) followed by once a week (for example, every Sunday). Additional contraceptive measures like condom is recommended in the first month.

Advantages: It has the following advantages:

- cheap and effective
- no side effects of COC pills like nausea, vomiting and weight gain
- no adverse effects on liver function, lipid profile and blood coagulation
- quicker return to fertility
- no adverse effects seen if pregnancies, accidental ones, continued
- useful in the treatment of dysfunctional uterine bleeding.

Disadvantages: Following are the disadvantages:

- no major side effects reported
- may cause delayed periods especially in the first three months of use
- scanty periods in some women
- initially may cause fluid retention, breast tenderness and acne
- difficulty in remembering the timing of the dose. Please add the following as the last point in
- Centchroman is a SERM and acts as contraceptive essentially by rendering the endometrium unfavourable for implantation.

KEY POINTS

- Hormonal contraception provides the combination of estrogen and progestogen or progestogen only in the form of oral pills, injectables, implants, vaginal rings, transdermal patches and intrauterine devices.
- Most modern pills contain the lowest possible dose of hormones to achieve reliability, cycle control and safety.
- Combined oral pills (COC or OCP) are the most common form of hormonal contraceptives.
- The progestogen-only pill (POP) is free of estrogenic side effects.
- Mala N containing 30 µg of ethinyl estradiol and 0.3 mg of levonorgestrel is provided by the National Family Planning programme of India.
- If properly used, the effectiveness of COCs is comparable to that of tubal ligation and its failure rate is 0.1% or 1% in 1,000 but is 1.8% in practice. The effectiveness of mini pills is 96.5%–99.5% and that of injectables is 99%–99.5%.
- Combined oral pills have many extra benefits in preventing anemia, ovarian cancer, endometrial cancer, functional ovarian cysts and benign breast disease.

QUESTIONS

Select the single most appropriate answer:

1. Which of the following is not a route of administration for hormonal contraception?
   a. nasal spray
   b. dermal patch
   c. vaginal ring
   d. intrauterine device
2. Hormonal contraceptives have been in use
   a. from ancient times
   b. for over hundred years
   c. for fifty years
   d. for two decades
3. Hormonal contraceptives act by all of the following mechanisms except
   a. inhibiting ovulation
   b. thickening cervical mucus
   c. decreasing libido
   d. making endometrium unfavourable for implantation
4. The most commonly used estrogen in combined pill is
   a. conjugated estrogen
   b. ethinyl estradiol
   c. mestranol
   d. estriol
5. The most commonly used progestogen currently in oral pill is
   a. norethisterone
   b. norethindrone
   c. medroxy progesterone
   d. levonorgestrel
6. Which of the following has the least androgenic properties?
   a. desogestrel
   b. medroxy progesterone
   c. norethisterone
   d. levonorgestrel
7. Which of the following has the least effect on water retention and body weight?
   a. norethisterone
   b. levonorgestrel
   c. drosperinone
   d. desogestrel
8. When properly used, the failure rate of oral pill (in HWY) is
   a. 0.1 c. 1.0
   b. 0.5 d. 1.5
9. All of the following are non-contraceptive benefits of oral contraceptives except?
   a. regularises menstrual cycles
   b. prevention of sexually transmitted infections
   c. decreases rheumatoid arthritis
   d. reduces functional ovarian cysts
10. The advantage of oral pill is that
    a. it has to be taken daily.
    b. it offers protection against sexually transmitted diseases.
    c. it can be used by mothers who are breastfeeding.
    d. it offers the woman control over her fertility.
11. A serious side effect of the combined oral pill is
    a. headache
    b. nausea
    c. thromboembolic phenomena
    d. mastalgia
12. Combined oral pill is contraindicated in all of the following except
    a. after an abortion
    b. severe migraine
    c. lactation
    d. unexplained vaginal bleeding
13. Which one of the following drugs is known to interact with hormonal contraceptives?
    a. analgesics
    b. antiepileptics
    c. antiinflammatory agents
    d. insulin sensitisers
14. The main action of progestogen-only contraceptives is
    a. spermicidal
    b. inhibiting ovulation
    c. inhibiting gonadotrophins
    d. thickening cervical mucus
15. The main disadvantage of progestogen-only pill is that
    a. It cannot be used in lactating women.
    b. It increases risk of thromboembolism.
    c. It causes irregular bleeding.
    d. It predisposes to pelvic infection.
16. An example of an injectable hormonal contraceptive is
    a. Implanon c. Nuva ring
    b. Norplant d. NET-EN
17. Injectable hormonal contraceptives preparations include all the following molecules *except*
    a. medroxy progesterone and ethinyl estradiol
    b. drosperinone

c. norethindrone enanthate
d. medroxy progesterone depot

18. Implanon contains
   a. 3-keto desogestrel
   b. levonorgestrel
   c. cyproterone
   d. medroxy progesterone
19. A dermal contraceptive patch contains
   a. estrogen and progesterone
   b. estrogen only
   c. progesterone only
   d. drosperinone
20. The National Family Planning Programme of Government of India ensures free availability of
   a. Novelon
   b. Yasmin
   c. Mala-N
   d. Ovral-L

64

Intrauterine Contraceptive Devices

Raksha Arora

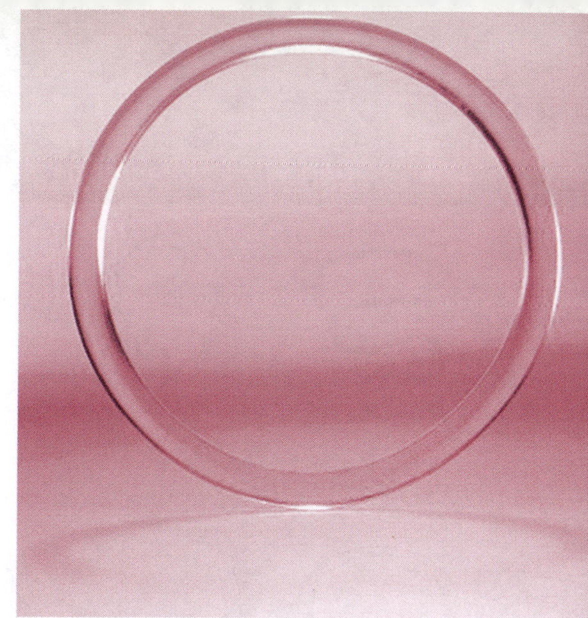

LEARNING OBJECTIVES

At the end of this chapter, the reader should be able to:

- define an IUCD
- enumerate the types of IUCDs
- describe their mechanism of action
- enumerate their advantages and disadvantages
- enumerate the indications and contraindications, and the complications for IUCD insertion
- list the criteria for the selection of a client for IUCD insertion
- describe the technique of insertion
- enumerate other uses of IUCDs

Introduction

Intrauterine contraceptive devices (IUDs or IUCDs) are small flexible devices made of plastic or metal or a combination of these materials, meant for insertion into the uterine cavity for contraception. They are preferred over other forms of contraception because they are effective and have a long duration of action.

The first widely used IUCD, introduced in Germany by Ernst Grafenberg, consisted of a ring of silkworm gut and silver wire. Lippes loop was the first modern IUCD introduced in the 1960s. By the early 1970s, medicated or chemically active devices were developed. All the frames of currently marketed IUCDs are made of polyethylene, except progestasert which was ethylene vinyl acetate. They are impregnated with barium sulphate to make them radio-opaque for easy location. The chemically active or medicated devices, contain copper or hormones. All the IUCDs have a 'tail', a nylon thread which helps to ensure that the device is in place.

Types of IUCDs

There are three generations of IUCDs. Those belonging to the first generation are unmedicated (Lippe's loop). The second generation IUCDs contain copper (CuT). The devices containing hormones belong to the third generation (Mirena and Progestasert).

Earlier, Lippes loop was the most popular; it is no longer in use (**Fig. 64.1**). Currently, chemically active IUCDs, which are more effective and safe, are recommended.

Copper IUCDs are of several types and are referred to by their shape and copper content. The number against the designation of each device denotes

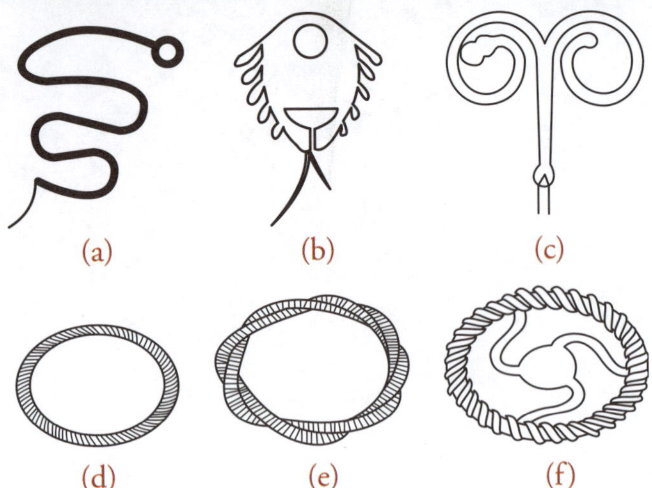

Fig. 64.1 Types of IUCDs a: Lippe's loop b: Dalkon shield c: Saf T coil d: Single coil ring e: Mahua ring f: Ota ring.

the surface area of copper in mm^2. There are two generations, and efficacy and lifespan are higher in the second generation.

The first generation copper IUCDs are Copper-T 200 and Multiload 250, and carry copper wire with a surface area of 200 mm^2 and 250 mm^2 each. The second generation copper IUCDs are Cu T-380, CuT-220C, Nova-T and Multiload 375. These have more copper wire on their sleeves and a silver core to the copper wire.

Currently, the IUCDs available in India are mainly the copper devices. They are Copper-T 200, 220C, 380A, Nova-T, Multiload 250 and 375. However, only Copper-T 220C and Copper-T 380A are available in the National Family Planning programme. The Copper-T devices including CuT-200 are effective for five years and Cu-380A for 10 years (**Fig. 64.2**).

Hormone-releasing devices

The addition of hormone in IUCDs is an advantage, as the device acts as a delivery system for the hormone. Currently, two IUCDs are available; however, they are not available through the National Family Planning programme of India. Hormonal IUCDs have the advantage of being beneficial to women with menorrhagia.

Progestasert: This is a T-shaped device, made of ethylene vinyl acetate copolymer impregnated with barium sulphate. The device is 36 mm long and 32 mm wide, and has a single blue/black thread at the lower end of the stem. The vertical shaft is fitted with a capsule

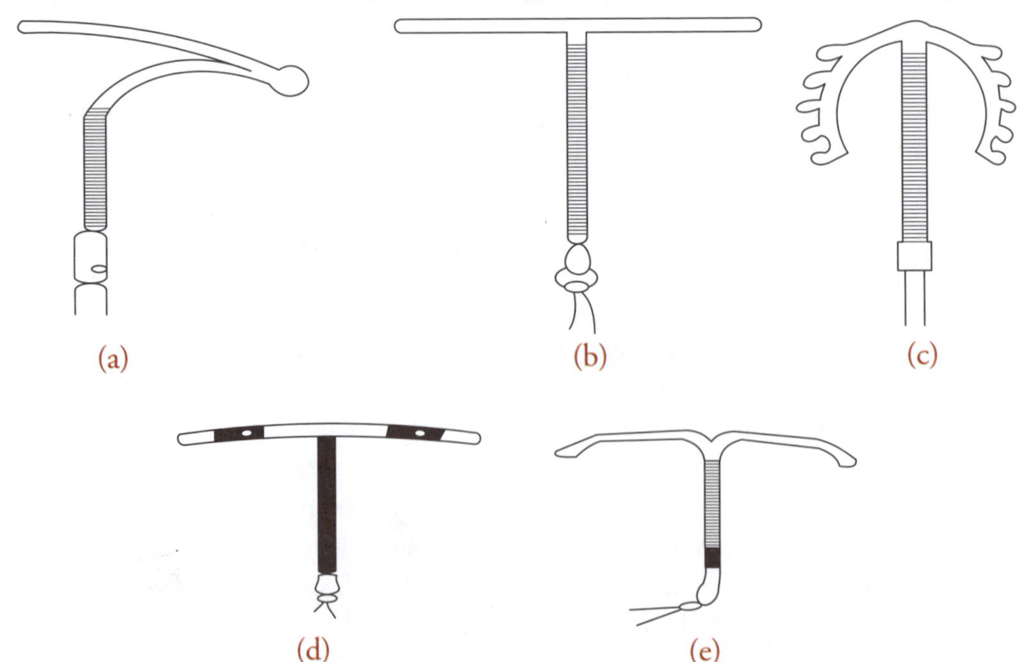

Fig. 64.2 Types of copper IUCDs a: Copper-7 b: Copper-T200 c: Multiload 375 d: Copper-T 380A e: Nova-T.

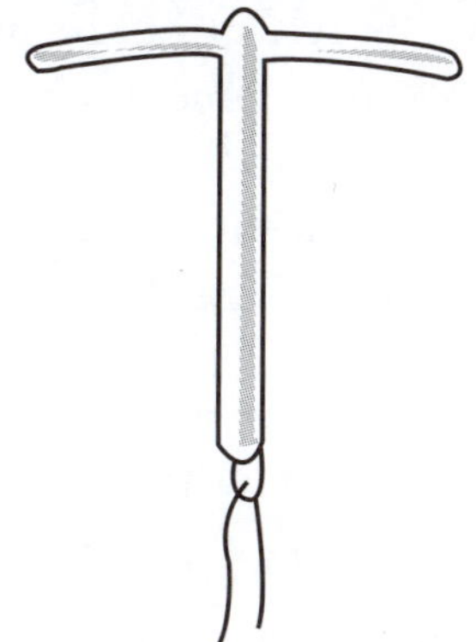

Fig. 64.3 Progestasert.

containing 38 mg of progesterone dispersed in silicone oil (**Fig. 64.3**). It delivers the hormone at the rate of 65 µg/day. It needs to be replaced every year and is suitable for women with heavy bleeding. It acts locally to make the endometrium nonconducive to implantation and also blocks sperm migration by thickening the cervical mucus. The disadvantages are intermenstrual spotting and increased risk of ectopic pregnancy.

Levonorgestrel devices: These are marketed as LNG 20, Mirena and Levonova (**Fig. 64.4**). This system delivers 20 µg of levonorgestrel per day. It is as effective as female sterilisation but unlike sterilisation, is easily reversible (0.1–0.2 per HWY).

Mechanism of action: IUCDs act in several ways.

- blocking sperm migration to the upper genital tract by thicken the cervical mucus
- spermicidal effect of lysosomal activation by intense local inflammatory action

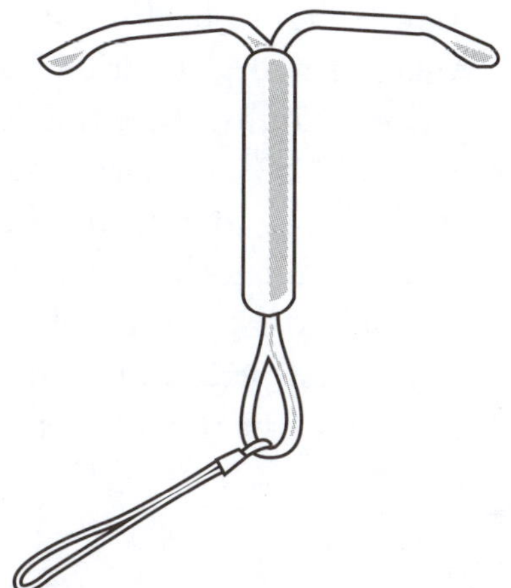

Fig. 64.4 Levonorgestrel IUCD.

- accelerated tubal motility
- endometrium hostile to implantation of the blastocyst

Effectiveness: Chemically active IUCDs are highly effective. In fact, the effectiveness of some IUCDs is comparable to female sterilisation. The failure rate for Cu-380A is 0.6–0.8 per HWY. Pregnancy during the first year of use for Multiload 250 and Cu-200 has been noted to be 1–3 per HWY.

Advantages: IUCDs have a number of advantages compared to other methods of contraception.

- They are effective soon after insertion.
- Their use is not linked to sexual activity.
- They do not interfere with sexual intercourse.
- There is no need for constant motivation and effort to use the method. The client can 'use and forget'.
- There is no risk of drug interaction.
- They do not affect breastfeeding.
- The removal of the device is easy.
- Return of fertility is noted soon after removal.
- There are no systemic side effects.

Disadvantages: IUCDs have a few disadvantages and these have to be kept in mind while providing an IUCD to the client.

- They do not protect against sexually transmitted diseases including HIV.
- They cannot be used by women who suffer from reproductive tract infections.
- They require a skilled provider.

Side effects and complications:

Expulsion: The device can be expelled any time after insertion, but expulsions occur in the initial cycles, or when inserted during menstruation or early in the postpartum period.

Menorrhagia and dysmenorrhea: Some women may suffer from menorrhagia and dysmenorrhea during the first few cycles. This can be overcome with couselling and by prescribing NSAIDs. If the symptoms persist or are severe, it is advisable to remove the IUCD.

Infection: This is a possible complication that should be prevented by selecting the client meticulously and observing aseptic and antiseptic techniques. The consensus is that there is no need for the use of prophylactic antibiotics.

Perforation of the uterus: This complication has declined remarkably with the use of newer IUCDs and with the 'withdrawal' technique of insertion.

Pregnancy with IUCD in situ: The presence of an IUCD in a pregnant uterus is dangerous for both the woman and the fetus. If the tail of the IUCD is visible, it should be removed so that subsequent complications like infection, abortion, preterm delivery and IUGR can be avoided. In case the tail is not visible, it may be left as it is.

Indications for IUCD insertion

- parous women in the reproductive age group for spacing of pregnancy
- breastfeeding women
- women in whom hormonal contraceptives are contraindicated
- as a postcoital contraceptive

Contraindications

- suspected pregnancy
- abnormalities of the genital tract
- pelvic inflammatory disease (PID)
- vaginitis or cervicitis
- genital bleeding of unknown cause
- uterine pathology such as leiomyoma
- severe anemia
- multiple sexual partners
- previous history of ectopic pregnancy

Relative contraindications: IUCDs should be inserted with caution in the following cases:

- Cesarean section done within the last three months
- Hyperinvoluted uterus which is soft and likely to be perforated.
- If IUCD has to be used in a patient with valvular heart disease, prophylactic antibiotics are administered and the threads are cut short.
- Many nulliparous women develop uterine cramps. Also the IUCDs increase the risk of PID and subsequent infertility.

Timing of insertion

The ideal time for Copper-T insertion is within seven days of the last menstrual period.

After delivery, the IUCD can be inserted after six weeks when the woman comes for a postnatal check-up. However, it can also be inserted immediately after delivery (post-placental insertion); the risk of expulsion is high in this case. It may also be inserted along with first trimester MTP.

Prerequisites for IUD insertion

Before to inserting the IUCD, one must take measures to minimise the complications and ensure continuation.

- Pre-insertion counselling
- Thorough clinical assessment to rule out contraindications
- Appropriate timing for insertion
- A pap smear must be done
- Adherence to guidelines for insertion
- Post-insertion follow-up and counselling

Technique of insertion

A pelvic examination is performed to ascertain the size and direction of the uterus; thereafter, the length of the uterus is measured. The flange is adjusted to that length. The device, inside the inserter is introduced into the uterus with the plunger in situ. Holding the plunger, the inserter tube is **withdrawn.** The tail is cut about 2–3 cm from the os (**Fig. 64.5**).

Post-insertion advice

The woman is informed that the device is effective immediately after insertion. She is warned that she may experience slight bleeding or spotting for a few days. Analgesics are prescribed as she may experience uterine cramps. Bleeding during the first 2–3 cycles could be excessive: she may need to take NSAIDs. She is advised to check for the thread of the device after each menstrual period to be sure that it is in situ. She is asked to return for follow-up after the first period or if she misses her periods or does not feel the thread, or has abnormal vaginal discharge.

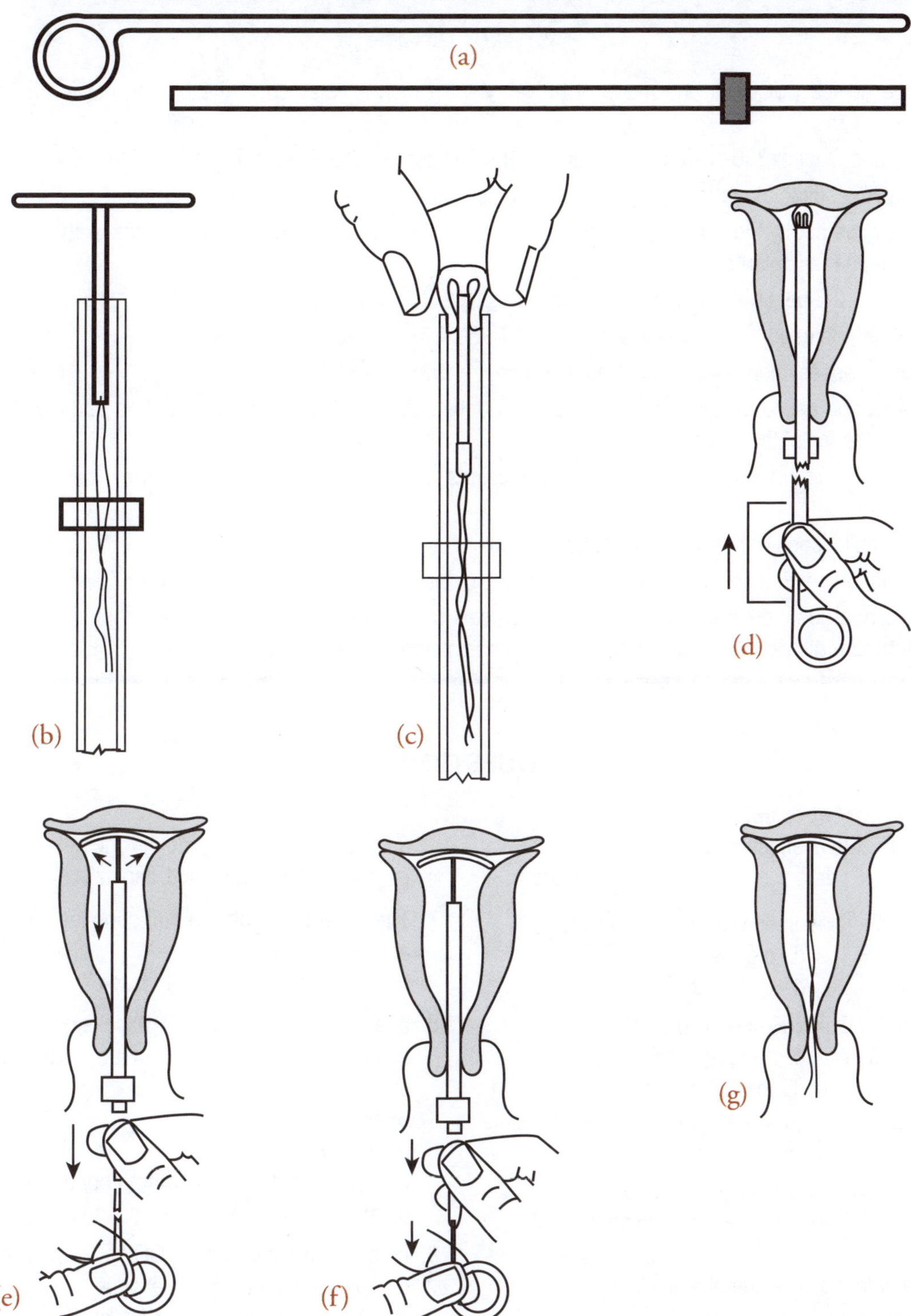

Fig. 64.5 Insertion of copper-T a: Flexible plastic inserter with plastic plunger. b–c: Cu-T is negotiated into the top end of the inserter d: Cu-T loaded inserter with plunger is introduced into the uterine cavity e: The inserter is retracted over the plunger leaving Cu-T inside the uterus f: The plunger and inserter are withdrawn g: Cu-T in position.

KEY POINTS

- An intrauterine device (IUCD) is one made of polyethylene which is retained in the uterine cavity for the purpose of contraception.
- Copper-T 200 and Copper 380-A are available in the National Family Planning Programme of India.
- The IUCD is a very suitable method for spacing pregnancies.
- Intrauterine devices act by blocking the migration of sperms, producing inflammatory changes in the endometrium and making it hostile to the implantation of the blastocyst.
- Failure rate is 0.6–0.8 per HWY in the first year of use.
- Copper-T 200 can be used for 3–4 years and Copper-T 350 A for 10 years.
- Thorough clinical assessment and counselling are essential prior to IUCD insertion.
- The woman must be asked to report in case she experiences abdominal cramps, amenorrhea and fever with chills or if she cannot find the tail of the device.
- Progestasert and Mirena contain progestogens; besides their contraceptive action, they can be used to treat menorrhagia.
- Overall, the complications with the newer IUCDs are fewer.
- Pre- and post-insertion counselling and proper technique of insertion minimise complications and ensure continuation.
- The IUCD is a near-ideal contraceptive as the woman can 'use and forget', the contraceptive action is immediate, it is effective, return to fertility occurs soon after removal, it has minimal side effects and costs less.

QUESTIONS

Select the single most appropriate answer:

1. The IUCD, CuT-380A is effective for
   a. 10 years b. 6 years c. 5 years d. 3 years
2. The IUCD suitable for women with menorrhagia is
   a. CuT- 220 c. progestasert
   b. multiload-375 d. CuT-380A
3. The failure rate for CuT-200 or Multiload-250 is
   a. 0.1–0.3 per HWY c. 1–3 per HWY
   b. 0.5–0.8 per HWY d. more than 3 per HWY
4. An IUCD prevents pregnancy by all of the following means *except*
   a. accelerated tubal motility
   b. making the endometrium hostile to implantation of blastocyst
   c. spermicidal effect by lysosomal activation
   d. inhibiting ovulation
5. The ideal time to insert an IUCD is
   a. premenstrual period
   b. two weeks after cesarean section
   c. postmenstrual period
   d. puerperium
6. All of the following intrauterine devices are made of polyethylene *except*
   a. copper T c. progestasert
   b. multiload device d. nova T
7. The intrauterine device that contains hormone is
   a. Lippe's loop c. multiload
   b. levonova d. nova T
8. If a woman reports with excessive, painful period one month after the insertion of an intrauterine device, she should be treated with
   a. dilatation-curettage
   b. removal of IUCD
   c. non-steroidal anti-inflammatory drugs
   d. antibiotics because the cause is infection
9. In a pregnancy with IUCD in situ all of the following complications may occur *except*
   a. malpresentations c. infection
   b. abortion d. preterm delivery

Select the appropriate answer using the following key:

a. if only responses 1, 2 and 3 are correct
b. if only 1 and 3 are correct
c. if only 2 and 4 are correct
d. if only 4 is correct
e. if all are correct

10. The advantages of IUCD are
    1. there is no drug interaction
    2. not linked to sexual activity
    3. does not affect breast feeding
    4. fertility returns soon after removal
11. The IUCD should never be inserted in a woman who has
    1. fibroid uterus
    2. genital tract infection
    3. malformation of the uterus
    4. had cesarean section
12. The complications that may be encountered in a woman with an IUCD are
    1. menorrhagia
    2. failure of lactation
    3. dysmenorrhea
    4. weight gain

In the following questions, there are two statements. Select the appropriate answer using the following key:

a. if both statements are true and causally related
b. if both statements are true but not causally related
c. if the first statement is true and the second is false
d. if the first statement is false and the second is true
e. if both statements are false

13. If pregnancy occurs in a woman with IUCD, it should be removed *because*
    A pregnancy with an IUCD in situ can lead to complications like infection.
14. A woman with multiple partners is advised against the use of IUCD *because*
    An IUCD does not protect against sexually transmitted diseases.

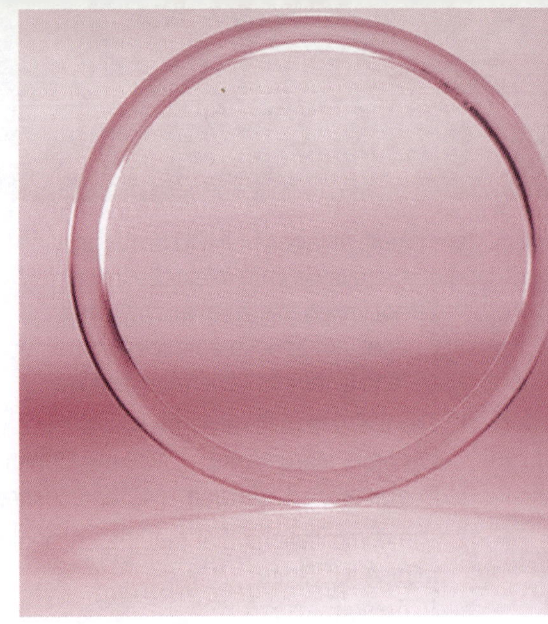

65

Surgical Contraception

C Ambuja

LEARNING OBJECTIVES

At the end of this chapter, the reader should be able to:

- define surgical contraception
- describe the principles of surgical contraception
- enumerate the elements that must be included in counselling
- appreciate of Government of India (MOHFW) directives in this regard
- list the criteria for selection of clients for sterilisation
- list the different approaches for performing tubectomy
- list the various methods of female sterilisation
- enumerate the steps of sterilisation by Pomeroy's technique
- list the complications of tubectomy
- explain the conventional method of vasectomy
- list the complications of vasectomy
- appreciate the advantages of non-scalpel vasectomy
- evaluate the possibility of reversal of surgical contraception

Introduction

Surgical contraception is the most effective and permanent method of birth control. In women the fallopian tubes are ligated and cut or occluded; this procedure is known as female sterilisation or tubectomy. In men, the vas is similarly ligated and cut or occluded and is known as vasectomy. While the surgery in men is much simpler and cheaper, female sterilisation continues to be the most widely used method. In India, female sterilisation accounts for more than 95% of all voluntary surgical contraception. One of the reasons is that women find it convenient to undergo the procedure as they are at the health facility for delivery or medical termination of pregnancy and men are reluctant to participate in contraceptive practice.

Definition and principle

Surgical contraception involves a surgical procedure, on the male or female, only for the purpose of contraception. It is a one-time method and does not need sustained motivation, as is needed in temporary methods.

The uterine tubes are paired structures situated in the upper free margin of the broad ligament. Each tube has two openings: a medial one communicating with the uterine cavity, and a lateral one communicating with the abdominal cavity. It is 10 cm long and is divided into four parts; from medial to lateral they are: the interstitial part measuring 1.25 cm, the isthmic part measuring 2.5 cm, the ampulla measuring 5 cm, and the infundibulum measuring 1.25 cm. The ovum, when released, is picked up by the infundibulum and enters the fallopian tube; the sperms swim up and fertilisation takes place. Thus, in order to prevent a pregnancy, cutting or ligating the fallopian tube produces discontinuity, preventing the union of sperm and the ovum.

In the male, each testis is filled with seminiferous tubules which drain into the epididymis, a crescent-shaped structure along the posterior border of the testis. The vas is a muscular tube of 2.5 mm diameter; it begins at the tail of the epididymis and courses upwards into the spermatic cord, passes through the inguinal canal into the pelvis to enter the seminal vesicle and ends in the ampulla. The contents of the ampulla of the seminal vesicle from either side pass into the ejaculatory duct through the prostate and empty into the prostatic urethra. In order to prevent pregnancy, the vas is divided and ligated so as to prevent the sperms from reaching the seminal vesicle.

Counselling

The following points must be included while counselling the couple regarding surgical sterilisation:

Permanent method of contraception: The couple must understand that tubectomy/vasectomy is a permanent method of contraception. It is possible to recanalise the tubes/vas but this does not ensure fertility. Therefore, the couple must make a considered decision before opting for surgical contraception. This is particularly true for areas where infant mortality is high; the couple should be advised to use a temporary method if tubectomy is requested in the immediate puerperium after the birth of a second child.

Risk of failure: It is accepted that there is a small risk of failure associated with surgical contraception whatever the technique used. The couple must understand this fact and report to the doctor if the woman misses her periods.

Complications of surgery and anesthesia: As in any surgical procedure, the client may suffer from consequences like hemorrhage, wound dehiscence and incisional hernia. It has been recorded that anesthetic complications are more frequent when general or regional anesthesia is administered.

It should be explained to male clients that vasectomy is not castration and that their sexual performance will not be affected. Their apprehensions regarding an increased risk of cardiovascular disease, cancer of the prostate and testis should be allayed.

An informed consent is obtained after reiterating the above points, in accordance with directives issued by the Government of India which include:

- Female sterilisation by minilaparotomy can be done by a trained MBBS doctor, but laparoscopic method can be performed only by a qualified gynecologist trained in laparoscopy. Conventional or non-scalpel vasectomy can be performed by a trained MBBS doctor.
- Every doctor should fill up a checklist before performing a sterilisation.
- An informed consent form should be signed by a client before the procedure.
- A Quality Assurance Committee has been set up by the state governments.
- An insurance policy has been introduced to improve acceptance, reduce malpractice suits and compensate for any untoward outcome arising due to the procedure.
- A compensation of at least ₹ 2,00,000 for death and ₹ 30,000 for failure and ₹ 20,000 for treatment of complications limited to actual cost of treatment has been suggested.

Female Sterilisation

Selection of clients

Thorough clinical examination is performed to detect any existing medical disorder. Laboratory investigations are requested to assess the general condition of the client and also to detect any complications/severity of an existing disease. **One must remember that surgery for contraception is not performed for any disease; on the contrary, it is only to control fertility.** Therefore, the procedure may be postponed and the client advised to opt for other methods of contraception if she/he is suffering from a medical disorder. The WHO and the MOHFW (2006) have laid down the following guidelines for ensuring safety of a client for surgical contraception.

The surgery is **postponed** if the client any of the following conditions:

- puerperal sepsis, acute pelvic infection, skin infection, upper/lower respiratory tract infection
- significant recent hemorrhage
- severe anemia, complicated valvular heart disease current cerebrovascular disease and acute liver disease.
- psychiatric disorders that impair decision-making.
- newborn who is ill

The client is referred to a health facility equipped to manage complications like:

- conditions that increase anesthetic risk like history of cardiovascular disease, hypertension (BP≥ 160/100 mm Hg), diabetes mellitus, thyroid disorders, moderate anemia and chronic liver disease
- conditions that increase surgical difficulties like previous complicated abdominal or pelvic surgery, marked obesity and coagulation disorders.

Timing

Technically, sterilisation may be performed at any time. In women, however, it is not advisable to perform the operation in the premenstrual phase as there is a risk that pregnancy may have already occurred. Female sterilisation should be performed whenever it is convenient for the client. However, there are some factors which govern the timing of the procedure.

During puerperium: In India, the majority of sterilisations are performed during the puerperium. There are three distinct advantages:

- The client is already in a health facility for her delivery.
- The uterus is an abdominal organ and the tubes are easily accessible.
- The puerperal and postoperative period coincide so that hospital stay is minimised.

Tubal sterilisation is usually performed 24–36 hours after delivery so that the woman has had some rest after delivery and the wellbeing of the newborn can be assessed better.

The Government of India recommendation to perform puerperal sterilisation stipulates that the operation be carried out 24 hours after delivery but within 7 days, or after 6 weeks.

Cesarean section: Whenever a woman requires CS and opts for sterilisation, tubal sterilisation can be performed along with CS.

Postabortal sterilisation: In this case the sterilisation is carried out laparoscopically or by minilaparotomy following evacuation of the uterus.

Interval tubectomy: This should be performed in the postmenstrual phase and laparoscopic approach is the best.

Concurrent sterilisation: This term is used when sterilisation is performed along with another surgery, such as abdominal surgery (ovariectomy) or vaginal surgery (Manchester operation).

Preoperative care for sterilisation

The following precautions must be adhered to meticulously:

- counselling of the couple
- selection of client
- taking an informed consent
- requisition of relevant laboratory investigation
- preanesthetic evaluation

Surgical technique

For female sterilisation, the tubes can be accessed through a conventional laparotomy, minilaparotomy, laparoscopy or transvaginally by colpotomy. Whatever the route, strict asepsis and antisepsis must be observed.

Conventional laparotomy: It can be performed under general, regional or local anesthesia. The abdomen is opened by a vertical or transverse incision, about 2 cm long, for puerperal sterilisation; the incision may be larger depending on the need. For interval sterilisation or concurrent with medical termination of pregnancy, a suprapubic incision is useful. **Minilaparotomy** is most useful when an interval tubal ligation is planned. One must ensure that the uterus is mobile. It is performed under local anesthesia: the woman is placed in a semi-lithotomy position, and the abdomen is opened as in conventional laparotomy till the peritoneum is reached. Then an assistant, using a uterine elevator, brings the fundus of the uterus at the incision and the peritoneum is opened. He manipulates the uterus so as to expose one cornu and then the other. Further exposure of the tubes is achieved by using small, angled retractors.

Colpotomy: The woman is placed in lithotomy position with head down, the posterior lip of the cervix is held with a vulsellum and pulled up. An incision is made in the posterior fornix including the peritoneum. The tubes are then accessed and ligated. Transvaginal sterilisation is rarely done as a primary procedure.

Tubal sterilisation

The following structures are seen (from anterior to posterior) at the cornual part of the uterus: round ligament, fallopian tube and ovarian ligament. Keeping this in mind, the fallopian tubes are picked up and identified by the presence of the fimbrial end. Once identified there are several methods of tubal ligation: the aim is to minimise the risk of spontaneous recanalisation and improve the efficacy. At the same time it is also advisable to adopt a method which, while being effective will also make subsequent surgical recanalisation effective. This is a significant point in areas where infant mortality is high.

Pomeroy's method: It is the simplest, the most frequently used and reasonably effective technique. The medial part of the tube is picked up with a Babcock's forceps to form a knuckle; then the base of the tube is ligated with 1/0 plain catgut and the knuckle cut. The rationale for using plain catgut is that on prompt absorption of the ligature, the cut ends of the tubes will separate adequately (**Fig. 65.1**). This technique is recommended by the MOHFW.

Parkland method: An avascular site in the mesosalpinx is perforated with an artery forceps and the tube is dissected from the mesosalpinx (about 2.5 cm). The tube is ligated proximally and distally with 1/0 chromic catgut; the segment is then resected and hemostasis ensured.

Irving's method: The tube is dissected from the mesosalpinx, ligated and divided. The distal end of the proximal segment is buried in a tunnel created on the posterior wall of the uterus. The proximal end of the distal part of the tube is buried in the mesosalpinx. This technique of tubal ligation is least likely to fail.

Uchida's method: Saline is injected into the serosa to produce ballooning locally, and the muscular layer of the tube is separated from the serosa. The mesosalpinx is then cut open, the tube is held to form a knuckle which is cut and ligated. The medial end is buried in the mesosalpinx, which is then sutured. After excising about 3–4 cm of the tube, the proximal end of the distal part is ligated and left outside the mesosalpinx. In this technique too there is hardly any failure and there are no menstrual abnormalities later.

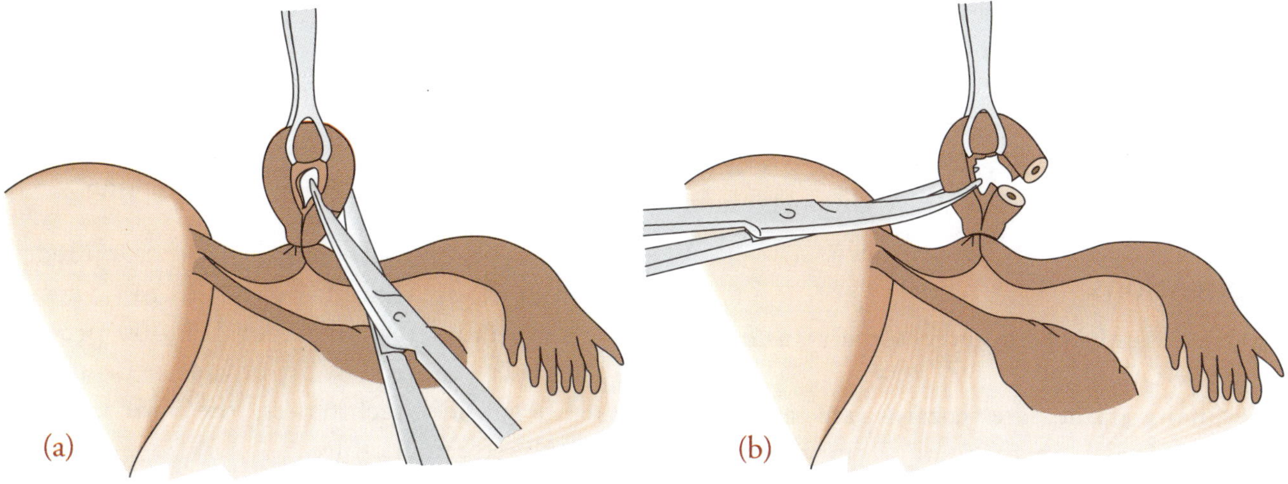

Fig. 65.1 Pomeroy method of tubectomy.

There are several other techniques like Madlener's method where the failure rate is high; in Kroener's method, fimbriectomy is done: it is not recommended since future recanalisation is likely to be unsuccessful if the fimbriae are lost.

Laparoscopic tubal ligation

Laparoscopic approach to tubal ligation has made the procedure of female sterilisation safe and acceptable. It can be performed through a single puncture or double puncture. The instrument consists of metal tubes as thin as 5–10 mm with a fibreoptic light bundle system to transmit cold light into the abdominal cavity. There are accessories like the lighting system, gas insufflator, intrauterine devices to manipulate the uterus during the procedure and ring or clip applicator or cautery forceps. The surgeon views the operating field directly or on a monitor. This procedure is contraindicated in women suffering from decompensated heart disease and severe respiratory disorders.

Preoperative preparation is carried out and aseptic and antiseptic measures are taken as discussed earlier. Under anesthesia, the client is placed in semi-lithotomy position at 30 degrees Trendelenburg position. A small skin incision is made below the umbilicus and the Veress needle is introduced into the abdomen; about 2 litres of carbon dioxide is insufflated to create pneumoperitoneum; the Verress needle is then removed. This is followed by a very careful introduction of the trocar; the obturator is removed and the telescope is introduced when the pelvic structures come into view (**Fig. 65.2a**). A double puncture laparoscope is more maneuverable. The tubes are identified, picked up and occluded with silastic rings, the most popular being the Falope rings (**Fig. 65.2b**). The scope is removed and the gas let out, and then the skin is closed using 1/0 chromic catgut.

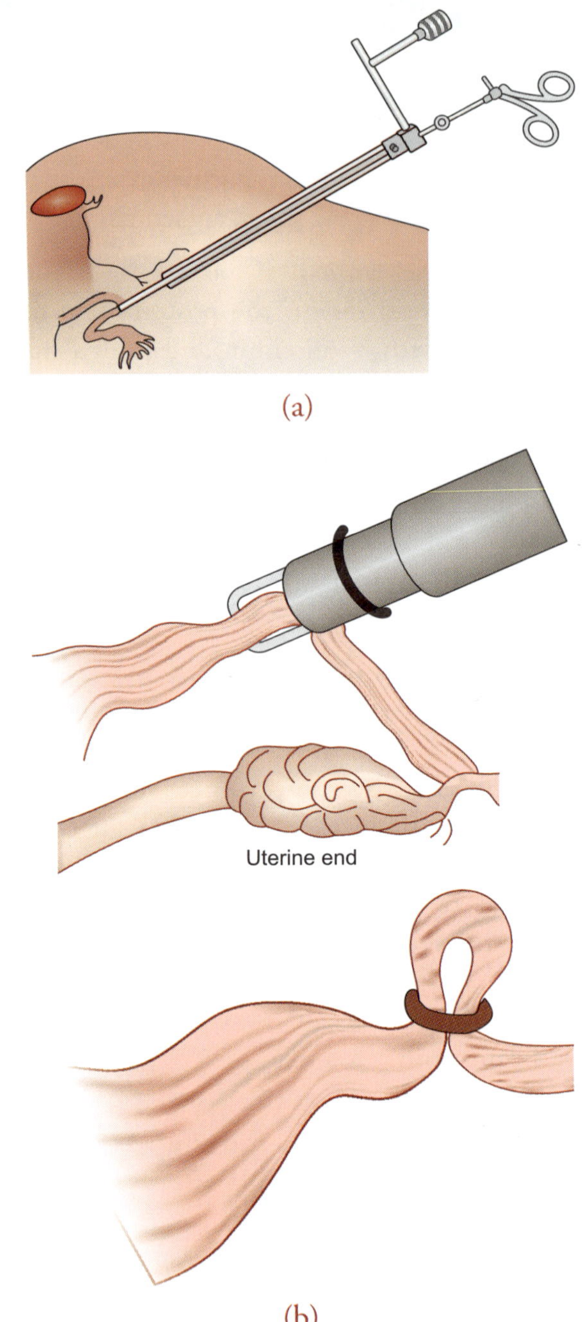

Fig. 65.2 a: Laparoscopic sterilisation
b: Laparoscopic sterilisation by silastic ring.

Complications

Female sterilisation, like any other surgery is associated with complications.

- The main immediate hazards are anesthetic complications, inadvertent injury to the intestines and urinary bladder, hemorrhage and infection. During laparoscopic tubal ligation, the major blood vessels may be injured; due precautions should be taken to avoid this. A mortality rate of 5 per 100,000 procedures has been noted. With advances in anesthetic and surgical techniques, the case fatality has declined remarkably.
- Failure of tubal ligation or failure to produce sterility is a complication of great concern. Failure

rates vary with the timing and the technique used for tubectomy; failure rates are highest when tubal ligation is performed with cesarean section and the ligation is done by Madlener's technique or by laparoscopy where the tube is not resected. On an average, the failure rates are 0.2%–1.3%.

- There is a significant association between tubal ligation and ectopic pregnancy. Of all the pregnancies that occur following tubectomy, 50% are in the fallopian tube. If a woman who has undergone tubectomy presents with symptoms of pregnancy, one must consider the possibility of ectopic pregnancy and investigate her accordingly.
- Pelvic infection was significant when transvaginal approach was adopted.
- Incisional hernia is a complication of conventional laparotomy.
- **Posttubal ligation syndrome** is characterised by vague pain or discomfort in the pelvis, cysts in the ovary and menorrhagia. However, recent studies have not reported any increase in menstrual blood flow as compared to non-sterilised women.

It is worth reiterating that tubal ligation is associated with complications, and hence every effort should be made to minimise the risk.

Reversal of tubal ligation

A health care provider must ensure during counselling that no woman opts for sterillisation because she can have her fertility restored by surgery or assisted reproductive techniques. The success rate of surgery for recanalisation is 75%, but could be much less despite improvement in microsurgical techniques. The results are best if tubal ligation was performed by Pomeroy's, Parkland's or Irving's technique, or when silastic rings are applied for laparoscopic tubal ligation. The rate of ectopic pregnancy is significantly high following tubal recanalisation.

Hysterectomy

Occasionally, there may be a demand for hysterectomy for sterilisation. However, it is important to remember that both morbidity and mortality are significantly high with this procedure and there is no justification to perform it only to achieve sterility.

Male Sterilisation

Male sterilisation or vasectomy is a permanent method of birth control. The lumen of the vas is disrupted to block the passage of sperms from the testes (**Fig. 65.3**). The operation is performed under local anesthesia through a small incision in the scrotum.

Technique

Under local anesthesia, a small incision is made on the scrotum. The vas deferens is identified in the spermatic cord and the sheath incised. A small segment of the vas is resected and the cut ends ligated. The procedure is repeated on the other side. A bandage applied for the wound also provides scrotal support.

Non-scalpel Vasectomy (NSV) is a simplified approach to vasectomy. The vas is fixed at the upper and middle third of the scrotum and a puncture is made in the midline. The vas is fixed with a specially designed ring forceps or with three fingers, and the skin is punctured with a sharp and pointed mosquito forceps. The vas on either side is dissected, ligated and a segment excised. The puncture in the skin needs no suturing.

Complications

These are hematoma, infection and formation of sperm granulomas although NSV has lowered their occurrence.

Advantages and disadvantages

Compared to tubectomy, vasectomy is easier, safer and less expensive. The only drawback is that sterility is not achieved immediately as it takes 6–12 weeks or 20 ejaculations for complete expulsion of sperms stored beyond the disruption of the vas. The couple must use a condom till semen analysis reveals azoospermia in two consecutive samples.

The failure rate for vasectomy is about 0.5%–1%; a higher failure could be attributed to unprotected coitus too soon after the operation.

An increased risk of cardiovascular disease, prostatic and testicular cancer is believed to be associated with vasectomy. There is no scientific evidence to support these fears. In some developing countries men have the

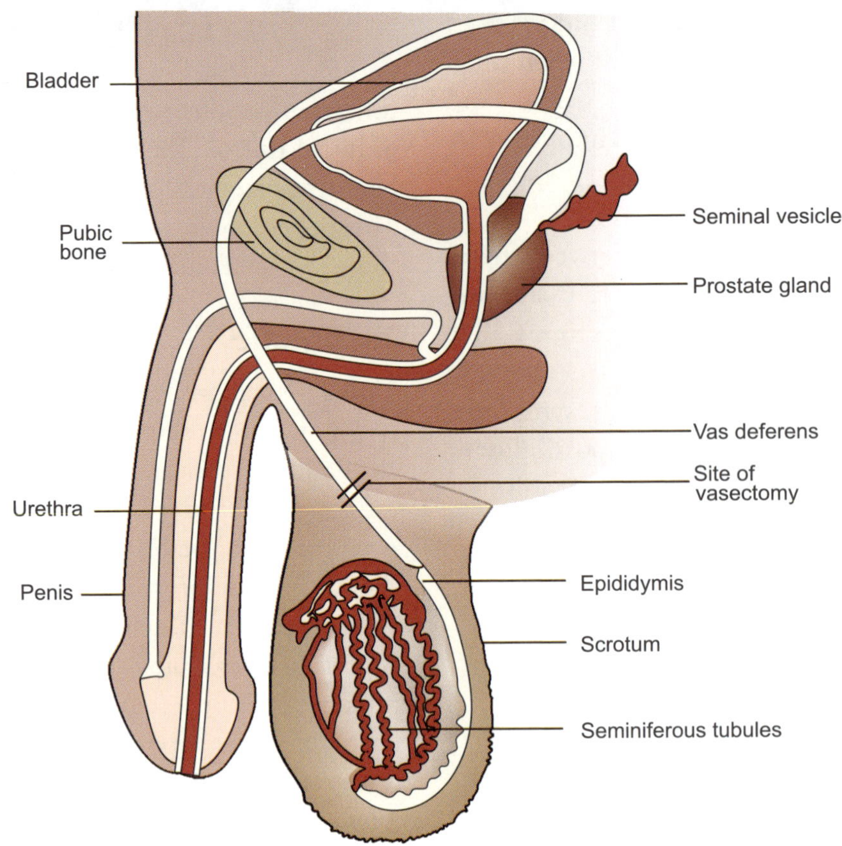

Fig. 65.3 Male reproductive organs showing area of vasectomy.

unfounded fear of losing their virility. The existence of a strong gender bias works on both men and women pushing women to opt for tubectomy. All these points need to be discussed with the couple during counselling.

Reversal of vasectomy has improved with the availability of microsurgery. Success depends on the length of time after vasectomy and the presence of sperm granulomas. The success rates are 50%–70%.

KEY POINTS

- Surgical contraception refers to creating disruption in the fallopian tubes or the vas deferens, and is referred to as tubectomy and vasectomy.
- During counselling the couple/client should be made to understand that sterilisation is a permanent method of birth control.
- The selection of clients must be done after thorough clinical evaluation; relevant laboratory investigations must be performed. It is mandatory to follow the guidelines for eligibility very meticulously as tubectomy and vasectomy are not performed for a disease.
- Technically tubectomy can be performed at any time. However, postpartum sterilisation should be done after 24 hours and upto 7 days after delivery. The approach to the tubes is through conventional laparotomy, minilparotomy or laparoscopy.
- Compared to tubectomy, vasectomy is an easier, safer and less expensive procedure. There is a need to stress on these points during counselling.
- The failure rate of tubal ligation varies with the technique used and is 0.2%–1.3%. It is 0.5%–1% for vasectomy.
- Hazards of tubectomy are anesthetic complications, hemorrhage and infection. Ectopic pregnancy is a late complication.
- Following vasectomy, hematoma, infection and sperm granulomas can occur.
- With improvement in microsurgical techniques the success of tubal or vas re-anastomosis is 50%–75%. However, a client should not opt for surgical contraception because facilities are available for recanalisation.

QUESTIONS

Select the single most appropriate answer:

1. Surgical contraception includes all of the following *except*
   a. laparoscopic tubal occlusion c. no scalpel vasectomy
   b. total hysterectomy d. puerperal sterilisation
2. Vasectomy should be preferred over tubectomy because
   a. It renders a man impotent.
   b. It is immediately effective.
   c. More men prefer to undergo the procedure.
   d. It is associated with fewer complications.
3. Tubectomy is said to be concurrent when it is done
   a. with the consent of the woman
   b. in the puerperium
   c. along with other surgical procedures
   d. after an abortion
4. Uterine elevator is used during
   a. minilap sterilisation c. puerperal sterilisation
   b. concurrent sterilisation d. vaginal tubectomy
5. The portion of the fallopian tube that is excised in tubectomy for sterilisation is
   a. interstitial part c. ampullary part
   b. isthmus d. fimbria
6. The most commonly performed technique of tubectomy for sterilisation is
   a. Uchida's method c. Pomeroy method
   b. Parkland method d. Kroener method
7. Conventional laparoscopic methods of tubal occlusion include all of the following *except*
   a. clip application c. tying the tube with an endosuture
   b. electrocoagulation d. ring application
8. The main risk associated with puerperal tubal sterilisation is
   a. injury to great vessels c. infection
   b. visceral injury d. anesthetic complications
9. Failure of tubectomy is highest when it is done
   a. laparoscopically c. after an abortion
   b. with cesarean section d. during puerperium
10. The failure rate of vasectomy is
    a. 0.5%–1% c. 2.5%–3%
    b. 1.5%–2% d. 3.5%–4%
11. The main disadvantage of vasectomy is
    a. It is technically more difficult.
    b. It is costlier.
    c. It is not immediately effective.
    d. It has more complications.
12. Success of reversal of tubectomy will depend on all of the following *except*
    a. duration after the tubectomy
    b. site of tubectomy
    c. technique of tubectomy
    d. simultaneously done with cesarean section

66

Emergency Contraception

S Soundara Raghavan

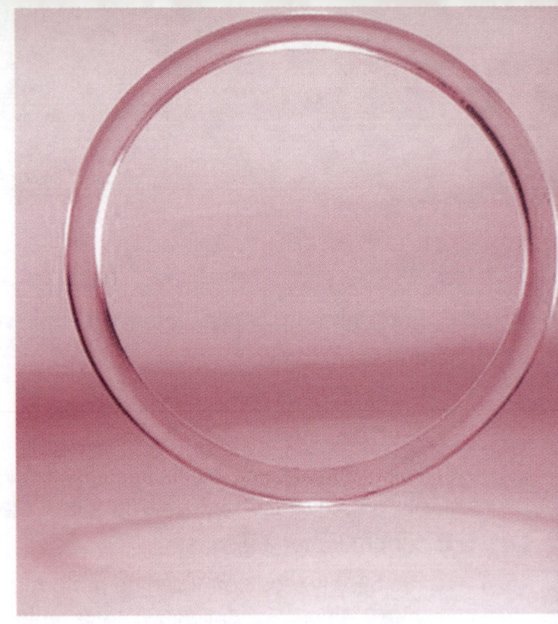

LEARNING OBJECTIVES

At the end of the chapter, the reader should be able to:

- define emergency contraception (EC)
- appreciate the need for emergency contraception
- appreciate circumstances in which EC should be advised
- enumerate various methods available
- explain the mechanism of action
- list the side effects and contraindications
- counsel couples about EC
- disseminate information about EC

Introduction

In India, the majority of pregnancies are unplanned. A vast proportion of these are continued and a good number end in termination of pregnancy; precise figures not available. It has been estimated that a single act of unprotected coitus will result in a pregnancy in 8% of women and two such acts on consecutive days in 30%. There were 1.75 million unintended pregnancies in 1995 in the USA. **Emergency Contraception** (EC) reduces the number of unintended pregnancies and the consequent need for abortion. EC is also important for a large number of women at risk of pregnancy but are not using a regular method. Emergency contraception does not protect against sexually transmitted infections, but reassures a large number of women using condoms in case of slippage or breakage. It may also provide a bridge to use an ongoing contraceptive method. Considering these factors, the Government of India has included EC as one of the components of National Family Welfare Program.

Definition

Emergency contraception (EC) is a method used before the missed periods but after an unprotected intercourse or where the regular method may be expected to fail.

The other names for EC include 'postcoital contraception' or 'morning after contraception'. **Intraception, interception** and **contragestion** are other terminologies used. The terms intraception or interception are used when an agent does not prevent fertilisation, but acts at the time of implantation or soon after. The term contragestion is used when it acts before or soon after missed periods. EC should not be confused with or considered to be early abortion, because pregnancy is defined to begin with implantation.

Situations where EC is useful

The provider should understand that EC cannot be relied upon as an ongoing method of contraception. When used in this way, the efficacy of the method decreases and the side effects increase.

Emergency contraception is useful after unprotected coitus in the following situations:

- couples having very infrequent intercourse
- unplanned single or occasional intercourse among adolescents
- breakage or slippage of condom or leakage while using diaphragm
- when oral pills have been missed
- sexual assault
- expelled IUCD
- premature ejaculation or ejaculation over external genitalia.

Methods of Emergency Contraception

Currently, combined oral contraceptive (COC), levonorgestrel and copper-containing IUCDs are well recognised for use as emergency contraception.

Combined oral contraceptive pills

The use of COC pills as emergency contraception is also known as **Yuzpe's method**. High-dose COC pills containing 50 μg of ethinyl estradiol and 500 μg of norgestrel are used. Two of these pills should be taken as soon as possible within 72 hours of intercourse, and two more, 12 hours later.

When low-dose pills with 30 μg of ethinyl estradiol and 150 μg of levonorgestrel are used, four tablets should be taken as the first dose within 72 hours followed by four more pills, 12 hours later. Four tablets should be taken as above, if triphasic pills are used.

Current evidence suggests that efficacy of the pill will decrease if the first dose is taken after 72 hours of intercourse. This does not mean a 100% failure. Similarly, the timing of the second dose may be altered to be user-friendly, but the efficacy may fall.

Mechanism of action: The COC pills prevent pregnancy by the following mechanisms:

- inhibition or delaying of ovulation in follicular phase
- impairing endometrial receptivity to implantation
- possible interference with corpus luteum
- possible thickening of cervical mucus with sperm trapping
- possible alteration of tubal transport of sperm, ovum or blastocyst
- possible direct inhibition of fertilisation

Efficacy: Approximately 8% of women can become pregnant from a single coitus. The use of COC as EC reduces the occurrence of pregnancy to 2%.

Side effects: The following side effects have been noted among women taking COC pills for emergency contraception:

- Nausea occurs in 60% of women.
- Vomiting occurs in 20%; both nausea and vomiting can be significantly reduced by using antiemetic medication. If the vomiting occurs within 1–2 hours of the first dose, it should be repeated.
- Early onset of menstruation or delayed menstruation
- Irregular bleeding
- Headache
- Dizziness and fatigue
- Mastalgia

Contraindications:

- A definite contraindication is pregnancy, though if taken inadvertently there is no risk of teratogenicity or adenosis in the offspring
- Active or crescendo migraine
- History of thromboembolism

Though a short duration of therapy for EC is unlikely to cause the last two conditions, it may not be appropriate to use COCs in such cases.

Progestogen-only emergency contraceptive pills

Levonorgestrel (LNG) is more effective than COC pills for emergency contraception and the side effects are definitely lower. Levonorgestrel is given in a dose of 750 μg as early as possible, within 72 hours of coitus and a second dose given after 12 hours. A recent WHO study has found that a single 1.5 mg dose of LNG is also as effective even up to five days after coitus.

LNG reduces the risk of pregnancy by 88% as compared to 75% with COC. The side effects are less pronounced; nausea decreases by 50% and vomiting by 70%.

Levonorgestrel is marketed in India in packs of two tablets of 750 μg each with the brand names of ECEE2 and NORLEVO exclusively for EC and a single dose of two tablets has been advocated within 72 hours of intercourse.

Copper intrauterine device

A copper bearing intrauterine device for emergency contraception has been used for over 30 years.

Mechanism of action: The copper intrauterine device acts as an EC by:

- prevention of implantation
- possible effect of copper on tubal function.

Time of insertion: In order to ensure effectiveness, it is recommended that the IUCD be inserted within five days of unprotected coitus. However, insertion within 10 days may still be effective.

Efficacy: The failure rate of copper IUCD is less than 1%. This method is 15 times more effective than the Yuzpe regimen.

Side effects: Bleeding, pain and expulsion are common when an IUCD is used as an ongoing method. There is an increased risk of infection, particularly in women who have multiple sexual partners or who have been sexually assaulted.

Advantage: Once inserted for EC, the IUCD can be left in situ for 5–7 years as an ongoing method.

Contraindications: An intrauterine contraceptive device should not be inserted in women who have contraindications for the use of IUCD.

Recent developments

Mifepristone (RU-486 an antiprogestogen) in doses of 600 mg is very effective as an EC with a failure rate of less than 1%. It also has fewer side effects. A recent WHO study has shown that mifepristone in a very low dose of 10 mg is as effective as levonorgestrel.

Problems of emergency contraception

The important technical problems of EC are high rate of side effects, need to start treatment within 72 hours and a small but important failure rate. Cost may also be a deterrent in the developing countries.

The other reasons for EC not being used widely are lack of awareness among providers as well as beneficiaries, poor availability and social inhibitions. Efforts to market EC products or to improve public awareness through campaigns should be initiated. Dissemination of information will definitely improve usage. Making EC available over the counter (OTC), providing routine information about EC to all couples and making it available in advance will also help.

EC is always cost-effective as it will prevent unintended pregnancies leading to births or abortions along their physical and psychological sequelae.

KEY POINTS

- Unplanned pregnancy is a major problem.
- EC prevents a majority of unintended pregnancies.
- There is a definite role for EC in the context of contraception.
- Hormonal methods and copper IUCDs are effective methods of EC.
- Appropriate use of the method will have optimum effect with minimum risk.
- EC has to be publicised in a very prominent way for it to be effective in developing countries like India.

QUESTIONS

Select the single most appropriate answer:

1. The possibility of pregnancy following a single unprotected intercourse is
   a. 2% b. 4% c. 6% d. 8%
2. The main advantage of emergency contraception is that it
   a. permits sexual freedom
   b. reduces unintended pregnancies and abortions
   c. can be used as a regular method
   d. protects against sexually transmitted infections
3. Emergency contraception is useful in all of the following situations *except*
   a. couples having regular intercourse
   b. after sexual assault
   c. breakage of condom
   d. unplanned single intercourse in an adolescent
4. Emergency contraception cannot be used
   a. post coitus
   b. morning after
   c. as an abortion method
   d. as an intrauterine contraceptive
5. After intercourse, to be most effective, an emergency contraceptive should be used within
   a. 24 hours c. 72 hours
   b. 48 hours d. 144 hours
6. Methods of emergency contraception include all of the following *except*
   a. combined pill
   b. progestogen-only pill
   c. intrauterine device
   d. female condom
7. Possible mechanisms of action of combined pill as emergency contraceptive are all of the following *except*
   a. decidual thrombosis
   b. making the endometrium unfavourable for implantation
   c. cervical mucus thickening and sperm entrapment
   d. alteration of tubal transport
8. The most effective method of emergency contraception is
   a. combined pill
   b. levonorgestrel
   c. intrauterine copper device
   d. mifepristone
9. If a woman requests contraception 6 days after intercourse, which of the following methods is most likely to prevent pregnancy?
   a. combined pill
   b. intrauterine copper device
   c. mifepristone
   d. levonorgestrel
10. The Yuzpe regimen involves the use of
    a. progestogen c. mifepristone
    b. ethinyl estradiol d. combined pill

Answer Key

Chapter 1: Obstetrics: An Overview

1. b, 2. d, 3. b, 4. d, 5. b, 6. a,
7. c, 8. a, 9. c, 10. c, 11. d, 12. d

Chapter 2: Ethical Issues

1. d, 2. c, 3. b, 4. d, 5. a, 6. c

Chapter 3: Gender Sensitisation

1. a, 2. d, 3. b, 4. b, 5. c, 6. d,
7. d, 8. c, 9. d, 10. a

Chapter 4: Reproductive and Child Health Programme

1. d, 2. d, 3. b, 4. c, 5. b, 6. d,
7. d, 8. c, 9. b

Chapter 5: Communication and Counselling

1. d, 2. d, 3. d, 4. b, 5. e, 6. c,
7. a, 8. d, 9a. T, 9b. F, 9c. F, 9d. T,
10a. T, 10b. F, 10c. F, 10d. F

Chapter 6: Elements of Reproduction and Embryology

1. c, 2. c, 3. a, 4. b, 5. b, 6. d,
7. b, 8. d, 9. b, 10. c

Chapter 7: Development of the Fetus and Placenta

1. c, 2. d, 3. b, 4. c, 5. c, 6. a,
7. c, 8. b, 9. b, 10. b

Chapter 8: Maternal Changes in Pregnancy

1. b, 2. c, 3. a, 4. c, 5. c, 6. b,
7. b, 8. a, 9. c, 10. d, 11. a, 12. b

Chapter 9: Diagnosis of Pregnancy

1. c, 2. d, 3. b, 4. c, 5. b, 6. d,
7. a, 8. c, 9. b, 10. e

Chapter 10: Antenatal Care

1. a, 2. b, 3. c, 4. d, 5. b, 6. a,
7. d, 8. c, 9. a, 10. d

Chapter 11: Nutrition in Pregnancy

1. b, 2. c, 3. a, 4. d, 5. a, 6. a,
7. d, 8. b, 9. e, 10. b

Chapter 12: Drugs in Pregnancy

1. a, 2. b, 3. a, 4. c, 5. d, 6. b,
7. c, 8. d, 9. c, 10. d

Chapter 13: Imaging in Obstetrics

1. c, 2. d, 3. a, 4. c, 5. b, 6. d,
7. c, 8. c, 9. b, 10. d

Chapter 14: Screening and Prenatal Diagnosis of Fetal Anomalies

1. a, 2. a, 3. d, 4. d, 5. b, 6. a,
7. b, 8. a, 9. c, 10. a, 11. b

Chapter 15: Antepartum Assessment of Fetal Wellbeing

1. d, 2. a, 3. c, 4. d, 5. a

Chapter 16: Abortion

1. d, 2. b, 3. d, 4. c, 5. b, 6. c,
7. a, 8. e, 9. a, 10. d

Chapter 17: Medical Termination of Pregnancy

1. b, 2. c, 3. c, 4. a, 5. c, 6. b,
7. d, 8. d, 9. a

Chapter 18: Ectopic Pregnancy

1. c, 2. a, 3. b, 4. d, 5. a, 6. c,
7. d, 8. a, 9. a, 10. b

Chapter 19: Gestational Trophoblastic Disease

1. c, 2. d, 3. d, 4. c, 5. b, 6. a

Chapter 20: Amniotic Fluid and its Abnormalities

1. d, 2. a, 3. d, 4. d, 5. b, 6. d,
7. c, 8. b, 9. b, 10. d, 11. a

Chapter 21: Anatomy of the Maternal Pelvis and Fetus

1. a, 2. d, 3. c, 4. b, 5. b, 6. F,
7. T, 8. F, 9. F, 10. F

Chapter 22: Physiology of Labour

1. c, 2. d, 3. d, 4. a, 5. b, 6. d,
7. d, 8. b, 9. b, 10. a

Chapter 23: Mechanism of Labour
1. d, 2. c, 3. a, 4. b, 5. b, 6. c,
7. c, 8. c, 9. d, 10. c

Chapter 24: Conduct of Normal Labour
1. d, 2. c, 3. a, 4. b, 5. c, 6. a, 7. F,
8. T, 9. F, 10. T, 11. T, 12. F, 13. F,
14. F, 15. F, 16. F, 17. T, 18. F, 19. F,
20. T, 21. T

Chapter 25: Analgesia and Anesthesia
1. b, 2. d, 3. a, 4. d, 5. c, 6. b, 7. d,
8. a, 9. c, 10. b, 11. d, 12. a, 13. c,
14. b, 15. d

Chapter 26: Prolonged Labour
1. b, 2. d, 3. c, 4. d, 5. a, 6. c, 7. d,
8. a, 9. b, 10. a

Chapter 27: Occipitoposterior Position
1. c, 2. c, 3. b, 4. c, 5. b, 6. a, 7. b,
8. b, 9. a, 10. a

Chapter 28: Breech and Shoulder Presentation
1. c, 2. a, 3. d, 4. a, 5. b, 6. d, 7. b,
8. a, 9. b, 10. e

Chapter 29: Multiple pregnancy
1. c, 2. b, 3. d, 4. c, 5. c, 6. a, 7. c,
8. a, 9. a, 10. c

Chapter 30: Induction of Labour
1. b, 2. c, 3. a, 4. b, 5. a, 6. c, 7. d,
8. d, 9. b, 10. d

Chapter 31: Vaginal Operative Delivery
1. a, 2. d, 3. d, 4. b, 5. c

Chapter 32: Cesarean Section
1. a, 2. c, 3. b, 4. b, 5. c, 6. b,
7. a, 8. a

Chapter 33: Complications of Third Stage of Labour
1. c, 2. b, 3. a, 4. c, 5. a, 6. d, 7. b,
8. d, 9. a, 10. e

Chapter 34: Care of the Newborn
1. c, 2. d, 3. a, 4. b, 5. c, 6. d, 7. a,
8. d, 9. c, 10. b, 11. d, 12. a

Chapter 35: Normal Puerperium
1. b, 2. b, 3. c, 4. d, 5. c,
6. d, 7. a, 8. c

Chapter 36: Lactation and Breastfeeding
1. a, 2. d, 3. b, 4. c, 5. b, 6. a,
7. c, 8. c, 9. a, 10. d

Chapter 37: Abnormal Puerperium
1. b, 2. d, 3. d, 4. d, 5. d,
6. a, 7. a, 8. a

Chapter 38: Hyperemesis Gravidarum
1. d, 2. c, 3. d, 4. a, 5. b

Chapter 39: Hypertensive Disorders
1. a, 2. b, 3. c, 4. a, 5. c, 6. b

Chapter 40: Antepartum Hemorrhage
1. d, 2. a, 3. b, 4. c, 5. c, 6. a,
7. e, 8. a, 9. c, 10. a

Chapter 41: Preterm Labour
1. a, 2. c, 3. a, 4. b,
5. c, 6. c, 7. d, 8. b, 9. b

Chapter 42: Prelabour Rupture of Membranes
1. b, 2. c, 3. d, 4. c, 5. d,
6. c, 7. b, 8. a, 9. a, 10. c

Chapter 43: Prolonged Pregnancy
1. c, 2. d, 3. d, 4. a, 5. d, 6. a, 7. b

Chapter 44: Rhesus Isoimmunisation
1. b, 2. d, 3. d, 4. b, 5. c, 6. c,
7. b, 8. a, 9. a, 10. e, 11. a

Chapter 45: Fetal Growth Restriction
1. b, 2. c, 3. b, 4. c, 5. b, 6. d,
7. c, 8. b, 9. a, 10. e

Chapter 46: Anemia in Pregnancy
1. a, 2. c, 3. b, 4. a, 5. c, 6. d, 7. b,
8. c, 9. d, 10. a, 11. c, 12. d, 13. d,
14. b, 15. a, 16. c, 17. d, 18. b, 19. d

Chapter 47: Cardiac Disease
1. a, 2. b, 3. c, 4. d, 5. b, 6. c, 7. b,
8. c, 9. a, 10. d

Chapter 48: Respiratory Disorders
1. a, 2. d, 3. b, 4. d, 5. d, 6. a,
7. d, 8. c

Chapter 49: Diabetes Mellitus
1. a, 2. c, 3. d, 4. c, 5. a, 6. d,
7. a, 8. c, 9. e, 10. a

Chapter 50: Thyroid Disease

1. d, 2. c, 3. b, 4. a, 5. c, 6. a, 7. e

Chapter 51: Urinary Tract Infections

1. c, 2. b, 3. c, 4. c, 5. b, 6. e, 7. b

Chapter 52: Sexually Transmitted Infections

1. d, 2. a, 3. c, 4. c, 5. d, 6. a,
7. a, 8. a, 9. e, 10. a, 11. a

Chapter 53: Tropical Diseases

1. T, 2. F, 3. T, 4. T, 5. T, 6. T, 7. F,
8. F, 9. F, 10. T, 11. F

Chapter 54: Epilepsy

1. a, 2. d, 3. d, 4. e, 5. a,

Chapter 55: Psychiatric Disorders

1. a, 2. d, 3. b, 4. d, 5. a, 6. d,
7. c, 8. b, 9. a, 10. d, 11. c, 12. b

Chapter 56: Liver Diseases

1. F, 2. T, 3. T, 4. F, 5. T, 6. F, 7. T,
8. T, 9. T, 10. F, 11. F, 12. F, 13. T,
14. T, 15. F, 16. T

Chapter 57: Common Surgical Causes of Acute Abdomen

1. b, 2. c, 3. a, 4. a, 5. c, 6. d,
7. d, 8. a, 9. a, 10. a

Chapter 58: Gynecological Disorders

1. d, 2. b, 3. c, 4. b, 5. a,
6. d, 7. d, 8. d

Chapter 59: Shock in Obstetrics

1. b, 2. c, 3. b, 4. c, 5. b, 6. a, 7. b

Chapter 60: Disseminated Intravascular Coagulation

1. b, 2. a, 3. a, 4. c, 5. c

Chapter 61: Demography, Population Control and Contraception

1. c, 2. b, 3. d, 4. a, 5. c

Chapter 62: Natural and Conventional Contraceptives

1. d, 2. c, 3. a, 4. b, 5. d, 6. c,
7. c, 8. a, 9. d, 10. c

Chapter 63: Hormonal Contraceptives

1. a, 2. c, 3. c, 4. b, 5. d, 6. a, 7. c,
8. a, 9. b, 10. d, 11. c, 12. a, 13. b,
14. d, 15. c, 16. d, 17. b, 18. a,
19. a, 20. c

Chapter 64: Intrauterine Contraceptive Devices

1. a, 2. c, 3. c, 4. d, 5. c, 6. c,
7. b, 8. c, 9. a, 10. e, 11. a, 12. b,
13. a, 14. a

Chapter 65: Surgical Contraception

1. b, 2. d, 3. c, 4. a, 5. b, 6. c,
7. c, 8. d, 9. b, 10. a, 11. c, 12. d

Chapter 66: Emergency Contraception

1. d, 2. b, 3. a, 4. c, 5. c,
6. d, 7. a, 8. c, 9. b, 10. d

Suggested Reading

1. **American College of Obstetricians and Gynecologists (ACOG)**. 2003. ACOG Practice Bulletin: Clinical Management Guidelines for Obstetrician–Gynecologists No. 43, Management of preterm labour. *Obstet Gynecol* 101(5): 1039–46.
2. **Arulkumaran S**, Ratnam SS and Bhaskar Rao K (eds). 1996. *Management of Labour*. Chennai: Orient Longman.
3. **Chaudhury SK**. 2008. *Practice of Fertility Control: A Comprehensive Textbook,* 7th ed. New Delhi: BI Publications.
4. **Colledge NR**, Walker BR and Ralston SH (eds). 2010. *Davidson's Principles and Practice of Medicine,* 21st ed. Philadelphia: Churchill Livingston.
5. **Cook GC** and Zumia AI (eds). 2009. *Manson's Tropical Diseases,* 22nd ed. London: Saunders.
6. **Creasy RK** and Resnik R (eds). 2004. *Maternal-Fetal Medicine,* 5th ed. New York: WB Saunders.
7. **Cunningham FG**, Leveno KJ, Bloom SI, Hauth JC, Rouse DJ and Spong CY. 2010. *Williams' Obstetrics,* 23rd ed. New Delhi: McGraw Hill.
8. **Government of India, Ministry of Health and Family Welfare (MOHFW)**. Manual for first trimester medical termination of pregnancy. New Delhi: MOHFW.
9. **Indian Council for Medical Research (ICMR)**. 1989. Nutrient requirements and recommended dietary allowances for Indians. New Delhi: (ICMR).
10. **James DK**, Steer PJ, Weiner CP and Gonik B (eds). 2006. *High-risk Pregnancy*, 3rd ed. Philadelphia: WB Saunders.
11. **National Family Health Survey (NFHS-2)**. 2000. India 1998–1999. International Institute for Population Sciences, Mumbai. Maryland: ORC Macro.
12. **National Family Health Survey (NFHS-3)**. 2007. India 2005–2006. International Institute for Population Sciences, Mumbai. Maryland: ORC Macro.
13. **Ong S** and Whittle M. 2005. Antenatal screening for Down syndrome. In *Recent Advances in Obstetrics and Gynecology* (eds) J Bonnar and W Dunlop. 23: 1–14.
14. **Oumachigui A**, Soundara Raghavan S and Habeebullah S. (eds). 2006. *Clinical Methods in Obstetrics and Gynecology: A Problem-based Approach,* 2nd ed. Chennai: Orient Longman.
15. **Park K** (ed). 2009. *Park's Textbook of Preventive and Social Medicine,* 20th ed. Jabalpur: Banarasidas Bhanot Publishers.
16. **Powrie R**, Green M and Camann W. 2010. *De Swiet's Medical Disorders in Obstetric Practice,* 5th ed. Wiley Blackwell.
17. **Ravindran TKS**, Savitri R and Bhavani A. 1999. Women's experience of utero-vaginal prolapse: A qualitative study from Tamil Nadu, India. In *Safe Motherhood Initiatives: Critical Issues,* (eds) Ravindran TKS and Berer M. London: Reproductive Health Matters.
18. **Royal College of Obstetricians and Gynecologists (RCOG)**. 2001. Guidelines for induction of labour. Evidence based clinical guidelines No. 9.
19. **Sadler TW**. 2009. *Langman's Medical Embryology,* 11th ed. New Delhi: Walter Kluwer.
20. **Sethuraman KR**. 2001. *Communication Skills in Clinical Practice: Doctor-patient Communication.* New Delhi: Jaypee Brothers Medical Publishers (P) Ltd.
21. **Sharp HT**. 2002. The acute abdomen during pregnancy. *Clin Obstet Gynecol* 45: 405–13.

Index